SPRINGER PUBLISHING

AF683097

GET THE MOST FROM YOUR BOOK

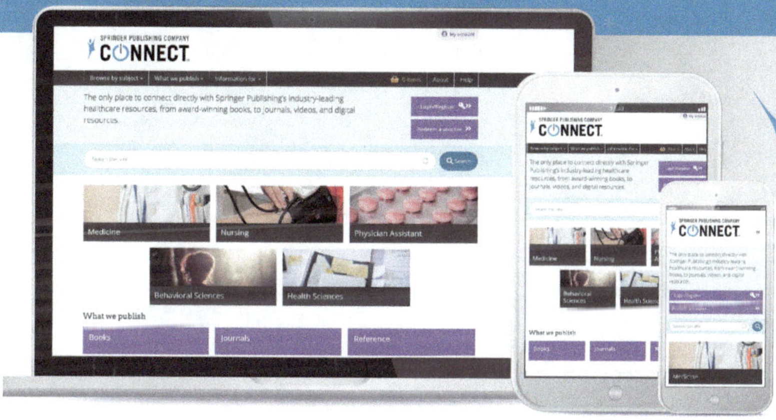

SPRINGER PUBLISHING
CONNECT™

VOUCHER CODE:

RXF5V6NJ

Online Access

Your print purchase of *Tappero & Honeyfield's Physical Assessment of the Newborn: A Comprehensive Approach to the Art of Physical Examination, Seventh Edition*, includes **online access via Springer Publishing Connect**™ to increase accessibility, portability, and searchability.

Insert the code at http://connect.springerpub.com/content/book/978-0-8261-4063-0 or scan the QR code and insert the voucher code today!

Having trouble? Contact our customer service department at ***cs@springerpub.com***

Instructor Resource Access for Adopters

Let us do some of the heavy lifting to create an engaging classroom experience with a variety of instructor resources included in most textbooks SUCH AS:

INSTRUCTOR MANUAL

POWERPOINTS

TEST BANK

Visit **https://connect.springerpub.com/** and look for the **"Show Supplementary"** button on your **book homepage** to see what is available to instructors! First time using Springer Publishing Connect?

Email **textbook@springerpub.com** to create an account and start unlocking valuable resources.

TAPPERO & HONEYFIELD'S PHYSICAL ASSESSMENT OF THE NEWBORN

Catherine L. Witt, PhD, APRN, NNP-BC, has been a neonatal nurse practitioner for over 30 years, working in both tertiary and community neonatal intensive care units. She is the previous coordinator of the Neonatal Nurse Practitioner Program at Regis University in Denver, Colorado, and currently serves as the dean of the Loretto Heights School of Nursing at Regis. She is past president of the National Association of Neonatal Nurses (NANN) and the National Certification Corporation (NCC)+. She also served as editor-in-chief of *Advances in Neonatal Care,* the official journal of NANN. She has authored many articles and book chapters and presented at local and national conferences.

Carol M. Wallman, DNP, APRN, NNP-BC, is a neonatal nurse practitioner with over 30 years of clinical experience in community and tertiary neonatal intensive care units and neonatal transport. She has been involved in the National Association of Neonatal Nurses (NANN) and the National Certification Corporation (NCC) in a variety of leadership roles including being a member on the board of directors for both organizations and the president of NCC. She is currently the coordinator of the Neonatal Nurse Practitioner Program at Regis University in Denver, Colorado. Her area of scholarship includes neonates born to mothers with substance use disorders and the impact of the legalization of marijuana on the developing fetus and neonate and late preterm infants. She has authored several articles and book chapters and presented nationally and internationally.

TAPPERO & HONEYFIELD'S PHYSICAL ASSESSMENT OF THE NEWBORN

A Comprehensive Approach to the Art of Physical Examination

SEVENTH EDITION

CATHERINE L. WITT, PhD, APRN, NNP-BC

CAROL M. WALLMAN, DNP, APRN, NNP-BC

Editors

SPRINGER PUBLISHING

First Springer Publishing edition 978-0-8261-2189-9 (2014); subsequent edition 2018.

Springer Publishing Company, LLC
902 Carnegie Center/Suite 140, Princeton, NJ 08540
www.springerpub.com
connect.springerpub.com

Senior Acquisitions Editor: John Zaphyr
Senior Director, Content Development: Taylor Ball
Production Manager: Kris Parrish
Compositor: Transforma

ISBN: 978-0-8261-4062-3
ebook ISBN: 978-0-8261-4063-0
DOI: 10.1891/9780826140630

SPRINGER PUBLISHING CONNECT™ | **A robust set of resources designed to supplement this text is located at http://connect.springerpub.com/content/book/978-0-8261-4063-0. Qualifying instructors may request access by emailing textbook@springerpub.com.**

LMS Common Cartridge ISBN (All Instructor Resources): 978-0-8261-4069-2
Instructor PowerPoints ISBN: 978-0-8261-4065-4
Instructor Image Bank ISBN: 978-0-8261-4066-1
Mapping to AACN Essentials ISBN: 978-0-8261-5329-6
Transition Guide to the Seventh Edition ISBN: 978-0-8261-8972-1

24 25 26 27/5 4 3 2 1

The author and the publisher of this Work have made every effort to use sources believed to be reliable to provide information that is accurate and compatible with the standards generally accepted at the time of publication. Because medical science is continually advancing, our knowledge base continues to expand. Therefore, as new information becomes available, changes in procedures become necessary. We recommend that the reader always consult current research and specific institutional policies before performing any clinical procedure or delivering any medication. The author and publisher shall not be liable for any special, consequential, or exemplary damages resulting, in whole or in part, from the readers' use of, or reliance on, the information contained in this book. The publisher has no responsibility for the persistence or accuracy of URLs for external or third-party internet websites referred to in this publication and does not guarantee that any content on such websites is, or will remain, accurate or appropriate.

Library of Congress Control Number: 2023031129

Contact sales@springerpub.com to receive discount rates on bulk purchases.

***Publisher's Note*: New and used products purchased from third-party sellers are not guaranteed for quality, authenticity, or access to any included digital components.**

Printed in the United States of America by Gasch Printing.

CONTENTS

CONTRIBUTORS

Trish L. Anderson, MBA, BSN, CPHQ, Senior Director of Safety and Quality, Washington State Hospital Association, Seattle, Washington

Christina Baxter, DNP, APRN, NNP-BC, MUSC Shawn Jenkin's Children's Hospital, Charleston, South Carolina

Beth Bohara, MSN, APRN, CPNP-PC, NNP-BC, Neonatal Nurse Practitioner, MUSC Children's Health, Medical University of South Carolina, Charleston, South Carolina

Terri A. Cavaliere, DNP, RN, NNP-BC, FAANP, Clinical Associate Professor, Graduate Department, School of Nursing, Stony Brook University, Stony Brook, New York

Bresney A. Fanning, MSN, APRN, NNP-BC, Medical University of South Carolina, Shawn Jenkins Children's Hospital, Charleston, South Carolina

Debbie Fraser, MN, NNP, CNeon(C), FCAN, Associate Professor, Faculty of Health Disciplines, Athabasca University, Athabasca, Alberta, Canada

Mary Ellen Honeyfield, DNP, RN, Kiowa, Colorado

Kimberly M. Horns, PhD, NNP-BC, FAANP, Retired Clinical Professor, Salt Lake City, Utah

Julie A. Javernick, DNP, CNM, Associate Professor and CHOICE Program Coordinator, Loretto Heights School of Nursing, Regis University, Denver, Colorado

Patricia J. Johnson, DNP, MPH, RN, NNP, Neonatal Nurse Practitioner Coordinator, Valleywise Healthcare, Phoenix, Arizona

Jacqueline M. McGrath, PhD, RN, FNAP, FAAN, Thelma & Joe Crow Endowed Professorship and Vice Dean for Faculty Excellence, University of Texas Health Science Center at San Antonio, San Antonio, Texas

Susan R. Meier, DNP, APRN, NNP-BC, Associate Professor, Rueckert-Hartman College for Health Professions, Regis University, Denver, Colorado

Erin Mestas, MSN, APRN, NNP-BC, ELBW-C, Children's Hospital Colorado, Aurora, Colorado

Ellen P. Tappero, DNP, RN, NNP-BC, Neonatal Nurse Practitioner, Phoenix, Arizona

Carol Wiltgen Trotter, PhD, RN, NNP-BC, Neonatal Nurse Practitioner, St. Louis, Missouri

Rebecca Vahle, MEd, Founder, Executive Director, Family to Family Support Network, Littleton, Colorado

Lyn Vargo, PhD, RN, NNP-BC, Faculty, University of Missouri-Kansas City, Kansas City, Missouri, Stonybrook University, Stony Brook, New York

Dorothy Vittner, PhD, RN, FAAN, Assistant Professor, Program Director Post Masters-DNP, Egan School of Nursing & Health Studies Fairfield University, Fairfield, Connecticut, Nurse Scientist, Greenwich Hospital Greenwich, Connecticut

Carol M. Wallman, DNP, APRN, NNP-BC, Associate Professor, Neonatal Nurse Practitioner Program Coordinator, Loretto Heights School of Nursing, Regis University, Denver, Colorado

Dixie K. Weber, MS, RN, National Advisor of Healthcare Programs, Family to Family Support Network, Littleton, Colorado

Catherine L. Witt, PhD, RN, NNP-BC, Dean, Loretto Heights School of Nursing, Regis University, Denver, Colorado

FOREWORD

The art and skill of physical assessment may be thought of as the foundation for all healthcare professionals no matter the age or diagnosis of the client. Development of specialized neonatal care, and training of the advanced practice providers required to deliver that care, began over 40 years ago. While there were texts that included physical assessment across the life span, there was only one specifically focused on neonatal assessment: *A System of Newborn Physical Examination* (Scanlon, JW, et al. 1979. Baltimore: University Park Press), a must-have text for students of neonatal care. That original text did not have a second edition. As national organizations embraced the specialty, the need for more formal education, certification of specialties, and current literature arose. The first edition of *Physical Assessment of the Newborn* was published in 1993 and remains the sole text purposely addressing newborn physical assessment. While the importance of systematic physical assessment has not changed, chapters were added with each edition to strengthen the text's currency with changing culture and knowledge.

Changing culture acknowledges how our healthcare systems have evolved as well as how societal changes may impact our communication with families. Operationally, providers transitioned from handwritten charting to computerized template charting. Some might say not without consequences. More recent staffing and financial pressures have sometimes changed delivery of care and the speed it requires to attend to necessary functions. Template charting may force the provider out of the objective, assessment/diagnosis, and plan mode that was traditionally taught.

This seventh edition marks an editorial transition. We as co-editors have turned those responsibilities over to the very capable hands of new co-editors, Catherine L. Witt and Carol M. Wallman. They, as well as previous and new chapter authors, have continued the tradition of updating new knowledge yet keeping to the same format of previous editions. This edition includes a timely new chapter addressing communication with families. As the face of society's family has changed, so has the need for healthcare providers to recognize and be respectful of those changes.

All of this does not diminish the philosophy and importance of newborn physical assessment. Technology has provided practitioners the ability to diagnose and anticipate neonatal care needs prenatally. These advances may lead to some level of complacency for providers. However, systematic early assessment of problems remains imperative and cannot be overemphasized. The chapters in this text follow a pattern of assessment intentionally. Principles, techniques, history taking, assessment of body systems, dysmorphia, pain, and the infant with antenatal exposure to drugs are addressed. One of the many strengths of this text are the illustrations, many color pictures, and diagrams that aid in differential diagnosis and how to perform specific examination techniques.

The text is an international resource to any student who cares for neonates, neonatal and pediatric nurses and practitioners, nurse midwives, residents, and both occupational and physical therapists. Additionally, the text has become a resource in both rural and larger volume newborn nurseries and intensive care settings. The content remains a constant to those care providers and the families of the newly born.

We are honored that our names will remain a part of the title of this book. The original purpose and intent has stayed true to our belief that physical assessment begins in the delivery room and continues each day, sometimes each hour, through to the discharge examination. We are confident the new editors will carry our legacy forward, and we congratulate their dedication to the education of future students and, most of all, to newborns and their families.

Ellen P. Tappero, DNP, RN, NNP-BC
Mary Ellen Honeyfield, DNP, RN

PREFACE

It is an honor for us to accept the opportunity to edit the seventh edition of *Physical Assessment of the Newborn*. Since the beginning, this book has been a resource for healthcare professionals who are responsible for the care of neonates and recognize that a complete assessment of every neonate is essential. We are fortunate to have a solid foundation built over the last 30 years since this book was first published.

For this edition, we have continued the intention of the original publication, to provide important aspects of a head to toe examination. Our focus continues to be on the "well newborn" with some variations for preterm or ill neonates. Early in our careers, we were educated with the idea that one must know normal and common in order to recognize the abnormal or uncommon. We also want to remember the importance of gathering neonatal and prenatal history and how that informs diagnosis and treatment.

In addition to these aspects, we realize the importance of timely interaction with parents and families. We have consequently added a new chapter on communication. As part of this addition, we recognize the importance of using inclusive language and working with diverse communities and populations. We have made every effort to include this perspective in all of our chapters, recognizing that there will be areas that we may have missed or that will continue to evolve.

Many of our chapter authors have been part of this publication since the beginning. Their ongoing expertise is invaluable. We thank them for their work in updating their information, reviewing references, and seeking new photographs and illustrations. It is also important to recognize that each author has their own voice and format, resulting in some variation in each chapter. We also have a number of new authors, and we are grateful for their willingness to accept the challenge. They have all put their own perspective into their chapters, and this makes for a richer narrative and expanded knowledge.

While this book is not intended to be an exhaustive review of every system, we have strived to include things that are commonly seen in the newborn period. Things that should alert the care provider to examine further are noted. It is intended to be an introduction and a reference for the foundation of neonatal physical examination and history.

In addition to being grateful to our authors, we would like to thank our publication team at Springer Publishing Company for their guidance and support throughout this process. They have been an invaluable resource and have been very patient in working with two new editors.

Catherine L. Witt
Carol M. Wallman

ACKNOWLEDGMENTS

It is an honor to assume the role of co-editor of *Physical Assessment of the Newborn*. Dr. Mary Ellen Honeyfield and Dr. Ellen Tappero created this book in the beginning, and following in their footsteps is a humbling experience. I am grateful to them for being our role models in this endeavor and in neonatal care as a whole. I have learned a lot from both of them over the years. My co-editor, Carol Wallman was a terrific co-editor and had excellent suggestions along the way. I also want to acknowledge the many neonatologists, neonatal nurse practitioners, neonatal nurses, and other healthcare professionals who taught me over the years about the importance of history and physical assessment. Its importance cannot be overstated in caring for all patients.

This would not be possible without the help and contribution of all of our authors and our colleagues who shared knowledge, pictures and illustrations, and encouragement. I must also thank the editorial staff at Springer Publishing Company who were a tremendous help to new editors!

Finally, I would like to thank my family. My husband, John, has provided unwavering support of all the things I undertake. My children have been constant cheerleaders. Lastly, my parents, who passed away this last year while I was working on this book, gave me the vision and opportunity to build a foundation for my career in nursing.

Catherine L. Witt

It is both an honor and a privilege to have the opportunity to follow in the footsteps of two giants in our field, Ellen Tappero and Mary Ellen Honeyfield, and prepare the seventh edition of *Physical Assessment of the Newborn*. I appreciate their insight from nearly 30 years ago when they recognized the need for this book. Since that initial musing, this book has grown and become a mainstay in many disciplines requiring an expertise in newborn physical examination.

My thanks to the authors and editors of both the previous and current editions, including those at Springer Publishing Company. Each have contributed important and timely information to provide the foundational knowledge to complete a thorough physical assessment of the newborn. Without each of you sharing your time and expertise, this book would not be the valued and respected book it is.

I also want to thank the many mentors, including my co-editor Catherine Witt, and colleagues I have had throughout my career as each of you have played an important role in my professional growth. Also, to the many newborns and families I have had the privilege of learning from throughout my career, thank you!

Additionally, I want to thank my husband, Elry Wallman, and my two now adult children, Bryan and Sarah, for their continuous support and encouragement of my many projects and commitments over the years. I could not have been successful without your love and support.

Finally, I want to dedicate this book to my mother, Claire R. Madsen, who passed away during the final editing phase of this seventh edition. She experienced nearly a decade of Alzheimer dementia yet continued to love, recognize, and support our family in all our endeavors.

Carol M. Wallman

SPRINGER PUBLISHING RESOURCES

SPRINGER PUBLISHING CONNECT™

A robust set of resources designed to supplement this text is located at http://connect.springerpub.com/content/book/978-0-8261-4063-0. Qualifying instructors may request access by emailing textbook@springerpub.com.

INSTRUCTOR RESOURCES

- **LMS Common Cartridge With All Instructor Resources With Instructions for Use**
- **Instructor PowerPoint Presentations**
- **Instructor Image Bank**
- **Mapping to AACN Essentials: Core Competencies for Professional Nursing Education**
- **Transition Guide: Sixth Edition to Seventh Edition**

SPRINGER PUBLISHING

Visit https://connect.springerpub.com/ and look for the **"Show Supplementary"** button on the **book homepage**.

1 PRINCIPLES OF PHYSICAL ASSESSMENT

Mary Ellen Honeyfield

The importance of approaching newborn physical examination with a sense of privilege and responsibility cannot be overemphasized. This first examination offers a unique opportunity for early recognition of any problems the infant may have. Seeing each infant as a mystery to be unraveled requires mindful curiosity from the examining clinician. The newborn's inability to provide verbal information tests the acuity of the examiner's skills. While most infants examined are normal, when the examiner views this responsibility as a diagnostic challenge, accurate newborn physical assessment provides parents information as well as personal and professional satisfaction for the examiner.

Initially, the inexperienced examiner finds physical assessment time-consuming. Both a lack of familiarity with essential tools and limited practice with basic techniques can slow assessment. Students often view the infant as a series of systems to be examined. Repetition and experience help the examiner learn to see the newborn as a whole and process multiple observations while examining individual systems. For example, if a previously quiet infant begins to cry during palpation of the abdomen, the experienced examiner continues the abdominal examination but also notes the quality of the cry, the infant's color while crying, respiratory effort, facial movements, tongue, intactness of the palate, and movement of the extremities.

Clinical expertise develops throughout a practitioner's career. With experience, each clinician develops their own unique approach to newborn physical assessment. The sequence of how the examination is performed is not as important as developing a consistent and organized approach. Consistency—performing the newborn physical assessment in the same organized manner every time—maximizes information gained from each examination performed, thus adding to the clinician's knowledge base and ensuring that portions of any individual examination will not be inadvertently omitted.

TECHNIQUES OF PHYSICAL ASSESSMENT

Observation

The most important part of newborn physical assessment begins with perinatal, delivery, and neonatal history. Historical data reviewed prior to examination may suggest the examiner focus on a particular system. Querying caregivers and family also adds to the examiner's database.

Observation, or inspection, is the next most important physical assessment technique for practitioners to master. Observation also is the most difficult skill for the fledgling examiner to incorporate into their clinical approach. Often the novice clinician's first instinct is to touch, talk, and unwrap the infant, thus possibly startling the infant and missing an opportunity to observe the infant's presenting status.

In 1860, Florence Nightingale wrote these thoughts about the art and skill of observation:

> In the case of infants, everything must depend upon the accurate

> observation of the nurse or mother. ... For it may safely be said, not that the habit of ready and correct observation will by itself make us useful..., but that without it we shall be useless with all our devotion.... If you cannot get the habit of observation one way or [the] other, you better give up..., for it is not your calling, however kind and anxious you may be.[1]

Using visual, auditory, and olfactory senses, the practitioner observes the infant, assesses, and makes decisions about what has been seen, heard, or smelled (i.e., in the presence of infection). A specific observation may alert the examiner to assess a particular system more thoroughly. For example, the observation of an active precordium (visual cardiac pulsations) directs the examiner to careful cardiovascular assessment. Auscultation may reveal a heart murmur. This finding may lead the examiner to palpate the precordium and peripheral pulses and obtain four extremity blood pressures, actions that are not normally part of the examination of an otherwise healthy-appearing newborn.

The practitioner can collect much of the information needed for a complete physical assessment solely through observation (Table 1.1).

Auscultation

Auscultation is the technique of listening to sounds produced by the body (e.g., the lungs, heart, and gastrointestinal tract). Direct auscultation involves application of the examiner's ear to the body surface being assessed. Some sounds, such as stridor, wheezing, and expiratory grunting, may be heard simply by being near the infant. Indirect (mediate) auscultation utilizes a stethoscope to listen to these same sounds.

Accurate indirect auscultation of the newborn requires a stethoscope fitted with a pediatric-sized, double-headed chest piece with an open bell and a closed diaphragm. The stethoscope should be placed firmly on bare skin rather than over the infant's clothes. A quiet infant and environment as well as a warm room and warm stethoscope facilitate auscultation.

Palpation

Palpation is a technique in which the examiner uses the sense of touch to assess both superficial and deeper body characteristics. During palpation, the tips, palmar, and lateral surfaces of the fingers of both hands are used to assess external structures (e.g., skin, hair texture), vibrations (e.g., peripheral pulses, precordial activity, point of maximal impulse of the heart against the chest wall), and internal structures (e.g., liver, spleen, and kidneys). One hand can be used, or a bimanual technique may enhance the palpation of deeper organs, such as the kidneys (Figure 1.1).

For accurate palpation, the infant ideally should be quiet and relaxed at the beginning of the abdominal examination. Warm hands, progressing from superficial to deeper palpation, and elevating the infant's hips off the bed keep abdominal muscles relaxed. Examiners should take care not to palpate too deeply for superficial abdominal organs, such as the liver and spleen, as the fingertips may instead palpate stool-filled intestine or abdominal wall muscle mass rather than the organ itself. In palpation of the extremities and genitalia, a grasping action of the fingers is used to evaluate accessible features such as skin texture, skin lesions, descent of testes into the scrotum, muscle mass, and muscle strength.

Percussion

Percussion refers to tapping or striking a part of the body to put underlying tissue into motion. This movement produces audible sounds and palpable vibrations, which are then assessed for quality and duration of their tone and notes.

Indirect (mediate) percussion is performed (for a right-handed person) by

TABLE 1.1: OBSERVATIONS FOR PHYSICAL ASSESSMENT

TO ASSESS	OBSERVE
Distress	Facial expression, skin color, respiratory effort, activity, and tone
Color	Tongue, mucous membranes (centrally pink vs. cyanotic), nail beds, hands, feet (peripherally pink vs. cyanotic), skin (jaundice, pallor, ruddiness, and mottling), perfusion, and meconium staining
Nutrition status	Subcutaneous fat, breast nodule
Hydration status	Skin turgor, anterior fontanel
Gestational age	Skin (smooth vs. peeling), ear cartilage, areola and nipple formation, breast nodule, sole creases, descent of testes, scrotal rugae, and labia
Neurologic status	Posture, tone, activity, response to stimuli, cry, state, state transition, and reflexes
Respiratory/chest status	Respiratory rate and effort, retractions, nasal flaring, grunting, audible stridor or wheezing, chest shape, nipples (number and position), and skin color
Cardiovascular status	Precordial activity, visible point of maximal intensity, and skin perfusion and color
Abdomen	Size (full, distended, taut, and shiny), shape (round, concave), distention (generalized or localized), visible peristaltic waves, visible bowel loops, muscular development/tone, umbilical cord, umbilical vessels, drainage from cord, and periumbilical erythema (redness)
Head	Size, shape, fontanels, suture lines, swelling, hair distribution, and condition of hair
Eyes	Shape, size, position, pupils, blink, extraocular movements, color of sclera, discharge, and ability to fix and follow
Ears	Shape, position, external auditory canal, and response to sound
Nose	Shape, nares, flaring, and nasal bridge
Mouth	Shape, symmetry, movement, philtrum, tongue, palate, natal teeth, gums, and jaw size
Neck	Shape, range of motion, webbing, and masses
Genitalia (male)	Scrotum, descent of testes, rugae, inguinal canals, foreskin, penile size, urine stream, meatus, perineum, and anus
Genitalia (female)	Labia majora, labia minora, clitoris, vagina, perineum, inguinal canals, and anus
Skin	Color, texture, firmness, vernix caseosa, masses, lanugo, and lesions (pigmentary, vascular, trauma-related, and infectious)
Extremities	Posture, range of motion (involuntary movement), digits, palmar creases, soles of feet, and nails

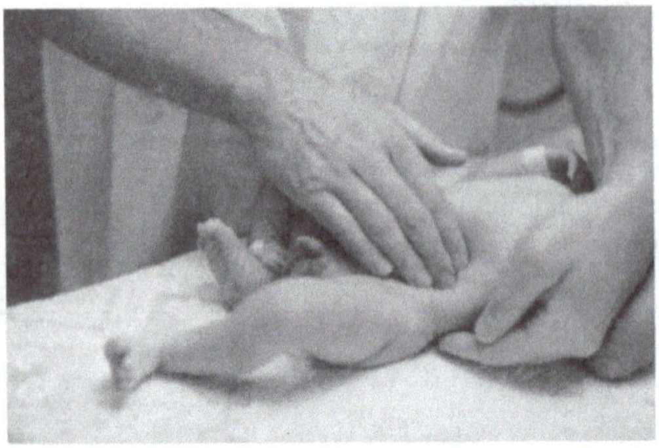

FIGURE 1.1 Bimanual inspection of the kidneys

Source: From Coen RW, and Koffler H. 1987. *Primary Care of the Newborn*. Boston, MA: Little, Brown, 30. Reprinted by permission.[2]

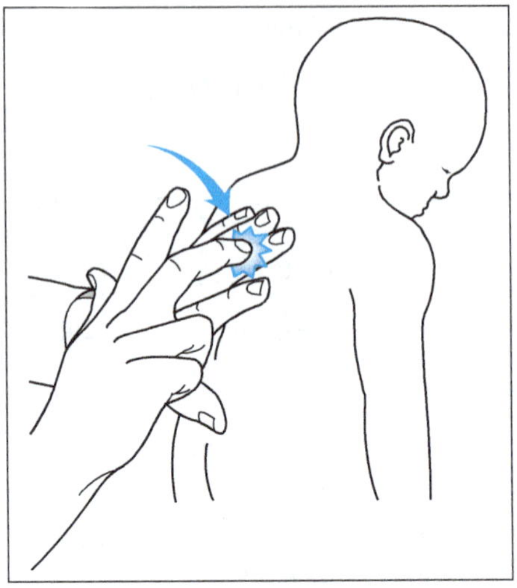

FIGURE 1.2 Indirect (mediate) percussion technique to assess underlying structures

Source: Adapted from Jarvis C. 2012. *Physical Examination & Health Assessment*, 6th ed. Philadelphia: Saunders, 117. Reprinted by permission.[3]

hyperextending the middle finger of the left hand and placing only the distal interphalangeal joint firmly on the part of the body to be percussed. Contact by any other part of the hand will alter the sounds produced. The right wrist is then hyperextended, and the middle right finger partially flexed and "cocked" upward so as to strike the middle left finger. With a quick downward motion of the wrist, the tip of the right middle finger strikes the left middle finger's distal joint (Figure 1.2). Vibrations are transmitted through the bones of this joint to the underlying tissue being percussed. Direct percussion is performed by directly striking the body surface to be assessed with the tip of the middle right finger.[4]

Translation of sounds heard during percussion into descriptive words is difficult at best. Practice and multiple examinations of normal infants and those with pathology are required to develop skill in describing percussed sounds.

Although the technique of percussion is commonly taught to students, in practice it is not a technique universally used on the newborn. When the examiner, using mediate percussion, suspects a pathology, such as pleural effusion or air leak, the common approach in the newborn is to confirm the suspected diagnosis by radiograph. A description of comparative sounds produced during percussion has therefore been omitted here.

Transillumination

Transillumination is the technique of applying a high-intensity light directly to a body part, such as the head, chest, or scrotum, and assessing the amount of pink light that can be seen as a corona (halo) around a cuffed flashlight or fiberoptic device (Figure 1.3). Transillumination of the enlarged scrotum of an infant with a hydrocele reveals a fluid filled mass that transmits light (Figure 1.4) rather than a solid mass that does not transmit light, as in the case of an inguinal hernia. As with other physical assessment techniques described, practice enables the examiner to recognize the difference between normal and abnormal halos of light.[4]

TIMING OF THE EXAMINATION

Timing of newborn physical assessment often depends on circumstance and hospital guidelines. A quick overall exam can be done in the delivery room unless the infant is clinically stable and has been placed with the mother. While disconcerting when parents are first to

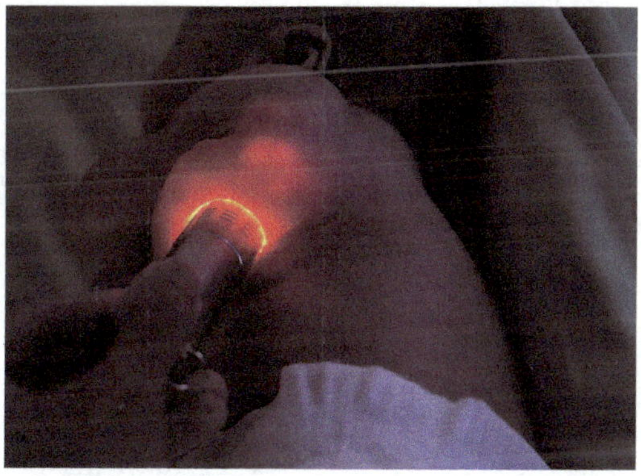

FIGURE 1.3 Transillumination

Source: Ho F-C, Chen H-L, Chung H-W. 2021. Axillary Cystic Hygroma. *The Journal of Pediatrics* 234: 273–274. doi: 10.1016/j.jpeds.2021.03.024

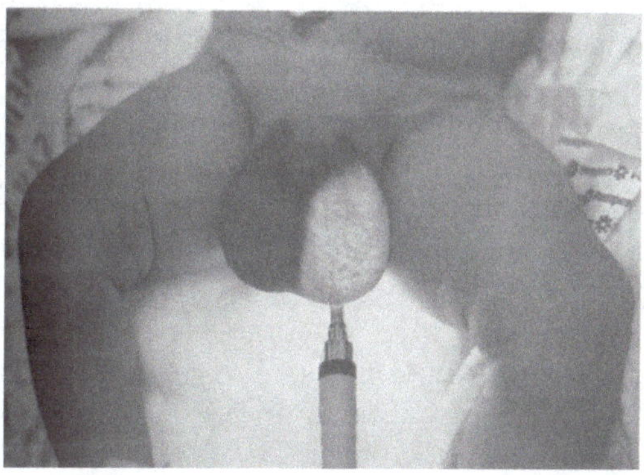

FIGURE 1.4 Transillumination of hydrocele

Source: From Coen RW, and Koffler H. 1987. *Primary Care of the Newborn*. Boston, MA: Little, Brown, 33. Reprinted by permission.[2]

discover a problem, the clinician is guided by hospital practice. A complete physical examination is done during the first few hours after birth when the infant becomes accessible.[5] Daily and discharge examinations are completed thereafter.

BASICS OF PHYSICAL ASSESSMENT

Certain themes recur throughout this text in discussions of assessments of each system. Repetition is intentional and reflects the importance of these activities. These basic principles of physical assessment include the following:

- **Review the perinatal history for clues to potential pathology.** The newborn's history begins with conception and includes events that occurred throughout gestation, labor, and delivery. The newborn is also affected by genetic histories of both parents and their families. For example, a maternal history that includes diabetes mellitus directs the experienced practitioner to carefully assess the extremities and cardiovascular and neurologic systems as infants of diabetic mothers show an increased incidence of abnormalities in these systems. Labor and delivery history may reveal the mother received medication for pain relief just before delivery; this could account for depression of the newborn's respirations and or muscular tone. With this knowledge, the examiner need not pursue a more serious etiology for the depressed respirations, as long as the respiratory pattern or muscle tone improves over time.
- **Assess the infant's color for clues to potential pathology.** The infant's color provides important information about several body systems. For example, very red, or ruddy, infants may have polycythemia and be more prone to complications such as respiratory distress or hypoglycemia associated with this phenomenon. The infant whose tongue and mucous membranes are pale or blue (central cyanosis) may be anemic, have a heart lesion, or have respiratory disease. Proper lighting is essential for accurate assessment of color. When the examiner is concerned about central color, pulse oximetry can aid assessment.
- **Auscultate in a quiet environment.** Assessing sounds produced by the body is difficult if there are noises, such as people talking or a radio/television playing, in the room. External

interferences impede accurate evaluation of heart, breath, and bowel sounds.

- **Keep the infant warm during examination.** After the infant is undressed, preventing heat loss is crucial to the infant's comfort, maintaining a normal temperature, and glucose homeostasis. An undressed infant is examined in a warm environment with an external heat source, such as an overhead radiant warmer. To keep from startling the newborn and maintaining a stable metabolic status, warming the stethoscope as well as the examiner's hands aids accurate assessment.
- **Have the necessary tools at hand.** A stethoscope, ophthalmoscope, and a tape measure are used in all comprehensive newborn examinations. Having these tools ready saves time.
- **Calm the infant before beginning the examination.** A quiet infant provides the best opportunity for data gathering. If a crying infant must be examined, patience—and possibly the aid of a second person to help calm the infant—are required.
- **Handle the infant gently.** The newly born infant is amazingly cooperative when the examiner is gentle. A soothing voice and a soft touch often allow the examiner to complete the entire physical assessment without disturbing the infant greatly or at all. If present, parents enjoy watching their infant interact with the examiner and appreciate a gentleness of touch. Certain portions of the examination cause the infant more distress than others. Examination of the hips, usually the most disturbing part of the examination, is therefore performed last.
- **Complete the examination.** Redress the infant to maintain a normal temperature. Document the examination findings in the medical record to notify the primary caregiver and team members the examination is over and of any abnormalities that were found or further observations that need to be made.

A SAMPLE APPROACH

One method of organizing examination of the newborn is described here as a guide for the inexperienced examiner. With practice, each examiner develops a personal style. It is assumed the infant is unclothed and supine under a radiant warmer.

Observation

It can be very difficult for a practitioner to just stand at a crib and observe the infant. The immediate inclination is to touch and talk to the infant. This natural response must be repressed until later in the examination, however, because observation alone produces important information about every organ system. These initial observations allow the examiner to develop a visual differential diagnosis before employing other assessment techniques (auscultation, palpation). Table 1.1 catalogs the many observations the skilled examiner must process in this initial assessment of the infant's status.

When multiple observations prove normal, the examiner is less likely to find a significant abnormality upon auscultation and palpation. Each observation of normality serves to reassure the examiner—just as an observation of abnormality should heighten the examiner's suspicion that further inspection is necessary.

Observation is not an isolated technique for use only at the outset of the examination. Although it is important to spend a moment or two at the bedside before touching the infant, observation of the infant's responses takes place throughout the examination. Depending on the infant's state and responses, all the observations listed in Table 1.1 can be made during the hands-on examination. The examiner must learn to take advantage of every opportunity the infant's behavior offers for observation. If, for example, the infant awakens spontaneously during the examination, the examiner should take advantage of that opportunity to examine the eyes.

Auscultation

After observing the infant closely, many examiners next auscultate the lungs, heart, and abdomen. Concentration allows the examiner to separate the sounds of the heart from those of the lungs. Listen first to one type of sound, then to the other. For example, listen first to the heart—its rate, rhythm, regularity, and any added sounds. Then listen to breath sounds, ignoring cardiac sounds.

Palpation

The examination continues with palpation. Palpating certain parts of the body disturbs the infant more than others. An ordered approach keeps the infant calm through much of the process. Because femoral pulses are difficult to assess in a crying infant, palpate them first, then palpate the brachial pulses. Next palpate the abdomen, beginning with the more superficial liver and spleen. (Learning to palpate the liver and spleen with the tips of the fingers as well as with the lateral edges of the index fingers facilitates examination from either side of the radiant warmer or bassinet.) Palpate for abdominal masses; then use deeper palpation for the kidneys. At this point, the infant may be disturbed and crying, but this will not impede the remainder of the examination.

Head-to-Toe Examination

After palpation, the examiner may then assess the infant from head to toe, examining the head and neck, upper extremities, lower extremities, back, and genitalia in sequence. This hands-on inspection also includes measurements and tactile examination of the skin. Maneuvers to assess symmetry and reflexes are also done.

The Integrated Examination

The skilled examiner integrates examination tasks. For example, after palpating the head, neck, clavicles, arms, and hands, the examiner can perform the pull-to-sit maneuver to assess palmar grasp, arm strength, and tone. At that point, the infant is being held in an appropriate position to elicit the Moro reflex. After progressing to the lower extremities, genitalia can be examined next. While the infant is positioned prone on the practitioner's hand to assess truncal tone and the truncal incurvation reflex, the back can be examined. These shortcuts facilitate multiple inspections and save time. Hips should be examined last as this procedure often causes the most stress to the infant.

Often it is not necessary to assess reflexes as a separate step. The examiner will likely have observed root and suck reflexes by this point. Moro and palmar grasp can be incorporated into the upper extremity examination, as just explained.

Although an extremely cooperative infant may sleep through the entire examination, assessment is not complete until the infant has been observed through various behavioral states. Facial asymmetry, for example, cannot be seen until the infant cries.

Ideally, the parents should observe the first complete examination. Parents appreciate demonstration of their infant's normality and uniqueness as well as early identification of unusual or abnormal findings.

EQUIPMENT

Ophthalmoscope

In addition to developing hands-on confidence with the newborn and performing the examination in the parents' presence, the student must become proficient with what may be unfamiliar equipment. Facility with the tools reduces stress to both infant and examiner. Again, practice is key.

If the ophthalmoscope is not already assembled, do so according to the manufacturer's instructions. Turn the ophthalmoscope on. To gain familiarity with the various apertures, rotate the aperture selection dial and project the light onto the palm of the hand or a piece of paper. The lens selector compensates for the visual acuity of the individual examiner. Adjust the lens selector dial to bring the structure being examined into focus.[4,6] The small and the large round beams are the two apertures used to assess the gemini choroidal light reflex (referred to as the *red reflex*) and pupillary response in the undilated eyes of the newborn. The most opportune time to examine a newborn's eyes is when the infant is in a quiet alert state. An infant who is in light sleep will often open the eyes if the room is darkened. To examine the infant's eyes, hold the ophthalmoscope in the right hand, with the viewing aperture as close as possible to the right eye, and use the right index finger to turn the lens selector dial to the appropriate lens for proper focus. While positioning the infant's head with the free hand, align the illuminating light along the infant's visual plane. If both the infant's eyes are open, the Bruckner test, a simultaneous bilateral red reflex test, may be performed. When using the large, full spot and holding the ophthalmoscope 18 to 20 inches (45–50 cm) from the infant's face, the light circle from the spot will cover both eyes. The examiner assesses symmetry and brightness of the red reflex as well as pupillary constriction.[6] The red reflex appears as a homogenous bright red-orange color. Any opacity along the central optical pathway will block all or part of the red reflex. Note that in infants with dark pigmentation, the reflex appears pale or cloudy rather than red.[6] Use the ophthalmoscope to observe pupillary constriction after assessing the red reflex.

Stethoscope

The acoustical stethoscope excludes environmental sounds, making it easier for the examiner to hear sounds coming from the infant; it does not magnify these sounds. The earpieces and connecting binaurals should be angled toward the wearer's nose to project sound onto the examiner's tympanic membrane. To minimize sound distortion, the tubing should be no longer than 12 inch. The chest piece of the stethoscope often has a double head: a flat, closed diaphragm and an open bell. The diaphragm is used to assess high-frequency sounds, and the bell, low frequency. Use the diaphragm to assess breath sounds by applying it firmly to the infant's skin so it moves with the chest wall. Both the diaphragm and the bell are used to assess heart sounds.[7] Do not compress the bell against the chest so firmly that it fills with tissue and acts like a diaphragm (see Chapters 7 and 8).

Otoscope

The infant's ears should be assessed for size, shape, and placement. The external auditory canals are examined for patency. Otoscopic examination is not normally done in the newborn period because the ear canals are often filled with vernix. For that reason, use of the otoscope is not described here.

SUMMARY

Each newborn examination is as different as each infant. This text explains basic techniques for examining each body system—to guide examiners with limited experience in performing a thorough newborn physical assessment. Only through experience, however, can practitioners develop clinical expertise. As experience and confidence grow, most examiners develop their own unique approach to physical examination, along with flexibility to adapt their approach to different situations. As long as the necessary equipment is available and basic principles are kept in mind, an infant can be examined in any setting.

ADDITIONAL RESOURCES

SPRINGER PUBLISHING CONNECT™

A robust set of resources designed to supplement this text is located at http://connect.springerpub.com/content/book/978-0-8261-4063-0. Qualifying instructors may request access by emailing textbook@springerpub.com.

REFERENCES

1. Nightingale F. 1969. *Notes on Nursing: What It Is and What It Is Not*. New York, NY: Dover, 112–113.
2. Coen RW, and Koffler H. 1987. *Primary Care of the Newborn*. Boston, MA: Little Brown, 30, 33.
3. Jarvis C. 2020. *Physical Examination & Health Assessment*, 8th ed. Philadelphia, PA: Saunders, 117.
4. Ball J, Dains J, Flynn J, Soloman B, and Stewart R. 2021. *Seidel's Guide to Physical Examination*, 9th ed. St. Louis, MO: Elsevier Mosby, 30–35, 42–43. Update pages.
5. Bickley L. 2020. *Bates' Guide to Physical Examination and History Taking*, 13th ed. Philadelphia, PA: Wolters Kluwer, 3–21, 779–926.
6. Wright K, and Strube Y. 2019. *Pediatric Ophthalmology for Primary Care*, 4th ed. Philadelphia, PA: Lippincott Williams & Wilkins, 35–45.
7. Orient JM. 2018. *Sapira's Art & Science of Bedside Diagnosis*, 5th ed. Philadelphia, PA: Lippincott Williams & Wilkins.

2 RECORDING AND EVALUATING THE NEONATAL HISTORY

Kimberly M. Horns

A comprehensive physical examination of the newborn, performed no later than 24 hours after birth by the physician, nurse practitioner, or physician's assistant, is a standard of perinatal care.[1] This applies to low-risk newborns; the high-risk newborn, however, requires an earlier comprehensive history and physical exam. Ideally, much of the history is obtained prior to the infant's birth. The physical examination must be preceded by a thorough review of the history of the current pregnancy; past obstetric history; intrapartum history; maternal medical, family medical, and social histories; and immediate neonatal adaptation history.[2] Admitting nursery personnel should evaluate the neonate's status and assess risks through a review of the history documented in the antepartum and intrapartum records no later than 2 hours after birth.[1]

Assessment is the gathering of accurate and comprehensive data and includes four components: (a) reviewing the history, (b) reviewing the results of the physical examination, (c) reviewing available laboratory or other data, and (d) formulating an impression (diagnostic differential). The practitioner then develops a plan of care and evaluates the newborn for actual or potential problems.

IMPORTANCE OF THE HISTORY

A comprehensive history is the prerequisite for adequate assessment. The newly born infant is a unique patient; no thorough history has ever been developed for this patient. When a newborn physical examination is performed without knowledge of the complete history, the information necessary for accurate formulation of an impression may be inadequate or incorrect.

The significance of the initial history and its thorough communication to the neonatal healthcare providers cannot be overstated. The newly born infant's history originates from the maternal records and includes the individual neonate's transitional experience. Neonatal healthcare providers commonly rely on a comprehensive maternal history; this history is often compiled from many sources and, perhaps, by many individuals. Communication with the obstetric healthcare provider, neonatal transport team members, and the parent(s) is essential to developing a thorough history. Written, faxed, or electronic information may be incomplete. The salient pertinent negatives and pertinent positives of a neonatal history are extremely important to develop the initial impression and diagnostic differentials.

Demonstrating knowledge of the perinatal history can also be useful in allaying parental anxiety when performing the initial physical examination. A prenatal ultrasound at 20 weeks gestation that revealed the possibility of the fetus having a fluid-filled gastrointestinal (GI) mass, but whose subsequent ultrasounds appeared to be normal, is likely to have increased parental concerns about the status of the neonate's GI tract. Knowledge of this pertinent history allows the examiner to emphasize the normal GI findings, discuss the history of the positive ultrasound findings, and reassure the parents.

The perinatal history also alerts the examiner to potential or suspected problems and may indicate the need for more frequent repeat examinations. For example, a cardiac murmur in a neonate with a history of maternal anticonvulsant use throughout pregnancy is of more concern than a murmur in a neonate with a negative history. Embryonic exposure to potential teratogens such as specific maternal anticonvulsant medications increases the risk for structural, congenital cardiac malformations.[3]

The history provides the context in which neonates with identified problems and disorders must be analyzed. Lack of a history or an incomplete history can lead to unnecessary testing or an incorrect impression or diagnosis. The following case exemplifies the need for obtaining an accurate history.

Case Example: The Need for an Accurate History

JM, a 36-week gestational age, 3-kg neonate, was admitted to the nursery at 1 a.m. following vaginal delivery to a 34-year-old, gravida 4, para 3 mother with a history of preeclampsia. JM's Apgar scores were 7 and 8 at 1 and 5 minutes, respectively. JM's admission was uneventful; physical examination revealed slightly decreased tone and spontaneous activity. Re-evaluation at 1 and 2 hours of age revealed continued poor tone and decreased spontaneous activity, with no other abnormal findings on the physical examination. At 2½ hours of age, an apneic episode was observed and noted. After being notified, the on-call healthcare provider requested blood for a complete blood count (CBC). On the neonate's next examination, the findings were consistent with decreased tone and activity. Blood and spinal fluid were obtained for culture and sensitivity, and antibiotics were started. The maternal chart with antepartum and intrapartum history was subsequently delivered to the nursery and revealed the mother had received bolus and maintenance doses of magnesium sulfate. The neonate's magnesium level was obtained and found to be elevated. Review of the history would have given a more accurate context in which to view this infant's poor tone and activity and would have led to an earlier identification of hypermagnesemia, perhaps avoiding unnecessary testing, or selecting specific other laboratory tests, such as an ionized calcium level.

The Supplemental Interview

Sometimes the birth parent or family may need to be interviewed for information not found in the record. Before approaching the parents, review all available medical records and identify the specific information needed. Remember that the first contact with the parent or family is one of the most important contacts. Introducing oneself, establishing a rapport, and defining the reason for one's questions will facilitate the interview. Asking a friendly question, such as what name has been chosen for the baby, helps establish a positive atmosphere.

Maintaining eye contact and presenting questions without reading them is important. Allow time for the parent to respond to your questions without interrupting them or checking your watch or the clock. Avoid technical language and the tendency to overexplain or lecture. If information must be recorded, remain engaged with the family to maintain effective communication.[4] Be an active listener. Show that the responses are understood, and request clarification when appropriate. Periodically, or at the end of the interview, summarize what the parents have shared. Evaluate answers to questions for content (what was said) and for affect or tone (how it was said). A parent who avoids answering a question or answers incompletely may not understand the question or may perceive the question as incriminating (such as questions involving substance use). When giving parents information about the neonate's health status, ask them to repeat at the end of the interview what they understand the neonate's health status or problems to be so any misunderstandings can be clarified immediately.

ELEMENTS OF A COMPLETE HISTORY

The historical information gathered must then be organized and presented in a systematic format commonly used by other professionals. The perinatal history may be hastily presented by healthcare providers when physical care of the infant is immediately warranted. The physical care of a newly born infant in transition often becomes the priority; however, a comprehensive history is equally important. This is especially true when infants are transported from one institution to another. A comprehensive history is imperative in these situations, and identification of potential problems during and after transport is the common goal. All pertinent information must be included. Elements of a complete history start with the identifying data, followed by the chief complaint, and then the interim history of the neonate or the history of the presenting problem or illness, if one exists. This is followed by the antepartum history; obstetric history; intrapartum history; and the maternal medical, family medical, and social histories. In most institutions, these data may be recorded by electronic medical record; in others, the data may be memorialized in a written or dictated history. After the history is compiled, the physical examination data are recorded, followed by any laboratory or radiology studies obtained. An impression and diagnostic differential of the neonate are then formulated, and a plan of care is outlined.

Identifying Data

The identifying data are the patients' names (mother and infant), birth dates, medical records, and referral sources. Both the referring obstetric care provider and the primary care pediatric provider should be listed so that they will have access to the admission history and physical examination. If the patient is admitted to the neonatal intensive care unit (NICU), contact information for the primary care providers should be included so that they can receive updates on the neonate's problems and progress. If the patient is transferred from another facility for care, the name of the referring healthcare facility should also be included.

Chief Complaint

The chief complaint in a neonate is often simply the identification, including age, sex, birth weight and current weight (if >1 day of age), gestational age by dates and examination, and any presenting clinical signs the infant exhibits. In the healthy newborn, the chief complaint might simply be stated as: "3-kg female, 41-weeks gestation by dates, appropriate for gestational age, now 2 hours of age." In an infant with complications, it may include identified problems, as in the following example:

1. 2.5-kg male, 42-weeks gestation by dates, small for gestational age, 3 hours of age
2. Hypoglycemia
3. Tachypnea: Pneumonia versus retained lung fluid
4. Suspected perinatal sepsis

Interim History

The interim history or history of present illness chronologically records the neonate's history from the time of delivery until the present time and, in the well newborn, should include data regarding temperature stabilization, feeding, voiding, stooling, and behavioral adaptation. In the neonate with identified problems, the sequence of the newborn's problem or problems is discussed, as are laboratory or x-ray findings, interventions, and responses to treatment. The age of the mother, type of delivery, neonate's birth weight and current weight, and Apgar scores are sometimes included to give a more comprehensive picture. Interim or monthly histories are often developed and documented when an infant is hospitalized for an extended length of time.

Antepartum History

The antepartum history includes specific historical data on the pregnancy: maternal age, gravidity, and parity; last menstrual period;

and estimated date of confinement (EDC) or estimated date of delivery (EDD). The EDD may be revised after serial ultrasound evaluation. The date and gestational age at which prenatal care began, who provided the care, and the number of prenatal visits should be recorded. Medical complications and high-risk pregnancy factors (Box 2.1), treatments, and monitoring are recorded. The antepartum history should also include information about fetal exposure to potential teratogens (Table 2.1).

BOX 2.1: CATEGORIZATION OF HIGH-RISK PREGNANCY FACTORS

SOCIOECONOMIC FACTORS

1. Inadequate finances
2. Poor housing–unhoused
3. Adolescent
4. Minority status
5. Nutritional deprivation
6. Parental occupation
7. Severe social problems—Inadequate Social Determinants of Health,[10] (economic stability, education, health and healthcare, neighborhood and built environment, and social/community context)

DEMOGRAPHIC FACTORS

1. Maternal age under 16 or over 35 years
2. Prenatal overweight or underweight
3. Height <5 feet
4. Maternal education <11 years
5. Family history of severe inherited disorders

MEDICAL FACTORS

a. Obstetric History

1. Infertility
2. Ectopic pregnancy or spontaneous abortion
3. Grand multiparity
4. Stillborn or neonatal death
5. Uterine/cervical abnormality
6. Multiple gestation
7. Premature labor/delivery
8. Prolonged labor
9. Cesarean section
10. Low-birth-weight infant
11. Macrosomic infant
12. Midforceps delivery
13. Baby with neurologic deficit, birth injury, or malformation
14. Hydatidiform mole or choriocarcinoma

b. Maternal Medical History/Status

1. Cardiac disease
2. Pulmonary disease
3. Metabolic disease—particularly, diabetes mellitus, thyroid disease
4. Chronic renal disease, repeated urinary tract infections, repeated bacteriuria
5. GI disease
6. Endocrine disorders (pituitary, adrenal)
7. Chronic hypertension
8. Hemoglobinopathies
9. Seizure disorder
10. Venereal and other infectious diseases
11. Weight loss >5 pounds
12. Malignancy
13. Surgery during pregnancy
14. Major congenital anomalies of the reproductive tract
15. Mental retardation, major emotional disorders

c. Current Maternal Obstetric Status

1. Late, inadequate, or no prenatal care
2. Rh sensitization

BOX 2.1: CATEGORIZATION OF HIGH-RISK PREGNANCY FACTORS (*continued*)

3. Fetus inappropriately large or small for gestational age
4. Premature labor
5. Pregnancy-induced hypertension
6. Multiple gestation
7. Polyhydramnios
8. Premature or prolonged rupture of membranes
9. Antepartum bleeding
   a. Placenta previa
   b. Abruptio placentae
10. Abnormal presentation
11. Postmaturity
12. Abnormality in tests for fetal well-being
13. Anemia

d. Substance use disorders including nicotine, alcohol, and prescribed and/or illicit drug use.

GI, gastrointestinal.

Source: Adapted from Healthy People.gov. *Healthy People 2030: Social Determinants of Health.*[10] Savich RD, and Famuyide M. 2021. Social and economic contributors to neonatal outcome in the United States. In *Fanaroff and Martin's Neonatal Perinatal Medicine*, 11th ed. Fanaroff RM, Fanaroff AA, and Walsh MC, eds. Philadelphia PA: Elsevier, 140–151.[11]

When reviewing the antepartum history, the examiner should note the results of all tests performed on the mother and/or fetus and understand their implications. Usual prenatal screenings may include the following tests: maternal blood type and Rh; antibody screen; serology; venereal disease research laboratory (VDRL) status; rubella immunity testing; cultures for *gonococcus, chlamydia, and Group B streptococcus, human papilloma virus*; hepatitis B surface antigen screening; alpha-fetoprotein; HIV testing; triple/quadruple screening; and ultrasound. Patients with specific high-risk factors for tuberculosis are tested. HIV antibody screening is now universally recommended in prenatal care.[5] Those who acquire HIV infection during pregnancy require more extensive evaluation.[5] If no HIV screening information is available, an HIV screen of the mother is recommended in labor or soon after delivery to facilitate early potential neonatal treatment.[5] Abnormal findings on routine screening tests will prompt follow-up or specialized screenings.

Fetal cells and cell-free nucleic acids originating from the placenta (trophoblast) are detectable in maternal blood as early as 5 weeks gestation, even before the establishment of fetal circulation. A noninvasive prenatal screening test utilizes this cell-free fetal DNA found in maternal blood to identify specific genetic disorders, including fetal sex, Rhesus blood group/type, hemoglobinopathies, fetal/neonatal alloimmune thrombocytopenia,[1] and genetic aneuploidies such at trisomies 13, 18, and 21 and microdeletions.[6]

A schedule for routine, general, and specific laboratory examinations during pregnancy appears in Table 2.2. Indications for antepartum fetal assessment are listed in Table 2.3. Appendix A explains many of the routine and some specialized antepartum screenings and indicates what the results mean.

Obstetric History

The maternal obstetric history is reviewed and recorded for the number of pregnancies, abortions, stillbirths, living children, types of deliveries, dates of birth or abortion, birth weights, and gestational ages at birth. Particular attention should be paid to serial ultrasound findings, biophysical profiles, and any nonstress or contraction stress tests. Any previous premature births, neonatal problems, or subsequent major medical problems of prior children should be noted. Previous placental pathology or previous neonatal asphyxia may be important for current pregnancy. The present age and health status of living children are recorded. If any child is deceased, the cause and date of death should be included.

TABLE 2.1: MATERNAL MEDICATIONS AND TOXINS: POSSIBLE EFFECTS ON THE FETUS AND/OR NEWBORN

MEDICATION/TOXIN	POSSIBLE EFFECT ON FETUS/NEWBORN
Analgesics and Anti-Inflammatories	
Aspirin	Hemorrhage, premature closure of ductus arteriosus, and pulmonary artery hypertension
Codeine	Neonatal abstinence syndrome
Ibuprofen	Reduced amniotic fluid volume when used in tocolysis, theoretic risk for premature ductus arteriosus closure
Indomethacin	Closure of fetal ductus arteriosus, pulmonary artery hypertension
Meperidine	Respiratory depression peaks 2 to 3 hours after maternal dose
Anesthetics	
General anesthesia	Respiratory depression of infant at delivery if anesthesia is prolonged before delivery
Lidocaine	High fetal serum levels cause CNS depression, accidental direct injection into fetal head causes seizures
Antibiotics	
Aminoglycosides	Ototoxicity reported after first trimester use of kanamycin and streptomycin
Streptomycin	Damage to the eighth cranial nerve, hearing loss
Vancomycin	Potential for ototoxicity
Cephalosporins	Some drugs in this group displace bilirubin from albumin
Isoniazid	Risk for folate deficiency
Sulfonamides	Some drugs in this group displace bilirubin from albumin
Tetracycline	Yellow-brown staining and caries of teeth
Trimethoprim	Folate antagonism
Anticoagulants	
Warfarin (Coumadin)	Warfarin embryopathy
Anticonvulsants	
Carbamazepine	Neural tube defects, midfacial hypoplasia
Phenobarbital	Withdrawal symptoms, hemorrhagic disease
Phenytoin	Hemorrhagic disease, fetal hydantoin syndrome
Trimethadione	Fetal trimethadione syndrome, cleft lip and palate, cardiac, and genital anomalies

(continued)

TABLE 2.1: MATERNAL MEDICATIONS AND TOXINS: POSSIBLE EFFECTS ON THE FETUS AND/OR NEWBORN (*continued*)

MEDICATION/TOXIN	POSSIBLE EFFECT ON FETUS/NEWBORN
Valproic acid	Myelomeningocele, facial, and cardiac anomalies
Antineoplastics	
Aminopterin	Cleft palate, hydrocephalus, myelomeningocele, and growth restriction
Cyclophosphamide	Growth restriction, cardiovascular, and digital anomalies
Methotrexate	Absent digits
Antithyroid Drugs	
Iodide-containing drugs	Hypothyroidism
Methimazole	Hypothyroidism, cutis aplasia
Propylthiouracil	Hypothyroidism
Antivirals	
Ribavirin	Teratogenic and embryolethal in animals
Zidovudine	Potential fetal bone marrow suppression, reduces perinatal HIV transmission
Cardiovascular Drugs and Antihypertensives	
Angiotensin-converting enzyme inhibitors	Neonatal bradycardia, hypoglycemia
ß-blockers (propranolol)	Neonatal bradycardia, hypoglycemia
Calcium channel blockers	If maternal hypotension occurs, could affect placental blood flow
Diazoxide	Hyperglycemia
Digoxin	Fetal toxicity with maternal overdose
Hydralazine	Maternal hypotensive risk with possible effect on placental blood flow
Methyldopa	Mild, clinically insignificant decrease in neonatal blood pressure
Diuretics	
Furosemide	Increases fetal urinary sodium and potassium
Thiazides	Thrombocytopenia
Hormonal Drugs	
Androgenics (danazol)	Masculinization of female fetus
Corticosteroids	Cleft palate reported in animals

(*continued*)

TABLE 2.1: MATERNAL MEDICATIONS AND TOXINS: POSSIBLE EFFECTS ON THE FETUS AND/OR NEWBORN (*continued*)

MEDICATION/TOXIN	POSSIBLE EFFECT ON FETUS/NEWBORN
Estrogens, progestins	Uncertain teratogenic potential, virilization of female fetuses reported with progestins
Tamoxifen	Increased risk of fetal anomalies
Sedatives, Tranquilizers, and Psychotropic Medications	
Barbiturates (short-acting)	Theoretic risk for hemorrhage and drug withdrawal
Benzodiazepines	Hypotonia, impaired thermoregulation, and drug withdrawal
Lithium	Cardiac anomalies (Ebstein's), diabetes insipidus, thyroid depression, and cardiovascular dysfunction
SSRI	Low birth weight, prematurity, hypoglycemia, respiratory problems requiring assisted ventilation, potential persistent pulmonary hypertension[12]
Tricyclic antidepressants	Association with limb-reduction defects
Tocolytics	
Magnesium sulfate	Transient respiratory depression, hypotonia, and hypermagnesemia
Ritodrine	Neonatal hypoglycemia
Terbutaline	Neonatal hypoglycemia
Vitamins and Related Drugs	
A	Excessive doses are teratogenic
D	Megadoses may cause hypercalcemia, lethargy, and poor feeding
Isotretinoin	Ear, cardiac, CNS, and thymic anomalies
Menadione (vitamin K_3)	Hyperbilirubinemia and kernicterus at high doses
Miscellaneous	
Antiemetics	Doxylamine succinate and/or dicyclomine hydrochloride with pyridoxine hydrochloride reported to be a teratogen (unproven)
Irradiation	Fetal death, microcephaly, and growth restriction
Methyl mercury	Mental retardation, microcephaly
Oral hypoglycemics	Neonatal hypoglycemia
Social and Illicit Drugs	
Alcohol	Fetal alcohol spectrum disorders or fetal alcohol syndrome
Amphetamines/ methamphetamines	Withdrawal, prematurity, fetal loss, infant death, low birth weight, and small for gestational age[13]

(*continued*)

TABLE 2.1: MATERNAL MEDICATIONS AND TOXINS: POSSIBLE EFFECTS ON THE FETUS AND/OR NEWBORN (*continued*)

MEDICATION/TOXIN	POSSIBLE EFFECT ON FETUS/NEWBORN
Cocaine	Decreased birth weight; microcephaly; prematurity; abruptio placentae with possible asphyxia, shock, cerebral hemorrhage, and stillbirth
Heroin	Increased incidence of low birth weight and small for gestational age, neonatal opioid withdrawal
Marijuana	Prematurity, lower birth weights, higher NICU admission rates, learning deficits and decreased executive functioning skills for school-aged children
Methadone	Neonatal abstinence syndrome
PCP	Irritability, jitteriness, hypertonia, and poor feeding
Tobacco smoking	Decreased birth weight; increased prematurity rate; increased premature rupture of membranes; jitteriness, hypertonicity, and decreased cognition in school-aged children

CNS, central nervous system; NICU, neonatal intensive care unit; PCP, phencyclidine; SSRI, selective serotonin reuptake inhibitors.

Source: Adapted from Levy J, and D'Harlingue AE. 2013. Recognition, stabilization, and transport of the high-risk newborn. In *Klaus and Fanaroff's Care of the High-Risk Neonate*, 6th ed. Fanaroff AA, and Fanaroff JM, eds. Philadelphia, PA: Saunders, 75–77. Reprinted by permission.

TABLE 2.2: RECOMMENDED INTERVALS FOR ROUTINE AND SPECIALIZED ANTEPARTUM TESTS

TIME (WEEKS)	ASSESSMENT
Initial (as early as possible)	CBC
	Urine culture and baseline protein screening
	Blood group and Rh type determinations
	Antibody screen
	Rubella antibody titer measurement
	Syphilis screen
	Cervical cytology—Papanicolaou test
	Hepatitis B surface antigen
	HIV testing/counseling
Optional labs	Hemoglobin electrophoresis
	PPD
	Chlamydia
	Gonococcus
	Trichomonas specialized genetic testing

(*continued*)

TABLE 2.2: RECOMMENDED INTERVALS FOR ROUTINE AND SPECIALIZED ANTEPARTUM TESTS (*continued*)

TIME (WEEKS)	ASSESSMENT
	Tay Sachs/other testing as indicated by history
	Hepatitis C testing when/if history suggests increased risk
8 to 20	Ultrasound
(Depending on test and maternal/fetal history)	Noninvasive prenatal screening DNA analysis
	Maternal serum alpha-fetoprotein
	Amniocentesis
	Chorionic villus sampling—karyotype, amniotic fluid alpha-fetoprotein
24 to 28	Diabetes screening
	Glucose tolerance testing if diabetes screen abnormal
	Repeat hemoglobin or hematocrit measurement
	Repeat antibody test for unsensitized Rh-negative patients
28	Prophylactic administration of Rho(D) immune globulin as indicated
32 to 36 (when indicated)	Ultrasound
	Testing for sexually transmitted disease
	Repeat hemoglobin or hematocrit measurement recommended
	Group B streptococcus culture at 35 to 37 weeks gestation

CBC, complete blood count; PPD, purified protein derivative.

Source: Adapted from American Academy of Pediatrics, American College of Obstetricians and Gynecologists. 2017. *Guidelines for Perinatal Care*, 8th ed. Elk Grove Village, IL: American Academy of Pediatrics, 347–408.[1]

Intrapartum History

The intrapartum history is evaluated for duration of labor, whether the labor was spontaneous or induced, medications and anesthetics used during labor and delivery, length of the first and second stages of labor, type of delivery, and whether delivery was spontaneous or required forceps or vacuum assistance. The time and duration of rupture of membranes, the use of amnioinfusion, and the status of the amniotic fluid volume and presence or absence of meconium are ascertained. Laboratory and monitoring data obtained during labor are reviewed and noted, as are any maternal complications that occurred during this period (such as fever, bleeding, or hypertension) and the treatment provided. The presentation of the neonate at delivery, the Apgar scores, any resuscitative interventions performed, and the response to resuscitation are documented. If resuscitation is required, the timing of the interventions is equally important. To ensure an objective determination of the fetal metabolic condition at the time of birth, umbilical cord blood sampling, including both arterial and venous blood, is indicated if there is any degree of

TABLE 2.3: MATERNAL AND FETAL INDICATIONS FOR ANTEPARTUM FETAL ASSESSMENT

MATERNAL	PREGNANCY RELATED
Antiphospholipid syndrome	Gestational hypertension, preeclampsia
Hyperthyroidism (poorly controlled)	Decreased fetal movement
Hemoglobinopathies (hemoglobin SS, SC, or S-thalassemia)	Abnormal amniotic fluid volume
Cyanotic heart disease	Growth restriction
Systemic lupus erythematosus	Isoimmunization (moderate to severe)
Chronic renal disease	Previous fetal demise (unexplained or recurrent risk)
Pregestational diabetes mellitus	Multiple gestation (with significant growth discrepancy)
Hypertensive disorders	

Source: Data from American College of Obstetricians and Gynecologists. 2021. *Antepartum Fetal Surveillance: ACOG Practice Bulletin 229.* Washington, DC: ACOG.[14]

perinatal depression.[7] Histologic findings of the placenta are an important part of the intrapartum history when defining and confirming perinatal depression.[8]

Maternal Medical History

The maternal medical history is reviewed for chronic health problems and for diseases or disorders treated in the past and/or during the pregnancy. Potential consequences of maternal medical problems for the fetus and/or newborn are listed in Table 2.4. Infections (past, present, and during the pregnancy) and surgical procedures and hospitalizations that occurred before or during the pregnancy are included. Maternal mental health history and treatment should be evaluated as well as risk for postpartum depression. Medication use, including herbal supplements and over-the-counter preparations, should be noted and potential impacts assessed.

Family Medical History

The family medical history is reviewed for ages of the infant's mother, father, and siblings; sexes of the other children; and any diagnosed chronic disorders, disabilities, or known hereditary diseases. A genetic history may be required if the neonate has dysmorphology, and further information should be sought regarding other family members affected with a similar disorder. Information about familial disease or disorders can be elicited by asking if anyone else in the immediate or extended family has the same or a related problem, or if any relative has a genetic abnormality or an unusual disease or disorder. A finding such as a head circumference several standard deviations above normal with normal weight and length percentiles may raise the possibility of an intracranial abnormality. Review of the family history should include questions regarding any similar finding in the baby's parents when they were children. A grandparent can often provide or confirm this information. The most common cause of a large head in an otherwise normal newborn is benign familial megalencephaly, and one of the parents, usually the father, generally had the same finding in infancy.[9] Preparation of a genetic pedigree chart (Figure 2.1) often helps clarify the relationships of affected family members when the history is positive for similar findings in relatives. The question of consanguinity (mating

TABLE 2.4: POTENTIAL EFFECTS OF MATERNAL MEDICAL CONDITIONS ON THE FETUS AND/OR NEWBORN

MATERNAL CONDITION	POTENTIAL FETAL/NEONATAL EFFECTS
Cardiopulmonary	
Asthma	Increased rates of prematurity, toxemia, and perinatal loss
Congenital heart disease	Effects of cardiovascular drugs (see Table 2.2)
Cystic fibrosis	Prematurity, IUGR, and fetal loss
Hypertension, preeclampsia	Premature delivery caused by uncontrolled hypertension or eclampsia; uteroplacental insufficiency, abruptio placentae, fetal loss; IUGR; thrombocytopenia; neutropenia
Endocrine/metabolic	
Diabetes mellitus	Hypoglycemia, hypocalcemia, macrosomia, polycythemia, hyperbilirubinemia, increased risk for birth defects, birth trauma, small left colon syndrome, cardiomyopathy, and RDS
Hypoparathyroidism	Fetal hypocalcemia, neonatal hyperparathyroidism
Hyperparathyroidism	Neonatal hypocalcemia and hypoparathyroidism
Hyperthyroidism (Grave's disease)	Fetal and neonatal hyperthyroidism, IUGR, prematurity, congestive heart failure, and tachycardia
Obesity	Macrosomia, birth trauma
Phenylketonuria (untreated pregnancies)	Intellectual disabilities, microcephaly, and congenital heart defects
Hematologic	
Fetal platelet antigen sensitization	Thrombocytopenia, CNS hemorrhage
Idiopathic thrombocytopenia purpura	Intracranial hemorrhage
Iron deficiency anemia	Potential teratogen
Rh or ABO sensitization	Hemolytic disease, jaundice, anemia, and hydrops fetalis
Severe anemia (hemoglobin <6 mg/dL)	Impaired oxygen delivery, fetal loss
Sickle cell anemia	Increased prematurity, IUGR, and fetal distress
Infections	
Chlamydia	Conjunctivitis, pneumonia
COVID-19	Respiratory problems requiring assisted ventilation, feeding and GI complications, prematurity, and fever[15]
Chorioamnionitis	Increased risk for neonatal sepsis, premature labor and delivery

(continued)

TABLE 2.4: POTENTIAL EFFECTS OF MATERNAL MEDICAL CONDITIONS ON THE FETUS AND/OR NEWBORN (*continued*)

MATERNAL CONDITION	POTENTIAL FETAL/NEONATAL EFFECTS
Cytomegalovirus	IUGR, microcephaly, cytomegalovirus inclusion disease, and hearing loss
Gonorrhea	Ophthalmia neonatorum
Hepatitis A	Perinatal transmission
Hepatitis B	Perinatal transmission, chronic hepatitis
Hepatitis C	Perinatal transmission, chronic hepatitis
Herpes simplex	Encephalitis, disseminated herpes (risk of neonatal disease is much higher when maternal infection is primary rather than recurrent)
HIV	Risk of infectious transmission
mPOX	Congenital defects, maculopapular lesions, hydrops, hepatomegaly, prematurity, neurological syndromes, and stillbirth[16]
Rubella	Rubella embryopathy, cataracts, and cardiac defects
Syphilis	Congenital syphilis, IUGR
Toxoplasmosis	IUGR, microcephaly, hydrocephalus, chorioretinitis, and myocarditis
Tuberculosis	Perinatal and postnatal transmission
Varicella	Congenital varicella syndrome, rash, pneumonia, myocarditis, and encephalitis
Zika	Maternal 3rd trimester rash, microcephaly, and 4-fold increase in neonatal mortality[17]
Inflammatory/Immunologic	
Inflammatory bowel disease	Increase in prematurity, fetal loss, fetal, and neonatal growth restriction
Systemic lupus erythematosus	Fetal death, spontaneous abortion, heart block, neonatal lupus, thrombocytopenia, neutropenia, hemolytic anemia, and endocardial fibrosis
Neuromuscular	
Maternal seizure disorder requiring anticonvulsants	Teratogenic effects of medications (see Table 2.2)
Myasthenia gravis	Transient neonatal myasthenia, preterm delivery
Myotonic dystrophy	Neonatal myotonic dystrophy
Seizure during pregnancy	Fetal hypoxia

TABLE 2.4: POTENTIAL EFFECTS OF MATERNAL MEDICAL CONDITIONS ON THE FETUS AND/OR NEWBORN (*continued*)

MATERNAL CONDITION	POTENTIAL FETAL/NEONATAL EFFECTS
Renal/Urologic	
Chronic renal failure	Prematurity, IUGR, and fetal loss
Transplant recipients	Prematurity, IUGR, possible effects of maternal immunosuppressive therapy, and mineral disorders
Urinary tract infection	Prematurity

CNS, central nervous system; GI, gastrointestinal; IUGR, intrauterine growth restriction; RDS, respiratory distress syndrome.

Source: Adapted from Bahadue FL, and Gecsi KS. 2020. Antenatal and intrapartum care of the high-risk infant. In *Klaus and Fanaroff's Care of the High-Risk Neonate*, 7th ed. Fanaroff AA, and Fanaroff JM, eds. Philadelphia, PA: Elsevier.[18]

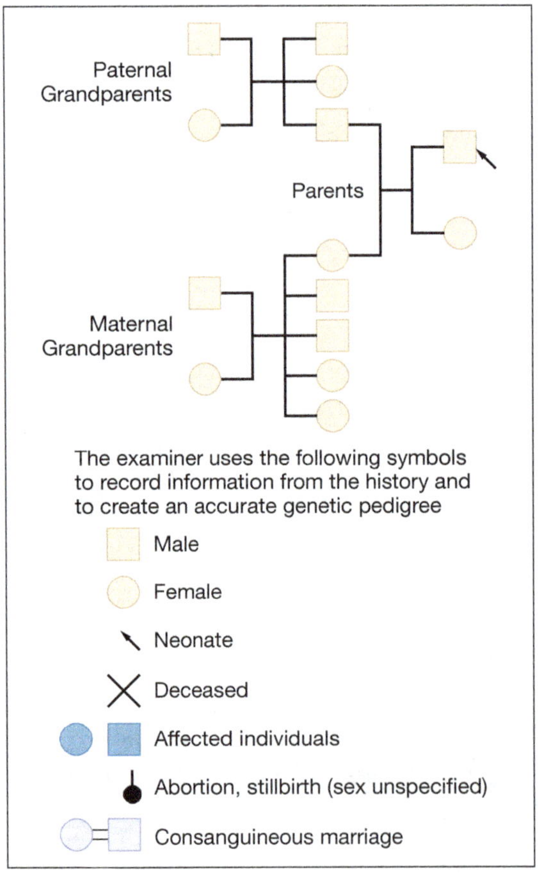

FIGURE 2.1 Genetic pedigree chart

of individuals related by blood) can be posed by asking the parents if they are related in any way besides by marriage and if there is anyone in the family who was related to both parents before their marriage.

Social History

The social history includes the marital status, presence, or support of the infant's other parent, and both parents' occupations and education. In addition to the mother's name, their sexual and gender identity, sexual orientation, and preferred pronoun(s) may be included. The family's sources of support in the financial, housing, and care areas are noted and number of people living in the home. The family's religious affiliation and cultural heritage are included. The family unit should be defined. The health status of all household members should also be ascertained. Identification of both formal and informal support systems including support agencies with which the family is working is important. Parental obligations outside the home should be identified to elicit plans for care of the infant after discharge. Information regarding frequent or recent family moves, deaths in the family, and job changes also gives an idea of the stressors affecting the family. This information will assist the examiner in establishing a safe discharge plan.

Remaining Elements

The physical examination is performed, and recorded, in the medical record. Laboratory or radiology data that have been obtained should be noted. An assessment or impression of the infant's status is then made, including a statement of suspected or potential problems. Here is an example for a neonate with identified problems:

1. 3.8-kg preterm female, 35-weeks gestation, born by cesarean section, large for gestational age, infant of a diabetic mother, now 4 hours of age
2. Hypoglycemia
3. Respiratory distress: tachypnea
4. Systolic cardiac murmur at upper left sternal border

An assessment statement for a well newborn with no complications might be similar to the following:

1. 3.5-kg term male, appropriate for gestational age, 4 hours of age
2. Teen parents with little social support

A plan addressing each identified problem or problems by system should then be developed and documented in the admission history.

SUMMARY

A thorough approach to neonatal history exploration, coupled with analysis of antepartum and intrapartum data, provides a comprehensive view of the neonate's present status and potential health problems. Taking the time to review perinatal history helps identify potential and actual problems in context and, with the physical examination findings, formulate care priorities and develop a comprehensive plan of care.

ADDITIONAL RESOURCES

A robust set of resources designed to supplement this text is located at http://connect.springerpub.com/content/book/978-0-8261-4063-0. Qualifying instructors may request access by emailing textbook@springerpub.com.

REFERENCES

1. American Academy of Pediatrics, American College of Obstetricians and Gynecologists. 2017. *Guidelines for Perinatal Care*, 8th ed. Elk Grove Village, IL: American Academy of Pediatrics, 347–408.
2. Dyet LE, and Crowley R. 2021. Physical assessment and classification. In *Avery & MacDonald's Neonatology: Pathophysiology and Management of the Newborn*, 8th ed. Boardman JP, Groves AM, and Ramasethy J, eds. Philadelphia, PA: Wolters-Kluwer, 215–237.
3. Thomas SV. 2008. Cardiac malformations are increased in infants of mothers with epilepsy. *Pediatric Cardiology* 29(3): 604–608.
4. Lee RV, Rosene-Montella K, Barbour LA, Garner PR, and Keely E. 2000. *Medical Care of the Pregnant Patient*. Philadelphia, PA: American College of Physicians, 727.
5. Centers for Disease Control and Prevention. 2022. *HIV Testing*. https://www.cdc.gov/hiv/testing/index.html
6. Kypri E, Ioannides M, Achillease A, Koumbaris G, Patsalis P, and Stumm M. 2022. Non-invasive prenatal screening tests: An update. *Journal of Laboratory Medicine* 46(4): 311–320.
7. ACOG Committee on Obstetric Practice. 2006. Opinion No. 348, November 2006: Umbilical cord blood gas and acid-base analysis. *Obstetrics and Gynecology* 108(5): 1319–1322.
8. Harteman JC, Nikkels PGJ, Benders, MJNL, Kwee, A, Groenendaal, F, and deVries LS. 2013. Placental pathology in full-term infants with hypoxic-ischemic neonatal encephalopathy and association with magnetic resonance imaging pattern of brain injury. *Journal of Pediatrics* 163(4): 968–995.
9. Goldbloom RB. 1997. *Pediatric Clinical Skills*. New York, NY: Churchill Livingstone, 51.
10. Healthy People.gov. 2020. *Healthy People 2030: Social Determinants of Health*. https://health.gov/healthypeople/priority-areas/social-determinants-health
11. Savich RD, and Famuyide M. 2021. Social and economic contributors to neonatal outcome in the United States. In *Fanaroff and Martin's Neonatal Perinatal Medicine*, 11th ed. Fanaroff RM, Fanaroff AA, and Walsh MC, eds. Philadelphia PA: Elsevier, 140–151.
12. Levy M, Kovo M, Miremberg Hl, Anchel N, Herman HG, Bar J, Schreiber L, and Weiner E. 2020. Maternal use of selective serotonin reuptake inhibitors (SSRI) during pregnancy—neonatal outcomes in correlation with placental histopathology. *Journal of Perinatology* 40: 1017–1024.
13. Anderson JM, Hoiseth G, and Nygaard E. 2020. Prenatal exposure to methadone or buprenorphine and long-term outcomes. *Early Human Development* 143. doi: 10.1016/j.earlhumdev.2020.104997

14. American College of Obstetricians and Gynecologists. 2021. *Antepartum Fetal Surveillance: ACOG Practice Bulletin 229*. Washington, DC: ACOG.
15. Giuliani F, Oros D, Gunier RB, Deantoni S, Rauch S, Casale R, Nieto R, Bertino E, Rego, A, Menis C, Gravett MG, Candiani M, Deruelle P, Garcia-May PK, Mhatre M, Usman MA, Abd-Elsalam S, Etuk S, Napolitano R, Liu B, and Villar J. 2022. Effects of prenatal exposure to maternal COVID-19 and perinatal care on neonatal outcome: Results from the INTERCOVID Multinational Cohort Study. *American Journal of Obstetrics and Gynecology* 227: 488.e1–488.e17.
16. Velasquez-Cervantes MA, Ulloa-Aguilar JM, and Leon-Juarez M. 2023. Mpox and pregnancy: A neglected disease and its impact on perinatal health. *Revista Clinica Espanola* 223: 32–39.
17. Velazquez-Cervantes MA, Ulloa-Aguilar JM, and Leon-Juarez M. 2023. Oliveira WK, et al. 2016 Congenital Zika virus syndrome in Brazil: A case series of the first 1501 livebirths with complete investigation. *Lancet* 388: 891–897.
18. Bahadue FL, and Gecsi KS. 2020. Antenatal and intrapartum care of the high-risk neonate. In *Klaus and Fanaroff's Care of the High-Risk Neonate*, 7th ed. Fanaroff AA, and Fanaroff JM, eds. Philadelphia, PA: Elsevier, 9–43.

3 COMMUNICATING WITH PARENTS

Dixie K. Weber, Trish L. Anderson, and Rebecca Vahle

Effective communication with families is an essential part of a newborn assessment. Whether sharing the good news of a family's newborn or discussing difficult topics if the infant is unwell, good communication skills are invaluable.

Considering the audience with whom one is speaking facilitates therapeutic conversations. Basic communication recommendations should be utilized for all patients. However, unique family and patient populations—such as those involved in adoptions, the LGBTQIA+ community, surrogacy arrangements, those with substance use disorder, and those in correctional care—require specific tools and intentional language in order to deliver respectful, neutral, and compassionate care.

CONCEPTS OF COMPASSIONATE COMMUNICATION

Body Language

Body language and nonverbal language play a large role in communication.[1] When a care provider enters a patient's room, the patient reads and interprets the provider's approach. Facial expression, a sense of avoidance, or a focus on other things may be interpreted as a lack of interest in the patient and family. It is important for providers to pay attention to their body posture and extraneous movements. Consider spacing an appropriate distance from the patient when communicating. An average distance of 1 meter (approximately 3 feet) from the care provider to the patient has been found to be an appropriate starting point; however, observe the patient's response to changes in physical proximity. Cultural norms and practices should be considered when establishing proximity for communication. Patients interacting with healthcare providers may have high anxiety or a sense of hypervigilance. The Egan model offers counseling and interaction methods in the SOLER approach: **S**it squarely, **O**penness, **L**eaning forward, **E**ye contact, and a **R**elaxed body form.[2] This framework provides the care provider an objective tool to "check" themselves and their approach.

Welcoming Ritual

A welcoming ritual lays the groundwork for effective communication with the patient and their family. First impressions are made in the initial seconds of a meeting, so including a smile, making appropriate eye contact, and sitting when possible are helpful in creating a collaborative environment.[3] A welcoming ritual should include introductions, including the provider's name and role on the care team, as well as how long one will be with the patient. It is important to ask the patient their name, and you may ask their pronoun preference. Instead of assuming who family members are, ask the patient who they consider to be close to them without assuming their biological family are the people in the room who they consider influential or "close as family." Care providers may ask, "What family members should I be aware of? Who are the support people you find helpful? What concerns do they have?" Additional questions may prompt for further information that the care provider may need to know. Talking *with* patients rather than *at* patients is most effective in establishing trust. Partner with the patient to assure expectations are clarified and needs are established.

The introduction will help establish successful two-way communication and will set the groundwork for safe patient care and optimal outcomes.[4] In the introduction, if directions are to be given, focus on the positive. Discuss what you would *like* the family to do, not what you *don't* want them to do. This positive approach can help facilitate ongoing interaction and deepen the relationship. Ask open-ended questions that allow the patient to discuss their needs. Utilizing the technique of repeat-back ensures understanding. Ask the patient to do the same.

When a patient has a history of trauma or a specific communication or listening style, they may not maintain eye contact during the welcoming introduction. This does not indicate that they are not listening. Direct communication can "feel intense" to some patients and, therefore, a patient may demonstrate avoidance or appear distracted to decrease the intensity of the interaction. They may avoid eye contact to lessen stimulation; they may look distracted on their phone or stare off into space.[5] Additionally, some cultures may regard direct eye contact as disrespectful; therefore, forcing direct eye contact to ensure the patient is listening is inappropriate. Cultural sensitivity also may include considering the intensity of facial expressions when communicating.[6] Culturally sensitive communication begins with understanding one's own cultural beliefs, attitudes, practices, and values. Adapting to cultural differences is key to creating an environment that encourages collaboration with patients and respectful interactions with their family.[7]

Correcting Misinformation

When a patient has misinformation, gently correcting or sharing accurate information without judgement is an important skill to ensure that trust between care provider and patient is developed. If clarifying information is necessary, care providers should provide patients with gentle corrections. Before correcting any misinformation a patient may have expressed, the care provider should assess their own emotions about the information, the source of that information if shared, and the patient's mind-set. If needed, validate how they are feeling. Correcting the information without validating the feelings associated with the information may cause the patient to feel unheard, and they may not share further information. Avoid blaming the patient or other care providers for the patient's confusion. If the patient continues to repeat their concerns, they likely are not feeling heard. Redefining an intervention and rationale may help them to feel heard and validated.

Both verbal and nonverbal clues are important aspects of communication. During primary care appointments, missed clues increase appointment times to 20.1 minutes compared to 17.6 minutes without missed clues. Missed clues in surgery visits increase appointment times from 12.5 minutes to 14 minutes.[8] Active listening, asking open-ended questions regarding concerns (e.g., "tell me more" or "help me understand"), and validating those concerns towards a solution will empower the patient to feel more connected to their care provider, and the care provider will be able to utilize the time more effectively.

Addressing the Patient and Their Family

With many unique family patient populations, calling the patient and their support person by their preferred first name can avoid misunderstandings about the role of the person giving birth. Therefore, asking rather than assuming will minimize mistakes. Calling a patient by their preferred first name avoids the question of the role they will play in the child's life.

The script of a care provider when caring for patients may routinely include titles like "Mom" and "Dad." While convenient, it can be impersonal and inaccurate in socially complex family models. The birthing person in the bed may or may not automatically be the newborn's "mom." Just as the care provider clarifies the names of the person giving birth and the support person who may be present, the care provider may also clarify the names of other family members in the room and follow the lead of the patient in using titles and roles designated within the family.

All people deserve person-first language. Person-first language and family-first language is when the person is addressed prior to a diagnosis or label. For example, there is not a "Down syndrome baby in Room 202," but instead "a baby who has Down syndrome." A patient who has diabetes should not be labeled "a diabetic." It is important that patients are respected as individuals and not defined by their ailment or condition. Labels can be hurtful and include assumptions and stereotypes. Patients should always receive respectful, individualized care that validates them as a person *first*, with the diagnosis *second*.

On July 11, 2006, The *People First Respectful Language Modernization Act of 2006* was enacted by the Council of the District of Columbia. This legislation provides a framework for person-first language and "requires the use of respectful language when referring to people with disabilities in all new and revised District laws, regulations, rules, and publications and all internet publications." Person-first language should be at the core of all interactions with patients, and should also be found in all healthcare policies, practices, and electronic health records. An example of non-person-first language would be describing a patient from the local jail as a "prisoner" instead of a patient in correctional care or a patient that is incarcerated.

Table 3.1 provides examples of ways to substitute person-first language for outdated and/or offensive terminology.

Effective Communication With *All* Families

Effective communication with all families of newborns is essential. Considering the audience with which one is speaking prepares the care provider for conversations that need to take place with the newborn's parent(s) or guardian(s). There is much to be considered

TABLE 3.1: EXAMPLES OF PERSON-FIRST TERMINOLOGY

OUTDATED TERM	REPLACE WITH
Disabled adults	Adults with disabilities
Disabled people	People with disabilities
Disabled child	Child with disabilities
Learning disabled	Person with a cognitive disability or has a learning disability
Handicapped parking	Accessible parking
Mentally ill person	Person with a mental health condition
Suffering from disability	Person who has a disability
Wheelchair user or wheelchair bound	Person who uses a wheelchair/mobility chair
Epileptic	Person who has epilepsy
Diabetic	Person who has diabetes

Source: People First Respectful Language Modernization Act of 2006.[9]

when crafting communication—the family's unique needs, characteristics, beliefs, and culture. Also, one must consider their own personal history and how their history may affect the interactions they have. Specific patient populations with unique needs should be considered in interactions with care providers. Families that consist of "mom, dad, and baby" are no longer the majority, and our understanding of different family needs and structures should reflect the patient populations we serve. Half of all current families do not meet the definition of a nuclear family. Families may consist of stepfamilies; single-parent families; families headed by two unmarried partners, either of different sex or the same sex; households that include one or more family members from a generation; adoptive families; foster families; and families where children are raised by grandparents or other relatives.[10] Nearly 2% of gestational carriers undergoing assisted reproductive technology (ART) are for the purposes of surrogacy, 1 out of 25 families are planning to adopt, and 3% of all live births result in adoption plans domestically.[10]

Examples of family structures that often have unique needs include the LGBTQIA+ community and those considering or pursuing adoption or surrogacy. Also, socially complex families, patients with a substance use disorder, or those in correctional care may need individualized family sensitive care. Often policies and procedures in traditional facilities do not specifically address the unique needs of differing patient populations. Updated policies, procedures, and workflows, coupled with updated language and terminology, can improve the continuum of care and patient experiences and outcomes. Clearly, all families are unique, and even "traditional families" of mom, dad, and baby can have unique needs that deserve individualized and sensitive care.

To offer respectful, neutral, compassionate care to the LGBTQIA+ community, it is important to understand the statistics related to their discrimination in healthcare. Transgender or gender nonconforming patients surveyed stated that 70% have experienced some type of discrimination in healthcare, 52% report they believe they would be refused medical services because of their LGBTQIA+ status, and 73% believe they would be treated differently by medical personnel because of their status. Of lesbian, gay, or bisexual patients surveyed, 56% have experienced some type of discrimination in healthcare and 29% report they believe they would be treated differently because of their lesbian, gay, or bisexual status.[11]

Establishing expectations with regard to preferred names and titles helps demonstrate the care provider is offering respectful, neutral, and compassionate care. When working with the LGBTQIA+ patient population, healthcare providers should ask their preferred pronouns. Care providers may also choose to introduce themselves with their preferred pronouns and then invite patients to share theirs.

An introduction with preferred pronouns may sound like, "My name is Karen and I'm going to be your nurse. I use the pronouns she, her, hers." A patient may say, "My name is Megan, and I use the pronouns they, them, theirs." Take note of pronouns within their medical record and share during report. A family may request that care providers use non-gender-identifying pronouns rather than he, him, his, or she, her, hers when speaking of their newborn or their child. In this situation, non-gender-identifying terms such as they, them, theirs may be utilized. Additionally, phrases like, "Have they eaten and have you changed them?" are non-gender-identifying. Alternatively, simply use the baby's name.

If incorrect pronouns are mistakenly used in discussion with patients and their families, care providers should simply apologize and correct themselves. For example, the care provider may state, "Sorry, I meant (insert correct pronoun)" and move on.[12] Misgendering someone with the wrong pronouns can make them feel dismissed, invalidated, disrespected, and/or dysphoric. "All major professional American psychological and psychiatric associations recognize that inclusive language usage for LGBTQ+ youth and adults drastically decreases experiences of depression, social anxiety, suicidal ideation, and other negative mental health factors."[13]

Comfort with updated terminology regarding gender identity, gender expression, biological sex, and sexual orientation allows care providers to communicate with patients in a sensitive, educated manner (Table 3.2).

TABLE 3.2: LGBTQIA+ AND TRANSGENDER BIRTHING PERSON TERMS

Ally	A person who confronts heterosexism, sexism, homophobia, biphobia, transphobia, and heterosexual privilege in themselves and others out of concern for the well-being of LGBTQIA+ people.
Asexuality	Generally characterized by not feeling sexual attraction or a desire for partnered sexuality. Asexuality is distinct from celibacy, which is the deliberate abstention from sexual activity.
Bisexual	A person whose primary sexual and affectional orientation is toward people of the same and other genders, or towards people regardless of their gender.
Cisgender	The prefix cis- means "on the side of" or "not across." A term used to call attention to the privilege of people who are not transgender.
Gay	A sexual orientation toward people of the same gender.
Gender	A social construct used to classify a person as a man, woman, or some other identity. Fundamentally different from the sex one is assigned at birth; a set of social, psychological, and emotional traits, often influenced by societal expectations.
Gender Expression	How one expresses oneself, in terms of dress, mannerisms, and/or behaviors that society characterize as "masculine" or "feminine."
Genderqueer	A person whose gender identity and/or gender expression falls outside of the dominant societal norm for their assigned sex, is beyond genders, or is some combination of them
Heterosexism	The assumption that all people are or should be heterosexual. Heterosexism excludes the needs, concerns, and life experiences of lesbian, gay, bisexual, and queer people while it gives advantages to heterosexual people. It is often a subtle form of oppression, which reinforces realities of silence and invisibility.
Heterosexuality	A sexual orientation in which a person feels physically and emotionally attracted to people of a gender other than their own.
Homophobia	The irrational hatred and fear of LGBTQIA+ people. Homophobia includes prejudice, discrimination, harassment, and acts of violence brought on by fear and hatred. It occurs on personal, institutional, and societal levels.
Homosexual/ Homosexuality	An outdated term to describe a sexual orientation in which a person feels physically and emotionally attracted to people of the same gender.
Internalized Homophobia	The fear and self-hate of one's own LGBTQIA+ identity occurs for many individuals who have learned negative ideas about LGBTQIA+ people throughout childhood. One form of internalized oppression is the acceptance of the myths and stereotypes applied to the oppressed group.

(continued)

TABLE 3.2: LGBTQIA+ AND TRANSGENDER BIRTHING PERSON TERMS (*continued*)

Intersex	People who, without medical intervention, develop primary or secondary sex characteristics that do not fit "neatly" into society's definitions of male or female. Many visibly intersex people are mutilated in infancy and early childhood by doctors to make the individual's sex characteristics conform to society's idea of what normal bodies should look like. Intersex people are relatively common, although society's denial of their existence has allowed very little room for intersex issues to be discussed publicly.
Lesbian	A woman whose primary sexual orientation is toward people of the same gender.
LGBT	Abbreviation for lesbian, gay, bisexual, and transgender. An umbrella term used to refer to the community as a whole.
Nonbinary	A gender identity that embraces full universe of expressions and ways of being that resonate with an individual. It may be an active resistance to binary gender expectations and/or an intentional creation of new unbounded ideas of self within the world.
Pansexual/ Omnisexual	Terms used to describe people who have romantic, sexual, or affectional desire for people of all genders and sexes.
Queer	This can include, but is not limited to, gay, lesbian, bisexual, transgender, intersex, and asexual people. This term has different meanings to different people. Some still find it offensive, while others reclaim it to encompass the broader sense of history of the gay rights movement. Can also be used as an umbrella term like LGBT, as in "the queer community."
Sex	A categorization based on the appearance of the genitalia at birth.
Sexuality	The components of a person that include their biological sex, sexual orientation, gender identity, sexual practices, and so forth.
Sexual Orientation	An enduring emotional, romantic, or sexual attraction. Sexual orientation is fluid. Asexuality is also considered a sexual orientation (see the definition of asexuality).
Transgender	Used most often as an umbrella term. Some commonly held definitions include the following: 1. Someone whose gender identity or expression does not fit (dominant-group social constructs of) assigned birth sex and gender. 2. A gender outside of the man/woman binary. 3. Having no gender or multiple genders.
Transphobia	The fear or hatred of transgender people or people who do not meet society's gender role expectations.
Transsexual	A person who lives full-time in a gender different than their assigned birth sex and gender. Some pursue hormones and/or surgery while others do not. Sometimes used to specifically refer to transgender people pursuing gender or sex confirmation.

Source: Gedzyk-Nieman SA, and McMillian-Bohler J. 2022. Inclusive care for birthing transgender men: A review of the literature. *Journal of Midwifery and Women's Health* 67(5): 561–568. doi: 10.1111/jmwh.13397 [28]

The Human Rights Campaign (HRC.org) provides the following definitions:[14,15]

- **Gender identity:** One's innermost concept of self as male, female, a blend of both, or neither—how individuals perceive themselves and what they call themselves. One's gender identity can be the same or different from their sex assigned at birth.
- **Gender expression:** External appearance of one's gender identity, usually expressed through behavior, clothing, body characteristics, or voice, and which may or may not conform to socially defined behaviors and characteristics typically associated with being either masculine or feminine.
- **Sex assigned at birth:** The sex (male, female, or intersex) that a doctor or midwife uses to describe a child at birth based on their external anatomy.
- **Sexual orientation:** An inherent or immutable enduring emotional, romantic, or sexual attraction to other people. Note: an individual's sexual orientation is independent of their gender identity.

KEY TOPICS IN FAMILY COMMUNICATION

Substance Use Disorder

Substance use disorder is common during pregnancy. The Centers for Disease Control and Prevention (2020) found that 10% of pregnant people reported current alcohol use and 40% went on to report other substance use such as tobacco and marijuana.[16,17] While verbal discussion is powerful when caring for those who have a substance use disorder, first and foremost a care provider must explore their own thoughts and feelings about those who struggle. This helps to ensure that one's body language and interactions with patients are compassionate and respectful. Language regarding substance use disorder has been updated to reflect that it is a medical diagnosis, not a behavioral issue or personality flaw.[16] Person-first language should be used with those with a substance use disorder. Words such as "the addict" or "the drug mom" should not be used to describe a patient. Utilizing respectful, neutral, compassionate language when interacting with the patient is necessary, and it is also important to use updated language in the charting for the patient and the infant.

Healthcare providers must also use updated language in describing the newborn and the effects of the substance. Newborns can be defined as either "substance exposed" or "substance affected" (Table 3.3).

Adoption

Adoption has been in practice since the beginning of time, yet without intentional, specific, and updated training on current practice and accurate adoption language, it can be difficult to offer compassionate communication and consistent care for those considering or pursuing adoption.

Changes in Adoption

Adoption practice has evolved from a closed, shame-based transaction for patients and families to an open interaction between those considering adoption and the family hoping to adopt. In the mid-1900s, patients involved in adoption were often treated poorly. Some birth parents delivered their babies with bags over their heads. Some did not know if they had a boy or a girl.[19] With such negative stigma, communication was limited between healthcare professionals and the patient. There was little concern for the patient's feelings as the birth was often perceived as a punishment for having sex out of wedlock. Toward the end of the 20th century, there was a shift to a more open model for infant adoption. Driven by the mothers who lost their children to adoption, then echoed by the adoptees who lost connection with their birth parents, sharing identifying information has been encouraged as the new norm. Mothers, and fathers if involved, transitioned to being in control of who was to parent their child in an open

TABLE 3.3: UPDATED TERMINOLOGY RELATED TO ADDICTION

OUTDATED TERM	REPLACE WITH
Abstinence-based or abstinence-only intervention	Not including medication
They are addicted	They have a chronic disease of addiction
Addict or junkie	Person with a substance use disorder; person with serious alcohol use disorder
Clean	Abstinent; abstaining from
Clean (urine test)	Negative for substance X; as expected
Dirty	Actively using; positive for substance use
Opioid replacement or opioid substitution therapy	Treatment that includes medication/ treatment with X (name of medication)
Sober	Well; healthy

Source: National Institute on Drug Abuse. 2022, April 10. *Words Matter—Terms to Use and Avoid When Talking About Addiction.* National Institute on Drug Abuse.[18]

adoption. Parents considering adoption are now encouraged to choose the parents for their child, and both parties now often share identifying information. This model has introduced potential adoptive parents into the healthcare space with the mother who is considering them to parent their child. This interaction during delivery has been referred to as a "wedding and a funeral in the same room."[20] Refining and updating our interactions as healthcare professionals within this dynamic is essential to ensure the patient has voice and choice throughout her hospital stay. It is also vital to be sensitive to a possible history of infertility or infant loss among potential adoptive parents. Also, prebirth matching, which means the expectant patient chooses the family to raise the newborn prior to the birth, is often occurring over the internet. This has introduced complexity for healthcare professionals in the continuum of the perinatal space.[21]

Patients considering adoption may now be accompanied by prospective adoptive parents in the healthcare setting, including at prenatal appointments and even at the hospital at the time of delivery. In other cases, the patient and the prospective family may have little face-to-face history if matching occurred via the internet. It is crucial for care providers to privately verify with the patient the level of their involvement with the prospective adoptive parents. Patients have full autonomy over decision-making throughout the adoption plan and may change the potential adoptive parents' level of involvement at any time.

Healthcare providers who care for those pursuing adoption are often left without clear and accurate practice guidelines as processes and standards become outdated.[22] Providers may lack accurate, updated adoption terminology to hold supportive dialogues with patients, thereby creating scenarios of uncertainty and ambiguity that do not optimize the therapeutic nurse–patient relationship and fail to provide comprehensive and respectful care.[23]

A patient's decision to make an adoption plan creates operationally and emotionally complex situations for the patient, the prospective adoptive parents, and the hospital staff. There is often ambiguous loss felt by all people involved in infant adoption, including the patient and prospective adoptive parents. There are two types of ambiguous loss: (a) when a person is physically missing but psychologically present, such as in divorce or adoption loss and (b) when a person is psychologically missing but physically present, such as with dementia or a traumatic brain injury.

The first type is very common in adoption as there is no "closure" per se—no concrete loss to grieve. Patients choosing adoption do not know what they are grieving, and potential adoptive parents who have faced infertility are grieving a child that they never met. Their loss is undefined and ambiguous, just like the parents of the child placed for adoption. In the future, the child will also grieve the future they did not have with their biological family. Their loss includes not only their parents, but possibly biological siblings as well. Universal training in bereavement and loss management can assist nurses and the multidisciplinary team as they guide the patient, parents, and family members through these emotions and prevent compassion fatigue.[24] Updated adoption language reflects neutral, compassionate care and creates an environment that encourages empowered decision-making and relationship development. Negative, stigmatizing language can inhibit open communication and can reflect outdated adoption practices (Table 3.4).

Surrogacy

Unlike adoption, surrogacy has a relatively short history. The first surrogate pregnancy was in 1976, and there were an additional 600 surrogate births between that year and 1988. Between 1988 and 1992, there were 5,000 births via surrogates. In 1976, we saw our first surrogacy legal agreement with the traditional surrogate.[25] On July 25, 1978, Louise Joy Brown was the first "test tube baby" (also known as *in vitro* fertilization [IVF]) born. Updated language is essential in caring for those involved in a surrogacy arrangement. "Traditional surrogacy" refers to a parent who uses their own egg during the surrogacy arrangement. The term "traditional surrogate" will rarely be heard because it is only used for a parent who donates their own egg and contributes DNA to the offspring. Historically, traditional surrogacies have been more legally complicated, and these situations sometimes resulted in a custody battle for a child.[26] Thus, traditional surrogacy is now very rare, and is most often used for altruistic surrogacy within families. Today, most surrogates or gestational carriers—these two terms can be used interchangeably—rarely utilize their own genetic material. In a surrogacy arrangement, intended parent(s) are often related to the embryo that is transferred to their gestational carrier. However, the infant(s) is not always genetically related to the intended parents. In a surrogacy arrangement, a donated egg, sperm, or embryo may be used in the fertility process. The family growing through surrogacy most often will have a history of infertility, so it is important for the care providers to be sensitive when interacting with the intended parent(s) involved in a surrogacy arrangement. As mentioned, embryos utilized in a surrogacy arrangement could have been created by utilizing a sperm donor, an egg donor, or both. In addition, it is possible

TABLE 3.4: UPDATED TERMINOLOGY FOR ADOPTION

OUTDATED TERM	REPLACE WITH
Real parent, natural parent	Birth parent, first parent, and biological parent
Give away, give up, or put up for adoption	Make an adoption plan
Keep the baby	Choose to parent
Adoption triad	Adoption constellation
Hard-to-place child	Child with special needs
Adopted child	Child who was/is adopted

to adopt embryos, and any of these options could provide genetic material to be utilized in a surrogacy arrangement. In this case, no one in the room is genetically related to the child being born. A "gestational carrier" does not use their own genetic material. They instead utilize an embryo conceived using the egg of the intended mother or an egg donor and sperm from the intended father or a sperm donor. The terms "surrogate mother" and "suro-mom" are both no longer appropriate. The gestational carrier or surrogate has never had the role of parent, and thus terms that define parenting, such as mother, should not be used. Calling them a surrogate or gestational carrier is perfectly acceptable.

How to Share Hard Information or Give Bad News

When caring for a pregnant patient or a family during the perinatal-neonatal period, an awareness about the ways in which difficult information is shared is important to the care provider and patient communication process. A therapeutic relationship is best established first, when possible. However, not all situations allow for time to develop the relationship before difficult information needs to be relayed.

Some specific considerations can be helpful when relaying difficult information. If possible, meet with the family in a private space where there is room for everyone to be seated. The provider should introduce themselves and explain their role. It may be helpful in some situations to ask the family what they understand about their infant's condition. In the delivery room, it is important to show the infant to the family and discuss any concerning findings. For example, if the provider notices an anomaly, it can be helpful to point it out to the family and let them know that further investigation will be done.

Speaking in plain language without medical terminology is not "dumbing down" one's message or "talking down" to a patient—it is communicating in a clear way that tells the patients exactly what they need to know without using unnecessary words or expressions. For example, if the patient's condition or the pregnancy necessitates a cesarean birth urgently or emergently, the care provider should provide clear anticipatory guidance and information about what will be happening in the coming minutes to hours. In addition, when giving instructions to the patient, the care provider should ensure they are providing the patient with clear, concise, and easy to follow instructions. If time allows, the care provider can best support the patient by sitting down next to them, speaking calmly while providing factual information, and answering the patient's questions. Utilizing common scripting when caring for patients during the grieving process may serve the care provider well when a patient is upset or going through a difficult situation. Examples of supportive phrasing may include, "Is there someone I can call for you?" or "I imagine this is difficult," and "Would you like me to contact the chaplain for you?" It can be difficult for families to give bad news to loved ones, so it may be helpful if the provider can call someone for the family.

Communicating with plain language and empathetic scripting will help provide neutral, compassionate care for patients during times of difficult information sharing. If the care provider has had a similar experience, they may feel comfortable sharing their own story with the patient; however, when discussing difficult scenarios or situations with patients, it is important to avoid burdening the patient with one's own personal emotions or stories. The patient should never feel obligated to comfort the care provider. Care providers should focus on the patient's needs, read their clues (verbal and nonverbal messages), and respond to their needs. If the care provider is focused on sharing their personal story with the patient, they risk missing vital pieces of information that the patient is sharing. By demonstrating a sincere intention to focus on the patient and listen attentively—being attuned to their attitudes and feelings—the care provider can demonstrate positive interactions by asking open-ended questions, speaking slowly, and using simple, nonmedical language.

Expect to repeat information more than once. It takes time to process difficult information. Parents and family members may not understand everything that is relayed to them, even when the information is simplified. Most people will need information repeated as it is difficult for families to understand or remember everything that is explained to them.

Feelings of guilt are common, and it is important to stress wherever possible that there is nothing the mother or other family member did to cause the issue. Clarifying facts and providing information is important. Facts are more valuable than speculation.[27]

Providing parents and families with choices wherever possible is important. In the case of a congenital anomaly or disability, spending time with the infant helps with gradual acceptance and adaptation to the situation. Chronic sorrow is a theory developed for explaining the responses of people experiencing situations of chronic illness, loss of a "perfect child," or ongoing caregiving responsibilities. It is often a loss of what "could have been" or the sometimes overwhelming responsibilities of caring for an ill or disabled child.[28] In the case of a stillborn, or infant death, allowing the family to spend as much time as they like with the infant is important. Consideration of cultural factors recognizes that there may be differences in what families want to do or what they consider appropriate. Therefore, being flexible and creative is essential. Ideally, a private and quiet environment provides room for families to be with their infant if they wish. Photographs and mementos are important to some families and should be offered. If families do not want these things initially, consider keeping them in a safe place in case they request to have them at a later time. Information on support groups, counseling, and other resources should be offered to the family.

SUMMARY

Effective communication skills are essential for creating a positive, attentive atmosphere for patients and for their families. Taking into consideration one's own thoughts and feelings upon entering a patient's space will empower the provider to set aside stress and distractions that may impede their ability to interact effectively. Patients and their experiences should be considered, validated, and valued, ensuring that all are treated with respectful, neutral, compassionate care.

ADDITIONAL RESOURCES

SPRINGER PUBLISHING CONNECT™

A robust set of resources designed to supplement this text is located at http://connect.springerpub.com/content/book/978-0-8261-4063-0. Qualifying instructors may request access by emailing textbook@springerpub.com.

REFERENCES

1. Mehrabian A. 1972. *Nonverbal Communication*. New Brunswick: Aldine Transaction.
2. Nandini. 2020, January–March. S.O.L.E.R way of communication in nursing Raipur. *Asian Journal of Nursing Education and Research* 10(1): 110–111. doi: 10.5958/2349-2996.2020.00025.7
3. TeamHealth. 2019, September 3. Nine ways to improve your patient communications. https://www.teamhealth.com/news-and-resources/featured-article/nine-ways-to-improve-your-patient-communications/?r=1
4. Agency for Healthcare Research and Quality. 2023. *Guide to Patient and Family Engagement in Hospital Quality and Safety*. Content last reviewed December 2017. Rockville, MD: Agency for Healthcare Research and Quality. https://www.ahrq.gov/patient-safety/patients-families/engagingfamilies/guide.html
5. Steuwe C, Daniels JK, Frewen PA, Densmore M, Pannasch S, Beblo T, Reiss J, and Lanius RA. 2012. Effect of direct eye contact in PTSD related to interpersonal trauma: An fMRI study of activation of an innate alarm system. *Social Cognitive and Affective Neuroscience* 9(1): 88–97. doi: 10.1093/scan/nss105
6. Uono S, and Hietanen JK. 2015. Eye contact perception in the west and east: A cross-cultural study. *PLoS One* 10(2): e0118094. doi: 10.1371/journal.pone.0118094

7. Brooks LA, Manias E, and Bloomer MJ. 2019. Culturally sensitive communication in healthcare: A concept analysis. *Collegian* 26(3): 383–391. doi: 10.1016/j.colegn.2018.09.007
8. Levinson W, Gorawara-Bhat R, and Lamb J. 2000. A study of patient clues and physician responses in primary care and surgical settings. *Journal of the American Medical Association*. 284(8): 1021. doi: 10.1001/jama.284.8.1021
9. ODR. n.d. *People First Language*. Retrieved October 30, 2022, from https://odr.dc.gov/page/people-first-language
10. HealthyChildren.org. n.d. *Types of Families*. Retrieved November 3, 2022, from https://www.healthychildren.org/English/family-life/family-dynamics/types-of-families/Pages/default.aspx
11. Lambda Legal. n.d. *When Health Care Isn't Caring*. Retrieved November 1, 2022, from https://www.lambdalegal.org/publications/when-health-care-isnt-caring
12. LGBTQ+ Resource Center. n.d. *Gender Pronouns*. Retrieved November 1, 2022, from https://uwm.edu/lgbtrc/support/gender-pronouns/
13. Katz-Wise SL. 2021, July 23. *Misgendering: What It is and Why It Matters*. Harvard Health. https://www.health.harvard.edu/blog/misgendering-what-it-is-and-why-it-matters-202107232553
14. Human Rights Campaign. 2023. HRC.org
15. Human Rights Campaign. n.d. *Sexual Orientation and Gender Identity Definitions*. Retrieved November 2, 2022, from https://www.hrc.org/resources/sexual-orientation-and-gender-identity-terminology-and-definitions
16. Centers for Disease Control and Prevention. 2022, September 19. *Polysubstance Use During Pregnancy*. https://www.cdc.gov/pregnancy/polysubstance-use-in-pregnancy.html
17. England LJ, Bennett C, Denny CH, Honein MA, Gilboa SM, Kim SY, Guy GP Jr., Tran EL, Rose CE, Bohm MK, and Boyle CA. 2020. Alcohol use and co-use of other substances among pregnant females aged 12–44 years—United States, 2015–2018. *Morbidity and Mortality Weekly Report* 69(31): 1009–1014.
18. National Institute on Drug Abuse. 2022, April 10. *Words Matter—Terms to Use and Avoid When Talking About Addiction*. https://nida.nih.gov/nidamed-medical-health-professionals/health-professions-education/words-matter-terms-to-use-avoid-when-talking-about-addiction
19. Fessler A. 2006. *The Girls Who Went Away: The Hidden History of Women Who Surrendered Children for Adoption in the Decades Before Roe v. Wade*. New York: Penguin Publishing Group.
20. Vahle R. 2013, June 6. *Supporting Adoption Placements in Hospitals*. Congressional Coalition on Adoption Institute. https://ccainstituteblog.org/2013/06/06/supporting-adoption-placements-in-hospitals/
21. Glaser G. 2021. *American Baby: A Mother, a Child, and the Shadow History of Adoption*. New York: Viking.
22. Smith KJ, and Brandon D. 2008. The hospital-based adoption process. *MCN: The American Journal of Maternal/Child Nursing* 33(6): 382–388. doi: 10.1097/01.nmc.0000341260.10922.4e
23. National Council for Adoption. 2020, November 17. *Using Accurate Adoption Language*. https://adoptioncouncil.org/article/using-accurate-adoption-language/
24. Esplen MJ, Wong J, Vachon MLS, and Leung Y. 2022. A continuing educational program supporting health professionals to manage grief and loss. *Current Oncology* 29(3): 1461–1474. doi: 10.3390/curroncol29030123
25. Malaj J. 2021, May 2. *The One With the Surrogate* [Video]. TEDxVienna Magazine. https://magazine.tedxvienna.at/2020/05/26/the-one-with-the-surrogate
26. Bewkes FJ. 2014. Surrogate or "Mother"? The problem of traditional surrogacy. *Tennessee Journal of Race, Gender, & Social Justice* 3(2): Article 3.
27. Flugelman MY. 2021. How to talk with the family of a dying patient: Anger to understanding, rage to compassion, loss to acceptance. *BMJ Supportive and Palliative Care* 11: 418–421.
28. Eakes GG, Burke ML, and Hainsworth MA. 1998. Middle-range theory of chronic sorrow. *Image: Journal of Nursing Scholarship* 30(2): 179–184. doi: 10.1111/j.1547-5069.1998.tb01276.x

4 GESTATIONAL AGE ASSESSMENT

Carol Wiltgen Trotter

A newborn's *gestational age* (GA) is defined as the number of completed weeks that have elapsed between the first day of the mother's last menstrual period (LMP) and the day of delivery. GA (or menstrual age) differs from the *postconceptional* or *conceptional age*, which is defined as the number of completed weeks from conception until delivery, because ovulation usually occurs about 2 weeks after the first day of the LMP. Defining GA using the menstrual age is more accurate because women typically know the date of their LMP and not the date of ovulation.[1] When a preterm infant is conceived using reproductive technologies that allow for identification of the date of conception, the GA is actually 2 weeks longer than the conceptional age.[1] Figure 4.1 summarizes the terminology used for age assessment in the perinatal period.

An accurate definition and assessment of GA is important to the examiner for two reasons. First, knowledge of the neonate's age and the growth patterns appropriate to that age aid in identification of neonatal risks and in development of management plans. This is particularly true for infants born at or near the limit of viability, as there are numerous medical, social, and ethical issues to consider for the clinician and family. Accurate assessment of GA is critical for determining morbidity and mortality risks that can be used to counsel families regarding treatment decisions. According to data collected on infant mortality for 2020, infants born at less than 28 weeks had the highest mortality rates. Short gestation was the second leading cause of infant death after congenital malformations.[2] The National Institutes of Health has published a tool that estimates outcomes for infants born extremely preterm.[3] The data is based on outcomes for infants born in the United States from 2006 to 2012. Such tools are helpful in evaluating the risk of death and disability based on cohort data using accurate GA assessment data. Using this calculator, a 22-week singleton male whose mother received antenatal steroids has an average survival of 23% and an average risk of moderate-severe developmental impairment ranging from 52% to 78%. If that same singleton male infant is born at 24 weeks, his average survival rate increases to 43% with a risk of moderate to severe developmental impairment decreasing to 37% to 52%.[3] Rysavy et al. (2020) have published outcome statistics for very preterm infants using an updated model which includes hospital of birth. Based on data collected on extremely preterm infants from 2013 to 2016, the survival rate for 22-week gestation infants who were treated at birth was 25%. The survival rate increased to 83% at 25 weeks.[4] The risks associated with the lowest GAs are clearly recognized, and identification of those risks requires accurate assessment of GA.

There are also risks associated with birth at higher GAs. Late preterm infants (34 0/7–36 6/7 weeks gestation) as well as early term infants (37 0/7–38 6/7 weeks) have a different set of problems, and these infants must be identified to improve their management. When compared to the full-term infant, these infants are at increased risk for temperature instability, hypoglycemia, respiratory distress, apnea, hyperbilirubinemia, and feeding problems.[5–7]

An accurate determination of GA is essential for the collection of reliable fetal and

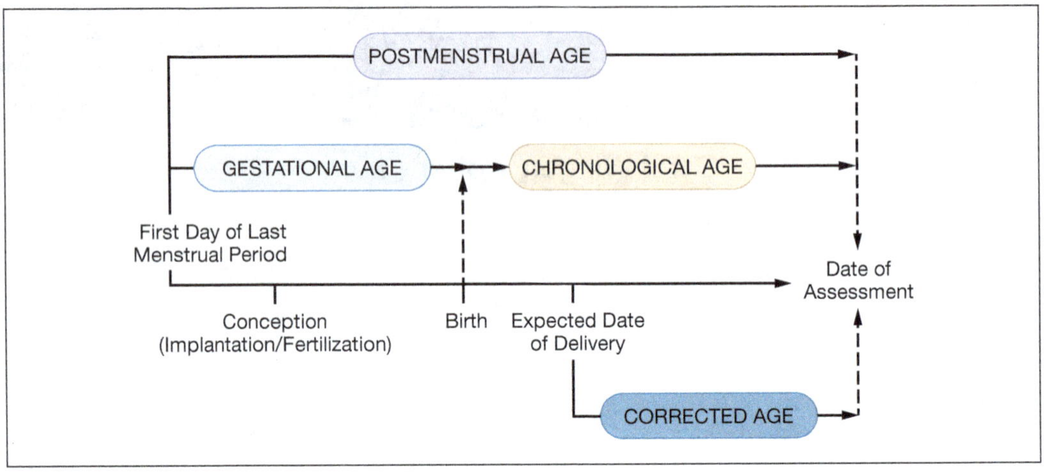

FIGURE 4.1 Age terminology during the perinatal period

Source: From American Academy of Pediatrics, and Committee on Fetus and Newborn. 2004. Age terminology during the perinatal period. *Pediatrics* 114(5): 1363. Reprinted with permission (Reaffirmed July 2021. https://www.pediatrics.aappublications.org/content/134/3/e920 and published in *Pediatrics* 134, 3, September, 2014).[1]

infant statistical data that will be used to improve perinatal outcomes.[8] It is also essential when conducting neonatal research and applying the findings to clinical practice. Gestational maturity is an independent predictor of outcome, so GA must be controlled for in clinical trials that evaluate new therapies. Accurate GA assessment is an important factor when comparing outcomes data from different neonatal care facilities.[1,9]

There are three general methods of determining GA in the newborn: (a) calculation of dates based on the mother's LMP, (b) evaluation of obstetric parameters obtained during the prenatal period, and (c) physical examination of the neonate. Although evaluations based on menstrual dates and obstetric methods are discussed briefly, this chapter focuses on determining GA through postnatal physical assessment.

The average pregnancy is usually described as lasting 280 days, or 40 weeks from the first day of the LMP.[10] The accuracy with which the estimated date of confinement (EDC) can be determined based on the LMP depends on the patient having regular menstrual cycles with ovulation occurring on the 14th day after the start of the LMP.[10] If the mother's menstrual cycles are irregular, ultrasound measurements provide the most accurate estimate of GA.

Obstetric methods for assessing GA include maternal physical examination and ultrasound measurements. Fetal ultrasound measurements are the most powerful methods for assessing GA. The best fetal parameters to measure by ultrasound depend on the timing of the exam.

In the first trimester, the embryonic pole and crown–rump lengths are the most accurate fetal measurements for determining GA but become less reliable with fetal flexion.[11] During the second and third trimesters, measurements of individual structures are used. The four most common measurements are biparietal diameter, head and abdominal circumferences, and femur length.[10,12] According to Lazebnik et al., the biparietal diameter obtained after week 12 is the most accurate measure in the second trimester. If there are alterations in skull shape, a head circumference may be an effective alternative.[11] Other measures used are the abdominal circumference, femoral length, and humeral and pedal lengths. Advances have been made in improving the accuracy of GA estimation by obstetric methods to such an extent that some healthcare professionals believe that formal assessment of GA is not required for routine newborn examination. The most accurate guide to GA is a combination of menstrual dates and early ultrasound measurements.[13] However, when these data are not known, or when there is a discrepancy with the antenatal dates and infant growth, a physical examination is appropriate.[13] When rapid assessment of GA is necessary, such as in the delivery room, a quick inspection of a few parameters will suffice. Physical assessment techniques used in the detailed examination of the neonate for GA, however, are inspection, palpation, and use of the ophthalmoscope.

HISTORICAL PERSPECTIVE

The GA assessment scoring system that provides the basis for many of the tools currently used was published in 1970 by Dubowitz et al.[14] The system is based on assessment of 11 external and 10 neurologic criteria. The external criteria were taken from characteristics defined by Farr et al.[15] According to Dubowitz, Dubowitz, and Goldberg, and Koenigsberger (as well as secondary sources), the development of neurologic criteria to assess GA originated in the work of the French schools in the 1950s under Andre Thomas and later, Madame Sainte-Anne Dargassies.[14,16] During the 1960s, a number of other investigators helped better define the neurologic criteria. Dubowitz, Dubowitz, and Goldberg selected criteria from the data published by Koenigsberger, Robinson, and Amiel-Tison to develop the neurologic portion of their scoring system.[14,16–18]

Since publication of the system devised by Dubowitz, Dubowitz, and Goldberg, many variations of the tool have been used.[19,20] In 1978, Capurro and coworkers published a simplified method of GA assessment using seven of the original variables defined by Dubowitz, Dubowitz, and Goldberg. These investigators identified five physical and two neurologic criteria that most accurately determine GA.[21] In 1979, Ballard, Novak, and Driver published a tool using six neuromuscular criteria and six physical criteria.[22] In addition, other investigators have published reports of determination of GA by measuring hand and foot length,[23–25] cerebellar vermis dimensions,[26] postnatal sonographic femur length,[27] and intermamillary distance.[24] Skin reflectance with an optical fiber spectrophotometer was also measured.[28]

Both the Ballard and the Dubowitz tools have been criticized for overestimating the actual GA by 2 weeks.[29,30] Therefore, Ballard et al. expanded their tool to achieve greater accuracy and to include the extremely premature neonate.[31] According to its authors, this tool, the New Ballard Score (NBS), overestimates GA by 0.3 to 0.6 weeks (2–4 days) at GAs less than 37 weeks. However, the NBS estimates of GA have been shown to exceed actual GA by 1.3 to 3.3 weeks in neonates less than 28 weeks.[32] Therefore, when assessing GA using the physical and neurologic criteria, it is important to note that accuracy is ±2 weeks and the scoring system may overestimate gestation age in extremely premature infants.[13] Healthcare professionals involved in making clinical decisions for extremely premature neonates must be cautious when applying the results of physical examination data. Because of this variability in accuracy of GA assessment, Jacob and Hulman developed an algorithm for GA determination (Figure 4.2).[9] They place an emphasis on accurate GA assignment for the purpose of comparing outcome data between institutions. The key component of this algorithm is the obstetrician's assessment of GA based on menstrual dates, ultrasound parameters, and maternal physical assessment. The algorithm recommends newborn assessment only if the obstetric parameters are uncertain. The limitations associated with the NBS for GA assessment must be kept in mind as it is used throughout this chapter to demonstrate assessment of the neuromuscular and physical criteria associated with various GAs.

PHYSICAL ASSESSMENT

There are two methods for determining GA by physical examination: (a) assessment of the anterior vascular capsule of the lens (AVCL) using the ophthalmoscope and (b) assessment of neuromuscular and physical criteria by inspection and palpation.

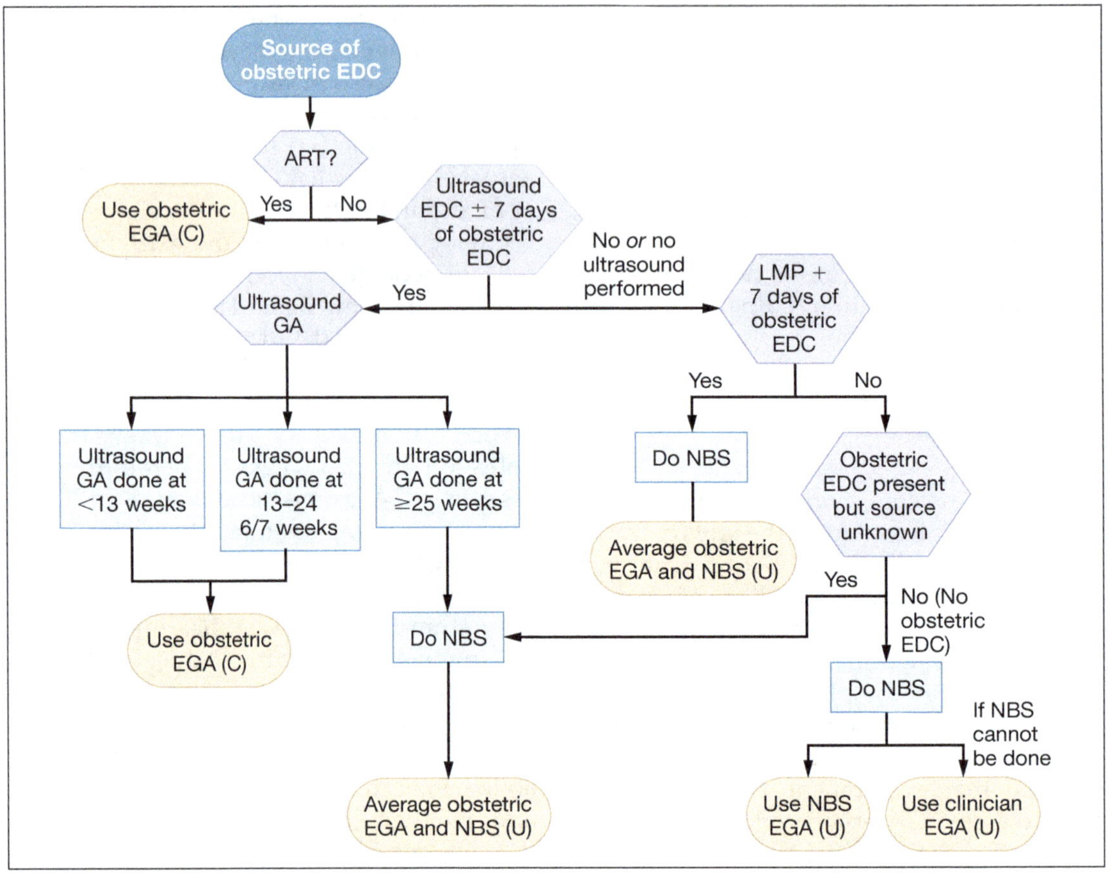

FIGURE 4.2 Algorithm for the assignment of gestational age

ART, assisted reproductive technology; C, certain; EDC, estimated date of confinement; EGA, estimated gestational age; GA, gestational age; LMP, last menstrual period; NBS, New Ballard Score; U, uncertain.

Source: Adapted from Jacob J, and Hulman S. 2006. A standardized method for assigning gestational age: A tool for measuring gestational age based newborn intensive care outcomes. *American Journal of Perinatology* 23(7): 399. Reproduced with permission of Thieme Medical Publishers via Copyright Clearance Center.[9]

Anterior Vascular Capsule of the Lens

The rationale and technique for examining the AVCL to determine GA were described in 1977 by Hittner, Hirsch, and Rudolph.[33] The hyaloid system and the tunica vasculosa lentis are transient embryologic vascular systems that invade the developing eye. The purpose of the vascular system is to nourish the eye during active growth. This system can be seen starting at approximately 27 weeks gestation; it then atrophies progressively until it is gone after week 34. Figure 4.3 depicts the developing eye from 5 weeks to term gestation. Early in fetal life, the lens is invaded by the tunica vasculosa lentis (Figure 4.3C). The hyaloid artery supplies the developing lens and the tunica vasculosa lentis until it disappears late in the fetal period. At that time, the tunica vasculosa lentis atrophies.[34]

To visualize the vessels, the examiner uses a direct ophthalmoscope set between +6 and +12. These settings allow the examiner's eye to focus on the lens rather than on the retina. To the novice practitioner, the image will initially appear blurry. As the ophthalmoscope is moved closer to the infant's eye (within 6–10 inches), the vascular system will come into view as the examiner focuses on the more anteriorly placed lens.

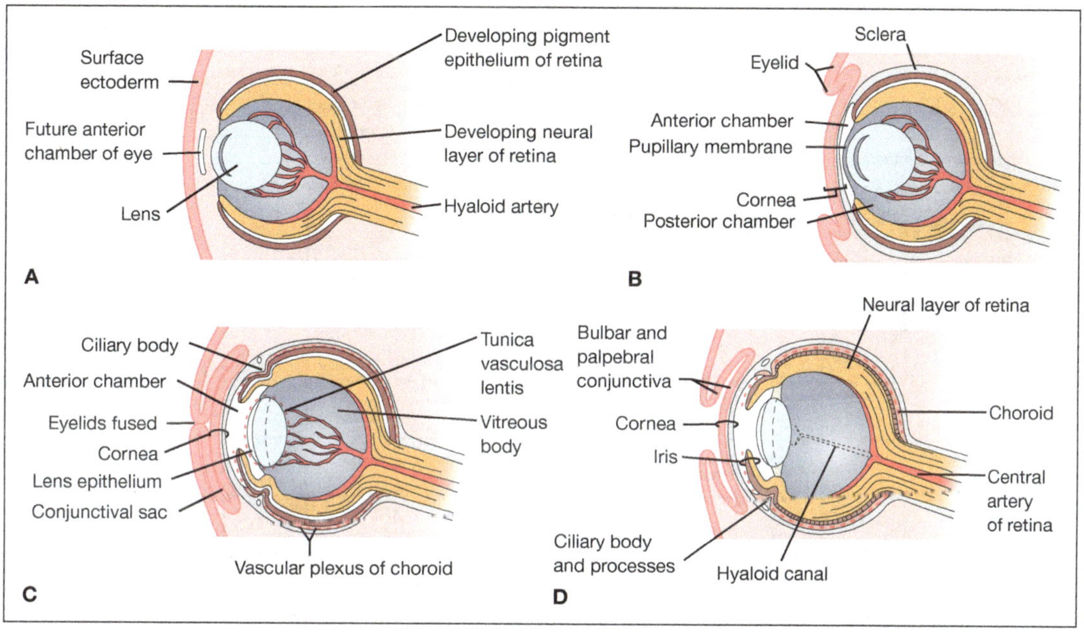

FIGURE 4.3 The sagittal sections of the eye, showing successive developmental stages of the lens, retina, iris, and cornea

Source: Adapted from Moore KL, Persaud TVN, and Torchia MG. 2020. *The Developing Human: Clinically Oriented Embryology*, 11th ed. Philadelphia, PA: Saunders, 402. Reprinted by permission.[34]

Figure 4.4 illustrates the grading system for GA assessment based on the pattern and presence of vessels noted. This examination must be performed within the first 24 to 48 hours of life because the vascular system atrophies rapidly after that period.[33] Although Dietz, Huppi, and Amato confirmed that the gradual disappearance of the AVCL is not impacted by maternal and neonatal risk factors, Hadi and Hobbs found that maternal chronic hypertension accelerates the atrophy of this system.[35,36] They suggest that chronic intrauterine stress may influence the maturation of this vascular structure.

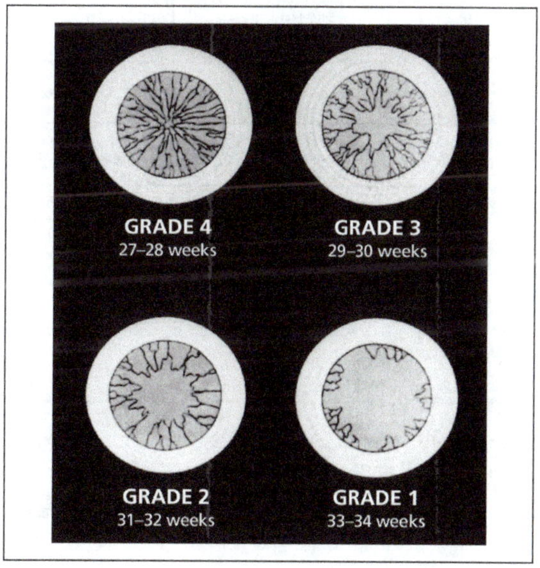

FIGURE 4.4 Gestational age assessment grading system: Anterior vascular capsule of the lens

Source: From Hittner HM, Hirsch NJ, and Rudolph AJ. 1977. Assessment of gestational age by examination of the anterior vascular capsule of the lens. *Journal of Pediatrics* 91(3): 456. Reprinted by permission.[33]

Neuromuscular and Physical Criteria

Ballard et al. have defined six neuromuscular and six physical criteria for evaluating GA in the newborn.[31,37] The criteria and the scoring tool are depicted in Figure 4.5. A discussion

Maturational Assessment of Gestational Age (New Ballard Score)

Name__________ Date/time of birth__________ Sex __________

Hospital no.__________ Date/time of exam __________ Birth weight __________

Race__________ Age when examined __________ Length__________

Apgar score: 1 minute __________ 5 minutes __________ 10 minutes__________ Head circ. __________

Examiner__________

Neuromuscular Maturity

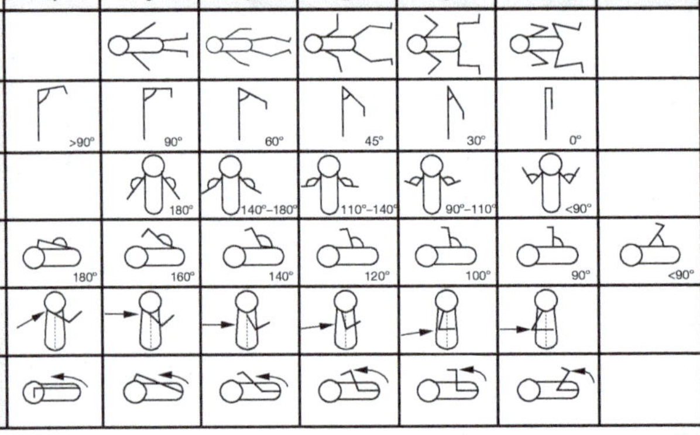

Neuromuscular Maturity Sign	Score -1	0	1	2	3	4	5	Record Score Here
Posture								
Square Window (Wrist)	>90°	90°	60°	45°	30°	0°		
Arm Recoil		180°	140°–180°	110°–140°	90°–110°	<90°		
Popliteal Angle	180°	160°	140°	120°	100°	90°	<90°	
Scarf Sign								
Heel to Ear								

Total Neuromuscular Maturity Score

Physical Maturity

Physical Maturity Sign	Score -1	0	1	2	3	4	5	Record Score Here
Skin	sticky friable transparent	gelatinous red translucent	smooth pink visible veins	superficial peeling and/or rash, few veins	cracking pale areas rare veins	parchment deep cracking no vessels	leathery cracked wrinkled	
Lanugo	none	sparse	abundant	thinning	bald areas	mostly bald		
Plantar Surface	heel-toe 40–50 mm:-1 <40 mm:-2	>50 mm no crease	faint red marks	anterior transverse crease only	creases anterior 2/3	creases over entire sole		
Breast	imperceptible	barely perceptible	flat areola no bud	stippled areola 1–2 mm bud	raised areola 3–4 mm bud	full areola 5–10 mm bud		
Eye/Ear	lids fused loosely: -1, tightly: -2	lids open pinna flat stays folded	slightly curved pinna; soft; slow recoil	well-curved pinna; soft but ready recoil	formed and firm; instant recoil	thick cartilage ear stiff		
Genitals (Male)	scrotum flat, smooth	scrotum empty faint rugae	testes in upper canal rare rugae	testes descending few rugae	testes down good rugae	testes pendulous deep rugae		
Genitals (Female)	clitoris prominent & labia flat	prominent clitoris & small labia minora	prominent clitoris & enlarging minora	majora & minora equally prominent	majora large minora small	majora cover clitoris and minora		

Total Physical Maturity Score

Score

Neuromuscular_____

Physical_____

Total_____

Maturity Rating

Score	Weeks
–10	20
–5	22
0	24
5	26
10	28
15	30
20	32
25	34
30	36
35	38
40	40
45	42
50	44

Gestational Age (weeks)

By dates_____

By ultrasound_____

By exam_____

FIGURE 4.5 Gestational age assessment scoring system: Neurologic and physical criteria (New Ballard Score)

Source: From Ballard JL, Khoury JC, Wedig KL, Wang L, Eilers-Walsman BL, and Lipp R. 1991. New Ballard Score, expanded to include extremely premature infants. *Journal of Pediatrics* 119(3): 418. Reprinted by permission.[31]

of each criterion follows, and photographs depicting assessment of the criteria accompany the text. Descriptions of the technique for assessment were taken from Dubowitz, Dubowitz, and Goldberg and from Ballard unless otherwise noted.[15,31,37,38]

Neuromuscular Criteria

Posture

Posture is an indicator of resting muscle tone. The infant is first allowed to assume a baseline position of comfort and is then observed in the supine position. A score is assigned based on the degree of flexion of the arms, knees, and hips. The degree of hip adduction/abduction is also noted. The neonate demonstrates increasing flexion and hip adduction with advancing GA; lower extremity flexion precedes flexion of the upper extremities (Figures 4.6–4.8).

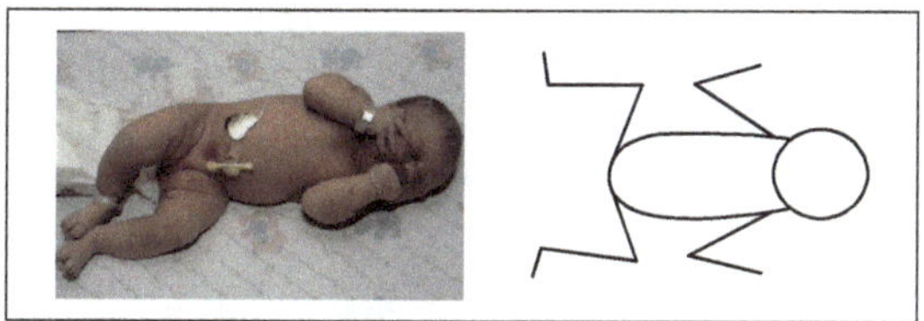

FIGURE 4.6 Full-term infant. Posture score=4

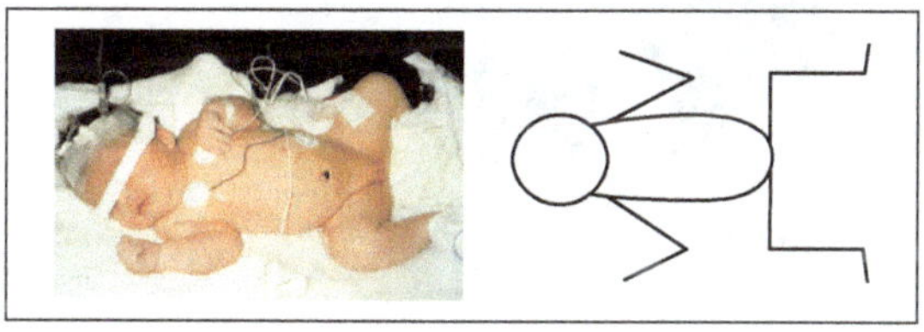

FIGURE 4.7 Preterm large-for-gestational-age female infant. Posture score=3

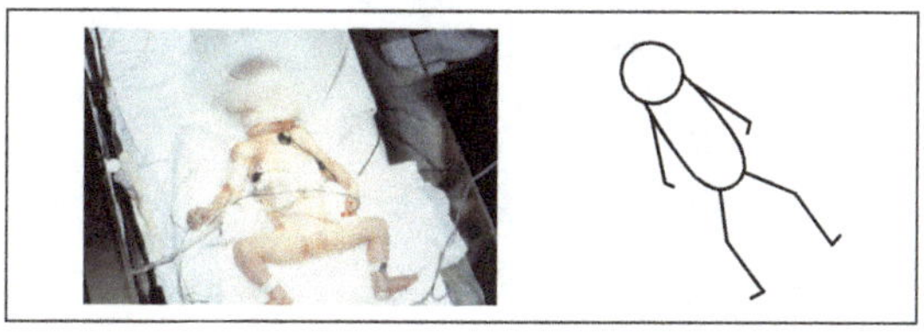

FIGURE 4.8 Preterm infant with no arm flexion. Posture score=1

Square Window

The infant's fingers are extended, and the hand is flexed to the forearm by applying gentle pressure on the dorsum of the hand. Enough pressure is applied to get as full a flexion as possible without rotating the wrist. The angle between the forearm and the palm is measured. The angle decreases with advancing GA (Figures 4.9–4.11).

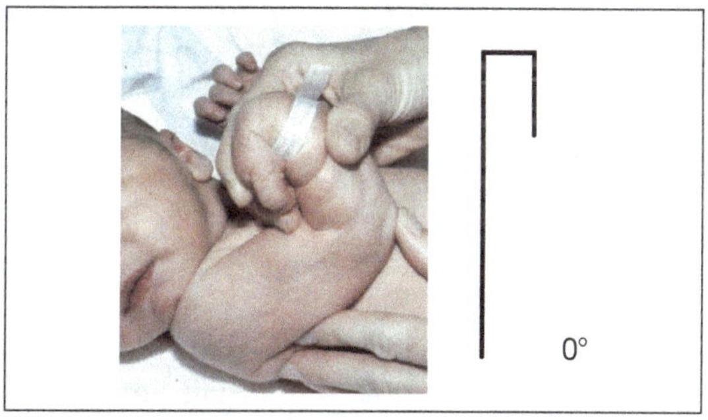

FIGURE 4.9 Square window in term neonate. Score=4

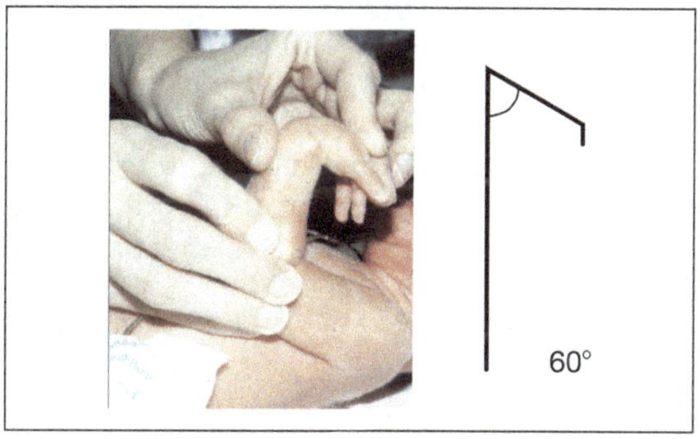

FIGURE 4.10 Square window in preterm infant. Score = 1

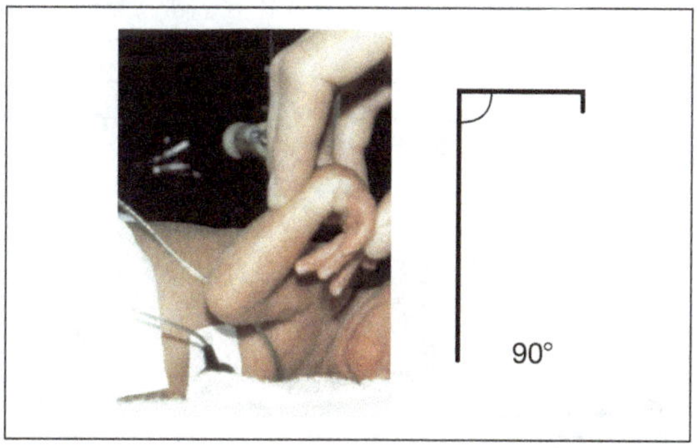

FIGURE 4.11 Square window in preterm infant. Score = 0

Arm Recoil

This criterion focuses on passive flexor tone of the biceps muscle. The neonate's arms are flexed for 5 seconds while in the supine position. The arms are then fully extended by pulling the hands and quickly releasing them. The examiner should avoid maintaining the extremity in the extended position for too long, thereby fatiguing the flexors. Degree of arm flexion and the strength of the recoil are scored. A sluggish response with little or no flexion receives a low score. A brisk, fully flexed response receives a high score. According to Ballard, a score of 4 requires that the fist come in contact with the face (Figures 4.12 and 4.13).[38]

Popliteal Angle

The popliteal angle maneuver evaluates passive flexor tone in the knee. The neonate should be in the supine position with the pelvis on the mattress. The untested portion of the extremity should be resting quietly on the supporting surface, and the thigh should be supported from the side without interfering with the flexor being tested.[38] With the thumb and index finger of one hand, the examiner holds the infant's knee and thigh adjacent to the chest/abdomen. At the same time, the examiner grasps the foot and extends the leg gently with the other index finger. The popliteal angle (the angle between the lower leg and thigh, posterior to the knee) is measured. This angle decreases with advancing GA (Figures 4.14–4.16).

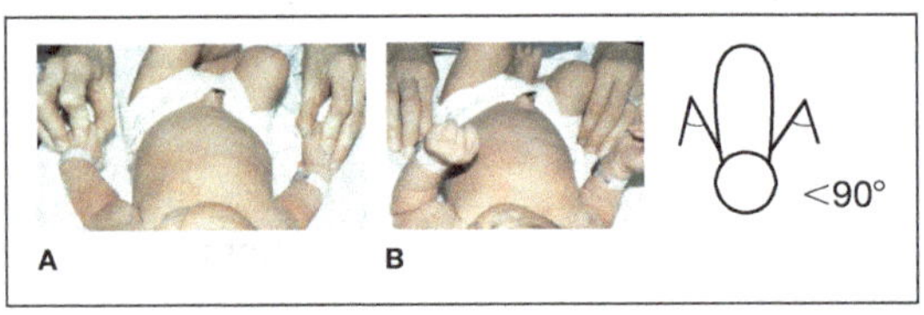

FIGURE 4.12 Eliciting arm recoil in a term infant. Score = 4

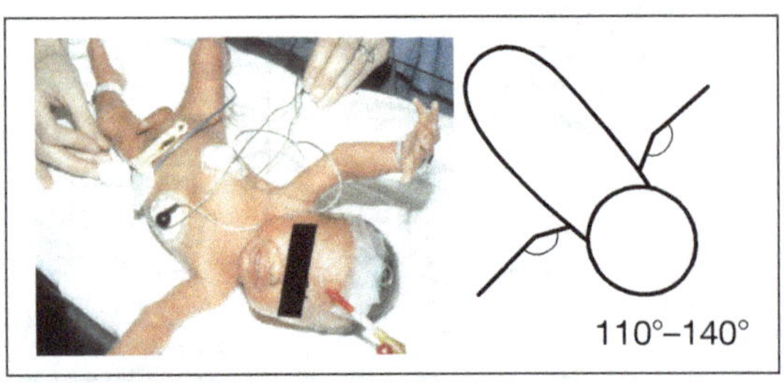

FIGURE 4.13 Arm recoil maneuver elicited Moro response in this preterm infant. Score = 2

Scarf Sign

With the neonate supine and the head in the midline position, the examiner grasps the infant's hand and pulls the arm across the chest and around the neck. The arm should be gently pulled across the chest and posteriorly as far as possible around the opposite shoulder. The examiner scores this item based on the relationship of the elbow to the midline of the body when the arm is pulled

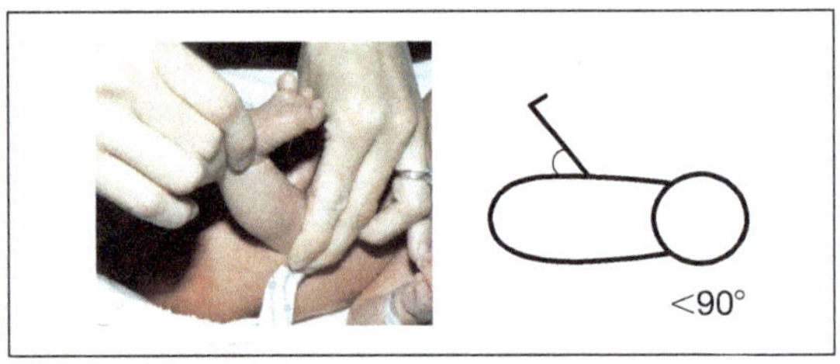

FIGURE 4.14 Popliteal angle in term infant. Score = 5

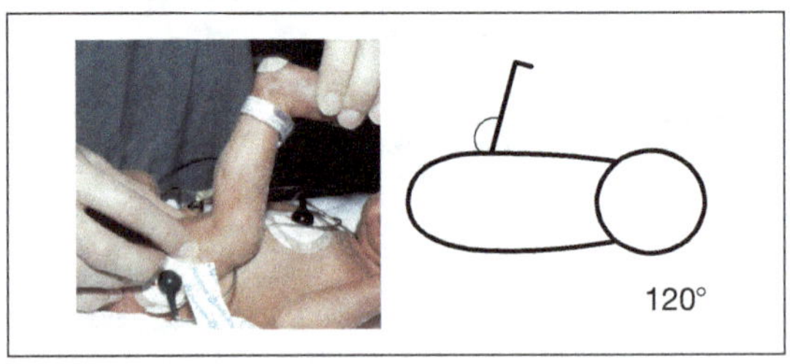

FIGURE 4.15 Popliteal angle in preterm infant. Score = 2

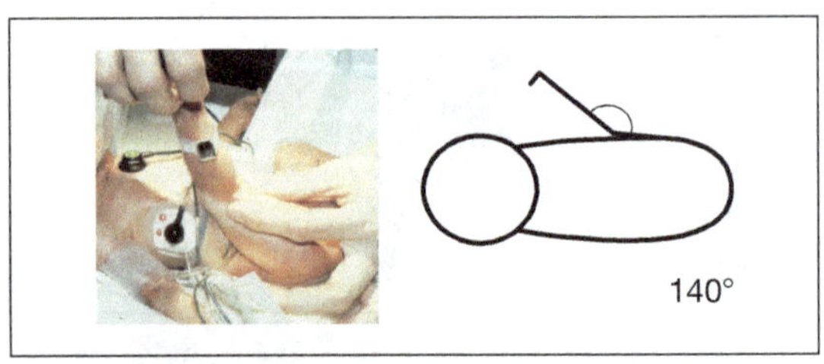

FIGURE 4.16 Popliteal angle. Score = 1

across the chest. The neonate demonstrates increasing resistance to this maneuver with advancing GA (Figures 4.17 and 4.18).

Heel to Ear

This maneuver evaluates passive flexor tone surrounding the pelvic girdle. With the infant supine and the pelvis flat on the table, the examiner gently grasps one foot with the thumb and index finger and draws the foot as near to the ear as possible without forcing it.[18] The thigh should be positioned along the side of the body. When significant resistance is detected, the examiner notes the distance between the foot and the ear, as well as the degree of knee extension. The location of the heel relative to the body landmarks is scored. The neonate demonstrates increasing resistance to this maneuver with advancing GA (Figures 4.19 and 4.20).

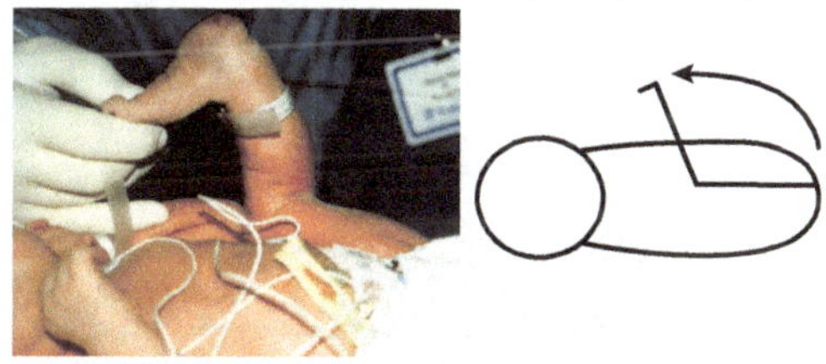

FIGURE 4.19 Heel to ear. Score = 2

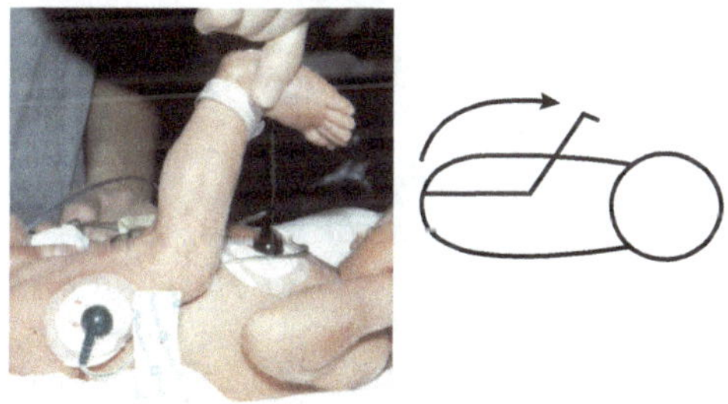

FIGURE 4.20 Heel to ear maneuver in preterm infant. Score = 1

Physical Criteria

Skin

The examiner assesses skin texture, color, and opacity. As the neonate matures, more subcutaneous tissue develops, and there is a gradual loss of the vernix caseosa. Veins become less visible, and the skin becomes more opaque (Figures 4.21–4.23).

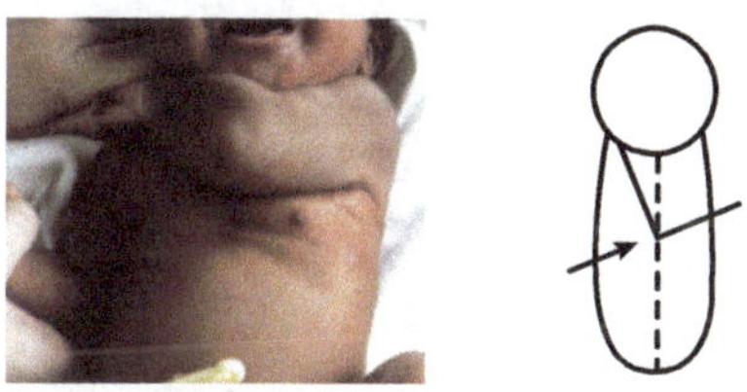

FIGURE 4.17 Scarf sign in term infant. Elbow drawn to midline of the body. Score = 2

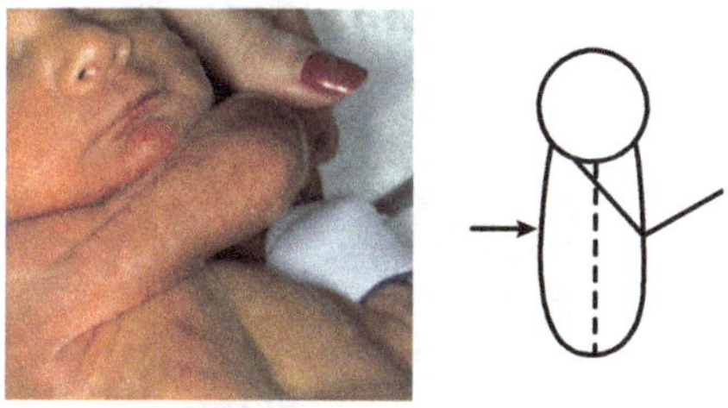

FIGURE 4.18 Scarf sign in preterm infant with elbow past midline. Score = 1

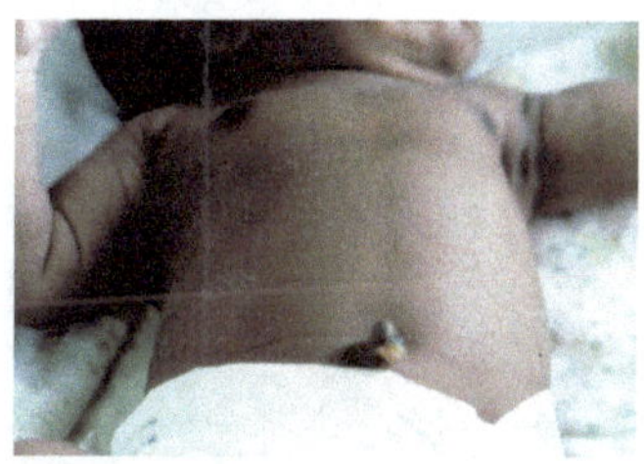

FIGURE 4.21 Skin of term infant. Score = 4

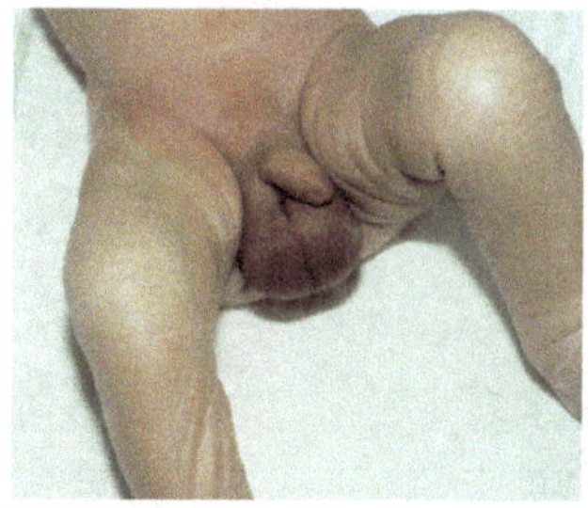

FIGURE 4.22 Skin of postterm infant. Score = 5

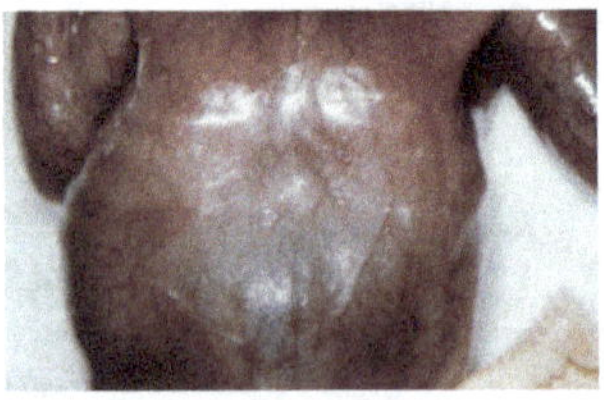

FIGURE 4.23 Friable, transparent skin of extremely preterm infant. Score = 1

Source: From Clark DA. 2000. *Atlas of Neonatology*. Philadelphia, PA: Saunders, 2. Reprinted by permission.[39]

Lanugo

Lanugo is the fine, downy hair present on the body of the neonate. Its production begins toward the end of the 12th week. Lanugo is most abundant over the back (particularly between the scapulae), although it will be noted over the face, legs, and arms as well. Thinning of lanugo begins on the back, and at term most of the lanugo on the back is gone (Figures 4.24–4.26).

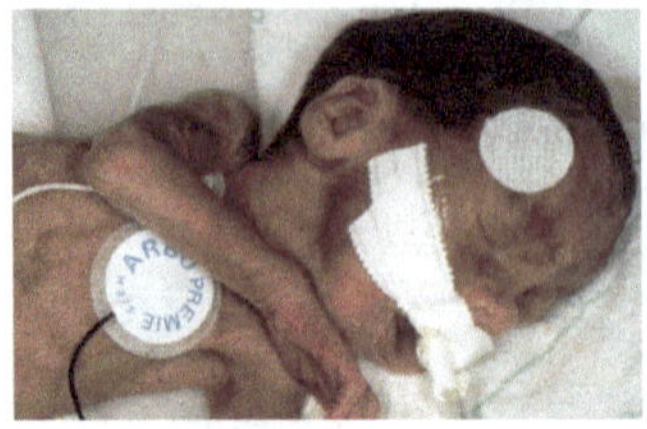

FIGURE 4.26 Lanugo noted over arm, shoulder, and face of preterm infant. Score = 1

Plantar Surface

In the extremely premature neonate, the examiner assesses the plantar surface of the foot for length and, as the neonate matures, for creases. Foot length is measured from the tip of the great toe to the back of the heel. Creases should appear between 28- and 30-weeks' gestation and should cover the entire plantar surface at or near term (Figures 4.27–4.29).

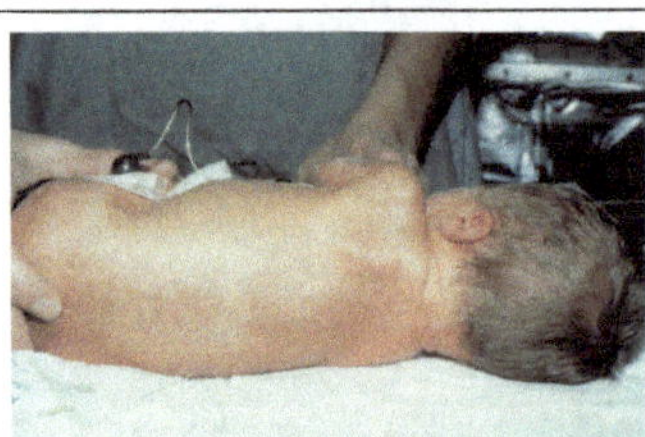

FIGURE 4.24 Lanugo over shoulders and cheek. Score = 3

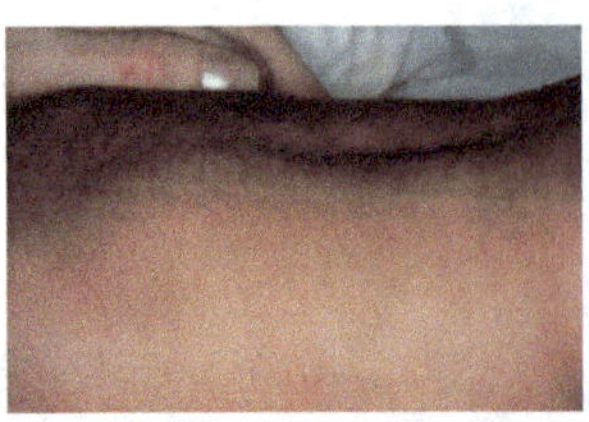

FIGURE 4.25 Lanugo over back of preterm infant. Score = 2

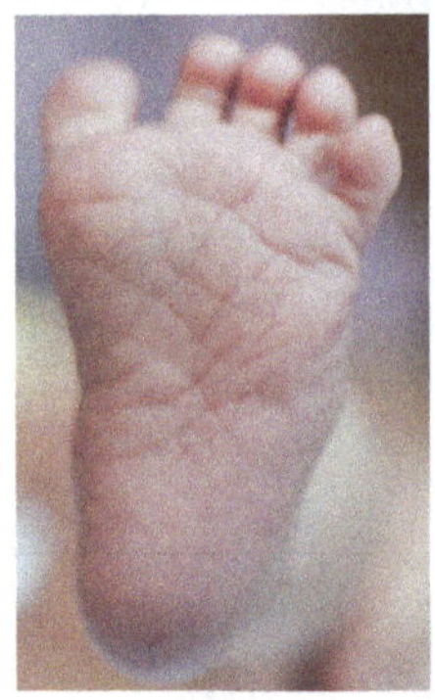

FIGURE 4.27 Sole creases covering the foot of a term neonate. Score = 4

Courtesy of Nancy Borowick.

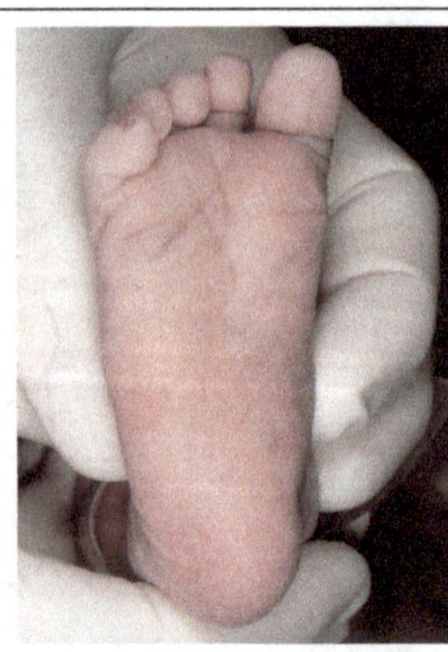

FIGURE 4.28 Sole creases covering the anterior two-thirds of the foot. Score = 3

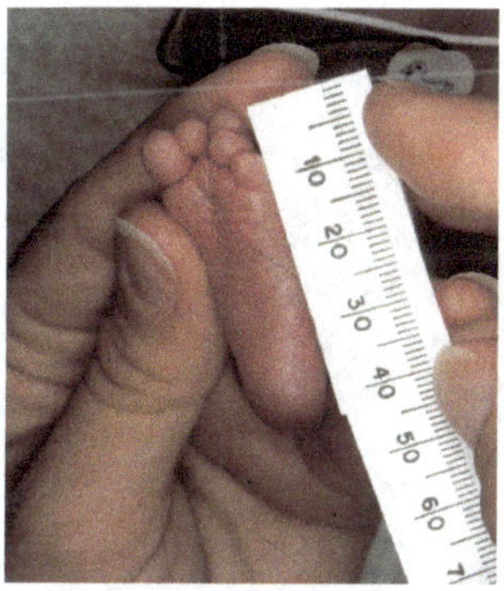

FIGURE 4.29 Faint red marks over the soles of the foot of a preterm infant. Score = 1

Breast

This is assessed by observing the size of the areola and for stippling, and it is palpated to determine the amount of breast tissue. Breast tissue is measured in millimeters. Breast tissue increases and areola development progresses with advancing GA, but the nutritional status of the fetus may affect the amount of breast tissue present (Figures 4.30–4.32).

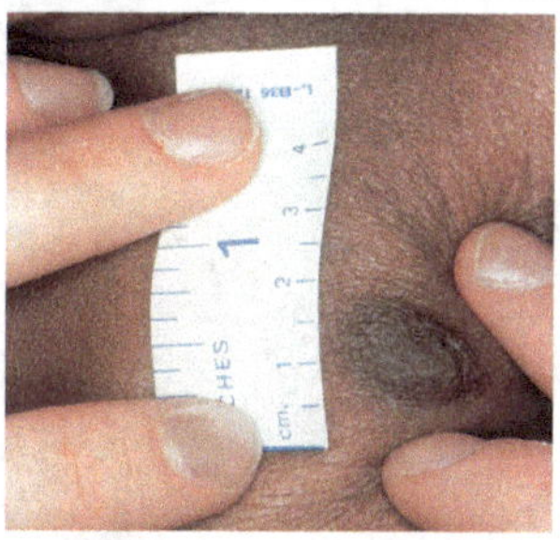

FIGURE 4.30 Evaluation of breast tissue in post-term infant. Score = 4

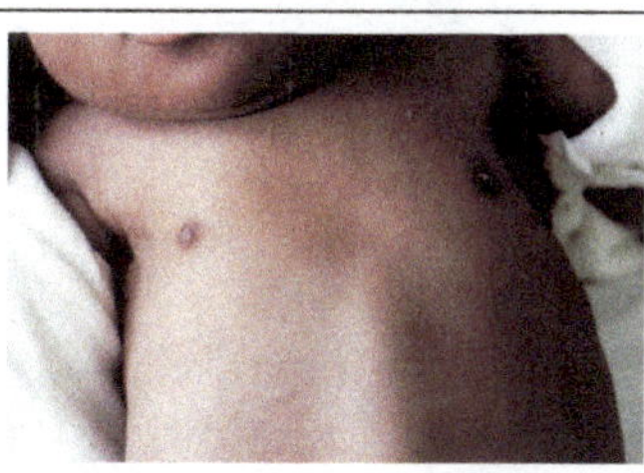

FIGURE 4.31 Breast tissue in a term neonate. The breast bud is 3 to 4 mm, and the areola is raised. Score = 3

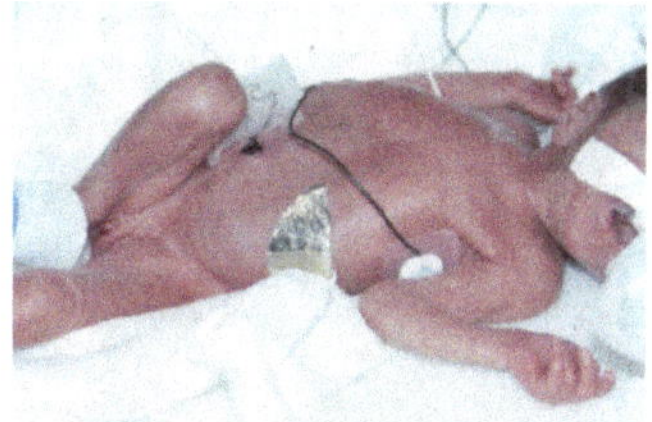

FIGURE 4.32 Breast tissue in a preterm neonate. There is no breast bud, and the areola is flat. Score = 0

Ear/Eye

The ear is assessed by observing its form, by palpating for the amount of cartilage present in the pinna, and for the recoil of the pinna when it is folded and released (Figures 4.33–4.35). In a mature neonate, the pinna will snap back rapidly when released. In a very immature neonate, there is a lack of cartilage in the pinna, so it may even remain folded when released. For an infant born at a very early gestation, the eyes are evaluated based on fusion of the eyelids, which occurs at approximately 9 to 10 weeks gestation. The eyelids open during the 26th to 28th week. Ballard and associates consider loosely fused lids (−1) as closed but able to be separated by gentle manipulation and tightly fused lids (−2) as unable to be separated with gentle manipulation.[31] They collected data on this criterion at gestational weeks 20–28. These data are depicted in Figure 4.36. All eyelids were fused at less than 23 weeks and open at 28 weeks. Between 23- and 27-weeks gestation, there is variability between the numbers of infants with tightly fused, loosely fused, and open eyelids. According to Ballard, the variability in eyelid fusion at each GA may be due to certain stress-related factors.[38]

Genitalia

The male genitalia are assessed for the presence of the testes, the degree of descent of the testes into the scrotum, and the development of rugae—creases that appear over the scrotum. Testicular descent from the peritoneal cavity begins at approximately 30 weeks gestation, and both testicles should be palpable

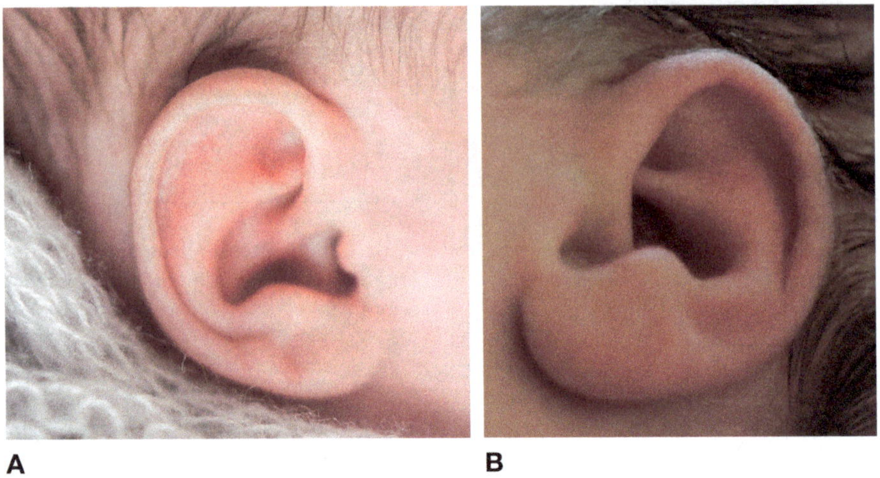

FIGURE 4.33 (A) Fully formed ear of term infant. Score = 4. (B) Well-curved pinna but not as complete and less cartilage when compared to (A). Score = 3

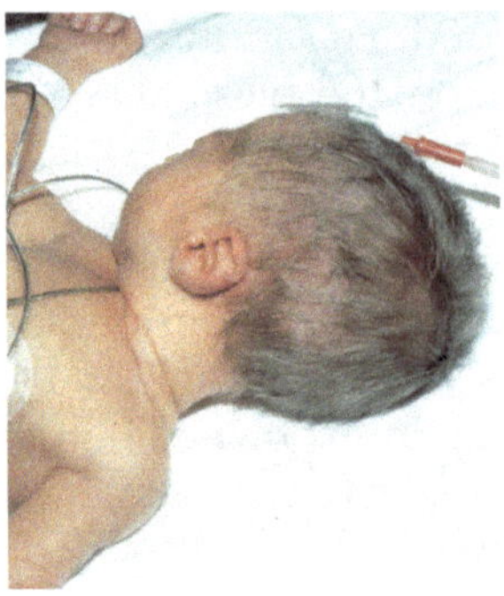

FIGURE 4.34 Ear of preterm infant with a partially curved pinna. Score = 1

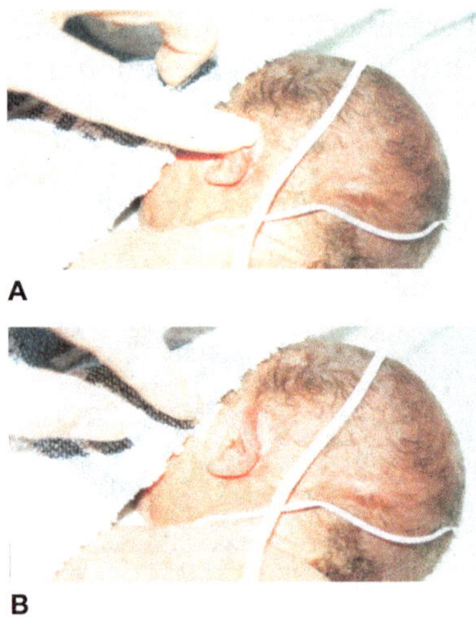

FIGURE 4.35 Eliciting recoil of pinna

in the inguinal canal by 34 weeks gestation. Rugae become more prominent as the scrotal sac thickens with advancing gestation (Figures 4.37–4.39).

The female genitalia are assessed with the hips abducted to about 45 degrees. Scoring is based on the prominence of the clitoris as well as the development of the labia minora and majora. With advancing GA, the labia majora and minora become more developed so that at term they completely cover the clitoris (Figures 4.40 and 4.41).

The labia majora contain fat; therefore, the nutritional status of the neonate will impact the size. The labia majora in neonates who have been nutritionally deprived in utero may be small relative to the clitoris and labia minora, causing the examiner to score the infant as less mature. The opposite is true for neonates who have been exposed to overnutrition in utero. According to Ballard, the criteria should be scored as observed, not as the examiner thinks it should be scored because of other influences (e.g., intrauterine nutritional status).[38] The total score will most

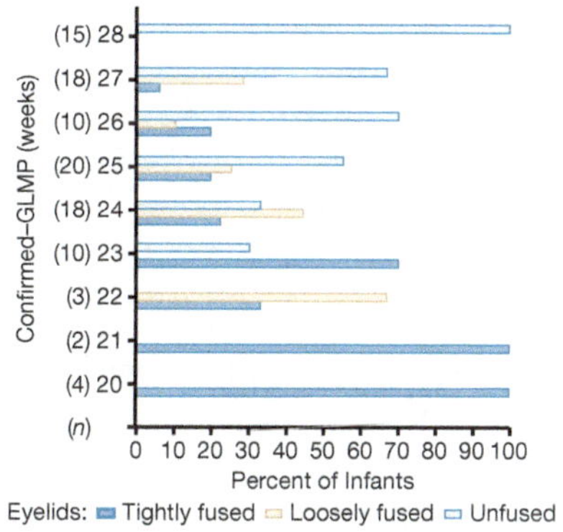

FIGURE 4.36 Eyelid fusion at gestational weeks 20 to 28 by C-GLMP

C-GLMP, confirmed-gestational age by last menstrual period.

Source: From Ballard JL, Khoury JC, Wedig KL, Wang L, Eilers-Walsman BL, and Lipp R. 1991. New Ballard Score, expanded to include extremely premature infants. *Journal of Pediatrics* 119(3): 422. Reprinted by permission.[31]

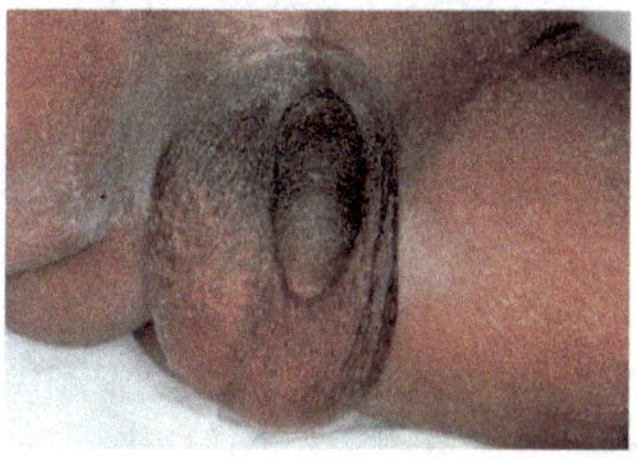

FIGURE 4.37 Male genitalia in postterm infant. Score = 4

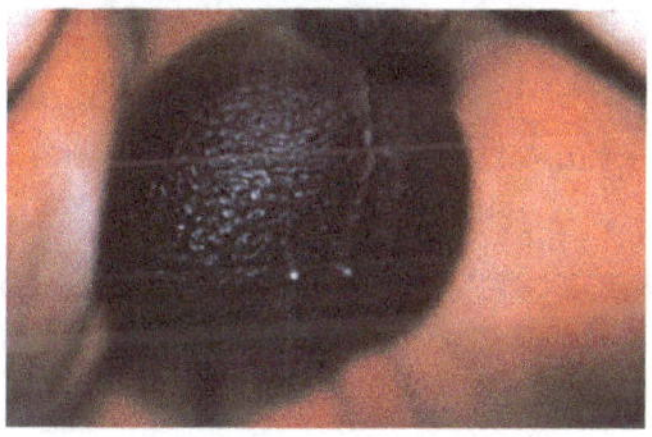

FIGURE 4.38 Deep rugae of male genitalia. Score = 4

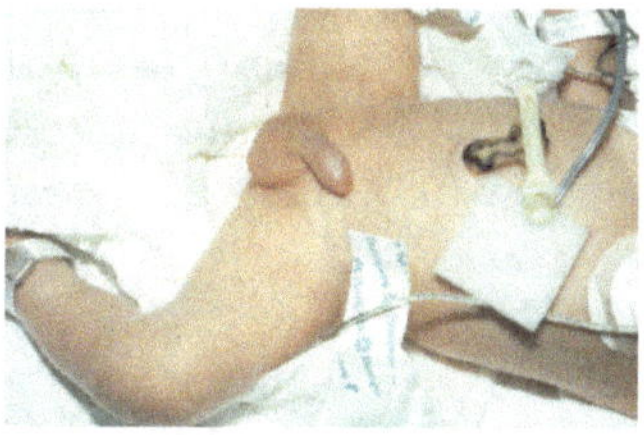

FIGURE 4.39 Male genitalia in preterm neonate. Score = 0

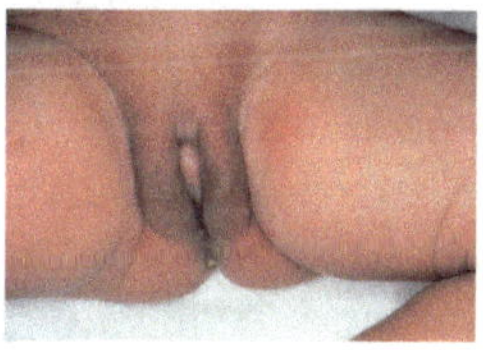

FIGURE 4.40 Female genitalia in term infant. Score = 3

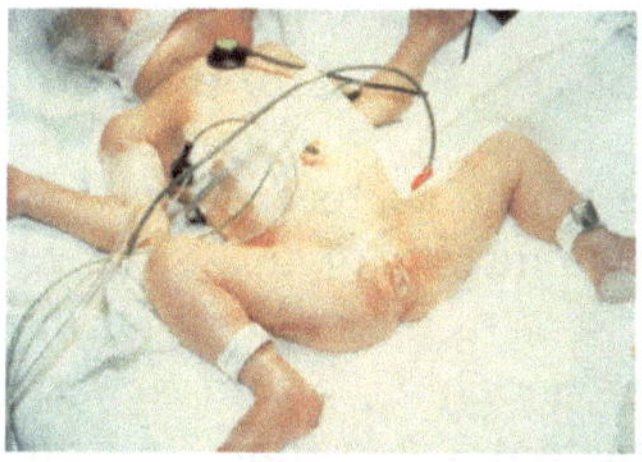

FIGURE 4.41 Female genitalia in preterm infant. Score = 0

likely be balanced out when the neuromuscular and physical scores are added together.

Scoring the Physical Examination

After the infant has been examined and a score assigned to each criterion, the score for each category, neuromuscular and physical, is determined. These two scores are added to obtain the final maturity rating score. As shown in Figure 4.5, the final maturity rating score (in the shaded area) is matched with the corresponding GA in weeks (in the unshaded column to the right). If the maturity rating score is 15, for example, the infant is assigned a GA of 30 weeks. The NBS authors do not give guidelines for what GA to assign when the maturity score falls between the numbers listed. In the experience of this author, a GA that most closely approximates the maturity rating is chosen. For example, if the maturity rating score is 23, a GA of 33 weeks is assigned. It is also appropriate to consider the GA determined by dates and obstetric measurements in making a final determination of GA.

Infants born before 37 completed weeks of gestation are considered preterm. Infants born between the beginning of week 38 and the completion of week 41 of gestation are considered term. Infants born at 42 weeks gestation or later are considered postterm. Recent terminology has focused on better defining these categories with an understanding that fetal and neonatal maturation is a continuous process. Duration of gestation is only one factor influencing fetal maturation. Other factors include the intrauterine environment; maternal diet, lifestyle, and medications; and fetal sex.[40] Figure 4.42 delineates the GA ranges of late preterm, early term, full term, late term, and postterm. Clinicians should understand that late preterm and early term infants experience increased morbidity and mortality and should be considered at-risk groups.[41,42]

Timing of the Physical Examination

There are no consistent, specific guidelines for optimal timing of the GA examination. Ballard and associates state that in extremely premature neonates, prompt examination at a postnatal age of less than 12 hours is essential to ensure validity of the examination.[31] Ballard, Novak, and Driver previously recommended examining all infants between 30 and 42 hours of age.[22] This short wait allows for stabilization and adjustment of the neonate to extrauterine life. Koenigsberger states that the neurologic examination is of little value during the first 48 hours of life because tone and reflexes change rapidly with extrauterine adjustment.[16] Amiel-Tison suggests repeating the examination performed on the first day of life again at 2 to 3 days of age because tone changes in the days following birth. Amiel-Tison also states that the optimal time for neuromuscular evaluation is 1 hour before feeding (when the infant is neither too sleepy nor too agitated) because both sleepiness and agitation affect tone.[18] When conducting their study, Dubowitz, Dubowitz, and Goldberg performed all assessments within 5 days of delivery. They found that when they did multiple assessments on 70 neonates, the assessments were as reliable during the first 24 hours as during the subsequent 4 days of life.[14]

Much of the concern regarding GA assessment and timing of the examination relates to neuromuscular adjustment following birth. This is further complicated by conditions altering neuromuscular function, such as asphyxia or medications administered during the pre- and postnatal periods. However, Ballard states that the items used to evaluate passive tone on the NBS are not affected by the perinatal events that profoundly affect active tone.[37] This may be the reason that Dubowitz, Dubowitz, and Goldberg did not find differences between the GA assessments performed on the first day of life and those done at 4 days of life.[14]

Still, controversy exists as to the optimal timing for the GA examination. In general, it is advisable that the initial examination be performed within the first 48 hours of life. Follow-up examinations may be indicated if

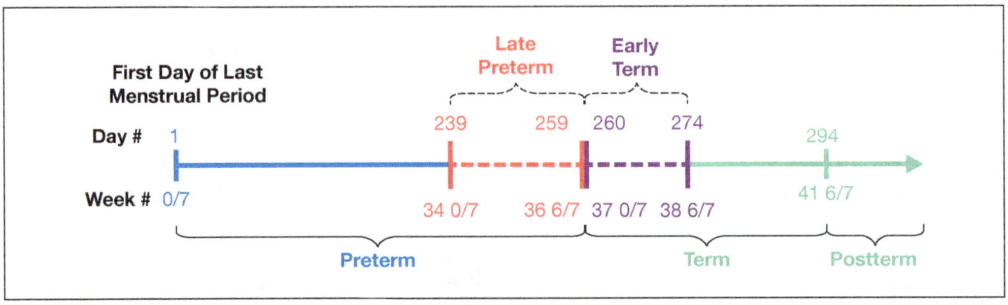

FIGURE 4.42 Definition of late preterm and early term

Source: From Engle WA, and Kominiarek MA. 2008. Late preterm infants, early term infants and timing of elective deliveries. *Clinics in Perinatology* 35: 326.[41]

the findings from the first examination disagree with GA assessments based on menstrual dates or obstetric methods. However, most healthcare professionals will assign the GA based on dates and obstetric measurements. When using the NBS tool, if the neuromuscular condition of the neonate is unreliable at birth, the examiner may assess the physical criteria, multiply the score by a factor of two, and then assign a GA based on this total score. Although the validity of this approach has not been addressed, it is based on the fact that Dubowitz, Dubowitz, and Goldberg, when analyzing their data, found that external characteristics scored collectively gave a better age index than did the neurologic criteria scored collectively.[14] However, the total score using both parameters was the most accurate.

EVALUATION OF GROWTH INDICES

When the GA of the neonate has been determined, the examiner plots the GA by the neonate's weight, length, and occipital-frontal circumference (OFC) on growth charts such as those seen in Figure 4.43.[43,44] For example, an examiner using the weight chart would define a neonate as being appropriate for gestational age (AGA) if the weight falls between the 10th and 90th percentiles. A small-for-gestational-age (SGA) neonate is one whose weight falls below the 10th percentile for GA. A large-for-gestational-age (LGA) neonate is one whose weight falls above the 90th percentile for GA. These classifications are depicted in Figure 4.43. On the basis of the relationship between weight and GA, each neonate will fall into one of nine categories: preterm SGA, AGA, or LGA; term SGA, AGA, or LGA; or postterm SGA, AGA, or LGA. These classifications are important because neonatal risk factors are identified based on intrauterine growth patterns and the GA of the neonate.

An intrauterine growth restricted (IUGR) neonate is one who has not grown at the expected in utero rate for weight, length, or OFC. Generally, an IUGR infant demonstrates restricted fetal growth subsequent to a pathophysiologic process occurring during the perinatal period. Box 4.1 and Figure 4.44 summarize the clinical features and complications of the IUGR infant.[45,46] The term IUGR has also been used interchangeably with SGA, which is not appropriate. Practically speaking, IUGR infants are often SGA, but this is not always the case. Some neonates may be growth restricted, yet not fall below the 10th percentile. For example, a 36-week-gestational-age infant with a birth weight of 2,000 g is well below the 50th percentile for weight on the graph depicted in Figure 4.43, which indicates a significant restriction of growth. However, this infant does not fall below the 10th percentile for weight so cannot be identified as SGA using this graph. Additionally, not all infants identified as SGA have experienced a pathologic process. They may simply be infants who are constitutionally small based on genetics, race, or ethnicity and represent one of the normal outliers for the newborn population. There are two types of IUGR patterns: symmetric and asymmetric. Generally, symmetric growth restriction involves the head, length, and infant's weight. Asymmetric growth restriction involves just the infant's weight. Table 4.1 summarizes the etiologies of these two types of growth patterns.[47] Generally, symmetric IUGR is caused by factors that produce a diminished overall growth rate and typically exert their effects early in gestation. Examples include congenital viral infections, single-gene defects, and chromosomal disorders. These conditions have a significant impact on cell replication and overall growth potential. Infants with asymmetric IUGR are typically those with normal OFC and length measurements, but who have a relatively low weight. These infants appear thin and wasted, with a head that is disproportionately large when compared with body size. This pattern of growth restriction is associated with poor placental perfusion or nutritional deficits to the fetus during the third trimester. Conditions predisposing the neonate to asymmetric growth restriction include maternal preeclampsia, poor caloric intake during pregnancy, and chronic fetal distress.

Classification of Newborns (Both Sexes) by Intrauterine Growth and Gestational Age

Name__________ Date of exam__________ Length __________

Hospital no.__________ Sex __________ Head circ.__________

Race__________ Birth weight__________ Gestational age __________

Date of birth__________

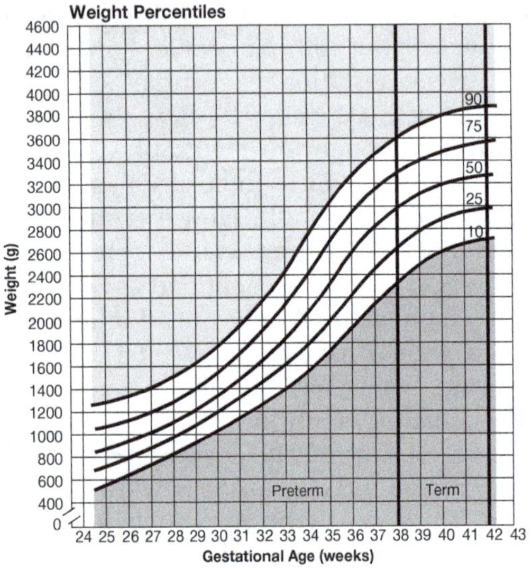

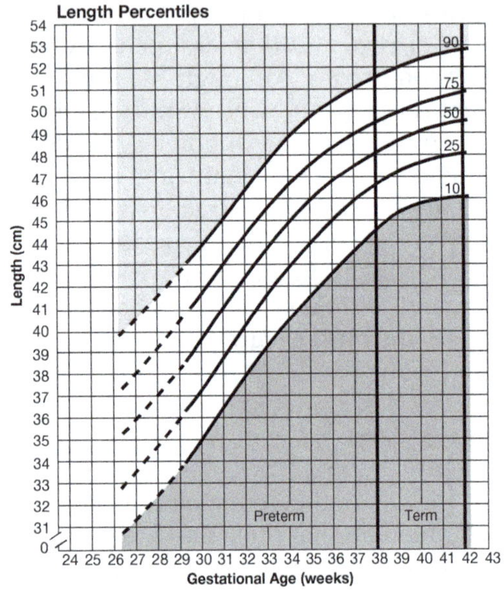

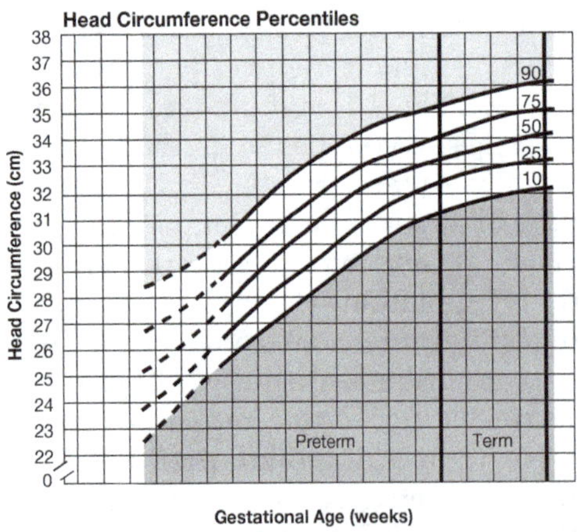

Classification of Infant*	Weight	Length	Head Circ.
Large for Gestational Age (LGA) (>90th percentile)			
Appropriate for Gestational Age (AGA) (10th to 90th percentile)			
Small for Gestational Age (SGA) (<10th percentile)			

*Place an "X" in the appropriate box (LGA, AGA or SGA) for weight, for length and for head circumference.

FIGURE 4.43 Intrauterine growth/gestational age charts

Source: From Ross Laboratories publication 10–91; (0.05) A-58560. Constructed from Battaglia FC, and Lubchenco LO. 1967. A practical classification of newborn infants by weight and gestational age. *Journal of Pediatrics* 71(2): 159–163[43]; Lubchenco LO, Hansman C, and Boyd E. 1966. Intrauterine growth in length and head circumference as estimated from live births at gestational ages from 26 to 42 weeks. *Pediatrics* 37(3): 404[44]. Reprinted by permission.

BOX 4.1: CLINICAL FEATURES OF INTRAUTERINE GROWTH RESTRICTION

- Relatively large head compared with whole body
- Shrunken abdomen with "scaphoid" appearance (must be distinguished from diaphragmatic hernia)
- Loose skin, sometimes dry, peeling, with the appearance of "hanging," occasionally meconium stained
- Long fingernails, especially in term and postterm infants with severe IUGR, occasionally meconium stained
- Face with shrunken appearance due to absence of buccal fat (old man look)
- Widened or overriding cranial sutures, anterior fontanel larger than usual
- Thin umbilical cord, sometimes meconium stained

Source: From Subhani M. 2005. Intrauterine growth restriction. In *Intensive Care of the Fetus and Neonate*, 2nd ed. Spitzer AR, ed. Philadelphia, PA: Mosby, 139. Reprinted by permission[45]; Sharma D, Shastri S, and Sharma P. 2016. Intrauterine growth restriction: Antenatal and postnatal aspects. *Clinical Medicine Insights: Pediatrics* 10: 67–83.[46]

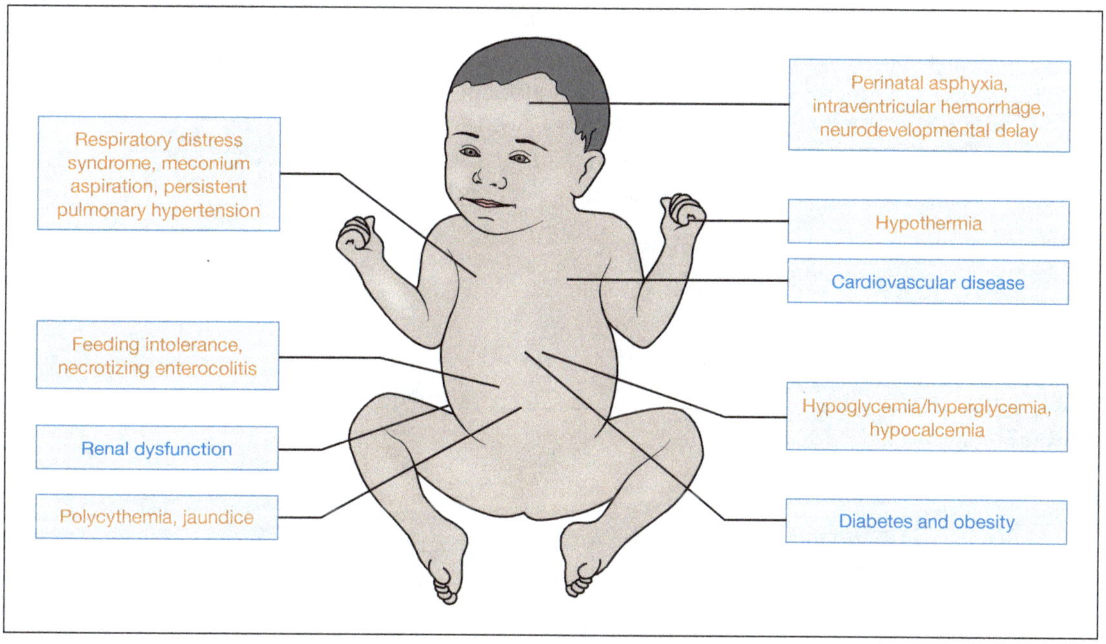

FIGURE 4.44 A schematic of complications of IUGR. Orange labels indicate short-term complications, blue labels indicate long-term complications

Source: Chu A, and Devaskar SU. 2020. Intrauterine growth restriction. In *Fanaroff & Martin's Neonatal–Perinatal Medicine: Diseases of the Fetus and Infant*, 11th ed. Martin RJ, Fanaroff AA, and Walsh MC, eds. Philadelphia, PA: Elsevier Saunders, 268.[47]

TABLE 4.1: ETIOLOGIES OF ASYMMETRIC AND SYMMETRIC INTRAUTERINE GROWTH RESTRICTION

	ASYMMETRIC IUGR	SYMMETRIC IUGR
Fetal	Genetics	Chromosomal disorders (e.g., trisomies 13, 18, and 21) Structural disorders (specific forms of congenital heart disease, gastroschisis)
Maternal	Age Parity Ethnicity Race Height Poor weight gain Short pregnancy intervals Medical conditions (pregestational diabetes, renal insufficiency, autoimmune disease, and cyanotic congenital heart disease) Diseases related to pregnancy (gestational hypertension, preeclampsia, and gestational diabetes) Thrombophilia (antiphospholipid antibody syndrome)	Advanced maternal diseases (e.g., severe hypertension, hemoglobinopathies)
Placental	Multiple gestation Placental insufficiency Placental disorders and umbilical cord abnormalities	
Environmental	Teratogen exposure (e.g., cyclophosphamide, valproic acid, and antithrombotic drugs) Substance use (alcohol, tobacco, cocaine, and narcotics) Altitude ART	

ART, assisted reproductive technology; IUGR, intrauterine growth restriction.

Source: Chu A, and Devaskar SU. 2020. Intrauterine growth restriction. In *Fanaroff & Martin's Neonatal–Perinatal Medicine: Diseases of the Fetus and Infant*, 11th ed. Martin RJ, Fanaroff AA, and Walsh MC, eds. Philadelphia, PA: Elsevier Saunders, 262.[47]

LGA infants are frequently born to diabetic mothers with poor glucose control. Maternal hyperglycemia results in fetal hyperglycemia and hyperinsulinemia. The high insulin levels act as a fetal growth hormone, causing macrosomia and resulting in hypoglycemia postnatally. The term macrosomia is frequently used interchangeably with LGA. A macrosomic infant is one who weighs more than 4,000 g at birth. Risks associated with macrosomic or LGA infants are typically related to difficult deliveries and the postnatal hyperinsulinemia that occurs after prolonged maternal hyperglycemia.

SUMMARY

Assessment of the neonate's GA is an essential component of the neonatal physical examination. Knowledge of GA and appropriate growth patterns assists the examiner in identifying potential risks to the neonate. With experience and a cooperative neonate, the examiner should be able to perform the GA examination in 5 minutes. Infants born with altered neuromuscular states may require an additional GA examination at a later date.

ADDITIONAL RESOURCES

SPRINGER PUBLISHING CONNECT™

A robust set of resources designed to supplement this text is located at http://connect.springerpub.com/content/book/978-0-8261-4063-0. Qualifying instructors may request access by emailing textbook@springerpub.com.

REFERENCES

1. American Academy of Pediatrics, and Committee on Fetus and Newborn. 2004. Age terminology during the perinatal period. *Pediatrics* 114(5): 1362–1364. (Statement reaffirmed July 2021) http://pediatrics.aappublications.org/content/114/5/1362.full.pdf+html. doi: 10.1542/peds.2021-054665
2. Ely DM, and Driscoll AK. 2022. Infant mortality in the United States. 2020: Data from the period linked birth/infant death file. *National Vital Statistics Report* 71(5): 1–18. https://www.cdc.gov/nchs/data/nvsr/nvsr71/nvsr71-05.pdf
3. National Institutes of Health. *Extremely Preterm Birth Outcomes Tool*. https://www.nichd.nih.gov/research/supported/EPBO/use (Accessed 10/12/2022)
4. Rysavy MA, Horbar JD, Bell EF, Li L, Greenberg LT, Tyson JE, Patel RM, Carlo WA, Younge NE, Green CE, and Edwards EM. 2020. Assessment of an updated Neonatal Research Network extremely preterm birth outcome model in the Vermont Oxford Network. *JAMA Pediatrics* 174(5): e196294. doi: 10.1001/jamapediatrics.2019.6294
5. Engle WA, Tomashek KM, and Wallman C. 2007. "Late preterm" infants: A population at risk. *Pediatrics* 120(6): 1390–1401.
6. American Academy of Pediatrics, and The American College of Obstetricians and Gynecologists. 2017. Care of the newborn. In *Guidelines for Perinatal Care*, 8th ed. Kilpatrick SJ, Papile LA, and Macones GA, eds. Elk Grove Village, IL: AAP, 347–408.
7. Stewart DL, Barfield WD, and Committee on Fetus and Newborn. 2019. Updates on an at-risk population: Late-preterm and early-term infants. *Pediatrics* 144(5): e210192760.
8. Barfield WD, and APP Committee on Fetus and Newborn. 2016. Standard terminology for fetal, infant, and perinatal deaths. *Pediatrics* 137(5): e20160551.
9. Jacob J, and Hulman S. 2006. A standardized method for assigning gestational age: A tool measuring gestational age based newborn intensive care outcomes. *American Journal of Perinatology* 23(7): 397–402.
10. The American College of Obstetricians and Gynecologists, Committee on Obstetric Practice, American Institute of Ultrasound Medicine, and Society for Maternal-Fetal Medicine. 2017. Methods for estimating the due date. *Committee Opinion Number* 700: 1–5. Reaffirmed 2022.
11. Lazebnik N, Judge NE, and Dar P. 2020. Perinatal ultrasound. In *Neonatal Perinatal Medicine. Diseases of the Fetus and Infant*, 11th ed. Martin RJ, Fanaroff AA, and Walsh MC, eds. Philadelphia, PA: Elsevier Saunders, 174–209.
12. American Institute of Ultrasound in Medicine. 2013. *AIUM Practice Parameter for the Performance of Obstetric Ultrasound Examinations*. Laurel, Maryland: AIUM, 1–17. Retrieved from http://www.aium.org/resources/guidelines/obstetric.pdf
13. Lissauer T, and Hansen A. 2020. Chapter 28: Physical examination of the newborn. In *Neonatal-Perinatal Medicine: Diseases of the Fetus and Infant*, 11th ed. Martin RJ, Fanaroff AA, and Walsh MC, eds. Philadelphia, Pennsylvania: Elsevier Saunders, 440–457.
14. Dubowitz LMS, Dubowitz V, and Goldberg C. 1970. Clinical assessment of gestational age in the newborn infant. *Journal of Pediatrics* 77(1): 1–10.
15. Farr V, Mitchell RG, Neligan GA, and Parkin JM. 1966. The definition of some external characteristics used in the assessment of gestational age in the newborn infant. *Developmental Medicine and Child Neurology* 8(5): 507–511.
16. Koenigsberger MR. 1966. Judgment of fetal age. Part 1: Neurologic evaluation. *Pediatric Clinics of North America* 13(3): 823–832.
17. Robinson RJ. 1966. Assessment of gestational age by neurological examination. *Archives of Disease in Childhood* 41: 437–447.

18. Amiel-Tison C. 1968. Neurological evaluation of the maturity of newborn infants. *Archives of Disease in Childhood* 43(227): 89–93.
19. Bhagwat VA, Dahat HB, and Bapat NG. 1990. Determination of gestational age of newborns: A comparative study. *Indian Pediatrics* 27(3): 272–275.
20. Eregie CO. 1991. Assessment of gestational age: Modification of a simplified method. *Developmental Medicine and Child Neurology* 33(7): 596–600.
21. Capurro H, Konichezky S, Fonseca D, and Caldeyro-Barcia R. 1978. A simplified method for diagnosis of gestational age in the newborn infant. *Journal of Pediatrics* 93(1): 120–122.
22. Ballard JL, Novak KK, and Driver M. 1979. A simplified score for assessment of fetal maturation of newly born infants. *Journal of Pediatrics* 95(5): 769–774.
23. Kumar GP, and Kumar UK. 1993. Estimation of gestational age from hand and foot length. *Medicine, Science, and the Law* 34(1): 48–50.
24. Amato M, Huppi P, and Claus R. 1991. Rapid biometric assessment of gestational age in very low birth weight infants. *Journal of Perinatal Medicine* 19(5): 367–371.
25. Van Wyk L, and Smith J. 2016. Postnatal footlength to determine gestational age: A pilot study. *Journal of Tropical Pediatrics* 62: 144–151. doi: 10.1093/tropej/fmv093
26. Anderson N, Wells E, Hay R, and Darlow B. 1996. Cerebellar vermis measurement at cranial sonography for assessing gestational age in the newborn weighing less than 2,000 grams. *Early Human Development* 44(1): 59–70.
27. Mackanjee HR, Iliescu BM, and Dawson WB. 1996. Assessment of postnatal gestational age using sonographic measurements of femur length. *Journal of Ultrasound in Medicine* 15(2): 115–120.
28. Lynn C, Saidi IS, Oelberg DG, and Jacques SL. 1993. Gestational age correlates with skin reflectance in newborn infants of 24–42 weeks gestation. *Biology of the Neonate* 64(2–3): 69–75.
29. Sanders M, Allen M, Alexander GR, Yankowitz J, Graeber J, Johnson TR, and Repka MX. 1991. Gestational age assessment in preterm neonates weighing less than 1,500 grams. *Pediatrics* 88(3): 542–546.
30. Alexander GR, de Caunes F, Hulsey TC, Tompkins ME, and Allen M. 1992. Validity of postnatal assessments of gestational age: A comparison of the method of Ballard JL, et al., and early ultrasonography. *American Journal of Obstetrics and Gynecology* 166(3): 891–895.
31. Ballard JL, Khoury JC, Wedig KL, Wang L, Eilers-Walsman BL, and Lipp R. 1991. New Ballard Score, expanded to include extremely premature infants. *Journal of Pediatrics* 119(3): 417–423.
32. Donovan EF, Tyson JE, Ehrenkranz RA, Verter J, Wright LL, Korones SB, Bauer CR, Shankaran S, Stoll BJ, Fanaroff AA, and Oh W. 1999. Inaccuracy of Ballard scores before 28 weeks' gestation. *Journal of Pediatrics* 135(2 Part 1): 147–152.
33. Hittner HM, Hirsch NJ, and Rudolph AJ. 1977. Assessment of gestational age by examination of the anterior vascular capsule of the lens. *Journal of Pediatrics* 91(3): 455–458.
34. Moore KL, Persaud TVN, and Torshia MG, eds. 2020. The eye and ear. In *The Developing Human: Clinically Oriented Embryology*, 11th ed. Philadelphia, PA: Saunders, 402.
35. Dietz U, Huppi P, and Amato M. 1993. Influence of perinatal risk factors on the involution of the iridopupillary membrane. *Journal of Perinatal Medicine* 21(1): 53–57.
36. Hadi HA, and Hobbs CL. 1990. Effect of chronic intrauterine stress on the disappearance of the tunica vasculosa lentis of the fetal eye: A neonatal observation. *American Journal of Perinatology* 7(1): 23–25.
37. Ballard JL. 1993. *New Ballard Score: A Maturational Assessment of Gestational Age*. Bethesda Hospitals, Clinical Staff Development, 619 Oak Street, Cincinnati, OH 45206.
38. Ballard JL. 1993. *New Ballard Score Maturational Assessment of Gestational Age (Video)*. Available at New Ballard Score Website (2019): https://www.ballardscore.com/CatalogView/Article/video-archive/ballard-score-assessment-demonstration. Chapters 1–5. (Accessed 10/24/2022).
39. Clark DA. 2000. *Atlas of Neonatology*. Philadelphia, PA: Saunders, 2. Reprinted by permission.
40. Raju, TNK. 2013. Moderately preterm, late preterm and early term infant: Research needs. *Clinics in Perinatology* 40(4): 791–797. doi: 10.1016/j.clp.2013.07.010
41. Engle WA, and Kominiarek MA. 2008. Late preterm infants, early term infants, and timing of elective deliveries. *Clinics in Perinatology* 35: 325–341. doi: 10.1016/j.clp.2008.03.003
42. Stewart DL, Barfield WD, American Academy of Pediatrics, and Committee on Fetus and Newborn. 2019. Updates on an at-risk population: Late preterm and early-term infants. *Pediatrics* 144(5): e20192760.
43. Battaglia FC, and Lubchenco LO. 1967. A practical classification of newborn infants by weight and gestational age. *Journal of Pediatrics* 71(2): 159–163.
44. Lubchenco LO, Hansman C, and Boyd E. 1966. Intrauterine growth in length and head circumference as estimated from live births at gestational ages from 26 to 42 weeks. *Pediatrics* 37(3): 404.
45. Subhani M. 2005. Intrauterine growth restriction. In *Intensive Care of the Fetus and Neonate*, 2nd ed. Spitzer AR, ed. Philadelphia, PA: Mosby, 135–148.
46. Sharma D, Shastri A, and Sharma P. 2016. Intrauterine growth restriction: Antenatal and postnatal aspects. *Clinical Medicine Insights: Pediatrics* 10: 67–83. doi: 10.4137/CMPed.S40070
47. Chu A, and Devaskar SU. 2020. Intrauterine growth restriction. In *Fanaroff & Martin's Neonatal–Perinatal Medicine: Diseases of the Fetus and Infant*, 11th ed. Martin RJ, Fanaroff AA, and Walsh MC, eds. Philadelphia, PA: Elsevier Saunders, 260–273.

5 SKIN ASSESSMENT

Catherine L. Witt

Assessment of the skin is an important element of the newborn physical examination. Valuable information regarding the newborn's health and well-being can be obtained by observing the color, integrity, and characteristics of the skin. Close examination can aid the practitioner in determining gestational age, nutritional status, functioning of organ systems, and the presence of cutaneous or systemic disease.

Newborn rashes, birthmarks, and lesions can be a source of questions and anxiety for parents. Those caring for newborns must be well versed in normal and abnormal variations, for both educational and diagnostic purposes.

A complete examination of the skin involves both inspection and palpation. Most skin variations can be noted by inspection alone, but palpation is essential to avoid missing less obvious problems. Palpation is also important for determining the thickness, turgor, and consistency of the skin.

ANATOMY AND PHYSIOLOGY

The skin serves several basic functions in the newborn. These include physical and immunologic protection, thermoregulation, sense perception, and self-cleaning. An understanding of the skin's structure is essential to careful examination and recognition of irregularities in appearance or function.

The skin consists of three layers: the epidermis, the dermis, and the subcutaneous layer (Figure 5.1). The epidermis, or outermost layer, is subdivided into five layers. The top layer is the stratum corneum, consisting of dead cells that are constantly being brushed off and replaced. Although the epidermis of a term newborn has the same number of layers as adult skin, it is thinner and does not function as well.[1,2] The epidermis is only about 0.01 mm to 0.05 mm thick. Close adherence of the stratum corneum cells to one another prevents chemicals and microorganisms from entering the body and prevents significant insensible water loss through the skin in the term newborn, child, and adult.[1,2]

The lower layers of the epidermis contain keratin-forming cells and melanocytes. Melanocytes are pigment-producing cells that provide protection from ultraviolet radiation. Different numbers of melanocytes are found in various regions of the skin, with more in the facial area than on the trunk.[2] The amount of pigmentation in the skin depends on the development of the melanocytes, with more advanced melanocytes producing and dispersing more pigment. Melanin production is immature in the newborn, increasing the newborn's sensitivity to sunlight.[2]

The dermis lies directly under the epidermis. The epidermis and dermis are attached by means of a basement membrane referred to as the *dermal–epidermal junction*. This junction consists of various structures that anchor and attach the epidermis to the dermis. This membrane is well established in the fetus in the third trimester, although the anchoring is less secure than in the adult.[1,2]

The dermis consists of fibrous and elastic tissues, sweat glands, sebaceous glands, and hair shafts, as well as blood vessels and cutaneous nerves. The fibrous, elastic tissues are what give the dermis its strength and elasticity. Sweat glands and blood vessels help to

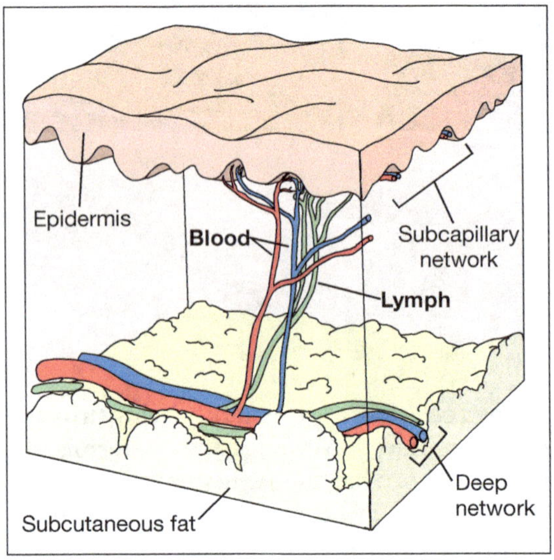

FIGURE 5.1 Cross section of human skin and the anatomic relationships among the various structures

Source: Adapted from Nasemann T, Sauerbrey W, and Burgdorf W. 1983. *Fundamentals of Dermatology*. New York, NY: Springer-Verlag, 11. Reprinted by permission.[3]

maintain body temperature, and cutaneous nerves protect the skin from injury and provide the sensations of touch, temperature, and pain.

The third layer of the skin consists of subcutaneous fat. This fat layer serves as insulation, protection for internal organs, and calorie storage. It is less developed in the preterm or low-birth-weight newborn.

The skin of the newborn is similar to that of the adult in its basic structure. As with any other organ, however, the less mature the newborn, the less mature the function of the skin.

The more immature the skin, the thinner and more permeable it is. Fibrils that connect the dermis and the epidermis are more fragile in the newborn's term and preterm skin than in adult skin, and the stratum corneum is thinner.[1,2] Sweat glands, although present at birth, do not reach full adult functioning until the second or third year of life.

Fetal skin is covered in utero with vernix caseosa, a greasy white or yellow material composed of sebaceous gland secretions, proteins, and exfoliated skin cells. Vernix becomes thicker during the third trimester and provides protection for the skin in utero. It gradually decreases as the fetus approaches 40 weeks gestation.[1,2]

The fetus is also covered with a fine, soft, and downy type of hair called *lanugo* while in utero. Lanugo first appears at approximately 20 weeks gestation and covers most of the body, including the face. Most of it disappears by 40 weeks gestation.

BEGINNING THE EXAMINATION

Several factors influence the appearance of the neonate's skin and affect the examiner's ability to note normal and abnormal variations. A consistent, systematic approach to examining the skin increases the likelihood of gathering all the information.

A family and maternal history and an account of the labor and delivery are useful to the examiner because they may highlight items that should be inspected with extra care. For example, a forceps or vacuum-assisted delivery may lead to disruption of skin integrity. A family history of neurofibromatosis would alert the examiner to search for café au lait patches.

Before beginning the examination, consider the newborn's environment. The amount and type of light and the temperature of the room will affect the appearance of the skin. Adequate lighting, preferably bright natural light, is important. Ideally, the newborn should be examined under a radiant heat source to allow for complete undressing and visualization. This allows the examiner to observe color and vascular changes.

To begin the examination, undress the newborn and inspect the general color, consistency (smooth, peeling), thickness, and opacity of the skin. Note the distribution of hair and any obvious markings or anomalies. Then begin a closer inspection of the newborn. It is important to follow the same pattern every time to avoid missing subtle deviations. Many examiners find it easiest to begin at the head and progress downward toward the feet. While looking closely at the skin, note the size, color, and placement of any discolorations, markings, or variations (Table 5.1). The newborn

TABLE 5.1: DERMATOLOGICTERMINOLOGY

When reporting skin irregularities, correct terminology facilitates accurate description of observations. The following terms are commonly used to define skin irregularities.	
Bulla	A vesicle >1 cm in diameter containing serous or seropurulent fluid
Crust	A lesion consisting of dried serous exudate, blood, or pus on the surface of the skin
Cyst	A raised, palpable lesion with a fluid- or semisolid-filled sac
Ecchymosis	A large area of subepidermal hemorrhage, initially bluish black in color, then changing to greenish brown or yellow; it does not blanch with pressure
Lesion	An area of altered or abnormal tissue
Macule	A discolored, flat spot <1 cm in diameter that is not palpable
Nodule	An elevated, palpable lesion with indistinct borders; some of the lesion is palpable below the skin outside the elevated area
Papule	An elevated, palpable lesion, solid and circumscribed, <1 cm in diameter
Patch	A macule >1 cm in diameter
Petechia	A small, purplish, hemorrhagic spot on the skin, the size of a pinpoint
Plaque	An elevated, palpable lesion with circumscribed borders >1 cm, or a fusion or coalescence of several papules
Purpura	A small hemorrhagic spot larger than a petechia, 1 to 3 mm in size
Pustule	An elevation of the skin filled with cloudy or purulent fluid
Scale	An exfoliation of dead or dying bits of skin; can also result from excess keratin
Vesicle (blister)	An elevation of the skin filled with serous fluid; <1 cm in diameter
Wheal	A collection of fluid in the dermis that appears as a reddened, solid elevation of the skin

should be turned over for a complete examination of the back. Inspect all skin crevices, including the axillae and the groin.

As stated earlier, palpation is an important aspect of the examination. It permits the examiner to assess the underlying dermis, thickness of the skin and subcutaneous fat, presence of edema, and any irregularities in texture or consistency. Palpation is also necessary to determine the size or configuration of certain lesions or variations that may be observed during the examination.

Note: It is important to describe the color of the lesion and its distribution. Lesions may be arranged in distinct patterns, such as linear or circular, or as distinct separate lesions.

Blanching of lesions can be assessed by pressing the pad of the thumb or finger against the lesion for a few seconds and observing for color changes when the pressure is removed. Hydration and nutrition can also be assessed by examination of the skin. Poor skin turgor or loose, hanging skin indicates dehydration or poor nutritional status. It is important to remember that poor skin turgor is a late sign of dehydration. Excessive fluid, or edema, can be noted by pressing the pad of the thumb into the skin and looking for pitting. Edema may be noted especially in dependent areas or on the scalp following delivery. Most newborns will have some edema around the face and eyes as a result of excess fluid volume after delivery.

To determine the amount of subcutaneous fat, the examiner pinches a skin fold between thumb and forefinger. Loose skin folds will be present in the term infant who has a decreased amount of fat—for example, the infant who has intrauterine growth restriction. Loose skin may also be seen in the post-term newborn who has lost weight in the week or 2 before delivery.

RECOGNIZING COMMON VARIATIONS IN NEWBORN SKIN

A number of changes occur in newborn skin during the first few days and weeks after birth. Most are benign, transient lesions that do not require therapeutic intervention. It is important to be familiar with these normal changes and to be able to distinguish them from signs of serious disease.

Color Variations

Acrocyanosis

Acrocyanosis refers to bluish discoloration of the palms of the hands and the soles of the feet. Most infants present with acrocyanosis at birth. It may persist for up to 48 hours after delivery and is exacerbated by low environmental temperatures. It is benign in the otherwise normal infant. Circumoral (around the mouth) cyanosis may also be present during the first 12 to 24 hours after birth. Acrocyanosis that persists beyond the first few days after birth, or circumoral cyanosis lasting longer than 24 hours should be investigated.

Plethora

Plethora describes the ruddy, or red, appearance present in some newborns. It may be indicative of a high hemoglobin level. The infant who is plethoric at birth and demonstrates clinical signs, such as hypoglycemia or respiratory distress, should have hemoglobin and hematocrit checked by heel-stick or central venipuncture. A newborn with a central hematocrit greater than 65% is considered polycythemic and should be watched closely for hypoglycemia, cyanosis, respiratory distress, or jaundice.[4]

Jaundice

Jaundice is the term used to describe a yellow coloring of the skin and the sclera. The color is caused by the deposit of bile pigment that is a result of hyperbilirubinemia, or excess bilirubin in the blood. The presence of jaundice in a newborn should be noted, with particular attention paid to the age of the newborn and the degree of jaundice present. As a general rule, jaundice first appears in the head or face, and then progresses head to toe as the bilirubin level rises. Because it is difficult, if not impossible, to estimate serum bilirubin levels on the basis of clinical appearance, transcutaneous or serum bilirubin levels must be obtained to determine the presence of hyperbilirubinemia. In darker skin, blanching may help decrease the effects of pigmentation to allow jaundice to be visible.

Cutis Marmorata

The bluish mottling or marbling of the skin seen in response to chilling, stress, or overstimulation is called *cutis marmorata*. It is caused by the constriction of capillaries and venules and usually disappears when the newborn is warmed. Persistent cutis marmorata may be seen in newborns and infants with trisomy 21, trisomy 18, and Cornelia de Lange syndrome.[5,6] Persistent, reticulated mottling that is associated with skin atrophy, ulcerations, or limb hypoplasia and does not respond to rewarming is more likely to be cutis marmorata telangiectatice congenita (CMTC). This usually improves over time without treatment.[7] Capillary malformations should be ruled out.

Harlequin Color Change

This phenomenon is seen only in the newborn period. When the newborn is lying on one side, a sharply demarcated red color is seen in the dependent half of the body, with the superior half appearing pale (Figure 5.2). If the newborn is rotated to the other side, the color reverses. The color change may last anywhere from 1 to 30 minutes and disappears slowly if the newborn is returned to the back or abdomen. This phenomenon occurs in both healthy and ill newborns and is of no pathologic significance.[7–9] It has been attributed to an immature autonomic vasomotor control.[9,11] This phenomenon can be observed in the first 3 weeks of life.

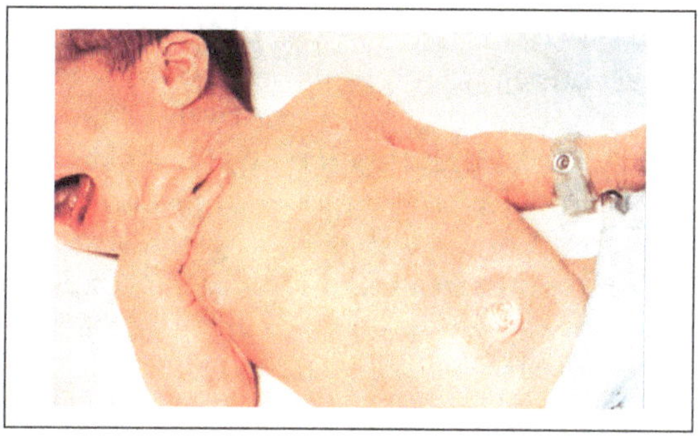

FIGURE 5.3 Erythema toxicum

Courtesy of Barbara Quissell, MD, Presbyterian/St. Luke's Medical Center, Denver, CO.

Common Newborn Skin Lesions

A benign rash, *erythema toxicum* is found in up to 70% of term newborns.[9] The rash consists of small white or yellow papules or vesicles with erythematous bases. It may be found on any part of the body, but it is most commonly seen on the face, trunk, and extremities (Figure 5.3). This rash often disappears and then reappears moments or hours later on a different part of the body. It may last anywhere from a few hours to several days. The peak incidence is from 24 to 48 hours of life, but it can continue to occur up to 3 months of age. The cause is unknown; however, it may be exacerbated by handling or chafing of linen. No treatment is necessary.[9]

Diagnosis is generally made by visual recognition of the eruption. A definitive diagnosis can be made by observation of the presence of numerous eosinophils in a smear of an aspirated papule.

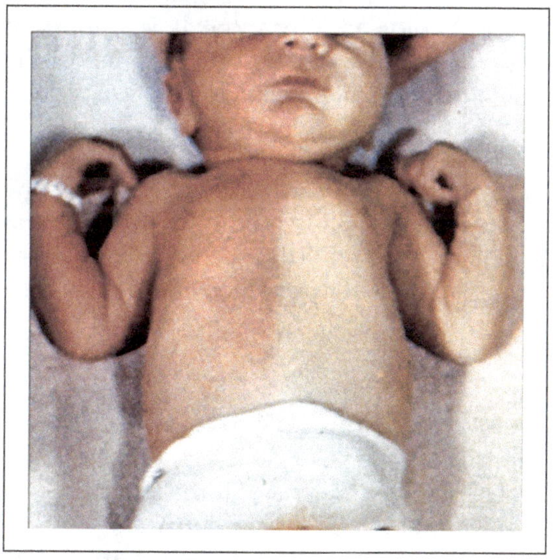

FIGURE 5.2 Harlequin color change

Source: From Solomon LM, and Esterly NB. 1973. *Neonatal Dermatology*. Philadelphia, PA: Saunders. Reprinted by permission.[10]

Milia

Milia are multiple yellow or pearly white papules about 1 mm in size (Figure 5.4). They are usually found on the brow, cheeks, and nose of up to 50% of newborns.[9] When found in the midline of the palate, they are called *Epstein pearls;* those found along the lingual and buccal parts of the dental ridges, away from the midline, are referred to as *Bohn nodules*. Milia are epidermal cysts caused by accumulation of sebaceous gland secretions. They resolve spontaneously during the first few weeks of life.

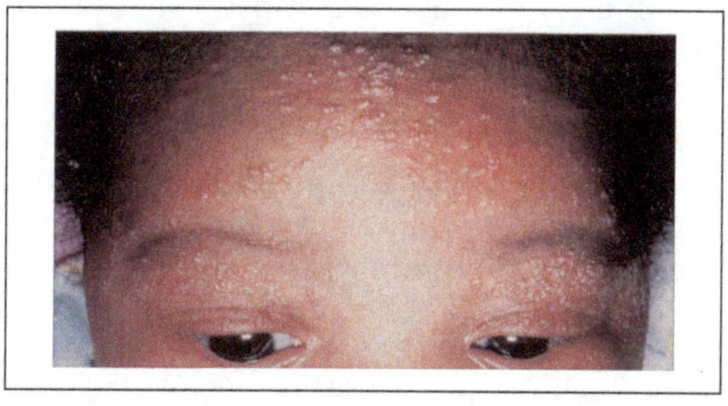

FIGURE 5.4 Milia

Source: From Cohen BA. 2013. *Pediatric Dermatology*, 4th ed. Philadelphia, PA: Saunders, 22. Reprinted by permission.[12]

Sebaceous Gland Hyperplasia

Sebaceous gland hyperplasia is characterized by numerous tiny (<0.5 mm) white or yellow papules found on the nose, cheeks, and upper lips. These enlarged sebaceous glands are caused by maternal androgenic stimulation and occur in approximately 50% of newborns.[9] They will spontaneously decrease in size after birth and require no treatment.

Miliaria (Heat Rash)

Miliaria is caused by obstruction of the sweat ducts as a result of an excessively warm, humid environment. This rash is seen primarily over the forehead, on the scalp, in skin creases on the neck or thighs, or in the groin area. Miliaria is classified as one of three types, depending on its severity.[9]

Miliaria crystallina consists of clear, thin vesicles, 1 to 2 mm in diameter, that develop in the epidermal portion of the sweat glands. The vesicles rupture about 24 to 48 hours after appearance, leaving a white scale.

Prolonged obstruction of the ducts of the sweat glands, leading to release of sweat into adjacent tissue, is termed *miliaria rubra* and is accompanied by a prickly sensation (prickly heat). Miliaria rubra appears as small erythematous papules about 2 to 4 mm in diameter. This rash is found most often in the neck, axilla, and groin areas, where sweat is likely to accumulate. Continued occlusion results in leukocyte infiltration of the papule. If the condition is not resolved, it can lead to a secondary staphylococcal infection of the deeper dermal portions of the sweat glands. This condition, termed *miliaria profunda*, is extremely rare and seen mostly in tropical locations.[7,9]

Treatment of miliaria consists of eliminating precipitating factors, such as excessive heat and humidity. Eliminating overheating and keeping the infant dry often cause the lesions to resolve within a few hours.

Sebaceous Nevus

Sebaceous nevus is a small yellow or yellowish-orange papule or plaque most often found on the scalp or face but may be seen on other parts of the body. It consists of immature hair follicles and sebaceous glands. The sebaceous nevus is devoid of hair when found on the scalp because of the rudimentary hair follicles found in the lesion. It may remain unchanged until puberty, when it enlarges and becomes thicker due to stimulation of the sebaceous glands found in the lesions. There is some risk for secondary tumors developing in these lesions, including basal cell or other neoplasms; therefore, surgical removal may be recommended.[8,9,12] Multiple sebaceous nevi may indicate epidermal nevus syndrome (Solomon syndrome), which can include skeletal, ocular, and cerebral anomalies.[7,9]

Common Pigmented Skin Lesions

Hyperpigmented Macule (Mongolian Spot)

The most common pigmented lesion in the newborn, the hyperpigmented macule is seen in up to 90% of African American, Asian, and Hispanic infants and up to 13% of Caucasian infants.[12] These large macules or patches are most commonly seen over the buttocks, flanks, or shoulders (Figure 5.5). They are gray or blue-green in color. Hyperpigmented macules may be mistaken for bruising because of their color and location. It is important to document the size and distribution of the lesion to avoid later suspicion of nonaccidental trauma.

Hyperpigmented macules are caused by melanocytes that infiltrate the dermis. The macules tend to fade gradually over the first 3 years of life and will become less apparent as the infant's skin darkens. Some may persist into adulthood.

Transient Neonatal Pustular Melanosis

Transient neonatal pustular melanosis begins with superficial, vesiculopustular lesions (Figure 5.6), often causing some alarm when present at birth. These vesicles rupture within 12 to 48 hours, leaving small, pigmented macules. The macules are often surrounded

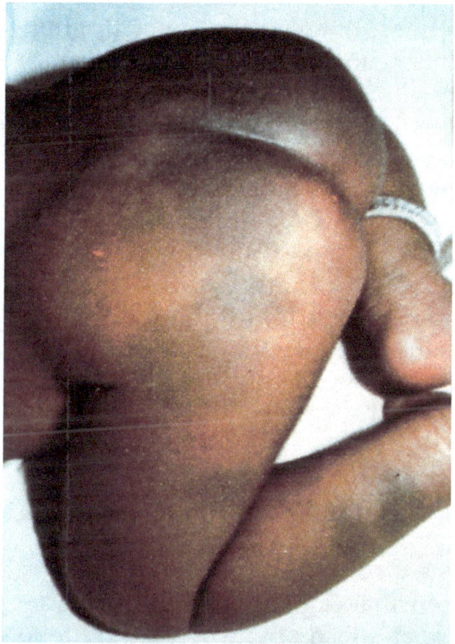

FIGURE 5.5 Hyperpigmented macule

Courtesy of Peter Honeyfield, MD, Presbyterian/St. Luke's Medical Center, Denver, CO.

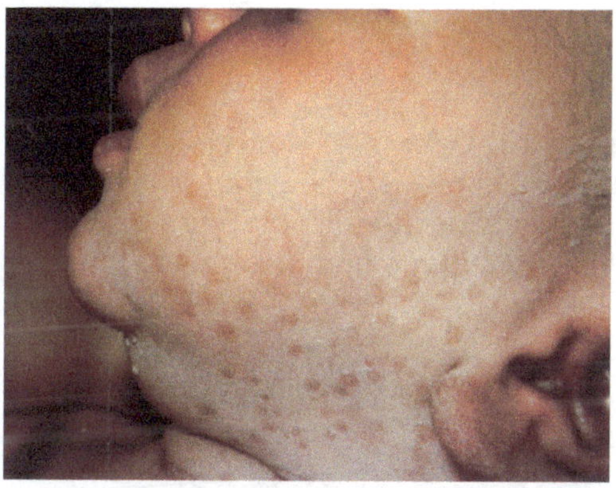

FIGURE 5.6 Multiple papules present in neonatal pustular melanosis

Source: From Clark DA. 2000. *Atlas of Neonatology*. Philadelphia, PA: Saunders, 261. Reprinted by permission.[13]

by a ring of very fine white scales. Any stage or combination of stages (vesicles, pustules, or scaling of ruptured vesicles) may be present at birth. These small hyperpigmented macules may remain for up to 3 months after birth. Transient neonatal pustular melanosis is benign, requiring no treatment. Aspiration of the vesicles reveals numerous neutrophils and almost no eosinophils. This skin lesion is found in up to 5% of African American infants and about .2% of Caucasian infants.[9,12]

Congenital Melanocytic Nevus (Pigmented Nevus)

A dark-brown or black macule, the congenital melanocytic nevus is caused by proliferation of melanocytes within the epithelial structures that sometimes extend into the subcutaneous fat. The pigmented nevus is most commonly seen on the lower back or buttocks but may occur anywhere on the body and is seen in all ethnicities.[10,13] The skin may be smooth over the lesion or may be nodular or irregular. Lesions range in size from less than 1 cm to more than 20 cm in diameter (Figure 5.7). Lesions may be with or without tufts of hair. Small- to moderate-sized lesions (<20 cm in diameter) are generally benign, but may pose a small risk for developing malignant melanoma and should be either excised or watched closely.[14–16] Two percent to 5% of larger lesions (>20 cm in diameter) can demonstrate malignant changes.[14–16] These larger lesions should be observed closely for changes in size or shape, and skin biopsies may be done.[14–16] Surgical excision may be considered depending on size and location of the nevus.[14–16]

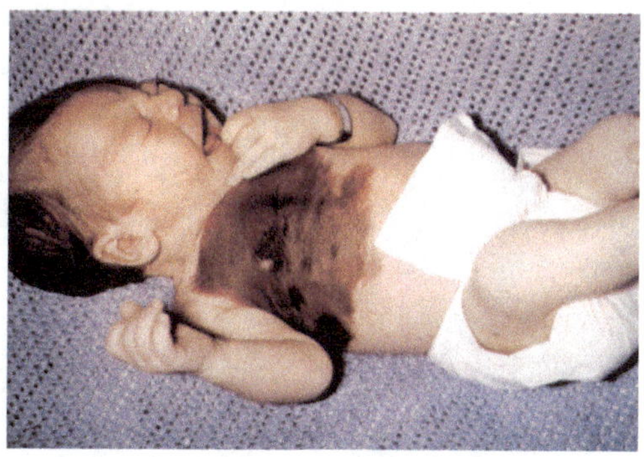

FIGURE 5.7 Congenital melanocytic nevi

Courtesy of Peter Honeyfield, MD, Presbyterian/St. Luke's Medical Center, Denver, CO.

Café au Lait Patch

A café au lait patch is a tan or light-brown, oval-shaped macule with a well-defined border (Figure 5.8). When less than 3 cm in length and less than 3 to 5 in number, they are of no pathologic significance. Up to 33% of normal children have one or more café au lait patches, with fair-skinned children often having multiple patches. The presence of six or more patches greater than 0.5 cm in length may indicate cutaneous neurofibromatosis, although they may occur in children without the disease.[1,7,17,18]

Neurofibromatosis (von Recklinghausen disease) is an autosomal dominant disorder in which tumors of various sizes form on peripheral nerves. Cranial nerves may also be affected. Ninety percent of patients with neurofibromatosis have café au lait patches.[7,17,18] Neurofibromas, small skin-colored nodules, may be present at birth or may not appear until adolescence in children with neurofibromatosis.

Tuberous Sclerosis

Tuberous sclerosis is a hereditary disorder characterized by cutaneous and central nervous system tumors resulting in seizures, developmental delays, and behavioral problems.[7,9] It presents with hypopigmented, white macules that may be thumb or leaf shaped. They are sometimes referred to as *ash leaf macules*. They may number up to 100 and are found anywhere on the newborn's skin, most often on the trunk and buttocks. Infants who present with unexplained seizures should be examined closely for these lesions. Most patients with tuberous sclerosis will have these macules at birth or soon afterward. Because of their light color, the lesions may not be readily apparent in fair-skinned infants. A Wood (ultraviolet) light may be helpful in illuminating white or hypopigmented lesions. Up to 5% of the population has one hypopigmented lesion.[13,21] If more than three are present, further evaluation is indicated.[9]

Skin Lesions Secondary to Trauma

Forcep Marks

Forcep marks may be seen on the cheeks, scalp, and face of newborns born following the use of forceps (Figure 5.9). The marks are generally red or bruised areas where the forceps were applied. The skin may also be abraded. The newborn should be examined for other complications of birth trauma, such as facial palsy, fractured clavicle, or skull fracture.

Subcutaneous Fat Necrosis

Subcutaneous fat necrosis consists of a subcutaneous nodule or nodules that are hard, nonpitting, and sharply circumscribed

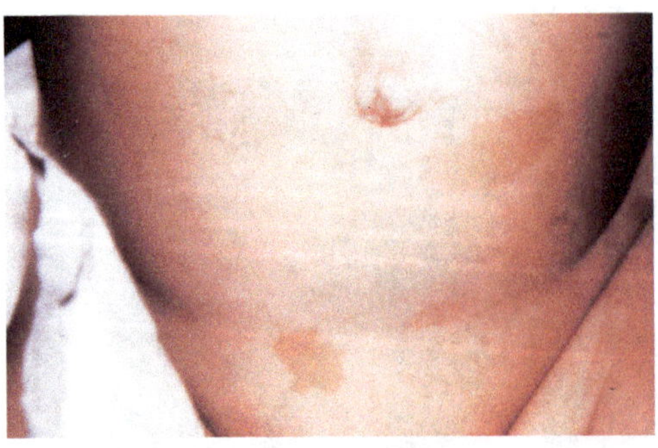

FIGURE 5.8 Café au lait patches

Courtesy of Eva Sujansky, MD, Associate Professor of Pediatrics, University of Colorado Health Sciences Center, Aurora, CO.

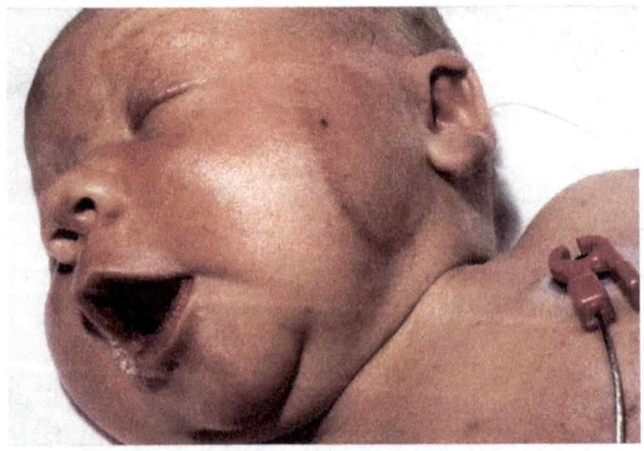

FIGURE 5.9 Forcep mark

Courtesy of Peter Honeyfield, MD, Presbyterian/St. Luke's Medical Center, Denver, CO.

(Figure 5.10). They may have a red or purplish color. They are more common in term newborns and are thought to be caused by trauma, cold, or asphyxia. It has been reported in some infants undergoing therapeutic hypothermia.[17,18] The nodules appear during the first weeks of life and are generally 1 to 2 cm in diameter. They may grow slightly larger over several days, and then resolve on their own over several weeks.[19,20] They may also be delayed or reoccur 2 to 3 weeks after resolution of the original nodule.[20] Occasionally, hypercalcemia may occur up to 6 months after presentation of the initial lesion. Serum calcium levels should be monitored, and intervention with fluids, calcium-wasting diuretics, and glucocorticoids may be necessary.[19,20]

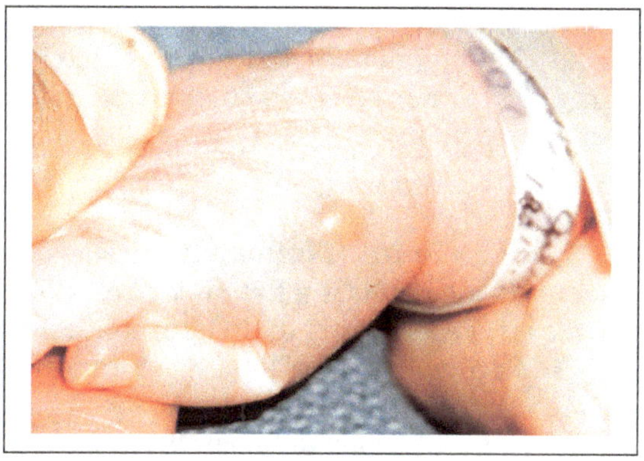

FIGURE 5.11 Sucking blister

Courtesy of Peter Honeyfield, MD, Presbyterian/St. Luke's Medical Center, Denver, CO.

Sucking Blister

A vesicle or bulla may appear on the lip, finger, or hand of a newborn as a result of vigorous sucking, either in utero or after birth. A sucking blister (Figure 5.11) may be intact or ruptured and requires no treatment.

Scalp Lesion

Scalp abrasions or lacerations may occur as a result of the insertion of a scalp electrode or trauma during delivery. Also, application of a suction cup for vacuum-assisted delivery may result in bruising or abrasions. Scalp pH measurements are used less often than in the past but may result in lacerations to the fetal scalp. Treatment of lacerations or abrasions consists of keeping the area clean and dry and observing for secondary infections. Facial bruising may also be significant following delivery.

Vascular Skin Lesions

Nevus Simplex

The *nevus simplex*, also called *salmon patch* or *stork bite*, is the most common of the vascular birthmarks. It is seen in over 40% of newborns.[9] Nevus simplex is an irregularly bordered pink macule composed of dilated, distended capillaries (Figure 5.12). The lesion is most often found on the nape of the neck, the upper eyelid, the bridge of the nose, or the upper lip. Nevi simplex blanch with pressure

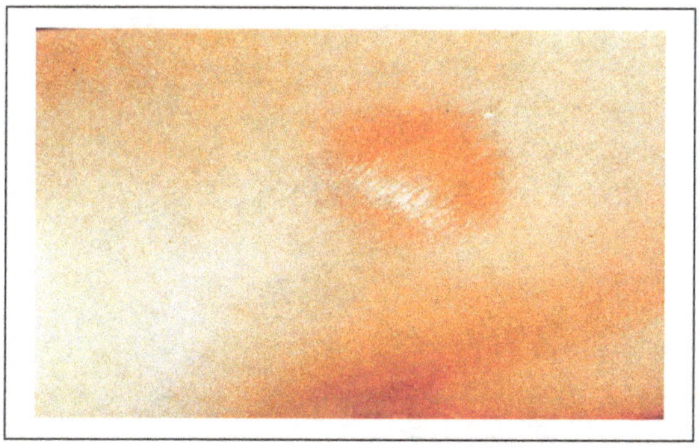

FIGURE 5.10 Subcutaneous fat necrosis

Courtesy of Barbara Quissell, MD, Presbyterian/St. Luke's Medical Center, Denver, CO. may persist.

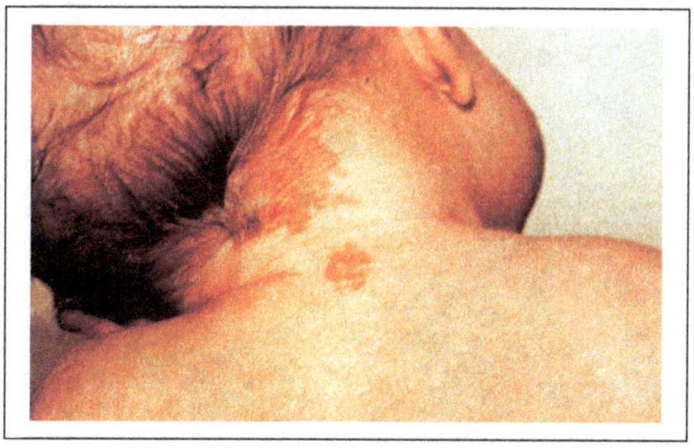

FIGURE 5.12 Nevus simplex

Courtesy of Barbara Quissell, MD, Presbyterian/St. Luke's Medical Center, Denver, CO.

and frequently become more prominent with crying. They generally fade by the second year of life, although those on the nape of the neck may persist.

Port Wine Nevus (Nevus Flammeus)

The port wine nevus is a flat pink or reddish-purple lesion consisting of dilated, congested capillaries directly beneath the epidermis. (In African American newborns, it is a jet-black color.) It has sharply delineated edges and does not blanch with pressure (Figure 5.13). The port wine nevus does not grow in size or spontaneously resolve. It may be small or may cover almost half of the body. It is usually unilateral but may occasionally cross the midline. Unfortunately, the lesion most often occurs on the face, but it may appear on other parts of the body.[9,21]

Temporary coverage can be obtained with the application of a water repellent cosmetic cream if desired. Flashlamp-pulsed dye laser therapy can be successful in eliminating or reducing port wine nevi. Pulsed dye laser works by photocoagulation and destruction of the blood vessels in the lesion without damaging surrounding healthy skin. The treatment is more effective in infants and young children because the lesion tends to become darker and thicker with time.[9,21] Despite reports of good results in the newborn period, up to 10% of port wine stains have been noted to recur 7 months to 15 years after treatment.[9,21]

Most port wine nevi are isolated, but those that follow a pattern similar to the branches of the trigeminal nerve (the forehead and upper eyelid) may be associated with Sturge–Weber syndrome. This disorder causes a proliferation of endothelial cells, particularly in the small blood vessels. Intracerebral calcifications and atrophic changes may be present.[9] Children with Sturge–Weber syndrome may present with seizures, developmental delays, hemiparesis, and glaucoma. The cause of this syndrome is unknown. It does not appear to be hereditary. An ophthalmologic examination is essential to monitor for glaucoma.

Infantile Hemangioma

Formerly called a *strawberry hemangioma*, the superficial infantile hemangioma is a bright red, raised, lobulated tumor that occurs on the head, neck, trunk, or extremities. It is soft and compressible, with sharply demarcated margins (Figure 5.14). The tumor may also occur in the throat (deep), causing airway obstruction.

Infantile hemangiomas are more common in Caucasian, female, and premature infants.[9,22] The lesion is caused by dilated capillaries, with associated endothelial proliferation in the dermal and subdermal layers. Most infantile hemangiomas have both superficial and deep components. It is not uncommon for an infant to have more than one of these lesions. The infantile hemangioma grows rapidly for approximately 6 months and then gradually begins to regress spontaneously. Complete regression

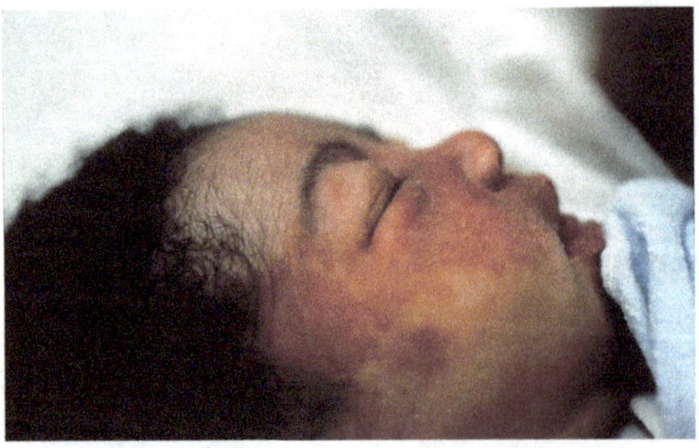

FIGURE 5.13 Port wine nevus

Source: From Clark DA. 2000. *Atlas of Neonatology*. Philadelphia, PA: Saunders, 267. Reprinted by permission.[13]

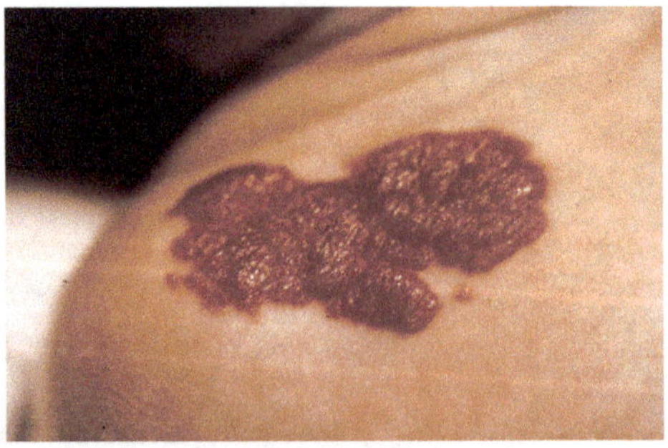

FIGURE 5.14 Infantile hemangioma

Source: From Clark DA. 2000. *Atlas of Neonatology*. Philadelphia, PA: Saunders, 265. Reprinted by permission.[13]

may take several years. Complications of infantile hemangioma include bleeding, ulceration, infection, or compression of vital organs or orifices. The preferred treatment is to allow natural spontaneous regression. If the lesion is interfering with vital functions (such as the airway or vision), treatment with systemic corticosteroids may be helpful. Propranolol has also been shown to successfully induce regression of infantile hemangiomas.[9,22,23] Pulsed dye lasers may reduce the extent of vascular proliferation and may increase healing in ulcerated hemangiomas or those likely to cause disfigurement.[9,22–24]

Deep Hemangioma

A deep hemangioma is similar to the infantile hemangioma, but consists of larger, more mature vascular elements lined with endothelial cells and involving the dermis and subcutaneous tissues. The overlying skin is bluish-red in color. On palpation, the deep hemangioma is soft and compressible, with poorly defined borders (Figure 5.15).

Like a superficial hemangioma, a deep hemangioma usually increases during the first 6 to 12 months of life and then involutes spontaneously. Treatment is unnecessary unless the lesion is interfering with vital functions. In those cases, treatment with propranolol or systemic corticosteroid therapy may be warranted.[9,23,24]

Two complications are related to vascular tumors. The first, Kasabach–Merritt phenomenon, is associated with sequestration of platelets, thrombocytopenia, and consumption of fibrinogen and coagulation factors. Mortality can be as high as 20% to 30%, usually resulting from infection, severe hemorrhage, or iatrogenic complications.[9] Treatment consists of supportive therapy, such as platelet transfusions and administration of corticosteroids. Angiogenesis inhibitors may restrain the growth of these tumors by inhibiting the growth of new blood vessels surrounding them.[23]

The second, Klippel–Trenaunay syndrome, consists of a vascular nevus with hypertrophy of the bone and soft structures of an extremity or other organs (Figure 5.16). The hypertrophy is probably the result of excess blood flow and malformed vessels.[9] This is a rare congenital anomaly, seen more frequently in males.[9] Prognosis depends on the severity of limb hypertrophy and other organ involvement.[9]

Infectious Lesions

Candida Oral Infection (Thrush)

A common infection in the newborn, thrush is an oral fungal infection caused by the organism *Candida albicans*. It appears as patches of white material scattered over the tongue and mucous membranes. The material is adherent and cannot be scraped off with a tongue depressor. Thrush is treated with an oral antifungal solution.[8,9]

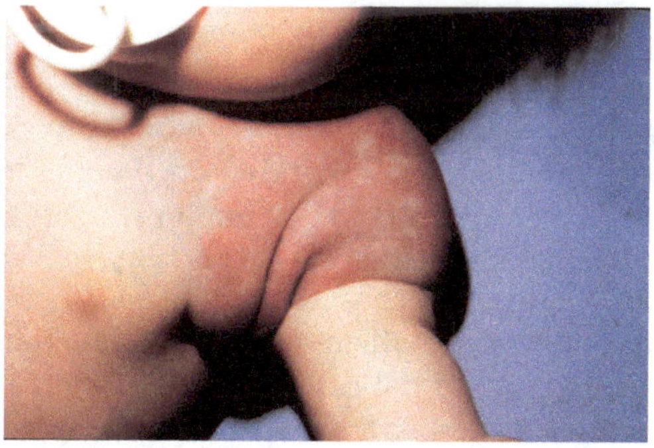

FIGURE 5.15 Deep hemangioma

Courtesy of Barbara Quissell, MD, Presbyterian/St. Luke's Medical Center, Denver, CO.

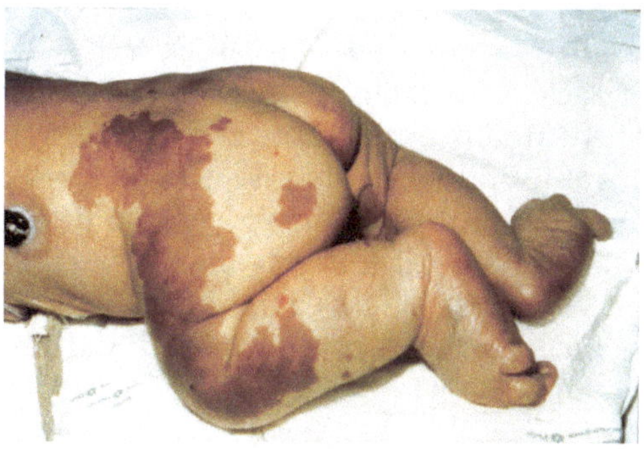

FIGURE 5.16 Klippel-Trenaunay-syndrome

Courtesy of Peter Honeyfield, MD, Presbyterian/St. Luke's Medical Center, Denver, CO.

Candida Diaper Dermatitis

Diaper dermatitis is common in newborns and generally needs no treatment other than frequent diaper changes and the diaper area kept clean and dry. Barrier ointments, such as petroleum or zinc oxide, help keep urine and feces away from the skin. Diaper dermatitis can be caused by *C. albicans*. This rash is a moist erythematous eruption with small white or yellow pustules. Small areas of skin erosion may also be seen. It is found primarily over the buttocks and perianal region, occasionally spreading to the thighs. Treatment consists of keeping the area clean and dry and applying an antifungal cream several times per day. If the rash is persistent or severe, an oral antifungal solution may be recommended to prevent reinfection resulting from Candida passing through the gastrointestinal tract.[25] Infants may present with both an oral Candida infection and Candida diaper dermatitis.

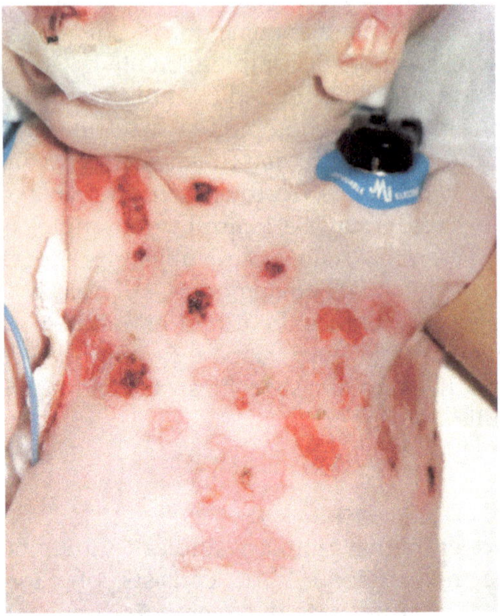

FIGURE 5.17 Blisters on trunk seen with neonatal herpes

Source: From Weston WL, Lane AT, and Morelli JG. 2007. *Color Textbook of Pediatric Dermatology*, 4th ed. Philadelphia, PA: Mosby, 130. Reprinted by permission.[30]

Herpes

Neonatal herpes is one of the most serious viral infections in the newborn, with a mortality rate of up to 40% in those newborns with disseminated disease.[26,27] Typically the infection appears as vesicles or pustules on an erythematous base (Figure 5.17). Clusters of lesions are common. The lesions ulcerate and crust over rapidly. Fifty percent to 70% of newborns with neonatal herpes eventually develop this characteristic rash, but not always before they exhibit other clinical signs.[26–28] Absence of vesicles does not rule out the presence of the disease.[26–28] However, if vesicles are seen, herpes should be suspected. Treatment includes use of an intravenous antiviral agent such as acyclovir. Topical ophthalmic antiviral therapy should be used if there is ocular involvement.[26–28] Other signs, such as seizures, should be treated as they occur. Precautions for blood and body secretions must be observed.[26–28]

Syphilis

Congenital syphilis is often asymptomatic at birth but can manifest as an erythematous maculopapular or bullous skin rash, mostly seen on the palms of the hands and the soles of the feet. The rash may spread to the extremities, trunk, and face (Figure 5.18). Rhinitis may accompany the rash and hepatosplenomegaly may be noted. Desquamation and crusting occurs as the lesions become copper colored.[26]

Staphylococcal Scalded Skin Syndrome

Staphylococcal scalded skin syndrome begins with a generalized, tender erythema, followed by bullous eruption and peeling of the epidermis, often in large sheets (Figure 5.19). The eruption is caused by a *Staphylococcus aureus* infection, which produces a toxin damaging to epidermal cell walls.[2,26,29] Treatment includes systemic antistaphylococcal antibiotics and isolation to prevent spread of the infection. There may be extensive insensible water loss, so fluids and electrolytes should be closely monitored.

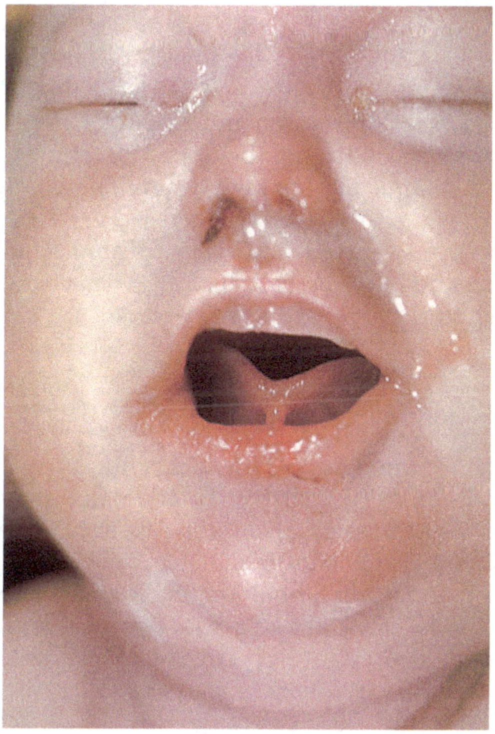

FIGURE 5.18 The face of a newborn infant displaying pathologic morphology indicative of congenital syphilis

Source: Centers for Disease Control and Prevention/Dr. Norman Cole.

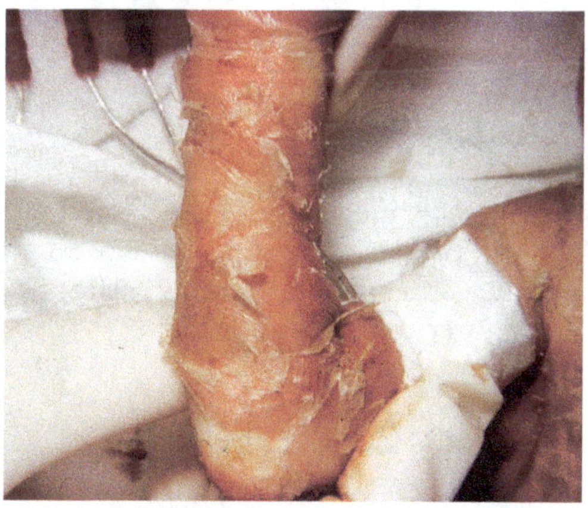

FIGURE 5.19 Scalded skin syndrome secondary to staphylococcal infection

Courtesy of Dr. David A. Clark, Albany Medical Center, Albany, NY, and Wyeth-Ayerst Laboratories. Philadelphia, PA. Reprinted by permission.

Neonatal Mastitis

Neonatal mastitis occurs most often in the first 2 months after birth. It is thought to be related to the physiologic breast hypertrophy resulting from maternal hormones.[31] *S. Aureus* is the most common cause, although other organisms such as Group B *Streptococcus* or gram-negative organisms may cause infection (Figure 5.20).

Neonatal mastitis is usually unilateral. It presents with swelling, erythema, induration, and tenderness. Fluctuation and nipple discharge may be seen if an abscess is present. Systemic signs of infection such as fever, irritability, and decreased feeding may be present.

Treatment includes a sepsis workup and intravenous antibiotics which cover staphylococcus. Consideration should be made for the possibility of methicillin resistant *S. Aureus*.

Other Dermatologic Congenital Viral Infections

Infections caused by cytomegalovirus, rubella virus, or enterovirus may present with

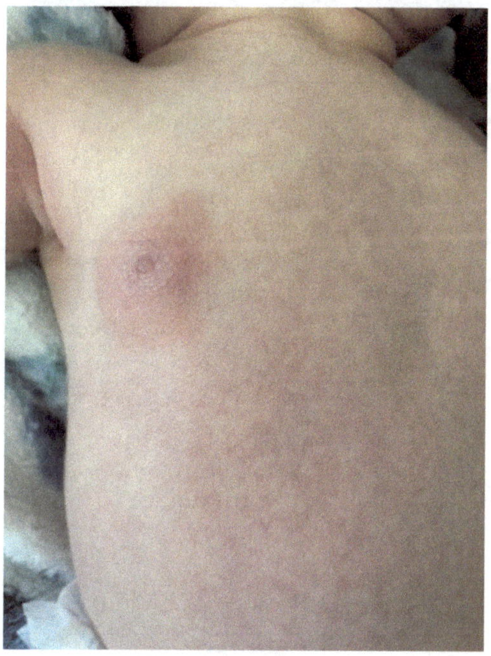

FIGURE 5.20 Neonatal mastitis

dermatologic findings. Most often, these consist of jaundice and petechiae or purpura seen on the head, trunk, and extremities. Often described as "blueberry muffin" spots, these lesions are caused by thrombocytopenia and dermal erythropoiesis. One associated finding is hepatosplenomegaly. Treatment depends on the specific viral agent present.[26]

Miscellaneous Skin Lesions

Aplasia cutis congenita (ACC) is a congenital abnormality characterized by the absence of some or all layers of the skin (Figures 5.21 and 5.22). It most often appears as an ulceration or scarred area on the scalp (on the parietal bones or near the sagittal suture), but it can occur on other parts of the body.

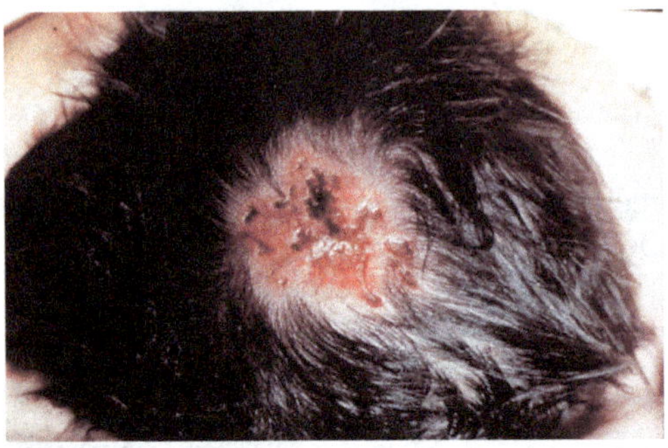

FIGURE 5.21 Aplasia cutis congenita

Courtesy of Peter Honeyfield, MD, Presbyterian/St. Luke's Medical Center, Denver, CO.

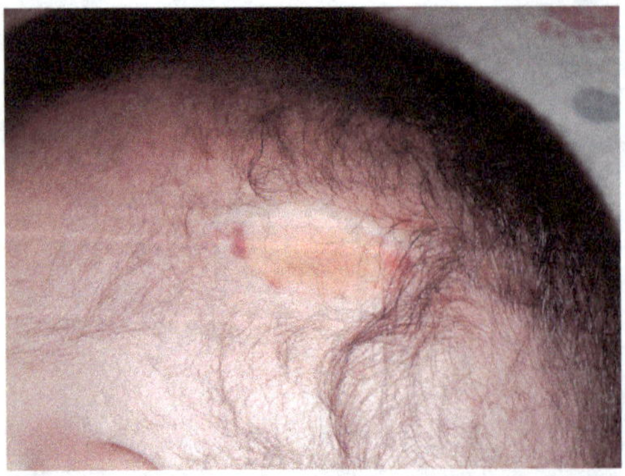

FIGURE 5.22 Aplasia cutis congenita

Courtesy of Mary Ellen Honeyfield, DNP, NNP, Sedalia, CO.

ACC may be an isolated defect, or it can be associated with other anomalies, such as midline defects and chromosomal disorders (trisomy 13).[6] The cause is unclear, but ACC may result from vascular disruptions, midline developmental disruptions, trauma, or uterine or amnionic abnormalities (amniotic disruption sequence). Treatment consists of keeping the area clean and dry. The use of antibacterial dressings may be helpful. Large defects may require surgery (see also Chapter 6).

INSPECTING THE NAILS

The examination of the skin is not complete without close attention to the nails on the hands and feet. The nail consists of hard keratin. Damage to the nail matrix can be caused by trauma, inflammation, or genetic abnormalities. This damage can appear as pits, ridges, aplasia, or hypertrophy.[6] Most defects in the neonatal period are congenital rather than traumatic in origin.

Absence or Atrophy of Nails

Absence or atrophy of nails is seen in several congenital syndromes, including trisomy 13, trisomy 18, and Turner syndrome.[6] Inherited ectodermal dysplasias and skeletal anomalies may also be seen with absent or dystrophic nails.[6]

Hypertrophy of Nails

Hypertrophic nails are rarely seen in the newborn period. They may occur in diseases such as congenital hemihypertrophy or familial onychogryposis.

Abnormally Shaped Nails

Spoon- or racquet-shaped nails may occur as a result of a congenital or hereditary anomaly. They may be associated with anomalies of the hair or skin. Spoon-shaped nails may also be a temporary finding in an otherwise healthy newborn.[6]

SUMMARY

Careful assessment of the skin gives the examiner insight into the overall health of the newborn as well as any underlying pathology. Although numerous other anomalies may occur in newborn skin, the most common variations presented here should aid the healthcare professional in performing a complete and thorough newborn skin examination.

ADDITIONAL RESOURCES

SPRINGER PUBLISHING CONNECT™

A robust set of resources designed to supplement this text is located at http://connect.springerpub.com/content/book/978-0-8261-4063-0. Qualifying instructors may request access by emailing textbook@springerpub.com.

REFERENCES

1. Association of Women's Health, Obstetric, and Neonatal Nurses. 2018. *Neonatal Skin Care, Evidence Based Practice Guideline*, 4th ed. Washington, DC: Association of Women's Health, Obstetric, and Neonatal Nurses, 4–6.
2. Narendran V. 2020. The skin of the neonate. In *Neonatal–Perinatal Medicine, Diseases of the Fetus and Infant*, 11th ed. Martin RJ, Fanaroff AA, and Walsh MC, eds. Philadelphia, PA: Elsevier, 1898–1932.
3. Nasemann T, Sauerbrey W, and Burgdorf W. 1983. *Fundamentals of Dermatology*. New York: Springer-Verlag, 11.
4. Diehl-Jones W, and Askin DF. 2021. Hematologic disorders. In *Core Curriculum for Neonatal Intensive Care Nursing*, 6th ed. Verklan MT, and Walden M, eds. Philadelphia, PA: Elsevier, 568–587.
5. Jones KL, Jones MC, and del Campo M. 2021. *Smith's Recognizable Patterns of Human Malformation*, 8th ed. Philadelphia, PA: Saunders, 1–70.
6. Jones KL, Jones MC, and del Campo M. 2021. *Smith's Recognizable Patterns of Human Malformation*, 8th ed. Philadelphia, PA: Saunders, 100–105.
7. Mancini AJ, and Krowchuk DP. 2021. *Pediatric Dermatology: A Quick Reference Guide*, 4th ed. Itasca, IL: American Academy of Pediatrics.
8. Habeshian KA, Choi HY, and Silverman RA. 2021. Dermatologic conditions. In *Avery and McDonalds's Neonatology: Pathophysiology and Management of the Newborn*, 8th ed. Boardman J, Groves A, and Ramasethu J, eds. Philadelphia, PA: Wolters Kluwer, 930–958.
9. Paller AS, and Mancini AJ. 2021. Cutaneous disorders of the newborn. In *Hurwitz Clinical Pediatric Dermatology: A Textbook of Skin Disorders of Childhood and Adolescence*, 6th ed. Paller AS and Mancini AJ, eds. Philadelphia, PA: Saunders, 11–37.
10. Solomon LM, and Easerly NB. 1973. *Neonatal Dermatology*. Philadelphia, PA: Elsevier.
11. Cohen BA. 2013. *Pediatric Dermatology*, 4th ed. Philadelphia, PA: Elsevier.
12. Kane KS, Nambudiri VE, and Stratigos AG. 2017. *Color Atlas and Synopsis of Pediatric Dermatology*, 3rd ed. New York, NY: McGraw Hill, 148–184.
13. Clark DA. 2000. *Atlas of Neonatology*. Philadelphia: Elsevier, 261, 265, 267.
14. Benjamin LT. 2013. Birthmarks of medical significance in the neonate. *Seminars in Perinatology* 37(1): 16–19.
15. Keim-Malpass J. 2021. Congenital melanocytic nevus: Considerations for neonatal clinicians and a parent perspective. *Neonatal Network* 40(1): 40–44.
16. Soong LC, Bencivengo A, and Fiorillo L. 2022. Neonatal curettage of large to giant congenital melanocytic nevi under local anesthetic: A case study with long-term follow-up. *Journal of Cutaneous Medicine and Surgery* 26(2): 149–155.
17. Simons EA, Huang JT, and Schimidt B. 2017. Congenital melanocytic nevi in young children: Histopathologic features and clinical outcomes. *Journal of the American Academy of Dermatology* 76(5): 941–947.
18. St. John S, Summe H, Csikesz C, Wiss K, Hay B, and Belazarian L. 2016. Multiple café au lait spots in a group of fair-skinned children without signs or symptoms of neurofibromatosis type 1. *Pediatric Dermatology* 33(5): 526–529.
19. Restrepo R, Inarejos-Clemente EJ, Corral G, Mas TA, Fenlon EP, and Jarmillo D. 2022. Subcutaneous fat necrosis of the newborn: A pictoral essay of an under-recognized entity. *Pediatric Radiology* 53(2): 313–323. doi: 10.1007/500247-05509-1
20. Rodd C, Schwieger-Briel A, and Hagmann C. 2021. Subcutaneous fat necrosis associated with hypercalcemia in neonates with neonatal encephalopathy treated with therapeutic hypothermia. *Seminars in Fetal and Neonatal Medicine* 26(4): 101269. doi: 10.1016/j.siny.2021.101269
21. Lederhandler MH, Pomerantz H, Orbuch D, and Geronemus MD. 2022. Treating pediatric port wine stains in aesthetics. *Clinics in Dermatology* 40(1): 11–18.
22. Darrow DH, Greene AK, Mancini AJ, and Nopper AJ. 2015. Diagnosis and management of infantile hemangioma. *Pediatrics* 136(4): e1060–e1104.
23. Ishikawa T, Seki K, and Uchiyama H. 2022. Efficacy of intravenous propranolol for life-threatening diffuse neonatal hemangiomatosis. *Pediatric Dermatology* 39: 613–615.

24. Miller AC, Gordon ES, Peterson CR, Cohen DJ, and Bowe AC. 2022. Benign neonatal hemangiomatosis. *Advances in Neonatal Care* 22(5): 408–412.
25. Cohen B. 2017. Differential diagnosis of diaper dermatitis. *Clinical Pediatrics* 56(55): 16S–22S.
26. Poinninti SG, and Kimberlin DW. 2021. Congenital infections. In *Avery and McDonald Neonatology: Pathophysiology and Management of the Newborn*, 8th ed. Boardman JP, Groves AM, and Ramasethu J, eds. Philadelphia, PA: Lippincott Williams & Wilkins, 748–766.
27. McPherson CC. 2020. Neonatal herpes simplex virus: The long road to improved outcomes. *Neonatal Network* 39(2): 92–98.
28. Rudd KM. 2021. Infectious diseases in the neonate. In *Core Curriculum for Neonatal Intensive Care Nursing*, 6th ed. Verklan MT, and Walden M, eds. Philadelphia PA: Elsevier, 588–616.
29. McKeown EK, and Baker RB. 2022. Staphylococcal scalded skin syndrome, identification and wound care. *Advances in Neonatal Care* 22(4): 325–332.
30. Weston WL, Lane AT, and Morelli JG. 2007. *Color Textbook of Pediatric Dermatology*, 4th ed. Philadelphia, PA: Mosby, 130.
31. Kaplan RL, Cruz AT, et al. 2021. Neonatal mastitis and concurrent serious bacterial infection. *Pediatrics* 148(1): e2021051322. doi: 10.1542peds.2021-051322

6 HEAD, EYES, EARS, NOSE, MOUTH, AND NECK ASSESSMENT

Patricia J. Johnson

Examination of the infant's head and neck requires visual inspection, obtaining measurements, palpation, use of an ophthalmoscope, brief auscultation, and, in rare cases, transillumination. After initial close observation, the examination should proceed from the top of the head down to the neck. Attention should be given to the infant's state, to facilitate optimal assessment with minimal discomfort. Portions of the examination may need to be postponed until the infant is in a more relaxed state. It is best to examine the eyes when the infant is in a quiet state and examine the oropharynx when the infant is crying.

Initial observations should include the infant's state; color of the skin and mucous membranes; size and symmetry of the head and face; and obvious deformations, malformations, or evidence of birth trauma. Minor anomalies of the head and neck are common. The initial inspection will provide important clues to possible congenital abnormalities as well as evidence of birth trauma and will often reveal important race-specific variations.

CRANIUM

Head Shape

The shape of the infant's head usually relates to molding of the skull during pregnancy, labor, and/or delivery (Figure 6.1). An infant delivered by cesarean section will usually have a well-rounded head. The breech position may cause the head to be molded posteriorly into an egg shape, with a prominent occiput. Prolonged diagonal pressure may cause the head to appear "out of round," or asynclitic, when viewed from above. Distortion of the skull due to positional, external pressures in utero or during labor can be expected to self-correct. Parents can be reassured that molding usually resolves within a few days to a few weeks after birth.[1–3]

Skull

Inspection and careful palpation of the infant's skull are necessary to identify bones, sutures (fibrous joints), and fontanels (Figure 6.2). Sutures separate bones, and fontanels occur where two or more sutures meet. The metopic suture extends midline down the forehead between the two frontal bones and intersects with the coronal suture, which separates the frontal and parietal bones. The anterior fontanel (AF) is formed at the intersection of the metopic, coronal, and sagittal sutures. The size of the AF varies from 0.6 to 3.6 cm across, and in Black infants, it is commonly larger—from 1.4 to 4.7 cm.[4] Fontanels are measured diagonally from bone to bone rather than from suture to suture (Figure 6.3). Because there is a wide variation in fontanel size at birth, the measurement may serve only as a baseline for serial comparison. Individual measurements are not useful as a single examination finding, have no clinical significance, and have limited reproducibility. The AF is normally described as flat and soft if assessed with the infant in a quiet state and held in the sitting position. A tense or bulging fontanel may be a sign of increased intracranial pressure or may occur when the infant is crying (Figure 6.4).[5,6]

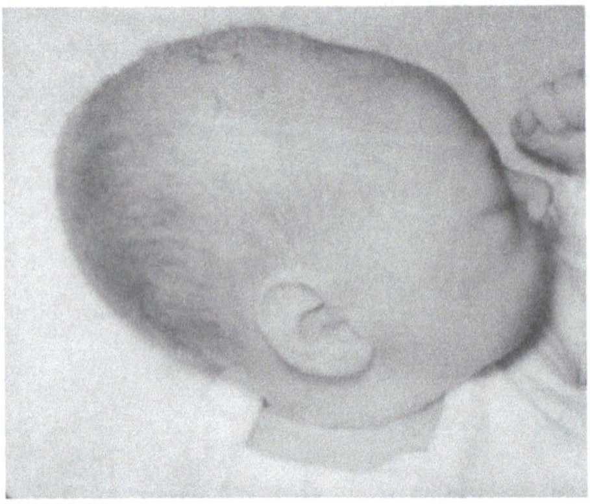

FIGURE 6.1 Head molding in the newborn infant

Courtesy of Dr. David A. Clark, Albany Medical Center, Albany, NY.

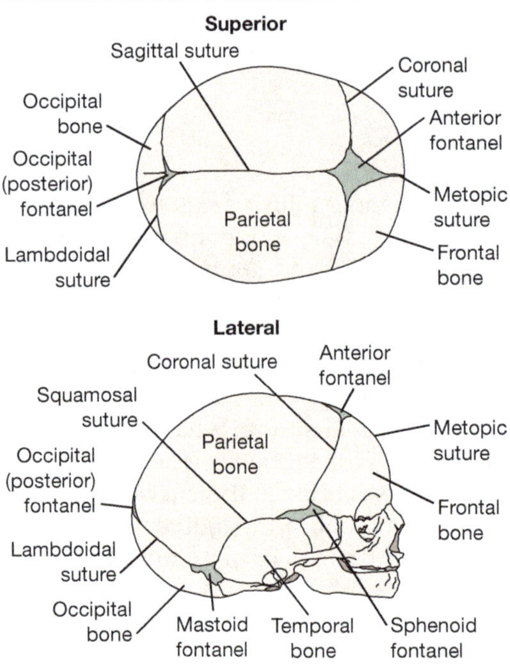

FIGURE 6.2 Sutures, fontanels, and bones of the neonatal skull

Source: Adapted from Scanlon JW, Nelson J, Grylack LJ, and Smith YF. 1979. *A System of Newborn Physical Examination*. Baltimore, MD: University Park Press, 47.[1]

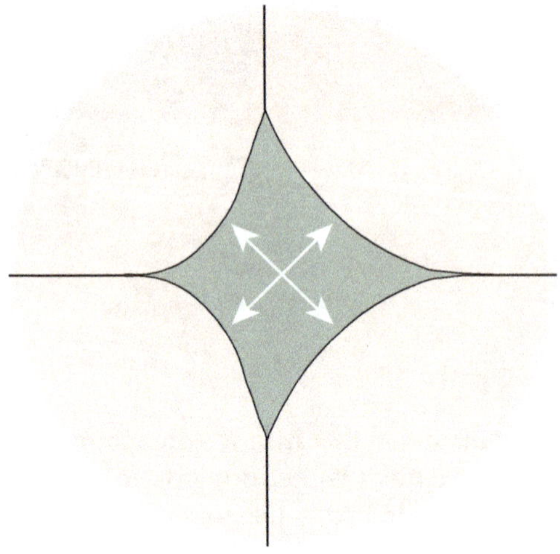

FIGURE 6.3 Measurement of the anterior fontanel: Bone to bone

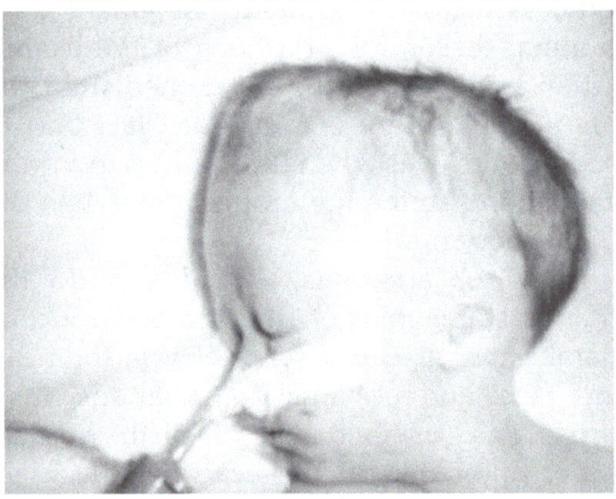

FIGURE 6.4 Bulging anterior fontanel

Courtesy of Dr. David A. Clark, Albany Medical Center, Albany, NY, and Wyeth-Ayerst Laboratories, Philadelphia, PA. Reprinted by permission.

If the examiner is uncertain whether the fontanel is flat or bulging, it should be palpated with the infant in an upright, sitting position. A sunken fontanel is a sign of severe dehydration and is rarely seen in the newborn nursery. However, it may indicate excessive or acute decompression in an infant with a newly inserted external ventricular reservoir, drain, or ventricular peritoneal (VP) shunt for treatment of hydrocephalus. A very large AF can be associated with hypothyroidism.[7] The AF normally closes by 6 to 24 months of age.[1,3]

Auscultation over the fontanels and lateral skull bones is performed during examination of the head and neck. Auscultation of the fontanels is specifically indicated in infants with multiple hemangiomas or heart failure.[4] In the otherwise normal infant, auscultation of a bruit (murmur-like sound) over the fontanels or the lateral skull can be a normal finding. Evidence of a bruit over the fontanel in an infant with suspected cardiac failure is associated with an intracranial arteriovenous malformation, which may be the cause of the congestive heart failure.[1,4,8]

The sagittal suture extends midline between the two parietal bones to the posterior fontanel (PF). This fontanel is formed where the sagittal suture meets the lambdoidal suture, which extends posterolaterally to separate the occipital from the parietal bones. The PF is usually small, 0.5 cm in diameter in Caucasian newborns and 0.7 cm in African American newborns and closes by approximately 2 to 3 months of age.[1,3,4] If palpable, the PF should be soft and flat. A third "fontanel" may occur along the sagittal suture between the AF and PF. This is really a defect of the parietal bone and not a true fontanel. It can be a normal variant or associated with Down syndrome or congenital hypothyroidism.[4,9]

The squamosal suture extends above the ear to separate the temporal bone from the parietal bone. This suture and the sphenoid and mastoid fontanels are usually apparent only when there is increased intracranial pressure, as with severe hydrocephalus, but may be palpable in the premature infant with rapid brain growth.[1]

Mobility of sutures is assessed by placing the thumbs on the bones on either side of the suture and gently pressing down alternately with one thumb and then the other. Normal sutures can be described as approximated and mobile. Sutures may be split (separated) up to 1 cm. More widely split sutures may indicate increased intracranial pressure and require further investigation. With molding, the edge of the bone on one side of the suture will feel as if it is on top of the edge of the opposing bone; these sutures are described as overriding (Figure 6.5). It is common for the lambdoidal sutures to be overriding, with the parietal bone on top of the occipital due to molding after birth or with a minor decrease in hydration.

It is important to differentiate an overriding suture from one that feels ridged and immobile. The suture that peaks and is immobile implies premature fusion of the suture, or craniosynostosis.[1,10] Premature closure of a suture stops bone growth perpendicular to the suture but allows continued parallel growth and compensatory expansion at the functional sutures, leading to abnormal head shape. Abnormal head shape resulting from craniosynostosis may be noted at birth, or the premature fusion may not be suspected until later in infancy (Figure 6.6).[11] Fused coronal sutures limit forward growth of the skull and lead to a broad skull (brachycephaly). Early closure of the sagittal suture limits lateral growth and results in a long, narrow head (scaphocephaly). Plagiocephaly is an asymmetric skull resulting from closure of the sutures on one side. The premature infant's head may develop the shape termed *dolichocephaly*, which is flattened side to side without craniosynostosis. Viewing the head from above may facilitate assessment of skull shape. Craniosynostosis may be primary (isolated), associated with a genetic syndrome, such as Apert or Crouzon, or the result of a metabolic disorder such as hyperthyroidism.[10,12,13] The incidence of isolated craniosynostosis in the United States is reported to be 0.4 to 1/1,000 live births.[10,13]

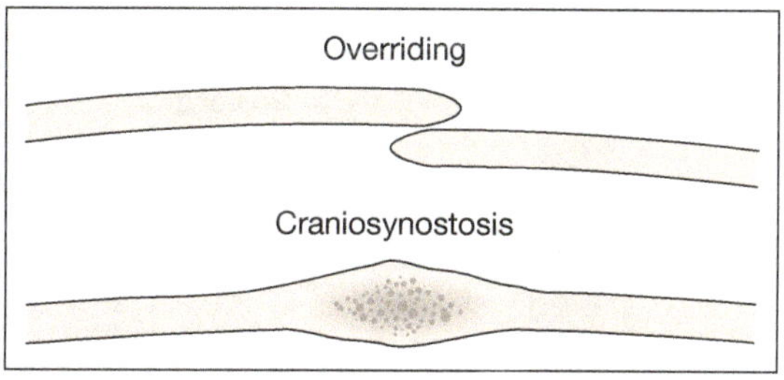

FIGURE 6.5 Cross-section of sutures

Palpation of the skull may reveal areas of soft or thinning bone, called *craniotabes.* Pressing on the bone elicits collapse with recoil of the underlying bone and a snapping sensation similar to pressing on a ping-pong ball. Craniotabes, an incidental finding evident upon palpation of parietal bones near the sagittal suture, is most often due to external pressure from prolonged vertex engagement or pressure of the fetal head on the uterine fundus with breech position. It is also seen in up to 30% of normal newborns, especially in premature newborns, and is associated with pathologic conditions, including rickets, osteogenesis imperfecta, congenital syphilis, and

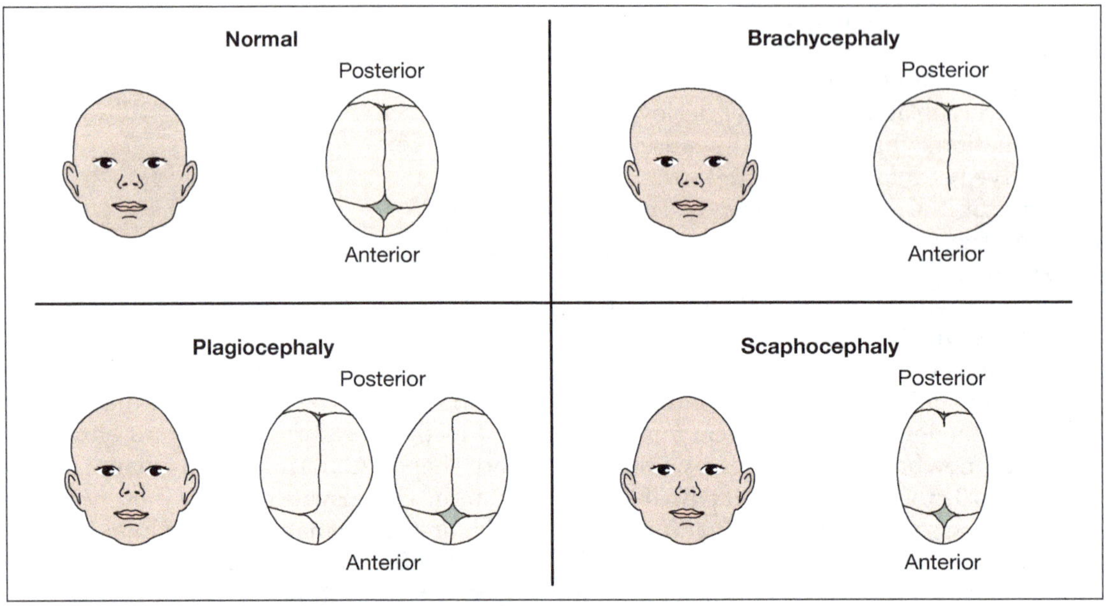

FIGURE 6.6 Normal skull and shapes that result from craniosynostosis

Source: From Disabato J, and Wulf J. 1989. Nursing strategies: Altered neurologic function. In *Family-Centered Nursing Care of Children*, Foster RL, Hunsberger MM, and Tackett JJ, eds. Philadelphia, PA: Saunders, 1731. Reprinted by permission.[11]

vitamin D deficiency.[14,15] Craniotabes may also be caused by internal pressure on the fetal head from hydrocephalus. When due to external pressures and not a metabolic or underlying disease process, craniotabes can be expected to resolve in a few weeks. If caused by hydrocephalus, resolution will depend on the degree and persistence of internal pressure causing the characteristic bone thinning.[1,3]

While palpating the skull, the examiner also inspects the scalp and head for evidence of birth trauma and other abnormalities. The most common form of trauma to the head is caput succedaneum (caput). This is edema of the presenting part of the scalp caused by pressure that restricts the return of venous and lymph flow during labor and delivery. It can be accentuated by vacuum-assisted delivery. The edema pits on pressure, usually crosses suture lines, and has poorly defined edges. Caput is noted immediately after birth and resolves within a few days, which can help differentiate it from a cephalohematoma (Figure 6.7).[1–3]

A cephalohematoma results from the collection of blood between the periosteum and the skull (Figure 6.8). It may not be evident at birth because of an associated caput. A cephalohematoma has clearly demarcated edges confined by suture lines. With time, it may liquefy and become fluctuant on palpation; it may take weeks or months to resolve completely. The most common locations for a cephalohematoma are the parietal and occipital bones. Associated depressed skull fractures are very rare.[1–3,11]

A subgaleal hemorrhage is the third and potentially most serious lesion resulting from birth trauma. It is most commonly associated with instrumented vaginal delivery, especially vacuum-assisted delivery. However, it has been reported with cesarean births or any maneuver during delivery that produces a shearing force to the scalp resulting in tearing of the large emissary veins. With a subgaleal hemorrhage, there is bleeding into the galea aponeurotica or subaponeurotic space, which extends from the orbital ridges to the nape of the neck and laterally to the ears (Figure 6.9). This potential space produces a large compartment capable of containing the total blood volume of an infant, and therefore a subgaleal hemorrhage has a 5% to 22% mortality rate if blood loss is extensive and undiagnosed.[16] It presents

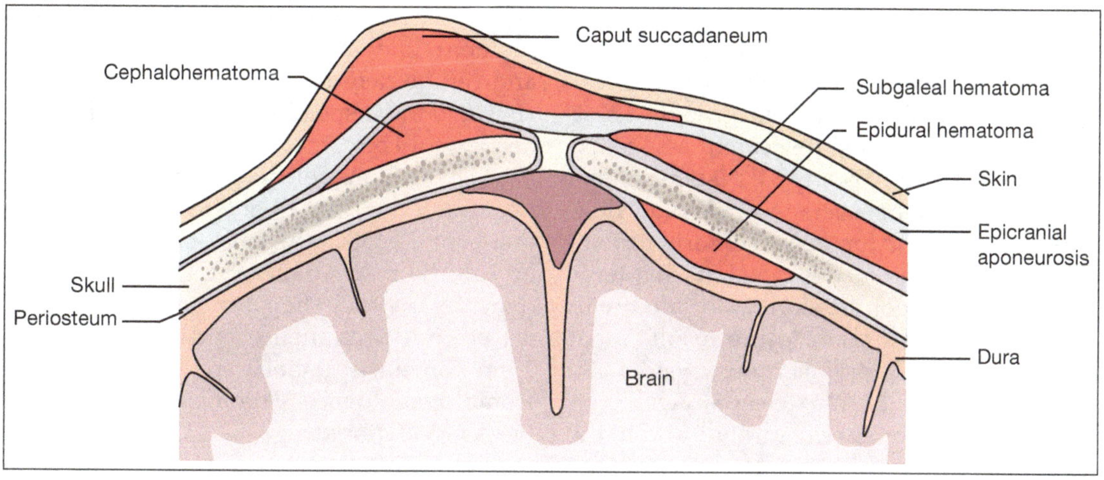

FIGURE 6.7 Areas of birth trauma

with generalized scalp edema, usually with ecchymosis, and often with bilateral or unilateral periorbital and periauricular edema. The ballotable fluid mass crosses the sutures and can be manually repositioned from the eyebrows to the nape of the neck, differentiating it from a large caput. If progressive, it can result in severe anemia, hypotension, and death unless diagnosed early. Effective treatment may involve volume resuscitation, blood replacement, and treatment of presenting clotting abnormalities.

Trauma to the scalp may include puncture from a scalp electrode; lacerations from fetal blood sampling or uterine incision; and bruises, abrasions, or subcutaneous fat necrosis from an instrument (forceps or vacuum) delivery.[2,5,17] The lesion should be described by its appearance, size, and location near sutures, fontanelles, or underlying bones.

Aplasia cutis congenita (see Figure 5.22) is an uncommon scalp lesion usually found on the parietal bones or near the juncture of the sagittal and lambdoidal sutures. This lesion is a hairless, circumscribed area of 1 cm or more, and its surface is often shiny, cicatricial, and flat or keloid in appearance. Occasional blistering or ulceration is evident

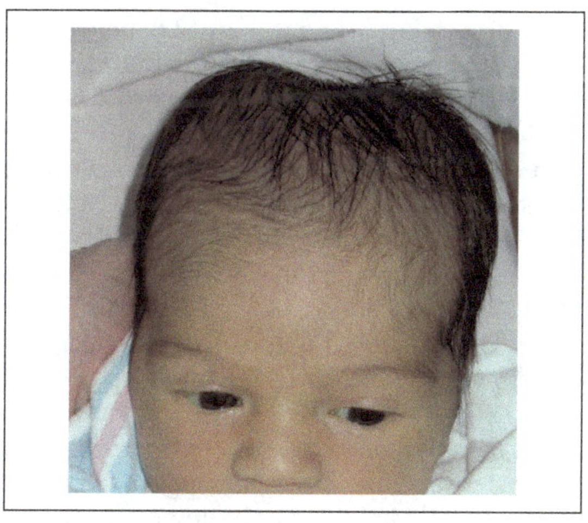

FIGURE 6.8 Bilateral cephalohematoma

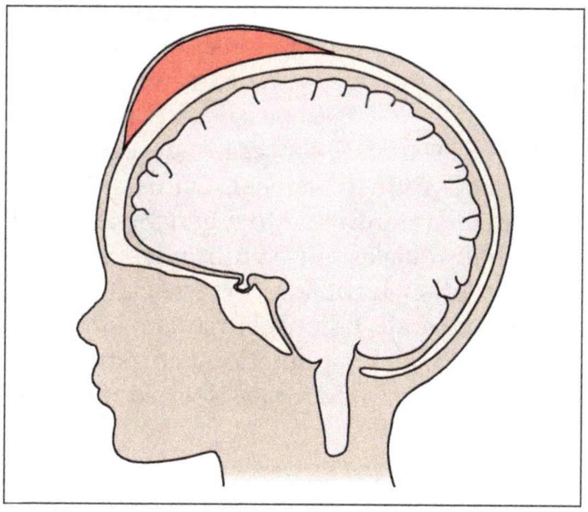

FIGURE 6.9 Subgaleal hemorrhage, sagittal vie

with serosanguineous exudate or fresh granulation. In most infants, the defect is an isolated finding that resolves with residual scar formation and absence of hair growth. There is a risk for underlying defect and associated major defects (e.g., trisomy 13) in some infants with this lesion, necessitating careful evaluation of the infant for major abnormalities.[18] Other skin lesions are described in Chapter 5.

Malformation of the skull associated with incomplete neural tube closure results in an encephalocele. Central nervous system tissue can protrude from a defect anywhere on the skull, most commonly midline and in the occipital area.[12]

Scalp Hair

Examination of the scalp should include assessment of the hair for quantity, texture, distribution, and hair whorls. Low hairline, increased quantity of hair, and brittleness may be associated with congenital anomalies. The slope of each hair follicle appears to be associated with the stretch of the skin during periods of rapid brain growth, particularly from weeks 10 to 16 of gestation.[7,19] One or two hair whorls can be normal. An abnormally placed whorl, absence of hair whorl, or unusual hair growth may be associated with aberrant brain growth and mental retardation.[7] Hair consistency, color, and growth patterns commonly reflect developmental, familial, and racial variations with no clinical significance.[19] Unusual hair growth patterns or presentation should be carefully described.

Alopecia is an abnormal deficiency of hair that is diffuse or focal. Diffuse alopecia is more commonly due to a genetic anomaly in the hair follicles or is syndromic. Focal alopecia is often traumatic or associated with underlying scalp lesions. Hirsutism, or excess hair growth, may be genetic, syndromic, metabolic, drug-induced, or an isolated finding.

Head Size

Measurement of the occipital–frontal circumference (OFC) is fundamental for adequate assessment of head size. Taking this measurement may be unsettling for the infant and can be deferred to the end of the exam. As such, the inspection and palpation of the head would be completed prior to measuring the OFC. A nonstretchable paper tape measure should be used to obtain three measurements of the OFC; the largest of these should be recorded. Accuracy of this measurement depends on encircling the head at the widest occiput prominence and anteriorly 1 to 2 cm above the glabella space at the largest frontal prominence. The average OFC at 40 weeks gestational age is 35 cm. The OFC ranges from 33 to 37 cm between the 10th and 90th percentile.[20] Before closure of the fontanels, the measurement of the OFC is an indirect measure of intracranial contents, including the brain, cerebrospinal fluid, cerebral blood volume, and bone.[21] The OFC is often misleading immediately after birth due to cranial molding, scalp edema, or hemorrhage under the periosteum. Subsequent measurement(s) should be obtained several days after birth once the initial distortions resulting from the birth process resolve. The OFC should be plotted on a standard growth chart and the gestation-specific percentile in which the measurement falls noted. The percentile of the OFC, along with those for weight and length for gestational age, are necessary to diagnose symmetric versus asymmetric growth restriction and micro- or macrocephaly.[1,22]

Microcephaly is defined as an OFC less than 2 standard deviations (SD) below the mean for gestational age or less than the 3rd percentile.[20] Microcephaly is usually associated with microencephaly and is caused by reduced brain growth.[20,21] With microcephaly, the sutures often become prematurely fused because the expansive force of brain growth that enlarges the cranial vault is lacking. Microcephaly can be an isolated finding, or it may be associated with a genetic syndrome or congenital infection.[1,12,21] As with the other growth parameters, OFC in the infant born prematurely tends to be lower than expected for gestational age. Discrepancies may be due to inaccurate dating or to biologic differences and/or maternal or neonatal pathology that results in growth restriction, which occurs more frequently than growth acceleration.[23] In addition, gender and racial variations have been reported. Females tend to have smaller head circumferences than males in most ethnic groups, and African American infants as well as most non-White groups have smaller head circumferences than White infants at the same gestation. These growth variations indicate the need for gender- and race-specific population growth references, which are currently not available, to minimize the potential of mislabeling infants as small for gestational age.[24,25]

Macrocephaly is diagnosed when the OFC is above the 90th percentile despite appropriate weight and length for gestational age. Macrocephaly may be familial, caused by hydrocephalus, or associated with dwarfism or osteogenesis imperfecta.[1,26] Familial macrocephaly is more often macroencephaly or large brain volume without hydrocephalus. Confirmation requires obtaining measurements of the parents' heads and plotting them on a Weaver curve.[27]

Transillumination of the skull is not part of the routine newborn physical exam, but it may be helpful when the infant's head has an unusual shape or size, or the neurologic examination is abnormal. A transilluminator or a flashlight with a rubber cuff may be placed flat against the infant's head in a dark room (see Figure 1.3). A ring of light more than 2 cm larger than the light source implies increased fluid or decreased brain tissue in the cranium. A false-positive transillumination may occur with a large caput because the scalp edema will transmit a halo of light. More definitive studies are necessary for diagnosis.[1] If the infant presents with a high level of suspicion for hydrocephalus, transillumination is often replaced by one of the more definitive studies, such as cranial ultrasound, CT, or MRI.

FACE

Examination of the face should begin with observation of the relationships among all the facial components: ears, eyes, nose, and mouth. The forehead of a newborn takes up the upper half of the face, reflecting the large cranial volume needed for rapid brain growth. In childhood, the growth of the mid- and lower face exceeds that of the upper face, eventually resulting in the face and skull shape of the adult.[12]

The shape and symmetry of the face, as well as evidence of trauma, should be noted. Face or brow presentation or the presence of a nuchal cord at delivery may cause facial bruising, petechiae, and progressive edema. Unusual flattening of facial features may occur as a result of prolonged intrauterine compression from oligohydramnios. Forceps application can cause bruises, abrasions, or subcutaneous fat necrosis.[3] The location and extent of any trauma should be carefully described. Other skin lesions that may be seen on the face are described in Chapter 5.

Many malformation syndromes have very distinctive facial features. Unusual facial characteristics may serve as aids in the diagnosis of a particular syndrome or may be familial.[7] Some syndromic facial features may not be evident in the prematurely born infant. Phenotypic presentation may be progressively evident when the infant's corrected gestational age (CGA) nears 40 weeks. Some features present later in infancy or childhood.

Facial movements during crying are assessed for symmetry. Damage to the facial nerve (seventh cranial nerve) prior to or during delivery can result in paralysis of the affected side of the face. Extensive damage can involve the entire side of the face innervated by the damaged nerve and cause drooping of the muscles on the affected side of the face. More common, the damage involves only the lower branch (mandibular branch) of the facial nerve, which controls the muscles around the lips. Evidence of this damage presents as a characteristic decreased movement on the affected side of the face when the infant cries, because the weakened facial muscles of the affected side allow the mouth to be pulled to the unaffected side ("drooping mouth" appearance; Figure 6.10). These infants often have loss of forehead,[28] wrinkling and nasolabial folds, and partial

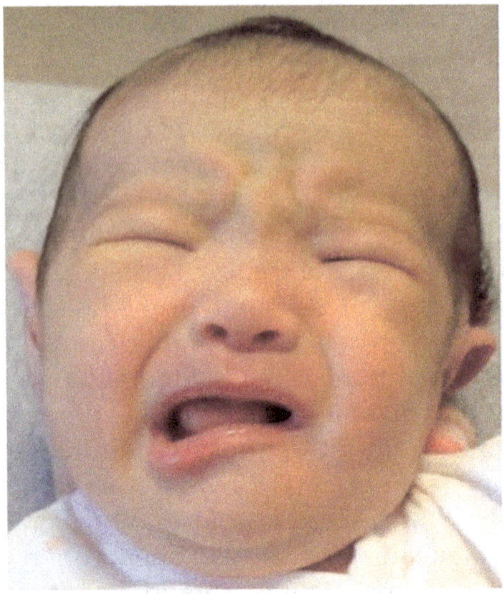

FIGURE 6.10 Facial asymmetry

Source: Ho K-Y, and Liang JN. 2019. Asymmetric crying facies syndrome. *The Journal of Pediatrics* 212: 235. doi: 10.1016/j.jpeds.2019.04.011

closing of the eye on the affected side, differentiating them from infants with congenital asymmetric crying facies (ACF). If the nerve damage is caused by pressure, then the facial effects resolve within hours to weeks after birth. Congenital facial palsy is often spontaneous but is also associated with difficult or instrumented delivery requiring forceps. A persistent palsy may be an indication of an underlying, more central abnormality. ACF, for example, is a congenital absence or hypoplasia of the depressor anguli oris muscle (DAOM) on one side. The DAOM controls frowning, with resulting asymmetry of the face with crying. There is an association with other anomalies, and further evaluation is warranted, especially for cardiovascular abnormalities.[10] (Chapter 12 provides guidelines for a complete neurologic assessment.)

Ears

Abnormal formation or placement of the ears can be associated with chromosomal anomalies and syndromes; however, a wide number of minor structural variations fall within the normal range. Ear anomalies are usually nonspecific and supportive of a diagnosis rather than presence of the anomaly being diagnostic in and of itself.[1–3,7] To describe abnormalities, the examiner should be familiar with the normal anatomy and descriptive nomenclature of the ear (Figure 6.11).[2] In a term infant, the pinna should be well-formed, with cartilage that recoils easily after folding (Chapter 4). Temporary asymmetry of the ears from unequal intrauterine pressure on the sides of the head is common.[1] Especially hairy ears, involving both the pinna and lobes, are familial, syndromic, or associated with infants of mothers with poorly controlled diabetes mellitus.

Minor malformations, such as pits and skin tags, may be familial or associated with other anomalies (Figure 6.12).[2,7] These minor malformations are usually located anterior to the tragus and are thought to be embryologic remnants of the first branchial cleft or arch. A preauricular sinus may be blind, or it may communicate with the internal ear or brain. Chronic infection could necessitate surgical removal of the entire sinus tract. Darwinian tubercle is a normal variant, appearing as a small nodule on the upper helix. A very poorly formed external ear should alert the examiner to a possible chromosomal anomaly or syndrome.[2,7]

The position of the external ear on the head can be assessed by extending a line from the inner to the outer canthus of the eye toward the ear (Figure 6.13). If the insertion of the ear falls below this line, it is low set. It is important to assess both ears because one may be

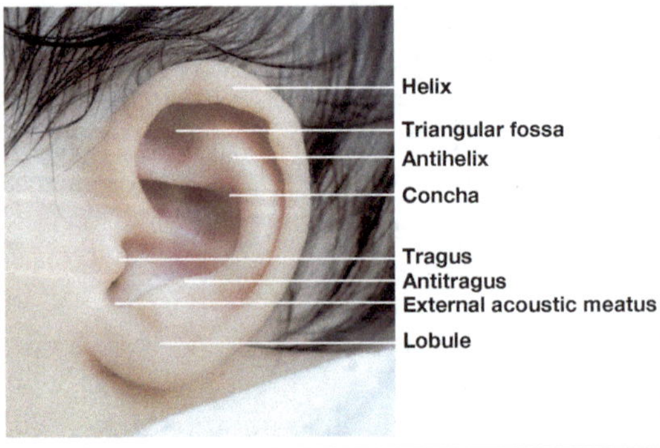

FIGURE 6.11 Normal external newborn ear (pinna)

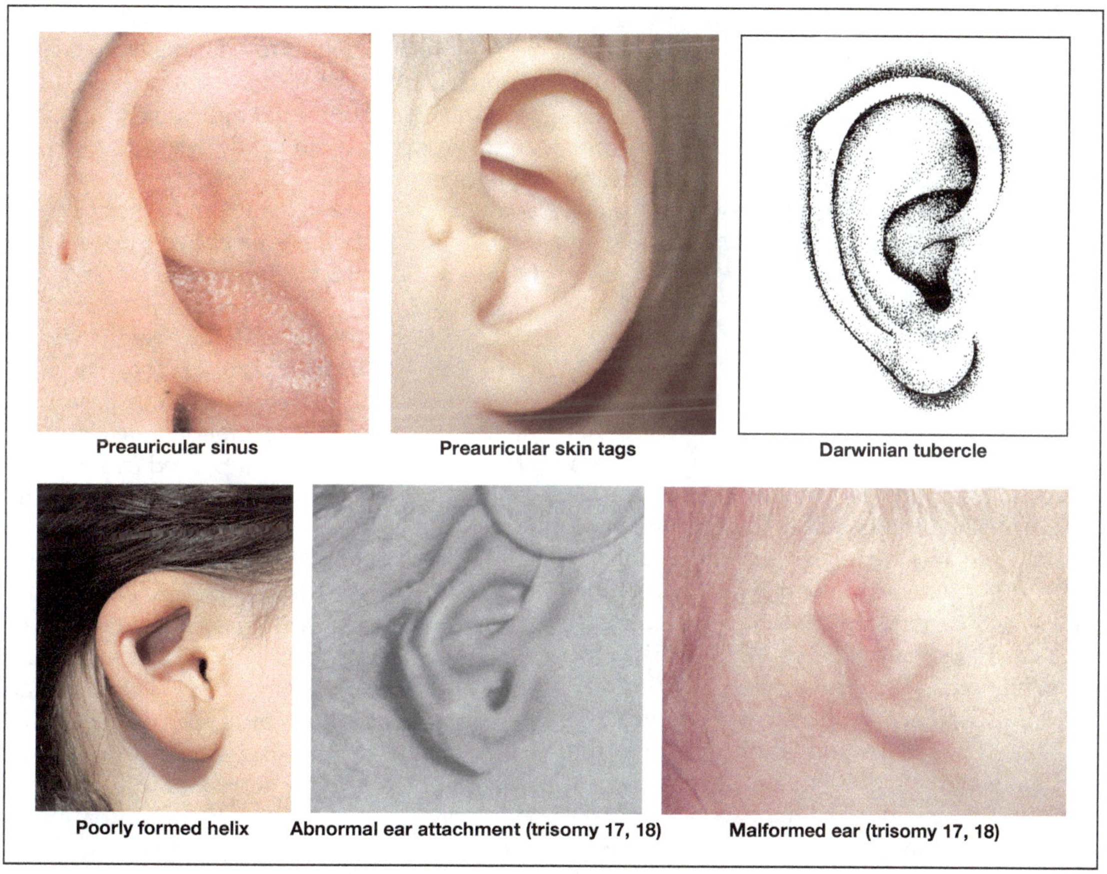

FIGURE 6.12 Variations and minor malformations of the ear

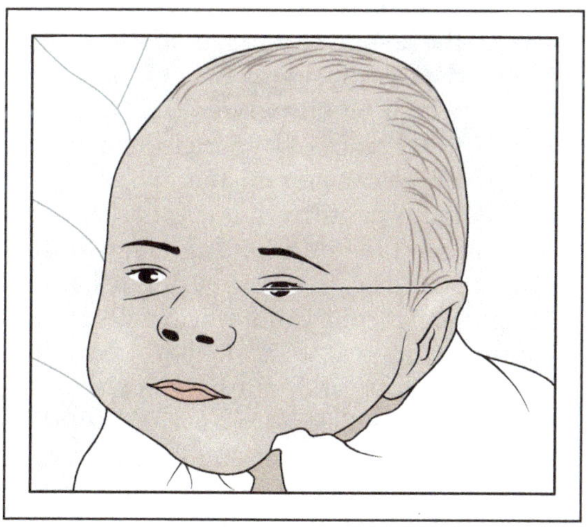

FIGURE 6.13 The normal ear position

posteriorly rotated and give the appearance of being low set.[2,5,7]

The ear should be inspected visually to assess the presence and patency of the auditory canal.[1,3,5] The newborn infant's external auditory canal is short and may contain vernix, intrapartum blood, or meconium debris, making otoscopic examination difficult. Otoscopic examination is not part of the routine newborn examination; it can be done later at the first well-baby visit.

Significant hearing loss is one of the most common major abnormalities present at birth.[29] Assessment of an infant's hearing during an examination, however, can be difficult. The infant should startle, cry, or stiffen at the sound of a loud noise or alert to the sound of a voice, but may be responding to air movement rather than noise and can quickly habituate to a repeated stimulus.[1,3] Any infant with a small or abnormally developed ear is at increased risk for hearing loss in that ear. Current recommendations endorse universal hearing screening of all newborns, with a goal of appropriate intervention by 6 months of age.[29,30]

Eyes

Eyes are usually a major area of interest when parents are viewing their newborn infant. It is important for the examiner to be familiar with the normal anatomy and descriptive nomenclature of the eyes (Figure 6.14). Parents will need reassurance about common eye trauma, such as bruises or edema of the eyelids and hemorrhages seen around the iris that can occur with a normal vaginal delivery. Conjunctival or subconjunctival hemorrhage results from rupture of a capillary in the mucous membrane that lines the eyelids and is reflected onto the eyeball (conjunctiva). It is seen as a bright-red area on the white part of the eye (sclera) near the iris and usually resolves within 1 week to 10 days without residual effects. Inflammation of the conjunctiva can be caused by debris from delivery or prophylaxis of the eyes with erythromycin ointment.[1] Malformation of the eyelids is uncommon, but coloboma (an absence or defect of some ocular tissue, including the eyelid) may be seen. Eyelid eversion with marked chemosis (swelling) of the palpebral conjunctiva is a rare, usually bilateral, abnormality seen more commonly in African American newborns at birth and may be seen with Down syndrome. This abnormality requires involvement of ophthalmology, but is often resolved without surgery.[31] Ptosis, a paralytic drooping of an eyelid when the lids are fully open, may also be seen. Nevus simplex is a common vascular birthmark seen on the eyelids and glabella (area above the nose and between the eyebrows).[2] (See Chapter 5 and Figure 5.12.)

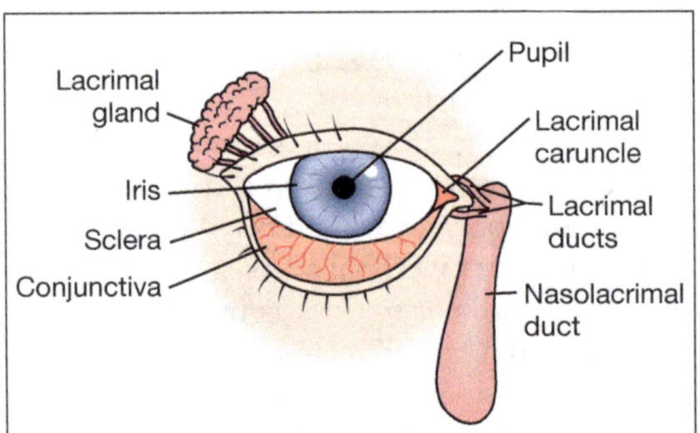

FIGURE 6.14 Anatomy of the eye

Tear formation does not usually begin until 2 to 3 months of age. The nasolacrimal duct is not fully patent until 5 to 7 months of age, and purulent or mucoid eye drainage is common. Unless accompanied by conjunctival inflammation with redness or swelling, this drainage can generally be treated by lacrimal massage and gentle cleansing with water and a cotton ball.[1,3,5] A rare obstruction of the nasolacrimal duct will develop cysts caused by distention of the lacrimal sac and duct. This is referred to as *dacryocystocele* and presents with a bluish bulge below the medial canthus. These infants require ophthalmology involvement due to risk of infection and recurrence but may respond to palpation of the lacrimal sac with mucoid discharge.[32]

Abnormal placement of the eyes or small palpebral fissures (eye openings) can alert the examiner to the presence of a syndrome or chromosomal anomaly. The distance between the outer canthi can be divided into equal thirds, with one normal palpebral fissure length fitting into the inner canthal distance (Figure 6.15).[31] Hypertelorism exists if the eyes are more widely spaced; hypotelorism is present if the eyes are more closely spaced. Small palpebral fissures can give the appearance of hypertelorism.[1,3,7]

If the outer canthus of the eye is higher than the inner canthus, the eye is said to be upslanting; if the outer canthus is lower than the inner canthus, the eye is downslanting. The epicanthal fold is a vertical fold of skin on either side of the nose that covers the lacrimal caruncle and, although a characteristic finding in Asians, occurs in 20% of non-Asians, usually disappearing by 10 years of age as the growth of the nasal bridge catches up to that of the medial canthal skin.[6,33] Epicanthal folds with upslanting palpebral

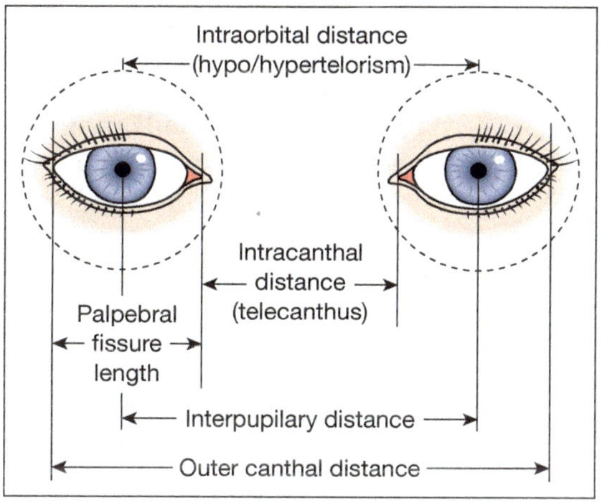

FIGURE 6.15 Eye measurements

Source: Adapted from Cheng KP, and Biglan AW. 2007. Ophthalmology. In *Atlas of Pediatric Physical Diagnosis*, 5th ed. Zitelli BJ, and Davis HW, eds. Philadelphia, PA: Mosby, 727. Reprinted by permission.[31]

fissures are common in infants of Asian descent. They may suggest Down syndrome in other ethnic groups, especially if associated with hypertelorism.[1,7]

An eyebrow normally extends above the eye in a curve approximately the length of the palpebral fissure. Eyebrows that meet at the glabella and abnormally long or tangled eyelashes are associated with some syndromes, such as Cornelia de Lange.[7] Examination of the eyes is much easier if the infant opens them spontaneously. At the beginning of the examination, the examiner can give an auditory stimulus, change the infant's position from supine to upright, gently swing the infant in an arc on the examiner's arm, or dim the lights. If the eyes are forcefully opened, the eyelids will often evert, making visualization impossible. The eye exam will be more difficult if attempted within several hours after eye prophylaxis.

A full ophthalmoscopic exam is not practical, so the examiner must be alert to obtain the information needed in a limited time.[3,5] The ophthalmoscope should first be adjusted for focus and then for supply of a small, round, and white beam of light. The examiner directs the light at the infant's pupils from a distance of about 6 inches to assess equality of pupil size and pupillary reflex (constriction with bright light). The notation "practical extraction report language (PERL)" can be used if "pupils are noted to be of equal size and react to light" by constricting. The examiner also seeks to elicit the retinal reflex (red reflex). When a bright light is directed at the newborn's lens, a clear red, orange, or yellowish color is reflected from the retina back to the examiner. Opacity of the lens or cornea interrupts the reflection (leukokoria or white retinal reflex); lack of the red reflex could imply congenital cataract, retinoblastoma, or glaucoma (Figure 6.16).[1,3,34] In dark-skinned infants, the red reflex pales from orange toward pale yellow to gray in the darkest pigmented infants. The lens vessels of the premature infant can be examined to help determine gestational age (Chapter 4). A keyhole-shaped pupil, also known as coloboma of the iris, may be associated with other anomalies, or it can be an isolated finding.[1,3,5]

The iris of a newborn infant is generally dark gray, blue, or brown at birth and will acquire final pigment color at about 6 months of age. Brushfield spots are white specks scattered linearly around the entire circumference of the iris. They are associated with Down syndrome but may be seen as a normal variant.[7] The sclera of a term infant is generally white to bluish white. A blue sclera is associated with osteogenesis imperfecta. The sclera may become jaundiced with hyperbilirubinemia. In a normal gaze, no sclera should be visible above the iris. The

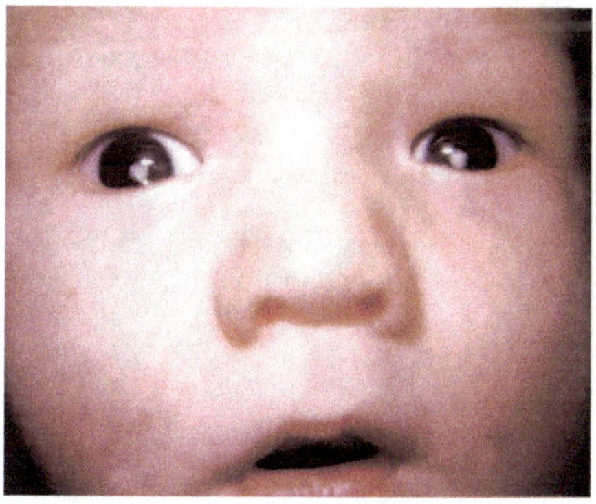

FIGURE 6.16 Congenital cataracts

Source: From Clark DA. 2000. *Atlas of Neonatology*. Philadelphia, PA: Saunders, 280. Reprinted by permission.[48]

"sunset sign" is often seen in infants with hydrocephalus, where there is lid retraction and a downward gaze.[1,3,5]

Observation of eyeball movements during neurologic assessment is discussed in detail in Chapter 12. Nystagmus is a rapid, searching movement of the eyeballs. Limited horizontal nystagmus may be elicited with rotational eye movement but disappears by 3 to 4 months of age. Spontaneous horizontal, vertical, or torsional nystagmus and persistent nystagmus are always aberrant and likely associated with visual and/or neurologic abnormalities. Strabismus results from muscular incoordination and gives the appearance of crossed eyes (Figure 6.17). Pseudostrabismus from a flat nasal bridge or epicanthal folds usually resolves by 1 year of age and is differentiated from strabismus by the presence of symmetric corneal light reflexes. Unusual protrusion (exophthalmos, proptosis), enlargement, or bulging of the eyeball is associated with hyperthyroidism, tumors, hemangiomas, and congenital glaucoma and can be associated with damage to the eye with hemorrhage into its orbit.[1,2,35,36]

Nose

The size and shape of the nose may be racially characteristic and familial, but the infant's nose is generally smaller and flatter than that of an adult. The nose should be symmetric and placed vertically in the midline. Nasal flaring is abnormal and is a sign of respiratory distress. Sneezing is common and normal unless excessive or continuous. Nasal stuffiness can be normal in the newborn period; however, chronic breathing difficulty or chronic nasal discharge is abnormal.[1,3,5,37] A very low nasal bridge with a broad base may be associated with Down syndrome.[3,7]

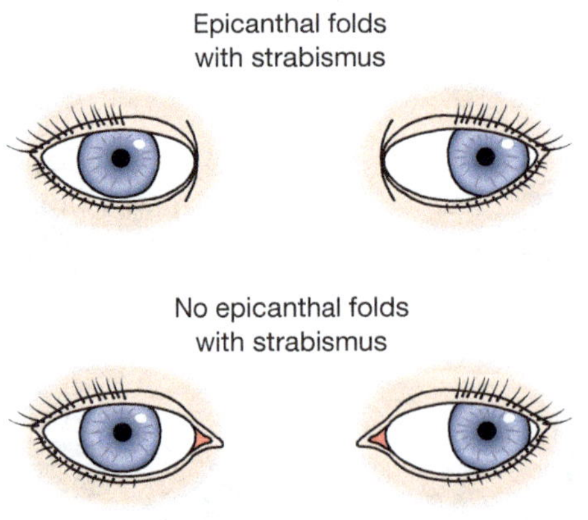

FIGURE 6.17 Strabismus

Source: Adapted from Alexander MM, and Brown MS. 1979. *Pediatric History Taking and Physical Diagnosis for Nurses*, 2nd ed. Philadelphia, PA: Mosby, 97. Reprinted by permission of the authors.[49]

Deviation of the nasal septum to one side may be a deformation from position in utero, or it may be caused by a dislocated septum. If the septum will not easily straighten and the nares remain asymmetric when the tip of the nose is pushed to midline, the septum is dislocated and will require treatment (Figure 6.18).[1,38] The examiner can elevate the tip of the nose slightly to view the nasal septum, the floor of the nose, and the turbinates.[38]

Nasal patency can be assessed by watching the infant breathe in a quiet state. Because infants are obligate nose breathers, bilateral choanal atresia (obstruction of the posterior nasal passages) will cause the infant to be cyanotic at rest and pink when crying and breathing through the mouth. If obstruction is suspected, a soft #5 French catheter can be gently passed through each nostril to assess patency. If an infant has noisy nasal respirations, a piece of cold metal can be held under the nose to observe for mist formation under both nares. If the turbinates are swollen from previous suctioning, passing a catheter to assess patency may only make the edema worse.[1,3]

Nasal occlusion can also be acquired from accumulation of secretions resulting in noisy respirations, feeding difficulties, respiratory distress, or apnea. Excessive bulb suctioning may aggravate the occlusive tendency; normal saline irrigation or intermittent installation of normal saline drops may facilitate resolution of obstruction from secretions.

With increased use of nasal continuous positive airway pressure (NCPAP) and nasal intermittent positive pressure ventilation (NIPPV) in premature infants and infants with respiratory distress, erosive trauma to the nasal labia, nasi columella, and nares is

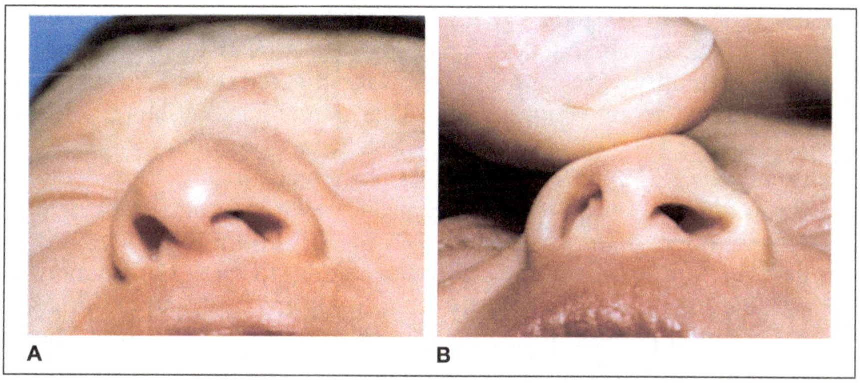

FIGURE 6.18 Nasal deformity. This infant incurred dislocation of the triangular cartilage of the nasal septum during delivery. Inspection of the nose reveals deviation of the septum to the right and asymmetry of the nares (A). When the septum is manually moved toward the midline, the asymmetry persists, confirming the dislocation (B).

Source: From Brozanski BS, Riley MM, and Bogen DL. 2012. Neonatology. In *Atlas of Pediatric Physical Diagnosis*, 6th ed. Zitelli BJ, McIntire SC, and Norwalk AJ, eds. Philadelphia: Mosby, 57. Reprinted by permission.

more common. Preventative and protective skin coverings can help, but monitoring the area for ulceration will minimize long-term disfigurement and scarring.

Major abnormalities of the nose, including clefts, single nares, masses, and partial or complete hypoplasia, are usually syndromic or associated with major central nervous system anomalies.

Mouth

The lips and mucous membranes of a healthy term infant should be pink. Mild circumoral cyanosis is normal during transition and with crying during the first few days.

Abnormal shape and size of the oral opening, lips, philtrum (midline groove between the nose and upper lip), and mandible may be associated with a syndrome. A small oral opening, known as microstomia, may be seen in some syndromes.[7] Macrostomia is seen with storage diseases such as the mucopolysaccharidoses. Lip thickness is related to racial and familial characteristics, and many infants have calluses on the lips from sucking in utero. Unusually thick or thin lips are abnormal and require further evaluation for trauma or an underlying mass. A thin upper lip with a smooth philtrum and short palpebral fissures may be seen in fetal alcohol syndrome. Cleft lip may be unilateral or bilateral and may be small or extend to the floor of the nose. Micrognathia, or abnormally small lower jaw, is seen in Pierre Robin sequence and some syndromes (Figure 6.19).[1,3,7,13]

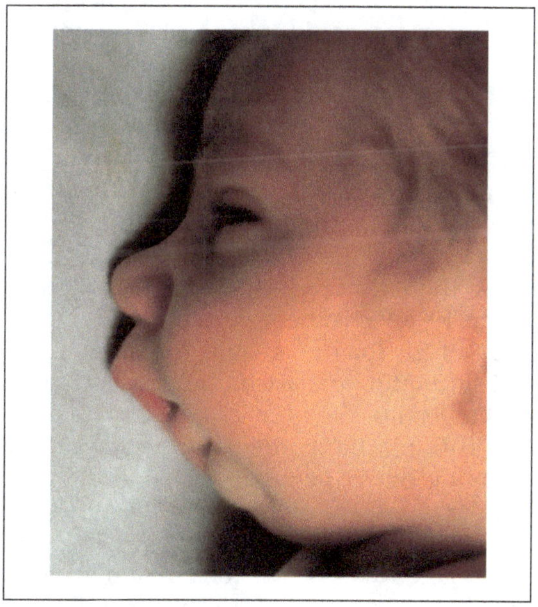

FIGURE 6.19 Pierre Robin sequence (micrognathia)

Source: From Clark DA. 2000. *Atlas of Neonatology*. Philadelphia, PA: Saunders, 144. Reprinted by permission.[48]

During the examination, assess the cry for quality, strength, pitch, and hoarseness or stridor. Inspect the symmetry of facial movements during the cry and assess rooting and sucking reflexes (Chapter 12).

Visual examination inside the mouth is easiest when the infant is crying. Use of a tongue depressor may stimulate a strong protrusion reflex, making assessment difficult. The mouth may be opened by gently pressing down on the chin. Abnormalities of the oropharynx are unusual, but a quick look is necessary to ensure absence of a structural anomaly or tumor. If possible, the uvula should be visualized at the back of the soft palate. A bifid uvula is often associated with submucosal cleft, notched hard palate, and muscular diastasis of the soft palate. It may be associated with other congenital anomalies.[3,7,39]

The tongue should fit well into the floor of the mouth and appear symmetric. A large tongue (macroglossia) impedes closure of the mouth and is associated with Beckwith–Wiedemann syndrome, hypothyroidism, and mucopolysaccharidosis. The tongue may *appear* large when the lower jaw is small (micrognathia). This is seen in Pierre Robin sequence, where there is hypoplasia of the mandible, the tongue is placed further back than normal (glossoptosis), and the palate is cleft.[7]

The frenulum (frenulum linguae) attaches the underside of the tongue to the floor of the mouth, usually midway between the tongue's ventral surface and tip. A very thick or prominent frenulum, or "tongue tie," is ankyloglossia. The incidence of ankyloglossia in the newborn has been reported to be 3% to 10%.[40–42] If the frenulum limits movement of the tongue or pulls the tongue to a "V" at the tip, it is abnormal and may limit suck effectiveness primarily for breast feeding. This may be an indication for frenotomy (clipping of the frenulum) or if severe may require frenuloplasty (surgical removal of frenulum).[40,42,43]

White patches on the tongue and mucous membranes may be from residual milk, and leukoplakia is normal in darkly pigmented infants. If the white coating cannot be easily removed with a tongue blade or cotton swab, it may be lesions of a candidal infection (oral thrush). A translucent or bluish swelling under the tongue is a mucocele or ranula. These mucous or salivary gland retention cysts usually resolve spontaneously.[2,3]

A gloved finger inserted into the infant's mouth with the finger pad up may be used to assess for continuity of the hard and soft palates, strength and coordination of suck, and for a gag reflex. A gloved finger can also be used to run along the gum line to assess for lumps or masses. Small whitish-yellow clusters of Epstein pearls may be seen at the junction of the hard and soft palates and on the gums. Epstein's pearls are epithelial inclusion cells and usually disappear by a few weeks of age. They are histologically the same as Bohn nodules found on the gums and milia seen on the skin.[1–3] The gums should be pink and smooth. Natal teeth are present at birth, and neonatal teeth erupt shortly after birth.[44] Natal teeth are rarely seen in Caucasian infants but are a common variant in Native American infants.[45] Teeth or eruption cysts with teeth appearing after birth (neonatal teeth) are usually seen in the lower incisor region. Natal and neonatal teeth are usually immature caps of enamel and dentine with poor root formation and may be very mobile. They may interfere with breastfeeding, may cause ulceration of the infant's tongue and pain with feeding, and there is a presumed risk of aspiration. For these reasons, removal is generally recommended, after consultation with a dentist and the family. If the tooth is firmly implanted, removal may result in hemorrhage and may impact future dentition, and the dentist may choose to leave it in place and do follow-up examinations, including x-rays, to assess for any complications.[2,3,44,46]

Excessive oral secretions requiring frequent suctioning are abnormal in the newborn infant. The etiology could be esophageal atresia or tracheal esophageal fistula, or poor swallow due to a neurologic abnormality. Strength and coordination of swallow should be assessed at every feeding. If there is concern, patency of the esophagus is assessed by passing a large-bore (usually #10 French) orogastric tube; an x-ray is done to confirm placement.[3]

NECK

The infant's neck is typically short, but severe shortness may be syndromic. To observe the shape and symmetry of the neck, elevate the shoulders, allowing the head to fall back slightly. Asymmetry is most likely the result of in utero positioning. The neck must be visualized and palpated anteriorly, laterally, and posteriorly. The thyroid gland is difficult to palpate unless it is enlarged. Goiter, caused by intrauterine deprivation of thyroid hormone, is very unusual.[3]

Cystic hygroma is the most commonly seen neck mass (Figure 6.20). It is caused by development of sequestered lymph channels, which dilate into large cysts. Cystic hygroma is soft and fluctuant, transilluminates well, and is usually seen laterally or over the clavicle. Its size can range from only a few centimeters to massive, and it may cause severe feeding difficulties or airway compromise. Very small lesions may regress spontaneously, but surgical resection is usually required.[1]

A mass high in the neck may be a thyroglossal duct cyst or a branchial cleft cyst. A branchial sinus may also be seen anywhere along the sternocleidomastoid muscle. It may communicate with deeper structures, and infection may necessitate surgical removal of the entire sinus tract.[47]

During palpation of the neck, note redundant skin or neck webbing. This is associated with Turner (Figure 6.21), Noonan, and Down syndromes.[1,5,7]

The clavicles should be palpated to assess for fracture, especially if there is a history of shoulder dystocia or macrosomia. Some infants present with nonrespiratory tachypnea caused by discomfort from the fracture. Movement of the bone ends and crepitus may be felt soon after birth, or a fracture may not be evident for weeks until a callus has formed and can be palpated as a mass over the clavicle. Fractured clavicles in the newborn heal spontaneously without treatment.

Assessment of neck reflexes, range of motion, and tone is described in Chapters 11 and 12.

SUMMARY

Careful examination of the head and neck is important because abnormalities presenting at birth in these regions are often indicative

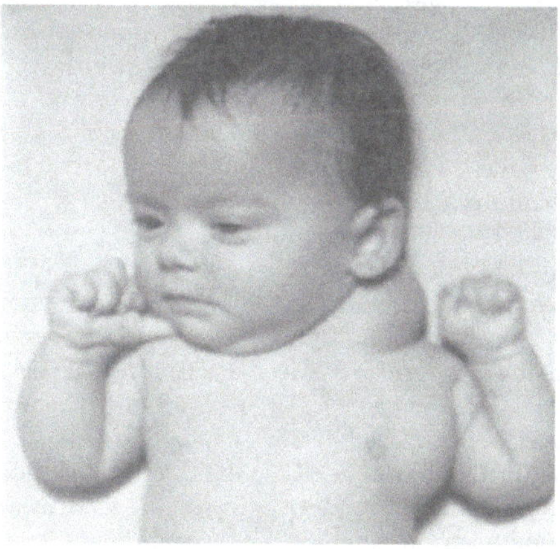

FIGURE 6.20 Cystic hygroma, with extension to the axilla

Source: From Koop CE. 1976. *Visible and Palpable Lesions in Children*. New York, NY: Grune & Stratton, 35. Reprinted by permission of the author.[50]

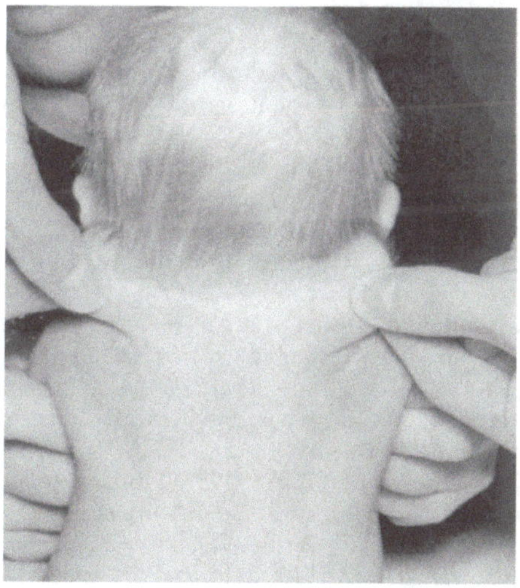

FIGURE 6.21 Neck webbing—Turner syndrome

Source: From Milner RDG, and Herber SM. 1984. *Color Atlas of the Newborn*. Oradell, NJ: Medical Economics, 102. Reprinted by permission of Blackwell Scientific Publications.[51]

of other anomalies or a specific syndrome. Examination of the eyes and mouth requires the infant's cooperation, and the examiner needs to be alert for opportune times. States are now adopting the current recommendation for universal hearing screening for all newborns. The states with statutes or other regulatory language related to universal newborn hearing screening can be found at www.infanthearing.org/legislation.[30]

ADDITIONAL RESOURCES

SPRINGER PUBLISHING CONNECT™

A robust set of resources designed to supplement this text is located at http://connect.springerpub.com/content/book/978-0-8261-4063-0. Qualifying instructors may request access by emailing textbook@springerpub.com.

REFERENCES

1. Scanlon JW, Nelson J, Grylack LJ, and Smith YF. 1979. *A System of Newborn Physical Examination*. Baltimore, MD: University Park Press, 45–60.
2. Mead Johnson. 1978. *Variations and Minor Departures in Infants*. Evansville, IN: Mead Johnson and Company.
3. Ball JW, Dains JE, Flynn JA, Solomon BS, and Stewart RW. 2023. *Seidels Guide to Physical Examination*, 10th ed. Elsevier Inc. ISBN: 978-0-323-76183-3, 209–229.
4. Kiesler J, and Ricer R. 2003. The abnormal fontanel. *American Family Physician* 67(12): 2547–2552.
5. Rennie JM. 2012. Examination of the newborn. In *Rennie & Robertson's Textbook of Neonatology*, 5th ed. Rennie JM, ed. Philadelphia, PA: Churchill Livingstone, 24.
6. McKee-Garrett TM. 2022. *Assessment of the New-Born*. UpToDate. Retrieved from www.uptodate.com/contents/assessment-of-the-newborn-infant
7. Jones KL, Jones MC, and Del Campo M, eds. 2022. Minor anomalies: Clues to more serious problems and to the recognition of malformation syndromes. In *Smith's Recognizable Patterns of Human Malformation*, 87th ed. Philadelphia, PA: Saunders, 955–972, 895–912.
8. Koenigsberg RA. 2011. *Brain Imaging in Arteriovenous Malformation*. Retrieved from https://emedicine.medscape.com/article/337220
9. Chemke J, and Robinson A. 1969. The third fontanelle. *Journal of Pediatrics* 75(4): 617–622.
10. Sheth RD. 2012. *Pediatric Craniosynostosis*. Retrieved from www.emedicine.medscape.com/article/1175957
11. Disabato J, and Wulf J. 1989. Nursing strategies: Altered neurologic function. In *Family-Centered Nursing Care of Children*, Foster RL, Hunsberger MM, and Tackett JJ, eds. Philadelphia, PA: Saunders, 1731.
12. Dirks PB, and Rutka JT. 2007. The neurogenetic basis of pediatric neurosurgical conditions. In *Principles and Practice of Pediatric Neurosurgery*, 2nd ed. Albright AL, Pollack IF, and Adelson PB, eds. New York, NY: Thieme Medical, 23–45.
13. Snively SL. 1987. Craniofacial anomalies. Part 2: Congenital syndromes and surgical treatment. *Selected Readings in Plastic Surgery* 4(25): 1–25.
14. Fox GN, and Maier MK. 1984. Neonatal craniotabes. *American Family Physician* 30(6): 149–151.
15. Yorifuji J, Yorifuji T, Tachibana K, Nagai S, Kawai M, Momoi T, Nagasaka H, Hatayama H, and Nakahata T. 2008. Craniotabes in normal newborns: The earliest sign of subclinical vitamin D deficiency. *Journal of Clinical Endocrinology and Metabolism* 93(5): 1784–1788.
16. Reid J. 2007. Neonatal subgaleal hemorrhage. *Neonatal Network* 26(4): 219–227.
17. Brozanski BS, Riley MM, and Bogen DL. 2012. Neonatology. In *Atlas of Pediatric Physical Diagnosis*, 6th ed. Zitelli BJ, McIntire SC, and Norwalk AJ, eds. Philadelphia, PA: Saunders Elsevier, 45–78.
18. Currarino G. 1976. Normal variants and congenital anomalies in the region of the obelion. *American Journal of Roentgenology* 127(3): 487–494.
19. Furdon SA, and Clark DA. 2003. Scalp hair characteristics in the newborn infant. *Advances in Neonatal Care* 3(6): 286–296.
20. Boom JA. 2022. *Macrocephaly in Infants and Children: Etiology and Evaluation*. UpToDate. Retrieved from www.uptodate.com/contents/etiologyand-evaluation-of-macrocephaly-in-infants-and children
21. Menkes JH, Sarnat HB, and Flores-Sarnat L. 2006. Malformations of the central nervous system. In *Child Neurology*, 7th ed. Menkes JH, Sarnat HB, and Maria BL, eds. Philadelphia, PA: Lippincott, Williams & Wilkins, 284–366.
22. Lissauer T, and Hansen, A. 2020. Physical examination of the newborn. In *Neonatal–Perinatal Medicine: Diseases of the Fetus and Infant*, 11th ed. Martin RJ, Fanaroff AA, and Walsh MC, eds. Elsevier, Inc., 440–457.
23. Blair EM, Liu Y, de Klerk NH, and Lawrence DM. 2005. Optimal fetal growth for the Caucasian singleton and assessment of appropriateness of fetal growth: An analysis of a total population perinatal database. *BMC Pediatrics* 5(13): 1–12.
24. Goldenberg RL, Cliver SP, Hoffman HJ, Cassady G, Davis RO, and Nelson KG. 1991. Black-white differences in newborn anthropometric measurements. *Obstetrics and Gynecology* 78(5 Part 1): 782–788.

25. Madan A, Holland S, Humbert JE, and Benitz WE. 2002. Racial differences in birth weight of term infants in a northern California population. *Journal of Perinatology* 22(3): 230–235.
26. Cole TR, and Hughes HE. 1991. Autosomal dominant macrocephaly: Benign familial macrocephaly or a new syndrome? *American Journal of Medical Genetics* 41(1): 115–124.
27. Weaver DD, and Christian JC. 1980. Familial variation of head size and adjustment for parental head circumference. *Journal of Pediatrics* 96(6): 990–994.
28. Ho K-Y, and Liang JN. 2019. Asymmetric crying facies syndrome. *The Journal of Pediatrics* 212: 235. doi: 10.1016/j.jpeds.2019.04.011
29. AAP.org. 2022. Early hearing detection and intervention: Resources. Retrieved from https://www.aap.org/en/patient-care/early-hearing-detection-and-intervention/early-hearing-and-detection-resources/
30. National Center for Hearing Assessment and Management. 2022. *NCHAM Book: A Resource Guide for Early Hearing Detection & Intervention*. Utah State University.
31. Cheng KP, and Biglan AW. 2007. Ophthalmology. In *Atlas of Pediatric Physical Diagnosis*, 5th ed. Zitelli BJ, and Davis HW, eds. Philadelphia, PA: Mosby, 727.
32. Paysse EA, and Coates DK. 2022. *Congenital Nasolacrimal Duct Obstruction (Dacryostenosis) and Dacryocystocele*. UpToDate. Retrieved from www.uptodate.com/contents/congeital-nasolacrimalduct-obstruction-dacryostenosi-and-dacryocystocele
33. Jarvis C. 2016. Eyes. In *Physical Examination and Health Assessment*, 7th ed. St. Louis, MO: Elsevier, 281–324.
34. Yanoff M. 2008. *Ophthalmic Clinical Advisor: Diagnosis and Treatment*, 2nd ed. Philadelphia, PA: Butterworth-Heinemann, 46, 47, 206, 254, 255.
35. Aase JM. 1990. *Diagnostic Dysmorphology*. New York, NY: Plenum, 34–118.
36. Gnanaraj L, and Rao VJ. 2000. Corneal birth trauma: A cause for sensory exotropia. *Eye* 14(Part 5): 791–792.
37. Perry S. 1991. Normal newborn. In *Essentials of Maternity Nursing*, 3rd ed. Bobak IM, and Jensen MD, eds. Philadelphia, PA: Mosby, 441–481.
38. Mangurten HH, Puppala BL, and Pazad PA. 2020. Birth injuries. In *Fanaroff and Martin's Neonatal–Perinatal Medicine: Diseases of the Fetus and Infant*, 11th ed. Martin RJ, Fanaroff AA, and Walsh MC, eds. Elsevier Inc., 458–488.
39. Shprintzen RJ, Schwartz RH, Daniller A, and Hoch L. 1985. Morphologic significance of bifid uvula. *Pediatrics* 75(3): 553–561.
40. Ballard JL, Auer CE, and Khoury JC. 2002. Ankyloglossia: Assessment, incidence, and effect of frenuloplasty on the breastfeeding dyad. *Pediatrics* 110: e63. Retrieved from www.pediatrics.org/cgi/content/full/110/5/e63
41. Messner AH, and Lalakea ML. 2002. Ankyloglossia: Controversies in management. *International Journal of Pediatric Otorhinolyrygology* 54: 123–131.
42. Knox I. 2010. Tongue tie and frenotomy in the breastfeeding newborn. *NeoReviews* 11(9): c513–c519.
43. Segal LM, Stephenson R, Dawes M, and Feldman P. 2007. Prevalence, diagnosis, and treatment of ankyloglossia. *Canadian Family Physician* 53: 1027–1033.
44. Mathewson RJ, and Primosch RE. 1995. Oral hygiene education. In *Fundamentals of Pediatric Dentistry*, 3rd ed. Mathewson RJ, ed. Chicago, IL: Quintessence Publishing, 89–104.
45. Adam M, and Hudgins L. 2003. The importance of minor anomalies in the evaluation of the newborn. *NeoReviews* 4(4): e99–e103.
46. Nik-Hussein NN. 1990. Natal and neonatal teeth. *Journal of Pedodontics* 14(2): 110–111.
47. Nicklaus PJ, and Kelley PE. 1996. Management of deep neck infection. *Pediatric Clinics of North America* 43(6): 1277–1296.
48. Clark DA. 2000. *Atlas of Neonatology*. Philadelphia, PA: Saunders, 280.
49. Alexander MM, and Brown MS. 1979. *Pediatric History Taking and Physical Diagnosis for Nurses*, 2nd ed. Philadelphia, PA: Mosby, 97.
50. Koop CE. 1976. *Visible and Palpable Lesions in Children*. New York, NY: Grune & Stratton, 35.
51. Milner RDG, and Herber SM. 1984. *Color Atlas of the Newborn*. Oradel, NJ: Medical Economics, 102.

7 CHEST AND LUNG ASSESSMENT

Debbie Fraser

Physical assessment of the lungs begins with a careful review of the infant's history. Physical findings vary greatly with the infant's gestational and postnatal age. Other important factors from the infant's prenatal, intrapartum, and postnatal history are outlined in Box 7.1.

Begin the physical examination of the chest with observation to avoid disturbing the infant before assessing breath sounds. Auscultation and palpation follow. Depending on the infant's physical condition, rest may be necessary between parts of the examination. Ensure the infant doesn't become cold during the examination; cold stress will precipitate or further aggravate respiratory distress.

LANDMARKS AND STRUCTURE

The chest cavity is surrounded by the sternum, 12 thoracic vertebrae, and 12 pairs of ribs. All 12 pairs of ribs are attached to the thoracic vertebrae posteriorly, while the upper seven ribs are attached to the sternum anteriorly (Figure 7.1). The 8th, 9th, and 10th ribs attach to the costal cartilages above them while the 11th and 12th attach posteriorly but not anteriorly.[1] The ribs in the neonate are much more cartilaginous than in the adult, accounting in part for increased chest-wall compliance and for retractions seen in the infant with respiratory distress. The lower boundary of the thorax is formed by the diaphragm, normally a convex muscular sheath. The diaphragm inserts on the sternum, the first three lumbar vertebrae, and the lower six ribs.

Other palpable thoracic landmarks include the suprasternal notch, found on the upper aspect of the sternum, and the xiphoid process, which protrudes below the sternum.

The clavicles and scapulae complete the bony structure of the chest.

The chest cavity consists of three spaces: the mediastinum and the right and left pleural cavities. The mediastinum contains the heart, esophagus, trachea, mainstem bronchi, thymus, and major blood vessels. The three lobes of the right lung and two lobes of the left lung are encased in serous membranes, which make up the visceral and parietal pleura (Figure 7.2).

Reference Lines

To aid in accuracy, use the following reference lines to describe the location of a physical finding during the examination of the chest and lungs (Figure 7.3):

- Anterior axillary line: Extends from the anterior axillary fold
- Midclavicular line: Vertical line drawn through the middle of the clavicle
- Midsternal line: Bisects the suprasternal notch
- Nipple line: Horizontal line drawn through the nipples

HISTORY

Prior to examining the newborn, review the maternal and newborn history. Check for any anomalies noted on the maternal ultrasound. In addition, note the infant's gestational age

BOX 7.1: HISTORY TO BE COLLECTED

PRENATAL/INTRAPARTUM HISTORY
Gestational age
Maternal drug ingestion
Fetal distress
Maternal health (e.g., diabetes, fever)
Prolonged rupture of membranes
Meconium-stained fluid
Delivery mode
Apgar scores

POSTNATAL HISTORY
Corrected age
Duration of mechanical ventilation
History of any respiratory diagnosis
Difficulty feeding
Apnea

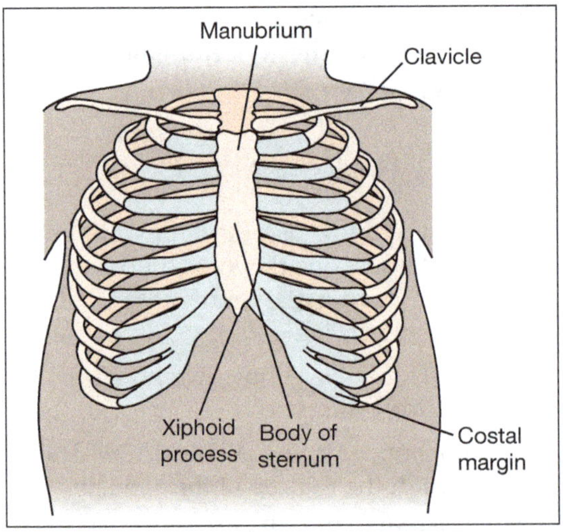

FIGURE 7.1 Bony structure of the chest

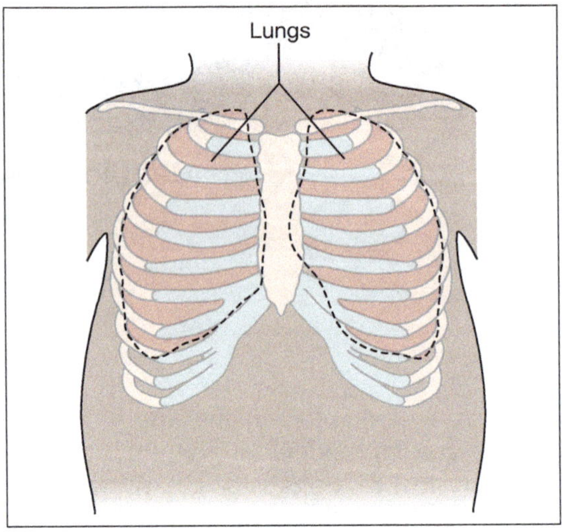

FIGURE 7.2 Internal structure of the chest

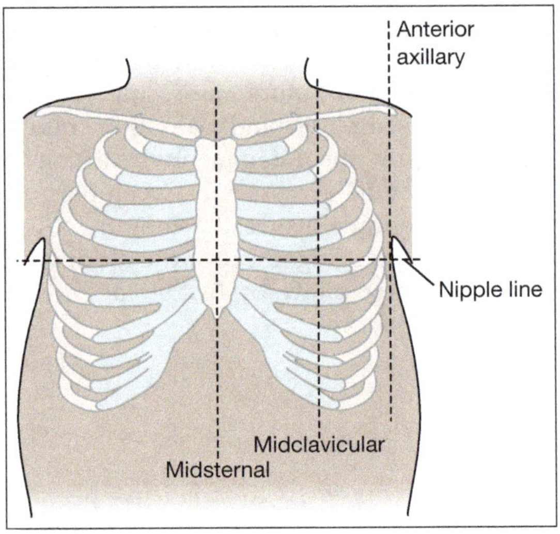

FIGURE 7.3 Reference lines

and any relevant maternal medical issues that may impact the infant's respiratory status. Depending on the age of the infant, note whether or not there has been any report of respiratory distress, increased work of breathing, or cyanosis. Note the infant's feeding pattern and any changes in color or respiratory effort associated with feeding.

INSPECTION

General

Begin the inspection with an overall assessment of the infant's color, tone, and activity. These findings provide clues to oxygenation and respiratory status.

Color

Observe the color of the infant's skin and mucous membranes. Normally the lips and mucous membranes should be pink and well perfused. Acrocyanosis (bluish coloration of the hands and feet) after birth is common and may persist during transition (up to 24 hours) following delivery.[2]

Color deviations might include cyanosis (either generalized or central [lips, tongue, and mucous membranes]) and acrocyanosis or mottling in the infant beyond transition. Other abnormalities in color, such as ruddiness and paleness, are discussed in Chapters 5 and 9.

Tone and Activity

Observe the infant's muscle tone and level and type of activity. Normal findings include flexed posture and active movement of all four limbs when awake. (Note the ability to attain and maintain flexion is decreased with prematurity.) Deviations include hypotonia and inactivity.

Respirations

Rate

Count the infant's respirations for 1 full minute. Normal findings are 30 to 60 breaths per minute, with wide variations. If the room is very warm or cool, the infant's respiratory rate can vary. Most infants experiencing temperature stress will be tachypneic (respirations >60 breaths per minute), but occasionally they may demonstrate bradypnea (respirations <40 breaths per minute). Because of the increased likelihood of retained fetal lung fluid, infants delivered by cesarean section have a higher incidence of transient tachypnea and respiratory distress.[2]

Although respiratory rates vary, tachypnea persisting beyond 2 hours of age may indicate underlying lung pathology (e.g., transient tachypnea of the newborn, respiratory distress syndrome [RDS], meconium aspiration, pneumonia, pneumothorax, or space occupying lesion), hyperthermia, or pain. Bradypnea and shallow respirations are associated with central nervous system (CNS) depression secondary to factors such as maternal drug ingestion, asphyxia, or birth injury.

Quality

Observe the general appearance of the infant. Relaxed, symmetric, diaphragmatic respirations are normal. The newborn infant uses the diaphragm as the primary muscle of respiration. For the diaphragm to work efficiently, the rib cage must be stabilized by the intercostal muscles and the abdomen by the abdominal muscles. Coordination of this activity is still developing in term infants; it is less well developed in preterm infants, especially during rapid-eye-movement sleep, when respiratory instability may be seen.[3] To compensate for chest-wall instability, the infant's diaphragm is situated higher in the chest and is more concave in shape than the adult diaphragm, allowing for more efficient contractions.[3]

Work of Breathing

During normal respiratory efforts in the neonate, the lower thorax pulls in, and the abdomen bulges with each respiration. Deviations include asymmetric chest movement and excessive thoracic expansion.

Infants are generally obligate nose breathers, so obstruction of the nasal passages is usually accompanied by respiratory distress.[4] Nasal flaring, grunting, or moaning may be noted immediately after birth as the neonate attempts to clear fetal lung fluid from the lungs. The sounds are created by exhalation against a partially closed glottis in an attempt to increase the functional residual capacity in the lungs and stabilize the alveoli. The presence of fetal lung fluid or lung pathology may decrease lung compliance and, coupled with a more cartilaginous rib cage, can result in visible retractions of the chest wall. Retractions may be seen above or below the sternum, under the rib cage (subcostal), or between the ribs (intercostal). Suprasternal retraction, especially if accompanied by gasping or stridor, is a sign of upper airway obstruction (laryngeal webs or cysts, tumors, or vascular rings). Severe respiratory distress

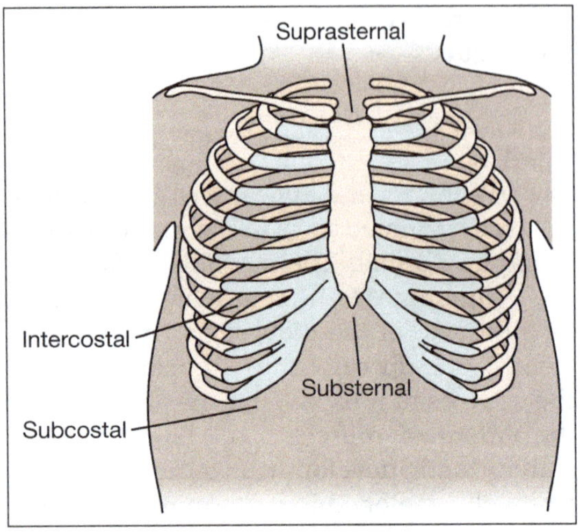

FIGURE 7.4 Sites of retractions

immediately after birth may signal an underlying condition such as diaphragmatic hernia or pneumothorax. Figure 7.4 illustrates the most common sites for retractions. Beyond the immediate newborn period, flaring, grunting, and retractions suggest respiratory pathology (e.g., transient tachypnea of the newborn, RDS, atelectasis, or pneumonia).

In 1956, Silverman and Andersen developed a scoring system to objectively measure respiratory distress; this system forms the basis of many of today's scoring systems.[5] This scoring system, shown in Table 7.1, can be used to quantify the extent of respiratory distress experienced by the infant at the time of examination.

Asymmetric chest movement is seen in the presence of conditions such as diaphragmatic hernia, cardiac lesions inducing failure, pneumothorax, or phrenic nerve damage. Sneezing is a common finding because it helps to clear the nasal passages. Coughing in the newborn is considered abnormal.

Pattern

While counting respirations, note the pattern (regularity) of inspiration. Normal newborns have an irregular pattern of respirations, which may vary with environmental temperature, sleep, and following a feeding. The less mature the infant, the more likely the breathing pattern is to be irregular. Periodic breathing (vigorous breaths followed by up to a 20-second pause) is common in preterm infants and may persist for several days after birth in term infants. For most preterm infants, the breathing pattern regularizes by the time they reach term gestation. In extremely preterm infants, cardiorespiratory events may not resolve until close to 44 weeks postconceptional age.[6]

Apnea of prematurity (AOP) is extremely common with the incidence increasing with decreasing gestational age at birth. A consensus definition of AOP is lacking;[7] with the most common definition being a cessation of

TABLE 7.1: ASSESSMENT OF RESPIRATORY DISTRESS

	SCORE		
CRITERION	**0**	**1**	**2**
Chest movement	Chest moves with abdomen	Chest sinks minimally as abdomen rises	Seesaw respirations; chest sinks as abdomen rises
Intercostal retractions	None	Minimal	Marked
Xiphoid retractions	None	Just visible	Marked
Expiratory grunting	None	Heard only with stethoscope	Audible with naked ear
Nasal flaring	None	Minimal	Marked

Note: The distress score is calculated by adding the values (0, 1, 2) assigned to each category. A score of 10 indicates maximum distress.

Source: Adapted from Silverman WA, and Andersen DH. 1956. A controlled clinical trial of water mist on obstructive respiratory signs, death rate, and necropsy findings among premature infants. *Pediatrics* 17(1): 1–10.[5]

breathing for more than 20 seconds or a cessation of breathing for 15 seconds when accompanied by bradycardia or cyanosis.[2] This condition, associated with prematurity, is gradually outgrown as the infant approaches 40 weeks postconceptional age. In extremely premature infants, periodic breathing may persist until 44 weeks postconceptional age.[8] Apnea in the term or close-to-term infant is considered abnormal and may indicate underlying illness (e.g., sepsis, hypoglycemia, CNS injury or abnormality, or seizures) or factors such as maternal drug ingestion.

Observe the quantity and quality of the infant's oral and nasal secretions. During transition, the appearance of oral and nasal secretions reflects the lungs' attempt to clear fetal fluid. Normal secretions are usually clear to white frothy mucus. Oral secretions will also reflect the stomach contents swallowed during delivery and therefore may be yellow or green in the presence of meconium, or blood-tinged if maternal blood was swallowed.

Deviations include excessive frothy oral secretions, which may indicate the presence of an esophageal atresia. Nasal stuffiness is associated with maternal drug use.[9] Snuffles (rhinitis) may be found with congenital syphilis.[10] Thick yellow secretions may be seen in the presence of a respiratory infection, and copious white nasal secretions are associated with respiratory syncytial virus (RSV) infection.

Components of the Chest and Respiratory System

Airways

The nasal portion of the airway is supported by bony and cartilaginous structures. The nasal passages are narrowed in the newborn; therefore, resistance to airflow in the nose contributes significantly to total pulmonary resistance. The pharyngeal component of the airway system is shorter in the infant than in adults and very compliant. In the absence of good muscle tone, the tongue can fall back against the soft palate and obstruct the airway, a process accentuated by neck flexion.[11] Look for the presence of nasal flaring or obvious signs of airway obstruction. In particular, infants with poor tone, a large tongue (macroglossia), or a small jaw (micrognathia) can experience upper airway obstruction.

Larynx and Trachea

In the newborn, the tracheal cartilages (hyoid, thyroid, and cricoid) are supported by superficial fascia. In premature infants, this fascia is underdeveloped, which increases the risk for airway obstruction.[3] The trachea and bronchi are supported by cartilaginous rings that are also less well developed than in the adult, increasing the risk for airway collapse and air trapping. Infants have the ability to alter laryngeal airway diameter by active movement of the vocal cords with breathing. Expiratory grunting in an infant with respiratory distress illustrates the infant's attempt to increase laryngeal airway resistance and ultimately to increase functional residual capacity in the lungs. Chemoreceptors in the larynx trigger reflex apnea to prevent entry of foreign substances.

On x-ray, the trachea is normally midline. Deviation suggests pneumothorax, a space-occupying lesion, or significant atelectasis. Rotation of the infant on the x-ray cassette may result in the false appearance of tracheal deviation.

Thorax

Observe the infant's chest and measure its circumference. The average chest circumference in term infants is 32.5 to 37.5 cm or 2 cm less than the occipital–frontal head circumference.[12] The difference between head and chest circumference is more exaggerated in premature infants and in those with intrauterine growth restriction, where the chest circumference will be small in comparison to that of the head.

In infants, the thorax is normally rounded rather than dorsoventrally flattened, as in older children. The ribs are oriented more horizontally, limiting the potential for expansion of the rib cage.[3] The soft cartilaginous structure of the newborn's chest results in a tendency for the chest wall to collapse inward in the presence of decreased lung compliance. To preserve end-expiratory lung volume, the infant compensates by increasing the respiratory rate, shortening the inspiratory time, and grunting.[13]

In neonates, the anterior–posterior (AP) diameter of the thorax is almost equal to the transverse diameter, giving the chest a round or boxlike appearance.[3,14] A small thorax is seen in pulmonary hypoplasia, and a bell-shaped thorax may be an indication of neurologic abnormalities or dwarfing syndromes.[15] A barrel chest, characterized by an increased AP diameter, is a finding characteristic of the air trapping seen in conditions such as transient tachypnea of the newborn, meconium aspiration, and overzealous mechanical ventilation. Sprengel deformity of the scapula occurs when the scapula fails to descend downward and becomes fixed to the cervical spine.[16]

Sternal deviations include protrusion of the sternum outward (pectus carinatum) or indented sternum (pectus excavatum; Figure 7.5). Pectus deformities occur in one per 400 newborns and are usually of cosmetic rather than medical significance. Severe cases may cause pain, cardiopulmonary dysfunction, increase work of breathing, and may restrict lung expansion.[17] The incidence of pectus carinatum is half that of pectus excavatum with a male predominance. About 25% of infants with pectus carinatum also have scoliosis. Pectus carinatum is associated with Marfan and Noonan syndromes, among other conditions.[17] Rib anomalies are relatively common and usually of no clinical significance. These anomalies may occasionally be noted on inspection or palpation but are more likely to be identified as an incidental finding on chest x-ray. Common anomalies include bifid ribs, rib agenesis, or bridging between the ribs. A cervical rib emanating from the seventh cervical vertebrae may cause compression of the brachial plexus or subclavian artery.[17] Eleven pairs of ribs may be seen in infants with Down syndrome or trisomy 18. Thin ribs are seen in infants with trisomy 13 or 18, and thickened ribs are a feature of thalassemia and mucopolysaccharidosis. Flaring of the lower ribs, known as *Harrison groove*, is another finding that may be normal or associated with rickets.[18] Abdominal distention may accompany hyperinflation as the diaphragm is pushed downward by air trapped in the lungs.

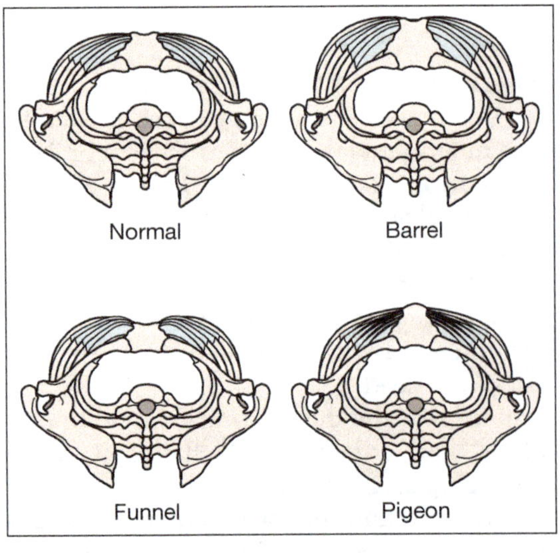

FIGURE 7.5 Different chest shapes

Muscle

Observe the chest for muscle development, symmetry, and bulges. The normal chest wall is symmetric and relatively smooth. Deviations include masses, atrophy, agenesis, and hypertrophy. Unilateral hypoplasia or absence of the pectoralis major muscle is a feature of Poland syndrome; other features of this syndrome include rib defects and upper limb hypoplasia.[19]

Cystic hygromas are benign tumors resulting from dilated lymphatic vessels and may be found in the neck, chest wall, or axillae. Hemangiomas may be seen in the neck or chest wall at birth or may develop over the first weeks of life.

Nipples

Observe the number, placement, shape, and pigmentation of the nipples. Also inspect the nipples for fissures and secretions. In the term infant, the areolae normally are raised and stippled, with 0.75 cm to 1 cm of palpable breast tissue. The distance between the nipples is normally less than 25% of the chest circumference.[20] The amount of breast tissue present at birth is also a useful indicator in gestational age assessment (Chapter 4).

In some infants, the influence of maternal estrogen results in breasts that are enlarged and engorged with a milky secretion, galactorrhea, also known as *witch's milk*. The effects of maternal hormones may last 1 to 2 weeks, and rarely, up to 2 months.[21] Rarely, newborn infants may develop mastitis, characterized by redness, tenderness, breast enlargement, and discharge of pus (see Chapter 5).

Wide-spaced nipples with hypoplastic areolae are features of Turner syndrome; associated findings include lymphedema and redundant skin at the nape of the neck (see Figure 6.21).[22] Supernumerary (accessory) nipples are most commonly seen as raised or pigmented areas 5 to 6 cm below the normal nipple but can be located anywhere on a vertical line drawn through the true nipple. Accessory nipples are more commonly seen in males and infants of African American descent than those of European descent.[21] Some studies have shown an association between supernumerary nipples and both congenital renal anomalies and an increased risk of genitourinary malignancies.[23]

AUSCULTATION

Breath sounds are louder and coarser in the neonate than in the adult because the infant has less subcutaneous tissue to muffle transmission. Sounds are very readily referred in the neonate's chest because of its small size; therefore, it is difficult to localize adventitious (abnormal) sounds. Breath sounds may be decreased but are seldom absent, even over areas of atelectasis or pneumothorax. Breath sounds are less readily transmitted if (a) the pleural space contains fluid or air, (b) a bronchus contains secretions or foreign bodies, or (c) the lungs are hyperinflated. Sounds are more readily transmitted in the presence of consolidation, for example, with pneumonia.

To auscultate breath sounds, use both the bell and diaphragm of a warmed neonatal

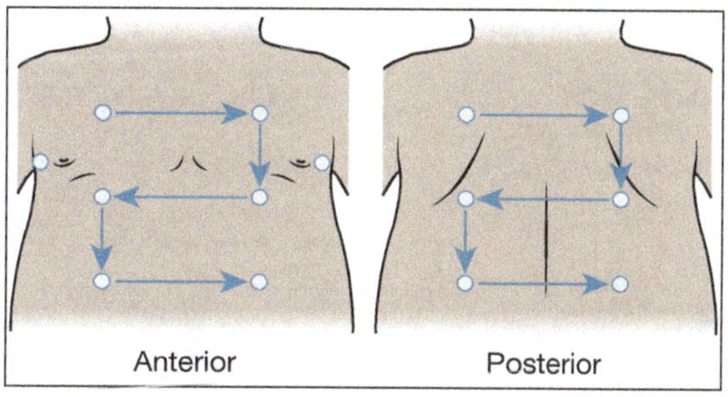

FIGURE 7.6 Sequence for breath sound auscultation: Anterior and posterior chest

stethoscope. Begin at the top of the chest and move systematically from side to side (Figure 7.6). Breath sounds in the lower lobes of the lungs can be assessed adequately only through the infant's back. Therefore, systematic auscultation of both the anterior and the posterior chest should be performed and one side of the chest compared with the other.

Normal Breath Sounds

Assess breath sounds for pitch, intensity, and duration. Normal breath sounds are described in adults and older children according to their location in the chest. As previously noted, localization of breath sounds in the neonate can be difficult. The following terms are sometimes used to describe normal sounds within the lungs. These terms are also listed in Table 7.2.

Vesicular Breath Sounds

Vesicular (from the Latin for *sac*) breath sounds are soft, short, and low-pitched during expiration and louder, longer, and higher pitched during inspiration. These sounds are normally found over the entire chest, except over the manubrium and trachea.

Bronchial Breath Sounds

The loudest of the breath sounds, bronchial sounds are characterized by a short inspiration and a longer expiration. In adults, these sounds are found over the trachea, but are not well-localized in neonates.[24]

TABLE 7.2: NORMAL BREATH SOUNDS

SOUND	CHARACTERISTICS	FINDINGS
Vesicular	Heard over most of lung fields; low pitch; soft, short expirations	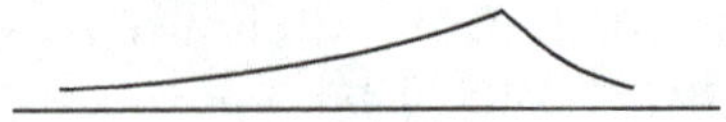 Low pitch, soft expirations
Bronchovesicular	Heard over main bronchus area and over upper-right posterior lung field; medium pitch; expiration equals inspiration	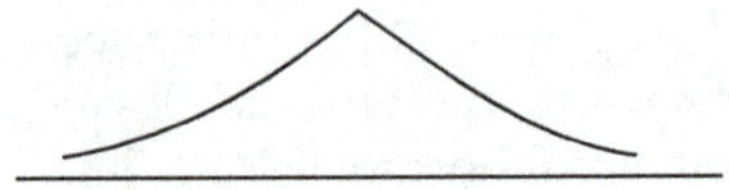 Medium pitch, medium expirations
Bronchial	Heard only over trachea; high pitch; loud and long expirations	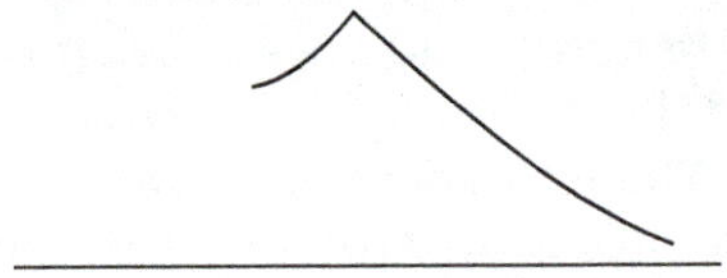 High pitch, loud expirations

Source: Adapted from Hagler DA, and Traver GA. 2002. Respiratory system. In *Mosby's Clinical Nursing*, 5th ed. Thompson JM, et al., eds. Philadelphia, PA: Mosby, 156. Reprinted by permission.[25]

Bronchovesicular Breath Sounds

Bronchovesicular sounds demonstrate an inspiration and an expiration that are equal in quality, intensity, pitch, and duration. Louder than vesicular but less intense than bronchial sounds, bronchovesicular sounds are normally found over the manubrium and intrascapular regions.

Adventitious Sounds

Adventitious breath sounds are usually a sign of disease and may be superimposed on normal breath sounds. Auscultation shortly after birth frequently demonstrates adventitious sounds resulting from the presence of fetal lung fluid. Adventitious sounds heard at the onset of inspiration are more likely to result from secretions in the larger airways; sounds heard at the end of inspiration represent distal disease. Take care to distinguish sounds arising in the lungs from those arising in the upper airway. Placing the stethoscope over the infant's nose and mouth helps to localize upper airway sounds. Suctioning will often clear the upper airway and assist in identifying the presence of referred sounds. Table 7.3 summarizes some adventitious breath sounds.

Crackles

Crackles are defined as a series of brief crackling or bubbling sounds, arising from a sudden release of energy—either an airway popping open or a liquid film breaking. In the past, this type of sound has also been referred to as *rales*.

Fine crackles can be simulated by rubbing together a lock of hair. These sounds commonly originate in the alveoli in the dependent lobes of the lung and are usually heard at the end of inspiration. Frequently heard in the first few hours after birth, fine crackles are also associated with RDS and chronic lung disease (CLD).

Medium crackles sound similar to the fizz of a carbonated drink. Believed to originate in the bronchioles, these sounds are associated with the passage of air through sticky surfaces, such as those found with pneumonia, pulmonary congestion, or transient tachypnea of the newborn.

Coarse crackles are loud and bubbly. These sounds are associated with significant accumulations of mucus or fluid in the larger airways.

Rhonchi

When distinguished from wheezes, rhonchi are described as lower in pitch. They are more musical in quality than crackles.

TABLE 7.3: ADVENTITIOUS BREATH SOUNDS

SOUND/CHARACTERISTICS	SIMULATION	PICTORIAL FINDINGS
Crackles: Discrete, noncontinuous sounds, sudden energy release		
Fine crackles (rales): High-pitched, discrete, noncontinuous crackling sounds heard during end of inspiration (indicates inflammation or congestion) (RDS)	Lock of hair	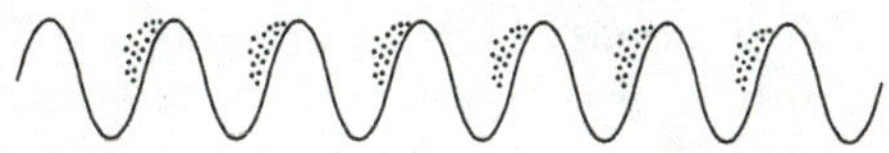
Medium crackles (rales): Lower, moister sound heard during midstage of inspiration; not cleared by a cough (edema, pneumonia)	Fizzy drink	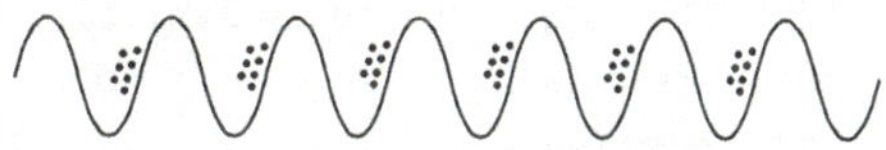
Coarse crackles (rales): Loud, bubbly noise heard during inspiration; not cleared by a cough		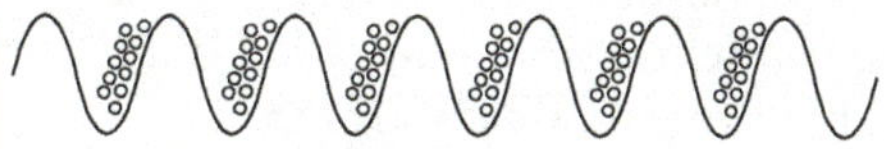
Rhonchi: Loud, low, coarse sound like a snore heard at any point of inspiration or expiration; coughing may clear sound (usually means mucus or foreign body in trachea or large bronchi)		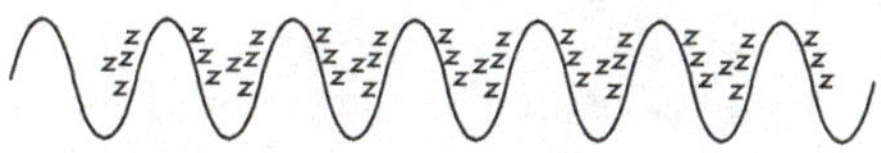
Wheeze: Musical noise sounding like a squeak; may be heard during inspiration or expiration; usually louder during expiration (CLD)		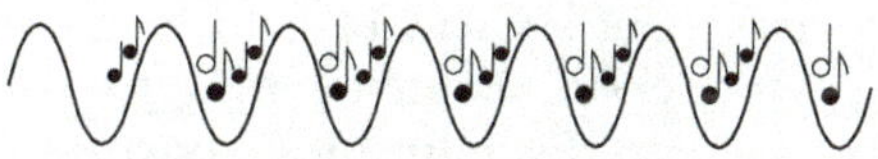
Pleural friction rub: Dry rubbing or grating sound, usually due to inflammation of pleural surfaces; heard during inspiration or expiration; loudest over lower lateral anterior surface (mechanical ventilation in RDS)	Rubbing cupped hand	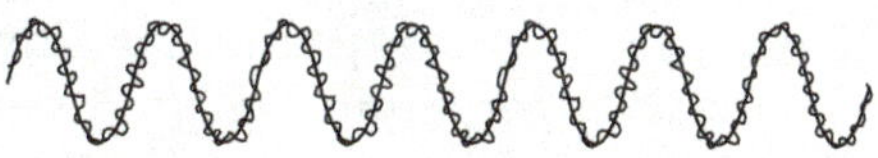

CLD, chronic lung disease; RDS, respiratory distress syndrome.

Source: Adapted from Hagler DA, and Traver GA. 2002. Respiratory system. In *Mosby's Clinical Nursing*, 5th ed. Thompson JM, et al., eds. Philadelphia, PA: Mosby, 156. Reprinted by permission.[25]

Rhonchi are seldom described in the neonate but may be heard when either secretions or aspirated foreign matter is present in the large airways.

Wheezes

Also referred to as *high-pitched rhonchi,* wheezes may be heard on inspiration or expiration, but are usually louder on expiration. Seldom heard in the newborn, wheezes may be audible in the infant with CLD because of narrowing of the airways or the presence of bronchospasm.

Rubs

Rubs can be simulated by holding a cupped hand to the ear and rubbing a finger over the cupped hand. Rubs are usually associated with inflammation of the pleura; however, in the neonate, this sound is frequently described during mechanical ventilation.

Stridor

Stridor is a high-pitched, hoarse sound produced at the larynx or upper airways during inspiration or expiration. In a newborn, this sound indicates a partial obstruction of the airway and should be investigated promptly. Stridor may also be heard post extubation in infants with edema of the upper airway.

Bowel sounds are occasionally auscultated over the lung fields. These may be referred sounds transmitted from the abdomen. If these sounds persist over the lung fields, especially on the left side, diaphragmatic hernia should be considered.

PERCUSSION

The small size of the neonatal chest relative to the examiner's hands makes percussion of limited value as a part of the neonatal physical examination. The infant's chest is normally hyperresonant because of the thin chest wall. The experienced examiner may find percussion useful in distinguishing between air and fluid or solid tissue in cases in which the infant is in distress and a pneumothorax, pleural effusion, or diaphragmatic hernia is suspected.

The technique for percussion involves placing one finger firmly against the chest wall and tapping that finger with the index finger of the other hand (see Figure 1.2).

A change in resonance indicates a change in the consistency of the underlying tissue.

PALPATION

After a thorough inspection of the chest, auscultation of breath sounds, and percussion, if necessary, the examiner next palpates certain areas of the infant's chest.

Clavicle

The clavicle is the bone most commonly fractured during the birth process, occurring in 0.2% to 2.9% of all live births.[26] Palpate the entire length of the clavicles. Suspect fracture if crepitus, swelling, or tenderness is present. An infant with a fractured clavicle may also demonstrate an incomplete Moro reflex on the affected side (Chapter 12). Absence of one or both clavicles results in hypermobile shoulders and is a feature of cleidocranial dysplasia, a rare genetic condition affecting teeth and bones. Other chest deformities may also be present in this condition.[27,28]

Breast Tissue

As indicated in the discussion of inspection, the breast buds should be gently palpated to determine the presence of hypertrophy, fissures, secretions, or masses.

Sternum and Ribs

Palpate the sternum and the ribs for crepitus or masses. Crepitus may indicate subcutaneous air from an underlying pulmonary air leak. A lump or mass should be investigated for the presence of an underlying fracture. The tip of the cartilaginous xiphoid process often protrudes anteriorly and may be movable with slight pressure.

Overall Structure

Palpate the costal cartilage between the ribs to assess for hypertrophy. The costal cartilages enlarge in rickets and can be palpated as a series of small lumps down the side of the sternum. This phenomenon is known as the *rachitic rosary*.[18]

TRANSILLUMINATION

Transillumination is a useful adjunct to physical examination when a pneumothorax is suspected. Place a high-intensity fiberoptic light source perpendicular to the neonate's chest. While moving the light source back and forth from side to side, compare the amount of transillumination between the left and right and the upper and lower aspects of the chest. In a darkened room, air pockets will present with a large halo of light.[29]

Subcutaneous edema or air may result in a false-positive reading. Chest-wall edema, dark skin, tape, and equipment may obscure transillumination and result in a false-negative finding. Diagnoses obtained by transillumination should be confirmed by chest x-ray or lung ultrasound.

ASSESSMENT DURING MECHANICAL VENTILATION

Conventional Ventilation

The use of mechanical ventilation necessitates increased vigilance in all aspects of physical assessment. Pay particular attention to assessing the adequacy and symmetry of chest expansion and auscultating breath sounds. Eliminate water in the ventilator tubing before assessing chest sounds because gas bubbling through water produces referred sounds.

Breath sounds may be altered by the presence of an endotracheal tube (ETT), which effectively narrows the neonate's airway, and by the flow of gases from the ventilator, which may increase turbulence. Wheezes and rubs are more common, and harsh or sandpaper breath sounds are often described in infants receiving mechanical ventilation for RDS. These sounds may result from the forced opening of atelectatic alveoli. Harsh breath sounds may also result from air leaking around the ETT. Listening with the stethoscope over the infant's mouth may be useful in differentiating sounds produced in the larynx from those produced in the chest. Air leaking around the ETT may produce a high-pitched sound heard during inspiration. Table 7.4 outlines some common concerns in the neonate receiving mechanical ventilation.

Patient-Triggered Ventilation

Ventilators that measure tidal volume allow the clinician to assess the neonate's ability to generate a spontaneous breath and to determine the relative size of that breath compared with the size of the breath generated by the ventilator. As the neonate's lung disease improves, larger tidal volumes will be generated, suggesting a readiness for weaning.

Ventilation in which a preset tidal volume is delivered results in breaths that require varying amounts of pressure to deliver the desired volume of gas. As the infant's lung compliance improves, less inspiratory pressure is required to deliver the same amount of volume. By monitoring the pressure used, the clinician can assess changes in the infant's lungs.

High-Frequency Ventilation

High-frequency ventilation techniques require several alterations in the traditional approach to physical assessment of the chest and lungs. The rapid rates used in high-frequency ventilation cause the infant to shake

TABLE 7.4: COMMON FINDINGS IN INFANTS RECEIVING MECHANICAL VENTILATION

FINDING	POSSIBLE CAUSE
Absence of air entry	Pneumothorax, blocked ETT, accidental extubation, space occupying lesion
Decreased or unequal air entry	Atelectasis, pneumothorax, intubation of right bronchus
Asymmetric chest movement	Pneumothorax, intubation of right bronchus
Increased chest excursion	Change in compliance resulting in overventilation
Decreased chest excursion	Underventilation, blocked ETT, accidental extubation, air leak

ETT, endotracheal tube.

or vibrate, making it impractical to count respiratory rates. Many infants on high-frequency ventilation will be apneic; however, spontaneous respirations that do occur can be recorded in the usual fashion.

The chest should be both observed and palpated to assess the symmetry and quality of vibrations. Excessive movement of the chest or abdomen may indicate overventilation. Decreased or asymmetric movement may indicate complications such as air leak or airway obstruction.

Breath sounds during high-frequency ventilation will be high pitched, with a jackhammer quality. Auscultation should be performed to assess changes in the pitch or quality of sound. Higher pitched or musical sounds may indicate the presence of secretions. Decreases in pitch may indicate the presence of a pneumothorax. Traditional breath sounds can be assessed during periods of manual ventilation or with sighs given during oscillation.

SUMMARY

The respiratory system undergoes rapid and significant changes during transition to extrauterine life. These changes leave the lungs vulnerable to both transient and more life-threatening maladaptations. Careful scrutiny of the respiratory system is required to identify potential problems requiring treatment. Findings from physical examination of the chest and lungs form the basis for further investigations. Findings should be documented using standard terms and reference points to permit comparison with subsequent assessments.

ADDITIONAL RESOURCES

SPRINGER PUBLISHING CONNECT™	**A robust set of resources designed to supplement this text is located at http://connect.springerpub.com/content/book/978-0-8261-4063-0. Qualifying instructors may request access by emailing textbook@springerpub.com.**

REFERENCES

1. Ball JW, Dains JE, Flynn JA, Solomon BS, and Stewart RW, eds. 2023. Chest and lungs. In *Seidel's Guide to Physical Examination*, 10th ed. Elsevier, 290–325.
2. Gardner SL, Enzman-Hines M, and Nyp M. 2021. Respiratory diseases. In *Merenstein & Gardner's Handbook of Neonatal Intensive Care: An Interprofessional Approach*, 9th ed. Gardner SL, Carter BS, Enzman-Hines M, and Niermeyer S, eds. Elsevier, 729–835.
3. Blackburn ST, ed. 2018. Respiratory system. In *Maternal, Fetal, & Neonatal Physiology: A Clinical Perspective*, 5th ed. Philadelphia: Elsevier, 297–346.
4. Kinghorn B, MacKintonsh EW, and Marshall SG. 2023. Upper airway obstruction. In *Nelson Essentials of Pediatrics*, 9th ed. Marcdante KJ, Kliegman RM, and Schuh AM, eds. Elsevier, 536–539.
5. Silverman WA, and Andersen DH. 1956. A controlled clinical trial of water mist on obstructive respiratory signs, death rate, and necropsy findings among premature infants. *Pediatrics* 17(1): 1–10.
6. Martin RJ. 2017. Control of ventilation. In *Assisted Ventilation of the Neonate*, 6th ed. Goldsmith JP, Karotkin EH, Keszler M, and Suresh GK, eds. Philadelphia: Elsevier, 31–35.
7. Gauda EB, and Martin RJ. 2018. Control of breathing. In *Avery's Diseases of the Newborn*, 10th ed. Gleason CA, and Juul SE, eds. Elsevier, 600–617.
8. Ahlfeld SK. 2020. Respiratory tract disorders. In *Nelson Textbook of Pediatrics*, 21st ed. Kliegman RM, St Geme JW, Blum NJ, Shah SS, Tasker RC, and Wilson KM, eds. Elsevier, 929–949.e1.
9. Anbalagan S, and Mendez MD. 2022, January. Neonatal abstinence syndrome. [Updated 2022 May 1]. In: *StatPearls* [Internet]. Treasure Island, FL: StatPearls Publishing. https://www.ncbi.nlm.nih.gov/books/NBK551498/
10. Kenner C. 2020. Fetal development: Environmental influences and critical periods. In *Comprehensive Neonatal Nursing Care*, 6th ed. Kenner C, Altimier L, and Boykova M, eds. New York, NY: Springer Publishing Company, 1–20.
11. Diu MW, and Walker KK. 2022. Pediatric diseases. In *Stoelting's Anesthesia and Co-existing Disease*, 8th ed. Hines RL, and Jones SB, eds. Elsevier, 663–696.
12. Ball, JW, Dains JE, Flynn JA, Solomon BS, and Stewart RW, eds. 2023. Growth and nutrition. In *Seidel's Guide to Physical Examination*, 10th ed. Elsevier, 110–132.
13. Di Fiore JM, and Carlo WA. 2020. Assessment of neonatal pulmonary function. In *Fanaroff and Martin's Neonatal-Perinatal Medicine*, 11th ed. Martin RJ, Fanaroff AA, and Walsh MC, eds. Elsevier, 1143–1158.

14. Tappero E. 2021. Physical assessment. In *Core Curriculum for Neonatal Intensive Care Nursing*, 6th ed. Verklan, MT, Walden M, and Forest S, eds. Elsevier, 99–130.
15. Fraser D. 2022. Assessment of the neonate. In *Goldsmith's Assisted Ventilation of the Neonate*, 7th ed. Keszler M, and Gautham KS, eds. Elsevier, 384–396.
16. Scott O, Stutz C, and Lake A. 2022. Disorders of the upper extremity. In *Tachdjian's Pediatric Orthopaedics*, 6th ed. Herring JA, ed. Elsevier, 300–421.
17. Going JJ, Fillmore EP, and Geddes D. 2021. Chest wall and breast. In *Gray's Anatomy*. Standring S, ed. Elsevier, 997–1019e3.
18. Greenbaum LA. 2020. Vitamin D deficiency (Rickets) and excess. In *Nelson Textbook of Pediatrics*, 21st ed. Kliegman RM, St Geme JW, Blum NJ, Shah SS, Tasker RC, and Wilson KM, eds. Elsevier, 375–385.
19. Fanaroff AA, Lissauer T, and Fanaroff JM. 2020. Physical growth: Physical examination of the newborn infant and the physical environment. In *Klaus and Fanaroff's Care of the High-Risk Neonate*, 7th ed. Fanaroff AA, and Fanaroff JM, eds. Elsevier, 58–79.e2.
20. Lopez VL, and Graziano PD. 2020. The neonatal physical exam. In *Neonatal Nurse Practitioner Certification Intensive Review*. Kohen AR, ed. Springer, 27–57.
21. Schechter M, and Rhim HJH. 2021. The pediatric patient. In *Textbook of Physical Diagnosis: History and Examination*, 8th ed. Swartz MH, ed. Elsevier, 535–600.
22. Styne DM. 2020. Physiology and disorders of puberty. In *Williams Textbook of Endocrinology*, 14th ed. Melmed S, Auchus RJ, Goldfine AB, Koenig RJ, and Rosen CJ, eds. Elsevier, 1023–1164.
23. Abidi NY, and Martin KL. 2020. Cutaneous defects. In *Nelson Textbook of Pediatrics*, 21st ed. Kliegman RM, St Geme JW, Blum NJ, Shah SS, Tasker RC, and Wilson KM, eds. Elsevier, 3456–3459.
24. Walker, VP. 2018. Newborn evaluation. In *Avery's Diseases of the Newborn*, 10th ed. Gleason CA, and Juul SE, eds. Elsevier, 289–311.
25. Hagler DA, and Traver GA. 2002. Respiratory system. In *Mosby's Clinical Nursing*, 5th ed. Thompson JM, McFarland GK, Hirsch JE, and Tucker SM, eds. Philadelphia: Mosby, 156.
26. Högberg U, Fellman V, Thiblin I, Karlsson R, and Wester K. 2020. Difficult birth is the main contributor to birth-related fracture and accidents to other neonatal fractures. *Acta Paediatrica* 109(10): 2040–2048. doi: 10.1111/apa.15217
27. Jirapinyo C, Deraje V, Huang G, Gue S, Anderson PJ, and Moore MH. 2020. Cleidocranial dysplasia: Management of the multiple craniofacial and skeletal anomalies. *The Journal of Craniofacial Surgery* 31(4): 908–911. doi: 10.1097/SCS.0000000000006306
28. Haddad GG, and Green TP. 2016. Diagnostic approach to respiratory disease. In *Nelson Textbook of Pediatrics*, 20th ed. Kliegman RM, Stanton BFMD, St. Geme J, and Schor NF, eds. Philadelphia: Elsevier Saunders, 1993–1998.
29. Kirkegaard E, and Damkjær, M. 2019. Transillumination—et diagnostisk værktøj ved neonatal pneumothorax. *Ugeskrift for Laeger* 181(29): V70439.

8 CARDIOVASCULAR ASSESSMENT

Lyn Vargo

Cardiovascular assessment of the newborn requires great skill in the techniques of inspection, palpation, and auscultation. Inspection of the general activity of the neonate, breathing patterns, presence or absence of cyanosis, and activity of the precordium are all important. Palpation of pulses, apical impulse, and thrills is also imperative. Auscultation, however, is the main focus of the cardiovascular examination. Through auscultation, the examiner assesses heart rate, rhythm, regularity, and heart sounds (especially murmurs). A pediatric or neonatal stethoscope with a diaphragm and a bell is very helpful for auscultation. The bell conducts sound without distortion (although it can be difficult to maintain an airtight seal). The bell is useful for low-pitched sounds. If properly sized, the diaphragm maintains its own seal and is useful for high-pitched sounds.

The dynamic properties of the newborn heart make cardiovascular assessment of the neonate challenging. The change from "fetal-placental" to "newborn-lung" circuitry means that the findings of the cardiovascular examination constantly change over the first few hours, days, and weeks of life. Those performing cardiovascular assessments must be aware of these alterations and their timing and incorporate this knowledge into their examinations.

Because changes in ductal flow, decreasing pulmonary vascular resistance (PVR), and increasing systemic vascular resistance occur over the first few hours and days of life, cardiovascular assessments ideally should be done shortly after birth, again at 6 to 12 hours of age, then at 1 and 3 days of age, and at regular intervals thereafter. Because this is rarely possible in the normal newborn, it is recommended that, at a minimum, examinations be done shortly after birth, at 1 day of age, and at regular pediatric office visits thereafter.

REVIEWING MATERNAL, FAMILY, AND BIRTH HISTORIES

The first step in a complete cardiovascular assessment is a thorough maternal history. Several maternal conditions can affect the neonate's cardiovascular system. These include maternal diabetes, systemic lupus erythematosus, and a maternal history of congenital heart disease (CHD). Maternal diabetes can increase the risk for CHD in the neonate to 3 to 4 times that of the general population.[1] The prevalence of CHD (for truncus arteriosus, ventricular septal defects [VSDs], atrial septal defects [ASDs], coarctation of the aorta [coarc], D-transposition of the great arteries [TGA], tetralogy of Fallot [TET], Ebstein anomaly, interrupted aortic arch, pulmonary atresia with intact septum, tricuspid atresia, total anomalous pulmonary venous return, double-outlet right ventricle, atrioventricular [AV] canal, and hypoplastic left heart syndrome [HLHS]) in national estimates for the United States between 1998 and 2005 was about 81.4/10,000 live births.[2] Septal defects (VSDs and ASDs), conotruncal abnormalities (transposition of the great arteries [TGA], truncus arteriosus, single ventricle [SV], and coarc), and dextrocardia are common defects seen in infants of diabetic mothers. There is also a specific cardiomyopathy, called *hypertrophic cardiomyopathy*, a thickening of the heart muscle, that is commonly found in infants of diabetic mothers.[3]

Systemic lupus erythematosus in the mother has been shown to increase the incidence of congenital complete AV block in the neonate.[4] These infants present with low resting heart rates, sometimes while in utero.

As patients with CHD are living longer and reaching childbearing age, new information has become available. It has been documented that there is up to a 15% risk for CHD in the offspring of birthing mothers with CHD.[5] Even though only a small percentage of CHD can be related to environmental factors, a history of the pregnancy (especially of the first 2 months, when the heart is forming) is important. Environmental factors known to increase the risk of congenital heart defects are listed in Table 8.1.[6] Drugs associated with congenital heart defects include amphetamines, alcohol, anticonvulsants (hydantoins, trimethadione, valproic acid, lithium, retinoic acid, angiotensin-converting enzymes), and possibly estrogen and progesterone.[5] In addition, viral infections during the latter part of pregnancy may cause myocarditis in the neonate.

Because of the influence of genetic factors, family history is an important feature of a cardiovascular assessment.[7] The examiner must gather details about other siblings with CHD. If one parent is affected or if an older sibling had a specific defect, there is a 3% to 5% risk for recurrence.[8] Approximately 30% of CHD occurs in association with a chromosomal or single gene disorder. The other 70% is likely to have a genetic component that is not yet identified (Table 8.2).[9]

Details of the labor and delivery history are also important to the cardiovascular examination. Knowledge of any causal factors, such as perinatal hypoxia, maternal infection, or drugs given to the mother during labor, will help the examiner determine whether CHD is a likely explanation for abnormal physical findings.

Finally, birth weight, gestational age, and gender must be taken into consideration. There is an increased incidence of CHD in low-birthweight infants, and premature infants have an increased risk for patent ductus arteriosus (PDA). Several congenital

TABLE 8.1: ENVIRONMENTAL FACTORS ASSOCIATED WITH CONGENITAL HEART DEFECTS

TERATOGENIC INFLUENCE	RISK OF CARDIAC DEFECT (%)	COMMON TYPES OF DEFECTS
Maternal rubella	35	PDA, PPS, and septal defects
Maternal diabetes	3 to 5	VSD, coarc, and complete transposition
Maternal phenylketonuria	25 to 50	TET
Systemic lupus erythematosus	20 to 40	Complete heart block
Maternal alcohol abuse	25 to 30	Septal defects
Hydantoin	2 to 3	Pulmonary and AS, coarc, and PDA
Lithium	10 to 20	Ebstein malformation, TA, and ASD
Retinoic acid	-	Defects of ventricular outflow tracts
Trimethadione	15 to 30	TET, complete transposition, and HLHS

AS, aortic stenosis; ASD, atrial septal defect; coarc, coarctation of the aorta; HLHS, hypoplastic left heart syndrome; PDA, patent ductus arteriosus; PPS, peripheral pulmonary artery stenosis; TA, tricuspid atresia; TET, tetralogy of Fallot; VSD, ventricular septal defect.

Source: Adapted from Burn J. 2002. The aetiology of congenital heart disease. In *Paediatric Cardiology*, 2nd ed. Anderson RH, et al., eds. New York, NY: Churchill Livingstone, 151. Reprinted by permission.[6]

TABLE 8.2: DISORDERS ASSOCIATED WITH CONGENITAL HEART DEFECTS

DISORDER	PATIENTS WITH CARDIAC DISEASE (%)	TYPES OF CARDIAC ABNORMALITIES
De Lange syndrome	30	VSD, ASD, PDA, AS, and EFE
Holt–Oram heart–hand syndrome	75	ASD-2, VSD or PDA in 2/3, conduction block, HLHS, TAPVC, and truncus arteriosus
Marfan syndrome	Up to 100	Aortic aneurysm, AR, MR, TR, and prolapse
Noonan syndrome	50 to 80	PS/dysplasia, hypertrophic cardiomyopathy, PDA, and coarc
Carpenter syndrome	29	PDA, PS, VSD, TET, TGA, ASD, and dextrocardia
Ellis van Creveld	80 to 90	ASD
Mucopolysaccharidosis type 1	50 to 60	Single atrium, primum ASD, coarc, and HLHS
Trisomy 21 (Down syndrome)	40 to 50	AV canal, VSD, PDA, ASD-1 and ASD-2, and TET
Trisomy 18 (Edwards syndrome)	90 to 100	VSD, polyvalvular disease, ASD, and PDA
Trisomy 13 (Patau syndrome)	80	PDA, VSD, ASD, coarc, AS, and PS
XO (Turner syndrome)	>50	Coarc, bicuspid aortic valve, aortic aneurysm, AS, and VSD
Beckwith–Wiedemann syndrome	15 (estimated)	Hypertrophic cardiomegaly, ASD, VSD, PDA, and TET
CHARGE association	44	TET, DORV, ASD, VSD, PDA, and PS
DiGeorge syndrome	>50	Interrupted aortic arch, TA, TET, and right aortic arch
VACTERL association	10	VSD, ASD, and TET
Williams–Beuren syndrome	75	Supravalvar AS, stenosis of left coronary artery, small aorta, multiple pulmonary arteries, cerebral and renal arteries, mitral valve prolapse, ASD, VSD, and MR
Cleft lip and palate	25	VSD, PDA, TGA, TET, and SV
Diaphragmatic hernia	25	TET

(*continued*)

TABLE 8.2: DISORDERS ASSOCIATED WITH CONGENITAL HEART DEFECTS (*continued*)

DISORDER	PATIENTS WITH CARDIAC DISEASE (%)	TYPES OF CARDIAC ABNORMALITIES
Omphalocele	20	TET, ASD
Intestinal atresia	10	VSD
Renal agenesis unilateral/ bilateral	17/75	VSD

AR, aortic regurgitation; AS, aortic stenosis; ASD, atrial septal defect; ASD-1, primum atrial septal defect; ASD-2, secundum atrial septal defect; AV, atrioventricular; CHARGE, coloboma, heart defect, atresia choanae, growth retardation, genital anomalies, ear abnormalities; coarc, coarctation of the aorta; DORV, double outlet right ventricle; EFE, endocardial fibroelastosis; HLHS, hypoplastic left heart syndrome; MR, mitral regurgitation; PDA, patent ductus arteriosus; PS, pulmonic stenosis; SV, single ventricle; TAPVC, total anomalous pulmonary venous connection; TET, tetralogy of Fallot; TGA, transposition of the great arteries; TR, tricuspid regurgitation; VSD, ventricular septal defect.

Source: Adapted from Blundell DF, Jones C, and Crossland. 2021. Structural cardiac disease and cardiomyopathies In *Avery's & MacDonald's Neonatology: Pathophysiology and Management of the Newborn*, 8th ed. Boardman JP, Groves AM, and Ramasethu J, eds. Philadelphia, PA: Wolters Kluwer, 461–462.

heart defects are more common in one gender than in the other.

OBSERVING APPEARANCE AND BEHAVIOR

Because of the central role the heart plays, a complete cardiovascular assessment encompasses most of the other systems. The cardiovascular examination cannot be considered in isolation from the neurologic, respiratory, abdominal, and skin examination.

The initial cardiovascular assessment of the neonate should include general observation of the infant's overall appearance and behavior. A newborn with CHD may exhibit decreased activity and/or appear flaccid. Notation of extracardiac anomalies is important because CHD is associated with such abnormalities in approximately 25% of infants.[10] Increased incidence of CHD is seen with neurologic and gastrointestinal anomalies, tracheoesophageal fistulas, renal irregularities, and diaphragmatic hernia.[5]

INSPECTING SKIN AND MUCOUS MEMBRANES

The next step in the neonatal cardiovascular examination is inspection of the infant's color. Accurate assessment of skin color depends on the observer's astuteness and on ambient temperature and lighting conditions.[11] A cyanotic Caucasian infant may look pink under bright lighting, and a centrally pink infant may look cyanotic under dim lighting. In a well-lit room, the infant should be centrally pink—that is, not only should the infant's general color appear pink, but the lips, tongue, earlobes, and (in males) scrotum should also appear pink. The best indicator to use to determine central cyanosis is generally the tongue and lips due to the rich vascular supply and lack of pigmentation. Sometimes detecting cyanosis can be difficult especially if the infant is cold or has polycythemia. However, the wide availability of pulse oximetry allows for rapid identification of an infant with true cyanosis.[3,5]

Polycythemia

Many infants appear pink at rest but become deep red to purplish with crying. This is usually related to polycythemia, a condition found when the infant's central hematocrit is greater than 65%. Although polycythemic/plethoric infants may appear cyanotic, as neonates, they rarely are. The ruddy or reddish color may be mistaken for cyanosis simply because newborns who have increased amounts of hemoglobin usually have a larger percentage of that hemoglobin unsaturated. This unsaturated hemoglobin masks the saturated hemoglobin, and the infants appear purplish in color.

Cyanosis

Central cyanosis refers to the bluish color of the skin, lips, tongue, earlobes, scrotum (in males), and nail beds seen in the neonate with significant arterial oxygen desaturation. Central cyanosis becomes visible when there are at least 5 g of hemoglobin not bound to oxygen/100 mL of blood.[9] Central cyanosis must be differentiated from peripheral cyanosis (acrocyanosis), which is blue color in the hands and feet, and circumoral cyanosis, which is blue color around the mouth. Peripheral cyanosis is normal in newborns until about 2 days of age and is thought to be caused by vasomotor instability. No treatment is necessary for peripheral cyanosis. When determining whether cyanosis is central or peripheral, check the infant's arterial saturation via a pulse oximeter.[5] Central cyanosis is difficult to detect unless the arterial desaturation is less than or equal to approximately 85% in an infant with a normal hemoglobin level.[5]

Cyanosis is one of the two best indicators of CHD (symptoms of congestive heart failure is the other). Central cyanosis can also be the result of lung disease, sepsis, persistent pulmonary hypertension, or neurologic disease. It is therefore important to carefully assess cyanosis and the infant's response to oxygen. Cyanosis that does not improve with administration of 100% oxygen or that increases with crying is most likely the result of a cardiac cause.[12]

Pallor/Mottling/Perfusion

Pallor and mottling of the skin should also be considered in assessing cardiac status, as should the infant's general overall perfusion. Infants with a compromised cardiac status may appear pale as a result of vasoconstriction and shunting of blood away from the skin to more vital organs. Mottling, if present, must be evaluated with any other signs and symptoms associated with it. It may be a sign of cardiogenic shock when associated with hypovolemia or decreased cardiac output. Mottling can also be seen in normal infants under certain circumstances, such as in the stressed or cold neonate, when it is then referred to as *cutis marmorata*. A hypoxic, anemic infant may not appear cyanotic because hemoglobin levels may be too low to produce a bluish color.[5,13]

Capillary filling time can give valuable information about the infant's cardiac perfusion to the skin and should be determined by pressing a finger against the infant's skin in both a central and a peripheral area. When blanching is noted, the examiner counts the seconds required for the color to return to the skin once the pressure is released. Capillary filling time of greater than 3 seconds is considered abnormal.[13]

Edema

In the infant, unlike in older patients, edema is rarely associated with cardiac problems. Isolated peripheral edema is a hallmark sign of Turner syndrome, however. Infants with this syndrome show a high incidence of coarctation of the aorta.

OBSERVING BREATHING PATTERNS

Respiratory activity must be observed in relation to the cardiac examination. Respiratory rate and effort should be documented (as addressed in Chapter 7). Signs of respiratory distress—such as grunting, nasal flaring, retractions, tachypnea, and crackles—may be signs of congestive heart failure. It is also important to keep in mind that a cyanotic infant with nonlabored respiratory effort may be cyanotic as a result of a congenital heart defect that restricts pulmonary blood flow.[14] Nonlabored tachypnea that occurs with central cyanosis is a result of a hypoxic respiratory drive.[12]

PALPATING PERIPHERAL PULSES

The character of the peripheral pulses should be assessed next. This is best done when the infant is quiet. Pulse rate, rhythm, volume, and character should all be examined. Pulses represent an approximate determination of cardiac output. The axillary, palmar, brachial, radial, femoral, popliteal, posterior tibial, and dorsalis pedis may be palpated using the index finger (Figures 8.1–8.4). (Note that the dorsalis pedis pulse may not be felt in newborns; this is considered normal.)

Pulse Rate/Rhythm

On initial palpation, the pulse rate should be noted. The significance of rate is discussed in

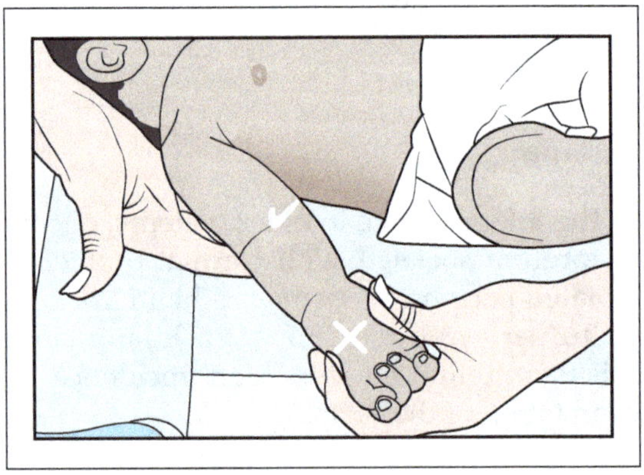

FIGURE 8.1 Radial and brachial pulses. Demonstrates the location of radial pulse (X), palpable on the flexor surface of the wrist just medial to the distal end of the radius. Demonstrates the location of the brachial pulse (✓) in and above the groove of the elbow, medial to the biceps muscle and tendon

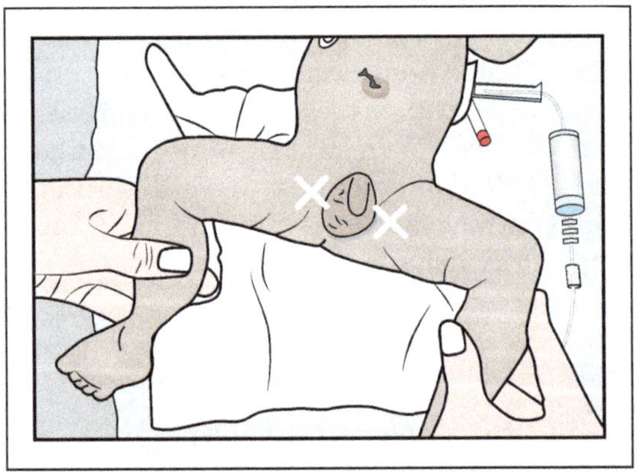

FIGURE 8.2 Femoral pulses. Demonstrates the location of the femoral pulses (X), palpable just below the inguinal ligament, an equal distance between the pubic tubercle and the anterior superior iliac spine

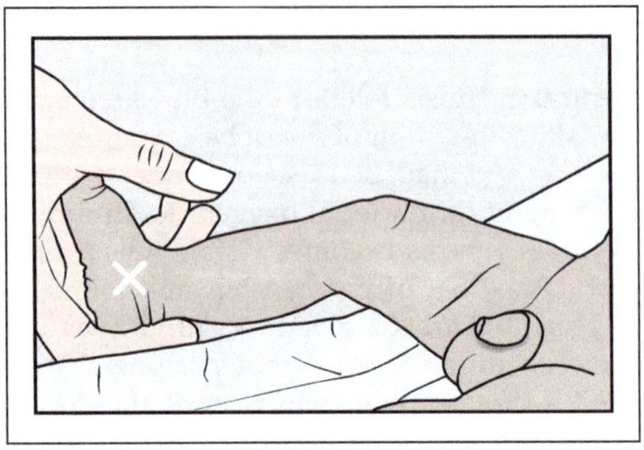

FIGURE 8.3 Posterior tibial pulse. Demonstrates the location of the posterior tibial pulse (X), palpable just behind and slightly below the medial malleolus

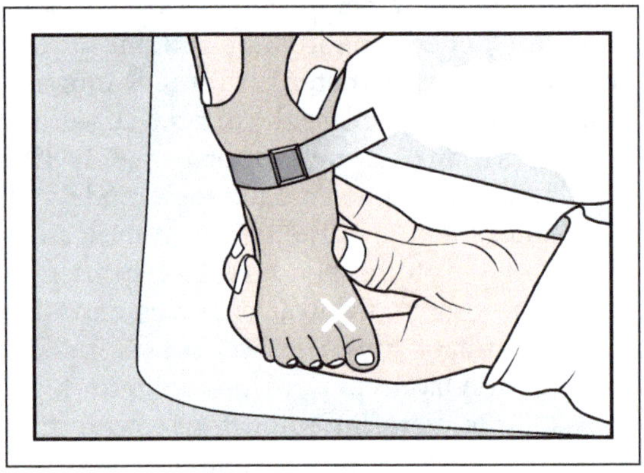

FIGURE 8.4 Dorsalis pedis pulse. Demonstrates the location of the dorsalis pedis pulse (X), palpable on the dorsum of the foot by following an imaginary line that traces the groove between the first and second toes

the Heart Rate section. After determining the rate, document any irregularities in rhythm or any skipped beats. A pulse deficit (the difference between the heart rate counted by auscultation and that counted with a pulse) is frequently seen with ectopic rhythms.

Pulse Volume/Character

Probably the most important determinations in neonatal pulse evaluation are those assessing volume and character. Volume of peripheral pulses is assessed on a scale of 0 to +3, with +3 being the strongest and 0 representing an absent or nonpalpable pulse. Pulses can be classified in the following way[15]:

- 3+ = Bounding
- 2+ = Brisk or normally palpated
- 1+ = Diminished or weaker than expected
- 0 = Absent or unable to palpate

It is imperative that the femoral and brachial pulses should be palpated bilaterally, and then one femoral and the right brachial should be palpated simultaneously.[5,12] (The right brachial should be palpated instead of the left because the right subclavian artery is always preductal, but the left subclavian artery may or may not be preductal.). Absent or weak femoral pulses or a brachial femoral delay—especially in comparison to the right brachial pulse—are abnormal and may indicate decreased aortic blood flow such as is seen with coarctation of the aorta, aortic stenosis (AS), interrupted aortic arch, and HLHS.[14]

Bounding pulses in any extremity should be noted. Bounding pulses are usually present with PDA and other aortic-runoff lesions (truncus arteriosus, aortic regurgitation (AR), and systemic arteriovenous fistula).[5,12] Typically it is easy to palpate peripheral pulses, in premature infants, but strong palmar or digital pulses indicate a wide pulse pressure such as that seen with PDA.[16] Weak or absent peripheral pulses occur in the presence of low cardiac output from any cause (e.g., shock and cardiac tamponade), but also occur in lesions with decreased systemic blood flow that rely on the ductus arteriosus for systemic blood flow, such as hypoplastic left ventricle.[17,18]

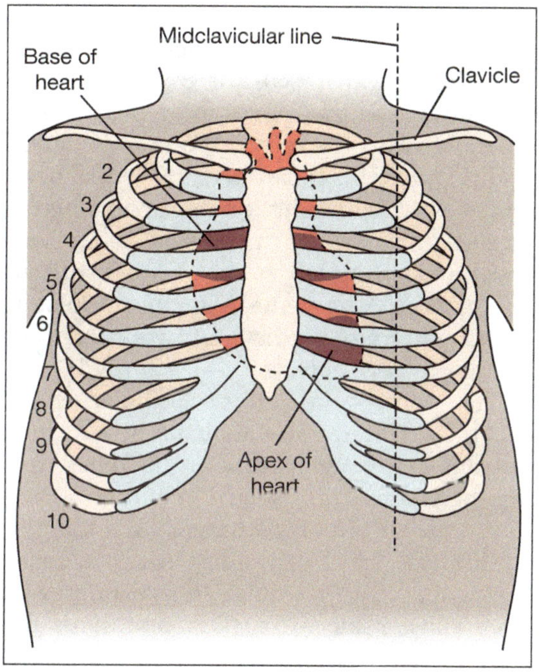

FIGURE 8.5 Position of the heart within the chest cavity and base and apex of the heart

INSPECTING AND PALPATING THE CHEST

Precordium

In the cardiac examination, assessment of the chest should begin with inspection of the precordium, the area on the anterior chest under which the heart lies (Figure 8.5). Generally, except during the first few hours of life, the precordium of a term neonate should be quiet. During the first few hours of life, there may be a visible impulse noted along the lower left sternal border in normal newborns because of the right ventricular predominance common to transitional circulation. As the transitional circulatory pattern changes, this sign will generally disappear in the normal newborn. The presence of a bounding or hyperactive precordium in a term neonate after the first hours of life is characteristic of heart disease, typically defects with increased ventricular volume, such as left-to-right shunt lesions (PDA or large VSD), or severe valvular regurgitation such as seen with mitral or aortic insufficiency.[5,18] Premature infants may be more likely to appear to have an active precordium because they have less subcutaneous tissue than the term newborn.

Apical Impulse

After general assessment of the precordium, the examiner should inspect for position and character of the apical impulse, the forward thrust of the left ventricle during systole. The apical impulse is usually seen in the neonate in the fourth intercostal space, either at or to the left of the midclavicular line (Figure 8.5). It can be further localized and examined with light palpation using the fingertips. An apical impulse placed downward and to the left suggests left ventricular dilation. A very sharp apical impulse is found with high cardiac output or left ventricular hypertrophy.

The point of maximum impulse (PMI) and the apical impulse are usually the same, but this is not always true in neonates during the first few hours to days of life. During that time, an impulse stronger than the apical impulse can be found in the fifth intercostal space at the lower sternal border or even substernally. This then represents the PMI and is normal because of the right ventricular predominance found in the newborn (Figure 8.6). The PMI or the apical impulse may be displaced in several situations, such as dextrocardia, tension pneumothorax, and diaphragmatic hernia.

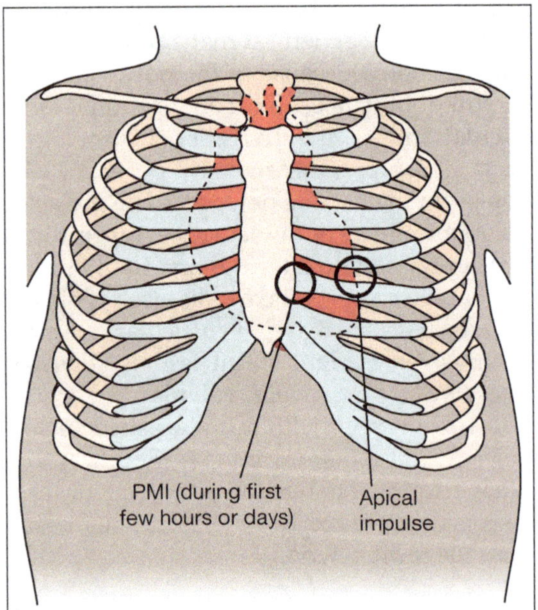

FIGURE 8.6 Areas of cardiac inspection and palpation

PMI, point of maximum impulse.

Heaves, Taps, and Thrills

Further palpation of the precordium may yield other valuable information. Heaves, taps, and thrills can all be palpated. These findings are usually best felt by palpating with the portion of the palm at the base of the fingers rather than with the fingertips. This is because certain parts of the hand are more discriminatory than others for specific sensations. Vibratory sensations are best felt with the ulnar surface of the hand.

A heave (or lift) is a PMI that is slow rising and diffuse. Heaves are associated with volume overload.[5]

A sharp, well-localized PMI is called a *tap*. Taps are usually associated with pressure overload.[5] Thrills are low-frequency, palpable murmurs that feel similar to touching a purring cat. On the chest they are best felt with the palm of the hand; a thrill is felt best with the fingertips when it is in the suprasternal notch or over a carotid artery. A thrill denotes a loud murmur (at least a Grade IV murmur). In the neonate, thrills are not common. When present, they can provide useful information about cardiac problems. A thrill in the upper left sternal border originates from the pulmonary valve or pulmonary artery and may be associated with pulmonary stenosis, or rarely, a PDA.[5]

AUSCULTATING TO ASSESS CARDIOVASCULAR STATUS

Expert auscultation of the neonatal heart requires much practice over time. An experienced mentor can help the fledgling examiner learn to identify and distinguish heart sounds. The neonatal heart should be auscultated with the infant inactive and quiet.

At a minimum, the four traditional auscultatory areas should be examined (Figure 8.7). These are the aortic area (second intercostal space, right sternal angle), pulmonic area (second intercostal space, left sternal angle), tricuspid area (fourth intercostal space, left sternal angle), and mitral area (fourth intercostal space, left midclavicular line). A more thorough examination is recommended,

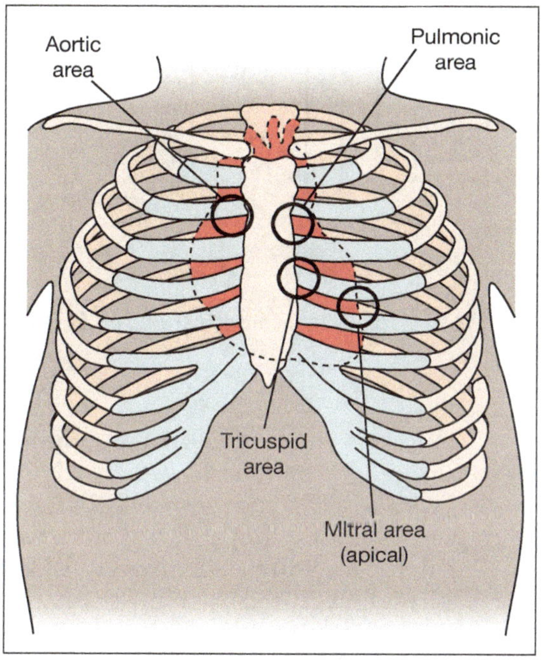

FIGURE 8.7 Four auscultatory areas of the heart

however. It should include the right and left infraclavicular areas, both sides of the back, the right anterior chest, both axillae, the anterior fontanel (examining for cerebral arteriovenous fistulas), and the liver (examining for hepatic arteriovenous fistulas).

Heart Rate

Heart rate should be auscultated first and counted. A term neonate's heart rate at rest should generally be 120 to 140 beats per minute (bpm), although fluctuations above and below these values can be anticipated in a normal newborn. That is, the heart rate may increase to ≥170 bpm with activity or crying, or it may decrease to 70 to 90 bpm in deep sleep.[17] Premature infants have a slightly higher mean heart rate than that seen in term infants.

Sinus bradycardia, or a heart rate less than normal for age (usually <80 bpm), is a common transient finding in both term and premature infants. The reason for this is the predominance of the parasympathetic system. Any stimulus—such as yawning, stooling, or suctioning—may result in vagal stimulation and subsequent bradycardia. These episodes are usually transient, require no treatment, and are self-correcting. Some episodes, especially in premature infants, may require stimulation or treatment of the underlying cause, such as treatment for apnea of prematurity with methylxanthines.

Sinus tachycardia is defined as a heart rate greater than normal for age (usually >180–200 bpm). It is generally considered the most common form of rapid heart rate in the neonate.[19] It normally occurs with any stimulus—such as crying, feeding, fever, or activity—that causes increased demands on the heart. Normally, with removal of the stimulus, the heart rate slowly returns to baseline. Sinus tachycardia rarely requires treatment.

Variation in the heart rate is normal among neonates and is seen as a positive sign of the infant's ability to react to the environment.[19] Infants who do not respond to stimuli with an increase in heart rate are clearly abnormal and should be observed very closely.

Although sinus tachycardia with rates up to 200 bpm can be tolerated by the neonate, sustained heart rates greater than 200 to 220 bpm or supraventricular tachycardia (SVT) cannot. SVT encompasses paroxysmal atrial tachycardia and atrial flutter and fibrillation. Figure 8.8 depicts a rhythm strip of SVT. In the neonate, persistent SVT represents a medical emergency and requires immediate intervention. At such rapid heart rates, cardiac output is extremely compromised because of short diastolic filling time. Without treatment, decreased cardiac output will cause congestive heart failure within 48 hours, and possibly death. Treatment for SVT depends on the cause, but the condition may respond to vagal stimulation (such as applying a cold washcloth or a small plastic bag or glove of ice to the face), medications, or cardioversion.

Cardiac Rhythm and Regularity

After assessing heart rate, evaluate cardiac rhythm and regularity. Listen carefully to the rhythm of the heart sounds and determine whether there is any irregularity. Noting

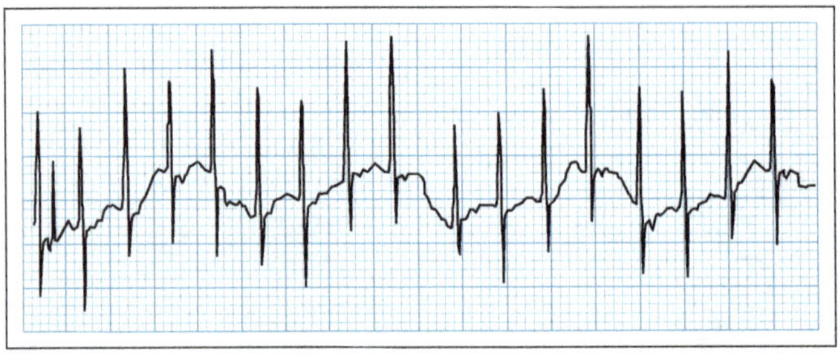

FIGURE 8.8 EKG rhythm strip of infant with supraventricular tachycardia with a ventricular rate of approximately 300 bpm

patterns and frequencies of the irregularity helps identify the type of arrhythmia. Whenever an arrhythmia is suspected, an EKG and/or continuous heart monitoring is indicated to establish a diagnosis. Arrhythmias are not uncommon in neonates. Fortunately, they are usually benign and require no treatment. Those most commonly found in the neonate include the following:

- *Sinus arrhythmia*: This is a very common, normal variant in most newborns. It is associated with respirations.[5] Sinus arrhythmia is characterized by irregularity of the R–R interval, with an otherwise normal cardiac cycle. No treatment is required for this rhythm.
- *Premature atrial contractions*: This arrhythmia is marked by an early beat arising from a supraventricular focus. Ventricular conduction is usually normal. The arrhythmia is almost always benign in the newborn, but can be abnormal when seen with CHD; sepsis; hypoxia; hyperthyroidism; cardiac tumors; myopathies; electrolyte abnormalities; digoxin toxicity; administration of caffeine, atropine, theophylline, or inotropic agents; irritation from a centrally placed catheter; and severe respiratory distress.[20] If significant, the underlying cause may require treatment (especially if related to digitalis toxicity), but these beats are usually well tolerated, and no treatment is indicated.[5]
- *Premature ventricular contractions*: With this early beat arising from an irritable ventricular focus, ventricular conduction will be abnormal, usually giving rise to a wide and bizarre QRS complex. The arrhythmia may result from acidosis, electrolyte abnormality, CHD, or irritation caused by an invasive catheter.[20] Treatment is unnecessary if the phenomenon is infrequent.

Heart Sounds

Traditional cardiac physiology teaches that the first heart sound (S1) is produced by closure of the mitral and tricuspid valves, and the second heart sound (S2) is produced by closure of the aortic and pulmonic valves. More recent literature debates this, however, and the true origin of heart sounds has been found to be the sudden slowing of blood flow following closure of the valves.[12] Despite this, the traditional concept is helpful in conceptualizing and learning to recognize heart sounds and therefore continues to be used.

S1

S1, if thought of as representing closure of the mitral and tricuspid valves at the onset of ventricular systole, should be heard most loudly *at the apex of the heart*, (See Figure 8.5 for the location of the apex and base of the heart.) Indeed, S1 is best heard *at the mitral or tricuspid area* (see Figure 8.7). S1 is usually loud at birth, decreasing in intensity during the first 48 hours of life. Any factor that increases cardiac output also increases the intensity of S1.

Splitting is defined as hearing two distinct components of a heart sound. It is caused by the asynchronous closure of the two valves that create the heart sound. The neonate's rapid heart rate usually makes splitting difficult to distinguish. Although some studies have documented splitting of S1 in the newborn, splitting is not commonly heard; S1 is usually described as being single.

S2

S2, if thought of as representing closure of the aortic and pulmonic valves, should be heard most loudly *at the base of the heart* (see Figure 8.5). Indeed, S2 is best heard *at the aortic or pulmonic area* (see Figure 8.7). S2 is usually single at birth, but by 1 to 2 days of age, splitting of the S2 with the infant's respirations should occur.[5] The trained examiner should be able to recognize, with practice, the splitting of S2 despite the infant's rapid heart rate.

Wide splitting of S2 should be considered abnormal in newborns. It can occur with ASD, pulmonary stenosis, Ebstein anomaly, partial anomalous pulmonary venous return, mitral regurgitation (MR), or right bundle branch block.[5,17]

S3

In addition to S1 and S2, extra heart sounds can potentially be heard in the neonate. Again, because of the infant's rapid heart rate, they may be difficult to distinguish. A third heart sound (S3) can occasionally be heard in infancy; if present, it is best heard *at the apex of the heart during early diastole* (see Figure 8.5). S3 most often signifies rapid or increased flow across the AV valves (rapid ventricular filling) and is commonly heard in premature infants with PDA. Rarely, it can be heard in the newborn with overt congestive heart failure.[21]

S4

A fourth heart sound (S4) should also rarely be heard in neonates. If present, it is heard *at the apex of the heart and is a low-pitched sound of late diastole* (see Figure 8.5). S4 is always pathologic and is heard in conditions characterized by decreased compliance (especially cardiomyopathy) or congestive heart failure.[5,14] The term *decreased compliance* refers to myocardium that is relatively stiff and therefore does not expand well as the blood enters the chambers. This affects the volume of blood that is ejected by the heart with contraction.

Ejection Clicks

Ejection clicks (snappy, high-frequency sounds) can, if they are present, best be heard just after S1. Ejection clicks occur at the time of ventricular ejection and resemble in timing, but not in quality, a widely split S1. Ejection clicks are occasionally heard during the first 24 hours of life and during that time are usually normal (related to the concurrent pulmonary hypertension). Ejection clicks are always considered abnormal after the first 24 hours of life. The most frequent findings associated with these clicks are aortic or pulmonic stenosis (PS), idiopathic dilation of the pulmonary artery, systemic or pulmonary hypertension, truncus arteriosus, or TET.[5,14]

Murmurs

Murmurs are caused by turbulent blood flow. They are often described as prolonged heart sounds. There are two kinds of murmurs: innocent and pathologic. Pathologic murmurs result from underlying cardiovascular disease; innocent murmurs do not.

Whenever an examiner detects a murmur, the question of its origin arises. The murmur must therefore be fully evaluated as to its timing, location, intensity, radiation, quality, and pitch. The neonate's age in hours and days is also especially significant because of the dynamic properties of the newborn heart. Putting all this information together with other findings of the physical examination should help the examiner determine the significance of the murmur.

The *timing* of a murmur is the first quality the examiner must listen for. To evaluate timing, the examiner must understand what is happening to the heart during systole and diastole. Systole is the period when the heart contracts and the heart chambers eject blood. Systole occurs following closure of the mitral and tricuspid valves, and its onset occurs just after S1. Diastole is the period when the heart is relaxed and the chambers are filling with blood. Diastole occurs following closure of the aortic and pulmonic valves, and its onset occurs just after S2. When establishing the timing of a murmur, the examiner must ask: "Does it occur in systole or diastole?" That is, does the murmur occur after S1 or after S2? Is the murmur early, mid, or late in systole or diastole? Does it occur throughout systole (holosystolic or pansystolic) or during midsystolic ejection? Continuous murmurs are heard through both systole and diastole.

Loudness, or intensity, of the murmur should be determined next. Murmurs are graded from I to VI, as follows:

> **Grade I:** Barely audible, audible only after a period of careful auscultation
>
> **Grade II:** Soft, but audible immediately
>
> **Grade III:** Of moderate intensity (but not associated with a thrill)
>
> **Grade IV:** Louder (may be associated with a thrill)
>
> **Grade V:** Very loud; can be heard with the stethoscope rim barely on the chest (may be associated with a thrill)
>
> **Grade VI:** Extremely loud; can be heard with the stethoscope just slightly removed from the chest (may be associated with a thrill)

Sometimes the intensity of a murmur will vary from examination to examination. The reason may be changing PVR or anything else that alters the status of cardiac output, such as anemia, activity, or changing ventilatory requirements.

Location of the place on the chest wall where the murmur is heard at maximum intensity is another important feature to evaluate. Location is usually described in terms of the interspace and the midsternal, midclavicular, or anterior axillary lines (see Figure 7.3), because the anatomic site of most murmurs is usually found at the location below where they are best heard. Describing murmurs in terms of aortic, pulmonary, tricuspid, or mitral areas is not recommended in neonates because malposition of valves and vessels may be found in CHD.

Document other locations where a murmur is heard. This is described as radiation or transmission of the murmur. Radiation from the normally positioned pulmonary outflow tract is to the left upper back; radiation from the normally positioned aortic outflow tract is to the carotid arteries.

Quality and *pitch* of the murmur are the final two features that should be assessed. Pitch is described as high, medium, or low. High-pitched murmurs occur when there is turbulence from a high-pressure area to a low-pressure area.[16] This can happen with aortic or mitral insufficiency. Low-pitched murmurs occur when there is a low-pressure difference in the turbulent flow. An example of this is mitral stenosis. Identifying the quality of a murmur (terms include *harsh, rumbling*, or *musical*) also helps to describe it.

Innocent Murmurs

During the first 48 hours of life, many newborns have murmurs, the majority of which are innocent. They are usually associated with the decreasing PVR occurring at this time and with the gradual closure of the PDA. Innocent murmurs, sometimes called *functional* or *flow murmurs*, are most often Grade I or II, are associated with normal pulses, normal EKG and chest x-ray findings, are usually systolic murmurs, and are not associated with any other symptoms.[22]

Some of the more common innocent murmurs heard during the first days to weeks of life include the following:

- *Pulmonary flow murmur of the newborn*: (also called *peripheral PS*, or *pulmonary branch murmur*): A systolic ejection murmur heard often in newborns, especially premature neonates, its intensity is usually Grade I to II/VI, and it is medium to high pitched. This murmur is best heard in *the upper left sternal border, with impressive wide radiation to both lung fields, axillae, and back.*[5,12] It presents within the first or second week of life.[23] The murmur can last for weeks to months, but generally disappears by 3 to 6 months of age.[5,12] The murmur results from turbulence produced at the relatively acute angle of the bifurcation of the pulmonary artery.[5,24]

- *Transient systolic murmur of PDA*: Caused by a closing PDA during the first days of life in a term infant. Usually a Grade I to II/VI murmur that is found at the upper sternal border and in the left infraclavicular area.[5]
- *Transient systolic murmur of tricuspid regurgitation (TR)*: Thought to be caused by a minimal tricuspid valve abnormality that causes TR in the presence of increased PVR and high right ventricle (RV) pressure in the first few days. The regurgitation and murmur will disappear as the PVR decreases.[5]

Pathologic Murmurs

Pathologic murmurs in the neonate occur at varying times, depending on the anatomic abnormality causing them and on normal changes associated with transitional circulation. For example, pathologic murmurs heard in the delivery room are almost always caused either by stenosis or by regurgitation; they are almost never the result of shunting because vascular resistances in the lungs and the body are equal at birth.[5] Many specific defects do not present with a murmur until 3 days (when the PDA is generally closing), 1 week, or 4 to 6 weeks of age, when the PVR has fallen sufficiently. ASDs sometimes do not present in the infant until 1 to 2 years of age.[5] The absence of a murmur does not rule out the potential for serious CHD. Many infants who have significant congenital heart defects do not have heart murmurs.[5] In fact, the absence of a murmur may be an ominous sign in both acyanotic and ductal-dependent lesions because it may indicate ductal closure.

Approach all murmurs cautiously. Soft murmurs heard in otherwise asymptomatic infants can be observed carefully by the experienced examiner for the first 48 hours of life. But any murmur that persists beyond this time, is louder than a Grade I or II, or occurs in a symptomatic neonate requires further investigation. The cardiovascular workup should include a chest x-ray, an echocardiogram, and a consultation with a cardiologist. Many cardiologists also believe that an ECG is an important component of a complete cardiac evaluation.

Pathologic murmurs are more difficult to categorize than innocent murmurs. The following commonly occur in the immediate neonatal period:

- *Loud systolic ejection murmur*: Usually Grade II to V, this murmur is audible immediately after birth and persists because it is not affected by PVR. It is almost always the result of aortic or pulmonary stenosis or coarctation of the aorta.[5]
- *Continuous murmur*: Heard both during systole and diastole in an older infant with PDA and often described as "machinery like." It is can also be heard after birth in an infant with an arteriovenous fistula.[5]
- *Systolic murmur of PDA in premature infant*: Unlike the continuous murmur of a PDA heard in an older infant with a PDA, the murmur of a PDA in a premature infant is usually a coarse systolic murmur best heard at the left sternal border.[25] This murmur may be difficult to hear in an infant being ventilated or on continuous positive airway pressure but may be accompanied by wide pulse pressure, bounding pulses, and an active precordium.[5,14]

In addition, pathologic systolic murmurs may occasionally be heard with mitral and tricuspid insufficiency of various causes (especially with left ventricular failure in infants with critical left ventricular outlet obstruction and TET).[5] Pathologic murmurs associated with VSD and PDA in term neonates do not present until PVR has fallen—often not until after discharge from the nursery or at several weeks of age.[5]

PALPATING THE LIVER

Palpation of the liver (described in Chapter 9) is a significant part of the cardiovascular assessment. The liver becomes engorged when central venous pressure increases. A liver located more than 3 cm below the right costal margin is a good indicator of right-sided heart failure in a term infant.

EVALUATING BLOOD PRESSURE

Evaluation of the neonate's blood pressure (BP) should be done with the infant quiet. This assessment should be left until the end of the examination because the pressure of the cuff inflating may make the infant cry. Although the American Academy of Pediatrics (AAP) does not recommend universal screening of BP, systemic BP should be measured in every neonate with suspected CHD, renal disease, or clinical signs of hypotension.[5,26]

A cuff of the proper size must be used when obtaining a BP measurement. Indeed, the most frequent reason for a hypertensive BP is the use of a BP cuff that is too small for the infant. Using limb length as the sole criterion for establishing cuff size for BP monitoring can be misleading. This method does not take into consideration large-for-gestational-age infants with excessive subcutaneous fat. These infants will show falsely elevated BPs if cuff size is inappropriate. It is therefore recommended that the cuff width (not the cuff length) be 40% to 45% (but less than 50%) of the circumference of the extremity. A cuff width 125% of the arm diameter equals to 40% of the arm circumference. Therefore, a practitioner should aim for a cuff width between 125% and 145% of the diameter of the limb being measured (Figure 8.9).[5] In addition, the cuff should be long enough to entirely encircle the extremity.[6]

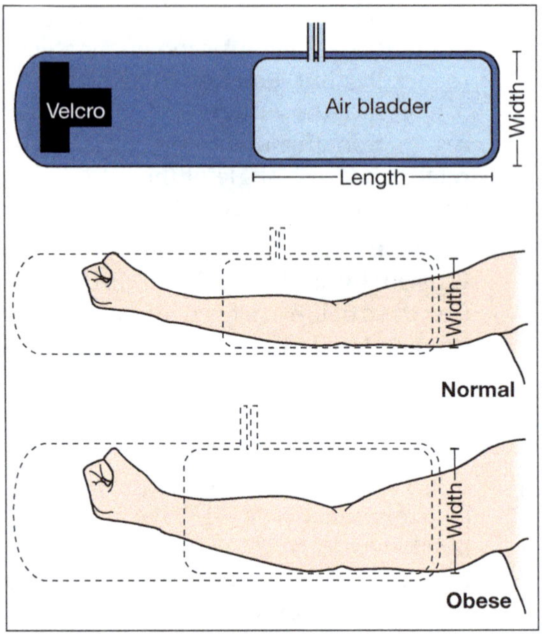

FIGURE 8.9 Diagram showing how to select accurate blood pressure cuff size

Source: From Park MK, and Salamat. 2020. *Park's Pediatric Cardiology for Practioners*, 7th ed. Philadelphia, PA: Elsevier, 15. Reprinted by permission.[5]

Monitoring Methods

There are several methods for monitoring systemic BP in neonates: flush, palpation, ultrasound Doppler, and oscillometric measurements. BP obtained by auscultation is not appropriate for neonates.

Flush

The flush method, now rarely used, is simple to do and can be useful in certain situations. With this method, the hand or foot is squeezed to blanch it, and the BP cuff is rapidly inflated. The pressure in the cuff is released, and the pressure point at which the extremity suddenly flushes is documented. The pressure obtained by this method represents the mean arterial pressure.

Palpation

BP can also be obtained by palpatory methods in infants. However, it is also very rarely used. While releasing the pressure in the cuff, the examiner palpates the pulse distal to the cuff. The pressure point at which the pulse reappears upon deflation approximates the systolic BP.

Doppler Ultrasound

A more accurate method, similar to the palpatory method of BP measurement, is done by Doppler ultrasound. Although an ultrasound can transmit images, a Doppler ultrasound can be used to measure blood flow. A transducer is placed over the artery distal to the BP cuff after a conductive gel is applied, and an audible pulse is listened for as the BP cuff is deflated. The pressure point at which the pulse is heard is documented. This method also approximates the systolic BP.

Oscillometric Measurement

Most centers now use oscillometric methods to document BP in neonates. Systolic, diastolic, and mean arterial BP and heart rate are all digitally recorded using special cuffs and oscillometric systems. These systems have been found to be fairly reliable.

Catheter

Finally, indwelling arterial catheters also provide systolic, diastolic, and mean BPs. These catheters provide minute-by-minute readings of BP values. Accuracy of this type of monitoring requires knowledge of the system and the variables that will affect it. Some of these variables include transducer position, air bubbles in the system, and equipment calibration.

Normal Values

Normal BP values in newborns vary, depending on body weight and postnatal age. In the first few hours of life, BP can be significantly affected by type of delivery, birth asphyxia, and placental transfusion. The newborn's initial BP decreases during the first 3 to 4 hours of life, presumably because of fluid shifts into and out of the vascular space.[21] The systolic pressure reaches a minimum at 3 to 4 hours of age and then gradually increases to reach a plateau at about 4 to 6 days of age to a level closer to the initial postpartum level.[27] BPs in neonates are also affected by activity, temperature, and behavioral state. Figure 8.10 documents confidence limits for newborns (based on birth weight) during the first day of life.[28] Whenever there is any question of CHD, if an examiner has difficulty obtaining BPs, if a murmur is heard, or if there is an absence of femoral pulses on the physical examination, four extremity BPs should be obtained. Pressures obtained in the legs are often slightly higher than those in the arms, but they can be equal or slightly lower in the neonate. A systolic BP in the upper extremities that is significantly higher than that in the lower extremities, especially with the combination of absent or weak femoral pulses, should increase suspicion of coarctation of the aorta.[29] This pressure difference can sometimes be masked in the left arm by a PDA that allows blood to pass around the restricted area; therefore, the right arm will yield the most valuable information because it is always preductal.

In addition to systolic, diastolic, and mean BP readings, the pulse pressure can provide additional valuable information. The *pulse pressure* is defined as the difference between systolic and diastolic BPs. Averages for term neonates are between 25 and 30 mmHg; for premature infants, they are between 15 and 25 mmHg.[21] Wide pulse pressures may be a sign of a large aortic runoff, as seen with PDA. Narrow pulse pressures are documented in neonates with peripheral vasoconstriction, heart failure, or low cardiac output.

SCREENING FOR CONGENITAL HEART DISEASE WITH PULSE OXIMETRY

Screening to detect CHD early, through the use of pulse oximetry during the immediate postnatal period, is an effective method for reducing mortality and morbidity in infants.[30] Screening and diagnostic follow-up of all infants should occur in the first 48 hours of life (Figure 8.11).[30] Oxygen saturation is measured using a pulse oximeter probe on the right hand and one foot either in direct sequence or in parallel in infants between 24 and 48 hours of age. The screen is considered positive if any of the following occur:

- Any oxygen saturation reading is less than 90%.

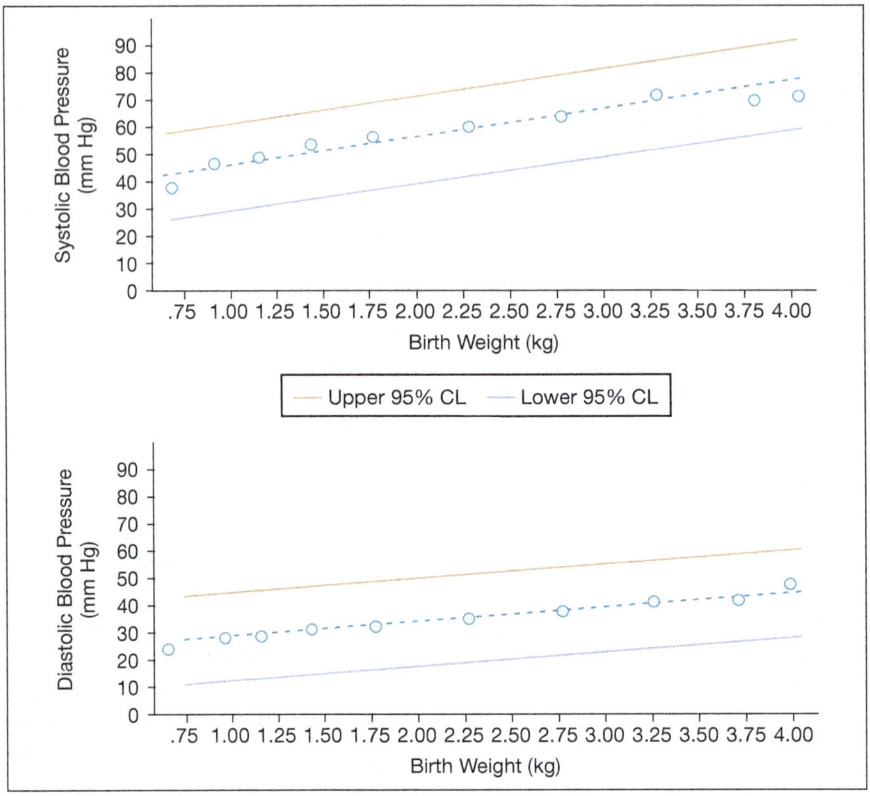

FIGURE 8.10 Systolic, diastolic, mean, and pulse pressures for newborns (based on birth weight) during the first 12 hours of life

CL, confidence limit.

Source: Redrawn from Zubrow AB, Kushner H, and Falkner B. 1995. Determinants of blood pressure in infants admitted to neonatal intensive care units: A prospective multicenter study. *Journal of Perinatology* 15(6): 472. Reprinted by permission.[28]

- The oxygen saturation is less than 95% in both extremities on three measures (each measure should be separated by 1 hour).
- There is a greater than 3% difference in saturation levels between the foot and right hand on three different measures separated by 1 hour.

Any newborn with a positive screen should have a comprehensive evaluation for the cause of the hypoxemia, and CHD should be excluded based on the results of an echocardiogram.[30]

Recently an expert panel recommended modification of the AAP algorithm to require an oxygen saturation of at least 95% in BOTH the upper and lower extremities (the initial recommendations were for EITHER upper or lower extremities) and require only one repeat screen (rather than two screens) for cases that neither fail nor pass initially.[31] However, the AAP has not yet endorsed this change.

SUMMARY

Properly executed, the cardiovascular assessment provides a great deal of information about the overall health of the newborn, as well as valuable information about congenital heart defects that might be present. Time, patience, and experience with inspection, palpation, and auscultation are all necessary to develop the skills essential to a thorough cardiac examination.

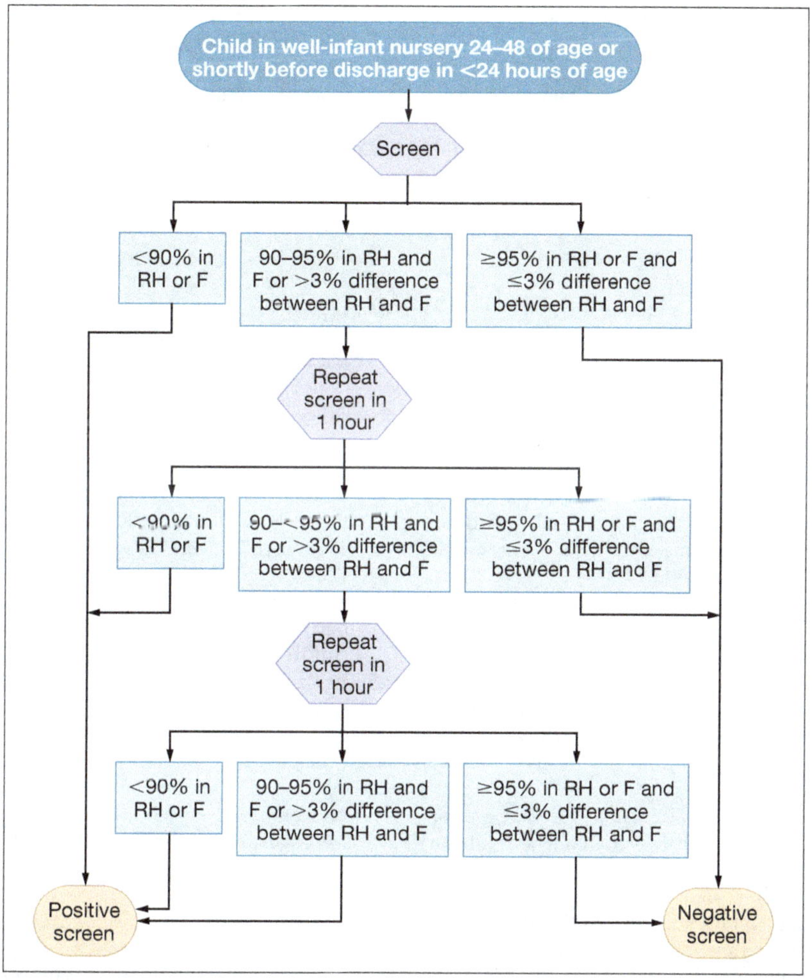

FIGURE 8.11 The proposed pulse-oximetry monitoring protocol based on results from the right hand and either foot

F, foot; RH, right hand.

Source: Adapted from Kemper AR, Mahle WT, Martin GR, Cooley WC, Kumar P, Morrow WR, Kelm K, Pearson GD, Glidewell J, Grosse SD, and Howell RR. 2011. Strategies for implementing screening for critical congenital heart disease. *Pediatrics* 128(5): e1259. Reprinted by permission.[30]

ADDITIONAL RESOURCES

SPRINGER PUBLISHING CONNECT™

A robust set of resources designed to supplement this text is located at http://connect.springerpub.com/content/book/978-0-8261-4063-0. Qualifying instructors may request access by emailing textbook@springerpub.com.

REFERENCES

1. Nora JJ, and Nora AH. 1978. The evolution of specific genetic and environmental counseling in congenital heart diseases. *Circulation* 57(2): 205–213.
2. Reller MD. 2008. Prevalence of congenital heart defects in metropolitan Atlanta, 1998–2005. *Journal of Pediatrics* 153(6): 807–813.
3. Blickstein I, Perlman S, Hazan Y, and Shinwell ES. 2020. Pregnancy complicated by diabetes mellitus. In *Neonatal and Perinatal Medicine*, 11th ed. Martin RJ, Fanaroff AA, and Walsh MC, eds. Philadelphia, PA: Elsevier, 304–311.
4. Hull D, Binns BA, and Joyce D. 1966. Congenital heart block and widespread fibrosis due to maternal lupus erythematosus. *Archives of Disease in Childhood* 41(220): 688–690.

5. Park MK, and Salamat M. 2020. *Park's Pediatric Cardiology for Practitioners*, 7th ed. Philadelphia, PA: Elsevier, 2–5, 6–30, 107–118, 155–183, 407–435.
6. Burn J. 2002. The aetiology of congenital heart disease. In *Paediatric Cardiology*, 2nd ed. Anderson RH, Baker EJ, Macartney FJ, Rigby ML, Shinebourne EA, and Tynan M, eds. New York, NY: Churchill Livingstone, 151.
7. Lacro RV. 2006. Dysmorphology and genetics. In *Nadas' Pediatric Cardiology*, 2nd ed. Keane JF, Fyler DC, and Lock JE, eds. Philadelphia, PA: Saunders, 49–72.
8. Boughman J, Berg KA, Astemborski JA, Clark EB, McCarter RJ, Rubin JD, Ferencz C, Opitz JM, and Reynolds JF. 1987. Familial risks of congenital heart defect assessed in a population-based epidemiologic study. *American Journal of Medical Genetics* 26(4): 839–849.
9. Blundell D, Jones C, and Crossland DS. 2021. Structural cardiac disease and cardiomyopathies. In *Avery's and MacDonald's Neonatology: Pathophysiology and Management of the Newborn*, 8th ed. Boardman JP, Groves AM, and Ramasethu J, eds. Philadelphia, PA: Wolters Kluwer, 459–490.
10. Greenwood RD, Rosenthal A, Parisi L, Fyler DC, and Nadas AS. 1975. Extracardiac abnormalities in infants with congenital heart disease. *Pediatrics* 55(4): 485–492.
11. Hazinski MF. 1984. Congenital heart disease in the neonate. Part 7: Common congenital heart defects producing hypoxemia and cyanosis. *Neonatal Network* 2(6): 36–51.
12. Spilman LJ, and Furdon SA. 1998. Recognition, understanding, and current management of cardiac lesions with decreased pulmonary blood flow. *Neonatal Network* 17(4): 7–18.
13. Cassidy SC, Allen HD, and Phillips JR. 2016. History and physical examination. In *Moss and Adams' Heart Disease in Infants, Children, and Adolescents: Including the Fetus and Young Adult*, 9th ed. Allen HD, Shaddy RE, Penny DJ, Feltes TF, and Cetta F, eds. Philadelphia, PA: Lippincott Williams & Wilkins, 249–260.
14. Phelps CM, Thrush PT, and Cua CL. 2020. The heart. In *Klaus and Fanaroff's Care of the High-Risk Neonate*, 7th ed. Fanaroff AA, and Fanaroff JM, eds. St. Louis, MO: Elsevier, 296–332.
15. Bickley LS, Szilagyi PG, Hoffman RM, and Soriano RP, eds. 2020. *Bates' Guide to Physical Examination and History Taking*, 13th ed. Wolters Kluwer, 753.
16. Moller JH. 1992. Physical examination. In *Fetal, Neonatal, and Infant Cardiac Disease*. Moller JH, and Neal WA, eds. Norwalk, CT: Appleton & Lange, 167–177.
17. Bernstein D. 2020. History and physical examination in cardiac evaluation. In *Nelson Textbook of Pediatrics*. Kliegman RM, Geme JW, Blum NJ, Shah SS, Tasker RC, and Wilson KM, eds. Philadelphia, PA: Elsevier, 2346–2354.
18. Zahka KG. 2011. Approach to the neonate with cardiovascular disease. In *Neonatal and Perinatal Medicine*, 9th ed. Martin RJ, Fanaroff AA, and Walsh MC, eds. Philadelphia, PA: Mosby, 1237–1245.
19. Theorell C. 2002. Cardiovascular assessment of the newborn. *Newborn and Infant Nursing Reviews* 2(2): 111–127.
20. Pilcher J. 2016. Cardiac rhythms and arrhythmias. In *Pocket Guide to Neonatal EKG Interpretation*, 3rd ed. Petaluma, CA: NICU INK, 15–40.
21. Johnson GL. 1990. Clinical examination. In *Fetal and Neonatal Cardiology*. Long WA, ed. Philadelphia, PA: Saunders, 223–235.
22. Lissauer T, and Hansen A. 2020. Physical examination of the newborn. In *Neonatal and Perinatal Medicine*, 11th ed. Martin RJ, Fanaroff AA, and Walsh MC, eds. Philadelphia, PA: Elsevier, 440–457.
23. Danford DA, and McNamara DG. 1998. Innocent heart murmurs and heart sounds. In *Science and Practice of Pediatric Cardiology*. Garson A, Bricker JT, Fisher DJ, and Reish SR, eds. Philadelphia, PA: Lea & Febiger, 2203–2212.
24. Danilowicz DA, Rudolph AM, Hoffman JI, and Heymann M. 1972. Physiologic pressure differences between main and branch pulmonary arteries in children. *Circulation* 45(2): 410–419.
25. Benitz WE, and Bhombal S. 2020. Patent ductus arteriosus. In *Neonatal and Perinatal Medicine*, 11th ed. Martin RJ, Fanaroff AA, and Walsh MC, eds. Philadelphia, PA: Elsevier, 1334–1341.
26. American Academy of Pediatrics, and Committee on Fetus and Newborn. 1993. Routine evaluation of blood pressure, hematocrit, and glucose in newborns. *Pediatrics* 92(3): 474–476.
27. Scanlon JW, Nelson T, Grylack LJ, Smith YF. 1979. *A System of Newborn Physical Examination*. Baltimore, MD: University Park Press, 67–73.
28. Zubrow AB, Kushner H, and Falkner B. 1995. Determinants of blood pressure in infants admitted to neonatal intensive care units: A prospective multicenter study. *Journal of Perinatology* 15(6): 472.
29. Hoschtitzky JA, Anderson RH, and Elliott MJ. 2010. Aortic coarctation and interrupted aortic arch. In *Paediatric Cardiology*, 3rd ed. Anderson RH, Baker EJ, Macartney FJ, Rigby ML, Shinebourne EA, and Tynan M. eds. Philadelphia, PA: Churchill Livingstone, 945–966.
30. Kemper AR, Mahle WT, Martin GR, Cooley WC, Kumar P, Morrow WR, Kelm K, Pearson GD, Glidewell J, Grosse SD, and Howell RR. 2011. Strategies for implementing screening for critical congenital heart disease. *Pediatrics* 128(5): e1259–e1267.
31. Martin GR, Ewer AK, Gaviglio A, Hom LA, Saarinen A, Sontag M, Burns KM, Kemper AR, and Oster ME. 2020. Updated strategies for pulse oximetry screening for critical congenital heart disease. *Pediatrics* 146(1): e20191650.

9 ABDOMINAL ASSESSMENT

Beth Bohara

Assessment of the newborn abdomen is best performed during the first few hours of life, when the bowel is not yet filled with gas. Ideally, the infant will be in a quiet state, with relaxed abdominal muscles. Techniques used in abdominal assessment include observation, auscultation, and palpation. Although percussion is used to examine the adult abdomen, it is of limited use when examining the newborn. The steps of abdominal assessment are discussed in this chapter as well as normal and abnormal findings that may be discovered during assessment.

REVIEW OF PREGNANCY AND DELIVERY HISTORY

Evaluation of the maternal history is discussed in Chapter 2; however, specific findings including abnormalities found on prenatal ultrasound and amniotic fluid volume are of particular interest when examining the abdomen and gastrointestinal (GI) tract of an infant. Such things as bowel obstructions, abdominal wall defects, and abnormalities of the genitourinary (GU) tract are now readily identifiable by fetal ultrasound. Any fetal abnormalities identified on prenatal ultrasound warrant close examination and follow-up postnatally.[1,2] The finding of polyhydramnios must also be evaluated as the risk for anomalies increase with increasing volume of amniotic fluid. *Polyhydramnios*, defined as an amniotic fluid volume of greater than 2,000 mLs, occurs in 1% to 3% of pregnancies. The prevalence of severe congenital abnormalities is as high as 75% in cases of severe polyhydramnios; fetal abnormalities include duodenal or esophageal atresia, tracheoesophageal fistula, gastroschisis, omphalocele, and diaphragmatic hernia.[1]

Reviewing an infant's delivery note is pertinent as well, as some immediate findings can correlate with specific abnormalities. The finding of an extremely large amount of amniotic fluid in the stomach at delivery with onset of bilious emesis within 24 hours of life in a well-appearing infant without abdominal distension may indicate the presence of duodenal atresia, which can often be confirmed after viewing an abdominal radiograph showing the "double-bubble" sign (Figure 9.1).[1,2] The presence of copious oral secretions and respiratory distress, along with the inability to pass a soft catheter to the stomach, may indicate an esophageal atresia, usually associated with a tracheoesophageal fistula (Figure 9.2).[1] Furthermore, the presence of any bilious gastric secretions at delivery is also abnormal and should alert the examiner to further evaluate for the possibility of intestinal obstruction.[1,3]

INSPECTION

Skin

The skin of a newborn's abdomen should be pink and intact, without rash or bruising, although occasionally newborn rash may be present as well as bruising from the delivery process. The skin's appearance varies based on gestational age. A preterm infant will have more visible vasculature, sometimes appearing more translucent, because of decreased subcutaneous tissue.[4,5] The postterm baby

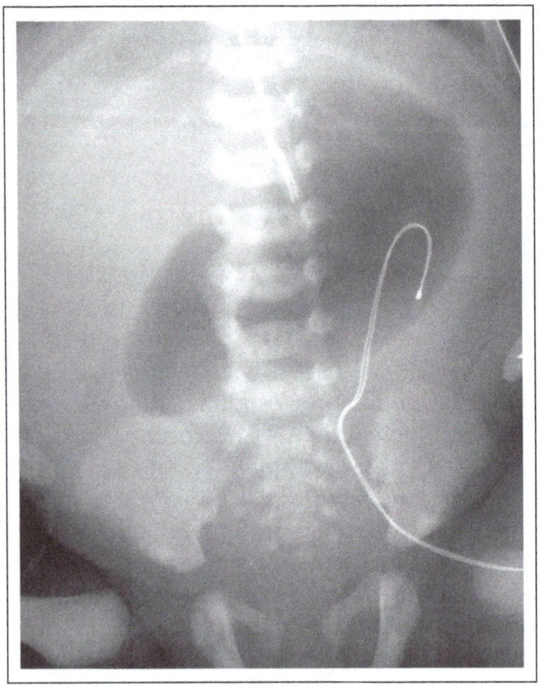

FIGURE 9.1 X-ray of "double-bubble" sign in duodenal atresia

Source: Wyllie R, Hyams JS, Kay M, and Wyllie R. 2021. *Pediatric Gastrointestinal and Liver Disease*, 6th ed. Hyams JS, and Kay M, eds. Elsevier, Figure 57.1.

may have superficial cracking and peeling of the skin over the abdomen.[1] A few large veins may be visible, especially on a light-skinned infant, but marked venous distention should not be present.[4] Any jaundice at birth is always abnormal.[5]

Shape

The normal shape of a term newborn's abdomen is soft and rounded without visible loops or masses, and with easy movements associated with respiration. The abdominal and diaphragmatic muscles work together during respiration, causing the chest and abdomen to move parallel with each other.[6,7] The shape of the abdomen should be symmetric, without obvious swellings or depressions. Diastasis recti is a midline separation of the rectus abdominis muscles and may be seen as a midline, elevated ridge extending from below the sternum to the umbilicus

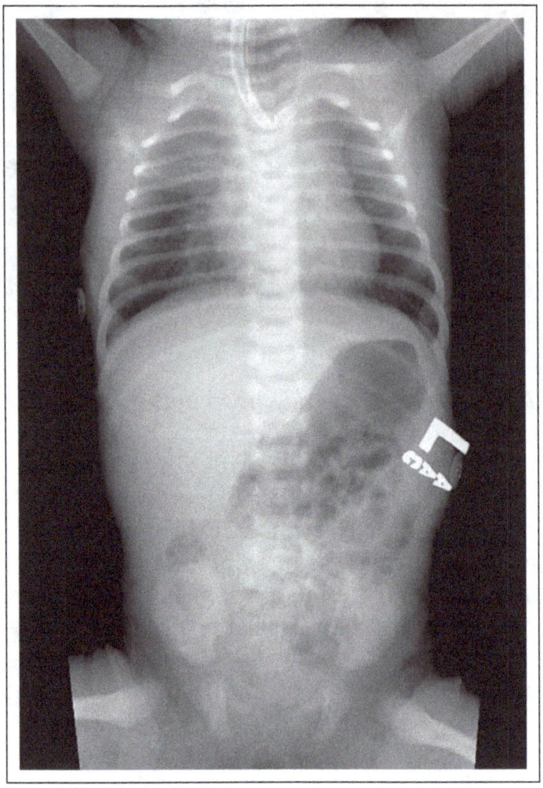

FIGURE 9.2 X-ray showing coiling of nasogastric tube in esophageal atresia. Tracheoesophageal fistula is present as air is shown distally in the stomach and intestines

Source: Holcomb GW, Murphy JP, St. Peter SD, Gatti JM, and Ashcraft KW. 2019. *Holcomb and Ashcraft's Pediatric Surgery*, 7th ed. Holcomb GW, Murphy JP, St. Peter SD, and Gatti JM, eds. Elsevier, Figure 27.2.

when the infant is crying (Figure 9.3). This is a normal finding and will resolve without intervention.[8]

Typically, abdominal girth is not measured, but there is some value in having a baseline girth for comparison when there is concern for new distension. The abdominal circumference measured at the greatest diameter (just above the umbilicus) is normally less than the head circumference up until 30 to 32 weeks gestational age. From 32 to 36 weeks gestational age, the abdominal and head circumferences will be equal. After 36 weeks gestational age, the abdominal circumference will be greater than the head circumference.[4] If serial abdominal circumferences are obtained, it is important to standardize the location of abdominal

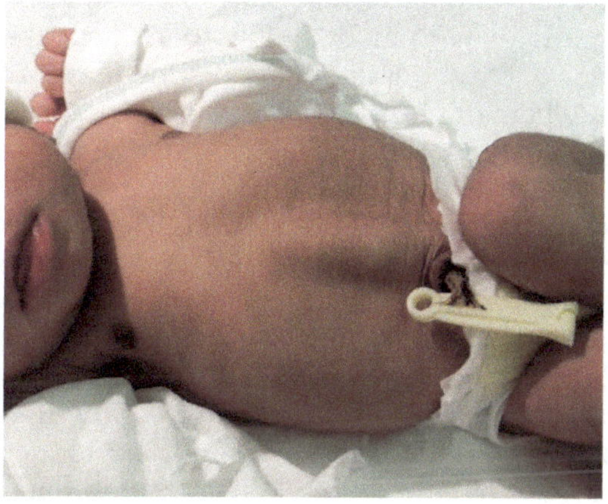

FIGURE 9.3 Diastasis recti

Source: Aby J. *Newborn Nursery at Lucile Packard Children's Hospital.* Stanford Medicine. https://med.stanford.edu/newborns/professional-education/photo-gallery/abdomen. Accessed 10/16/2022.

measurement as measurements can vary greatly whether taken above or below the umbilicus. Measurement should be taken at 1 cm above the umbilicus while an infant is supine. A change of >2 cm in abdominal girth on serial assessments is concerning and may be considered abnormal, although many variables can affect girth including if the infant has recently eaten and when the infant has last stooled. Preterm infants have been found to have abdominal circumferences varying up to 3.5 cm with one feed and still be considered normal.[8]

The abdomen of a normal preterm infant may appear distended because of lack of muscle tone.[8] Occasionally, a loop of bowel may be visible beneath the surface but is only of concern when it remains fixed in one spot or is associated with generalized distention and symptoms of bowel obstruction.[4] Fixation can be monitored via serial abdominal x-rays. A fixed bowel loop raises concern for a bowel without normal peristalsis, often leading to diagnoses of necrotizing enterocolitis (NEC), bowel obstruction, or bowel ischemia.[9]

Umbilical Cord

The umbilical cord of the healthy newborn is gelatinous, moist, and bluish white in color.[10] A yellow or green cord may be seen when meconium staining has occurred prior to delivery.[8] The average width of the umbilical cord is 1 to 2 cm at the base and is comprised of Wharton's jelly, which protects the umbilical vessels.[10] It also serves as an indicator of the infant's nutritional status.[11] A thick cord is often seen in large-for-gestational-age infants, whereas a small, thin cord is often seen in infants who are small for gestational age or affected by placental insufficiency.[10] Any unusual bulging or herniation in the cord requires further investigation and could indicate the presence of a small omphalocele.[11] If abnormalities are noted, the cord should be clamped and cut distal to the areas to avoid damage to any structures that might be present within the cord.[10]

When the cord is cut, the internal vessels should be visible. The umbilical cord contains one vein and two arteries.[6] The vein is large, thin walled, and open. The paired arteries are small, thick walled, and constricted.[8] Absence of one of the arteries is seen in approximately 0.4% of infants and may be associated with fetal abnormalities including chromosome abnormalities and congenital malformations, especially of the GU and cardiovascular systems. Although a single umbilical artery is associated with increased risk of morbidity and mortality, it can also be an isolated finding in an otherwise normal baby.[1,7] The cut surface of the cord may initially ooze a small amount of clear, sticky fluid, but it will dry quickly. In normal situations, the cord will begin to dry soon after birth and will shrivel and fall off in 7 to 10 days.[8]

AUSCULTATION

Auscultation should be performed with a warmed stethoscope before palpation as palpation can interfere with normal bowel sounds[12] and cause the infant to become agitated. While the infant is quiet, the examiner should patiently listen to all four quadrants of the abdomen. Bowel sounds should be present within a few hours of birth.[12] The presence, quality, and intensity of bowel sounds should be noted. Normal bowel sounds have a metallic, tinkling quality and are heard every 15 to 20 seconds.[6] If bowel sounds are infrequent, the examiner should listen for a full 5 minutes before diagnosing them as absent.[12] Maternal history of medications given prior to delivery, such as magnesium sulfate, must be noted as this can cause decreased GI motility and thus result in hypoactive bowel sounds in the infant.[8] Hyperactive bowel sounds in a healthy-appearing neonate who has just fed may be normal. The same finding in an ill-appearing infant with a distended abdomen is abnormal and could indicate obstruction, thus auscultation of bowel sounds must be correlated with other clinical exam findings.[4]

Breath sounds may be audible when the upper abdomen is auscultated. This is a normal finding as sounds transmit easily throughout an infant's body. In contrast, vascular sounds are not normally appreciated. Rarely, the sound of blood flow through a restricted or tortuous vessel, known as a bruit, may be heard.[13] The sound is similar to the swooshing of a cardiac murmur. Vascular sounds over the renal arteries can indicate renovascular hypertension, warranting further investigation. The exact position to auscultate the renal arteries is dependent on the size of the patient, but typically the location is about 2 cm above the umbilicus and 1 to 2 cm to the right and left of this location.[6]

PALPATION

Palpation can be performed with the infant in any state, but it is easiest when the infant is quiet. Palpation is the last step in the abdominal examination because it often results in agitation. If the infant is fussy, flexing the hips to relax the abdominal muscles or providing a pacifier during the examination may help.[6,12]

Normal newborn infants have soft rounded abdomens, and the skin of the abdomen should be warm and have brisk capillary refill.[12] Low abdominal tone can be a normal finding in the premature infant.[11] Otherwise, low abdominal tone may be present after birth due to maternal medications with depressant effects that pass to the infant or in infants with globally low tone.[4] Increased tone of the abdominal musculature may indicate pain or peritoneal irritation.[6]

Palpation should begin with the superficial structures and then progress to the deeper organs (Figure 9.4). Light and deep palpation are an extremely important part of the abdominal exam. Tender areas can be identified through light palpation, and deep palpation is used to assess deeper organs for size and consistency, including the liver, spleen, and kidneys.[6] It is important to identify normal structures first in the abdomen if palpable.[14] The liver is the easiest organ to palpate, followed by the right kidney. The left kidney is more difficult to assess, and the spleen is usually not palpable.[12] It is important to assess all four abdominal quadrants in a stepwise fashion, starting in the right upper quadrant and assessing the liver first.[14] The liver is a superficial organ and occupies a wide area of the upper abdomen in the normal newborn, extending well into the left upper quadrant.[11] To palpate, the examiner should begin just above the iliac crest on the

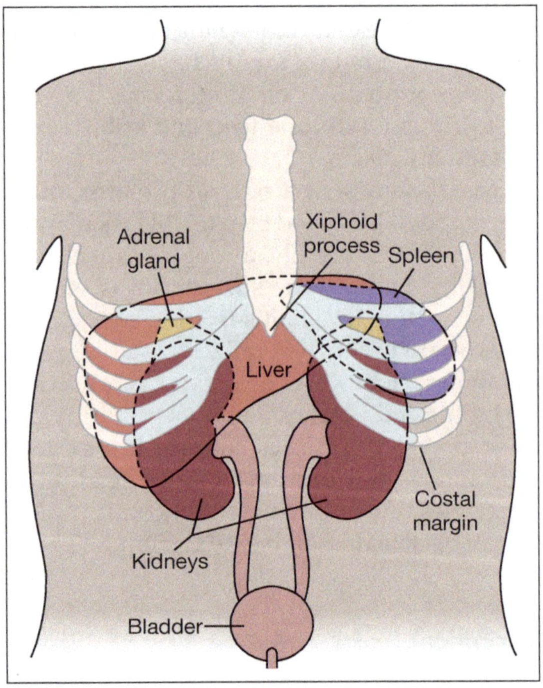

FIGURE 9.4 Abdominal organs of the infant

right in the midclavicular line.[12] Using the palmar surface of the fingers parallel to the costal margin, the examiner gently palpates in a progressively caudal fashion. The abdomen should be depressed 1 to 2 cm and care should be taken not to lift the hands completely off the abdomen as this may result in missing the edge of an enlarged liver.

The liver normally extends 1 to 2 cm below the right costal margin,[12] and the edge is smooth, firm, and sharp.[11] A boggy liver is a sign of congestion and may indicate congestive heart failure.[11] A hard or nodular liver edge is also abnormal.[4] If the liver extends greater than 3 cm below the right costal margin, hepatomegaly is of concern[12] and further evaluation is needed.

Using the technique described earlier, the left side of the abdomen is examined for the spleen in the left midclavicular line. The tip of the spleen may be felt, but in most cases, it is not palpable at all.[12] A spleen that is palpable more than 1 cm below the costal margin may be enlarged and warrants further investigation.[11] Rarely, situs inversus is present, where the liver will be found on the left and the spleen on the right.[1]

Palpation of the kidneys can be difficult, but it is easiest when done early in the first few days of life.[11] The kidneys are found using deep palpation at a 45° angle lateral to and below the umbilicus.[12] This can be most easily accomplished with one hand under the infant's back and the other hand's finger-tips pressing downward on the abdomen with deep palpation in the right upper quadrant to the right of midline.[12] Similarly, repeat this technique in the left upper quadrant to the left of midline. The normal newborn kidney is 4.5 to 5 cm from the upper to lower pole.[11] On examination, the kidneys feel firm, smooth, and round.[12] The right kidney is normally situated slightly lower than the left[14] due to its position below the right liver lobe.[12] A very easily palpated kidney is usually enlarged and may indicate hydronephrosis[4] or a cystic kidney.

The bladder can be palpated in the midline and is located 1 to 4 cm above the symphysis pubis.[11,12] If bladder distension is present, one must differentiate between causes including physical obstruction, neurogenic bladder, or acute urinary retention from things such as side effects of medication.[12]

Once the abdominal organs have been palpated, the entire abdomen should be palpated for masses. In a systematic fashion, the examiner should explore each quadrant using first light and then deeper palpation. Normal findings include stool in the colon, palpated as a sausage-shaped mass in the left lower quadrant.[12] Gaseous distention may also be palpated in an infant who has swallowed air. Serial examinations will differentiate between normal stool in the colon that progresses and an abnormal mass that is fixed. Neoplasia is very rare in the newborn.[4] Most abdominal masses present in the newborn involve the urinary tract and are cystic or solid feeling on examination.[4] A firm, olive-shaped mass may be felt in the right upper quadrant with pyloric stenosis,[6] although this does not usually present in the newborn period.

Groin and Perineum

Lastly, the groin and femoral regions should be inspected and palpated as well as the perianal area examined. Ideally, the groin and femoral regions should be evaluated while the infant is quiet and again while crying. The groins are normally flat and should be observed for bulges in the inguinal and femoral areas.[2] Palpation of a bulge in this region may indicate an inguinal hernia.[2] A visible femoral pulse may be present in a preterm infant, or thin term infant. The femoral artery pulses must also be palpated and their character evaluated. The pulses should be compared bilaterally and with the brachial pulse. Any difference in quality should be noted. An absent or weak femoral pulse may be noted with coarctation of the aorta.[8] Full and bounding femoral pulses may indicate a patent ductus arteriosus.[8] Complete evaluation of pulses is discussed in detail in Chapter 8.

The perianal area should be inspected for presence and placement of the anus, for anal sphincter tone, and for abnormalities such as fistulas. Sphincter tone can be assessed by gently stroking the anal area and eliciting an anal wink. Absence of an anal wink suggests a lower spinal cord lesion.[15] If very small dots of meconium appear in an infant's diaper and the rectal exam reveals a small, tight anus, this could indicate the presence of anal stenosis.[8]

If the anus is completely absent, or imperforate (see later, Figure 9.10), this may be evident immediately; however, atresia and stenosis can occur at any level of the anorectal canal.[1] Digital examination of the rectum or the insertion of instruments is not recommended because of the risk of damage to the anal canal. Patency of the anus cannot be established until the passage of meconium occurs. In otherwise asymptomatic infants, investigation is not warranted until an infant has not passed meconium by 48 hours of life. Passage of meconium usually occurs within 24 hours of birth, often within 12 hours, but a normal infant may not stool up until 48 hours.[8] Continued absence of stool warrants further investigation.

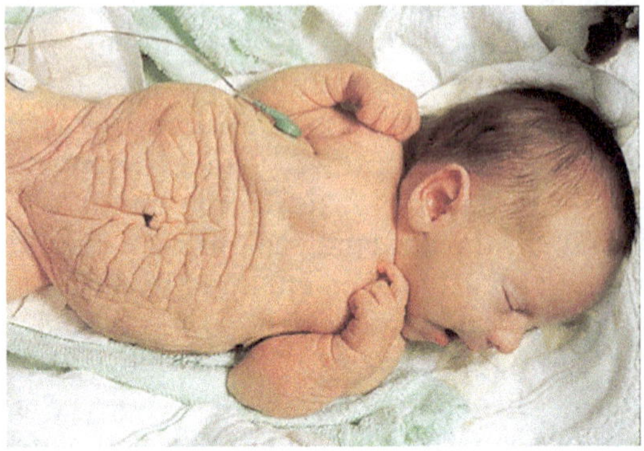

FIGURE 9.5 Prune belly syndrome or "Eagle–Barrett syndrome" with abnormal abdominal musculature

Source: Zitelli BJ, McIntire SC, Nowalk AJ, Garrison J, and Davis HW. 2022. *Zitelli and Davis' Atlas of Pediatric Physical Diagnosis*, 8th ed. Zitelli BJ, McIntire SC, Nowalk AJ, and Garrison J, eds. Elsevier.

ABNORMALITIES OF THE ABDOMEN

Shape Abnormalities

A sunken or scaphoid abdomen at birth can be indicative of a diaphragmatic hernia due to displacement of abdominal contents up into the chest.[8] This is easily distinguished from the flaccid, lumpy abdomen of the infant with congenital absence of the abdominal musculature, known as prune belly syndrome or *Eagle–Barrett syndrome* (Figure 9.5).[16] This rare syndrome, discussed further in Chapter 10, occurs mostly in males, and is associated with severe renal and urinary tract abnormalities.[16] A markedly distended abdomen in any infant warrants further investigation. Isolated distention of the lower abdomen may be associated with bladder distention.[11] Bowel obstruction typically presents with generalized abdominal distension, along with vomiting, the timing and character of which vary depending on the location of the obstruction. Obstructions of the upper GI tract, such as esophageal and duodenal atresia, tend to present with excessive salivation[16] and emesis that may or may not be bilious. As the level of obstruction progresses down the intestinal tract, abdominal distention and bilious emesis are hallmark symptoms. Bilious emesis is the result of obstruction beyond the level of the ampulla of Vater, where bile from the gallbladder enters the small intestine.[3] The presence of bilious emesis in any infant, with or without abdominal distention, requires immediate investigation to rule out a malrotation with midgut volvulus. A malrotation results from abnormal fixation of the intestine in the abdomen; midgut volvulus is the abnormal rotation of the bowel around the mesentery and subsequent obstruction of blood flow to the bowel. This is one of the most urgent emergencies in neonatal surgery. Immediate intervention is required to avoid irreversible infarction of the intestine.[1]

Meconium ileus needs to be considered as a diagnosis when the term infant has abdominal distension, emesis, and has not passed meconium by 48 hours of life.[2] There may or may not be a known family history of cystic fibrosis (CF) as well. Meconium ileus often results from the presence of thicker meconium due to abnormal pancreatic enzyme function and often is the first presenting symptom leading to the diagnosis of CF.[2,3] Of note, preterm infants may take longer than 48 hours to pass meconium depending on how much they have been fed enterally or if they have remained nothing by mouth (NPO) for a period of time.[8]

Abnormalities of the Umbilical Cord and Umbilicus

Purulent drainage from the umbilical cord may indicate the presence of an abscess. Excessive amounts of clear drainage may indicate the presence of a patent urachus, a persistent embryologic connection from the bladder to the umbilicus.[16] Ileal contents leaking through the umbilical cord indicates an omphalomesenteric duct, a persistence of the embryologic tract connecting the ileum to the umbilicus.[12]

Most often, as stated earlier, a green coloration of the umbilical cord is usually related to meconium staining, but rarely it may be an indicator of infection. Redness encircling the cord and extending onto the abdomen can be a sign of omphalitis (infection of the umbilical cord). Although the incidence is low, less than 1% in developed countries, it may be as much as six times greater in home births. Omphalitis must be treated promptly and properly because it can spread rapidly to underlying structures, causing severe systemic disease and even death.[1]

Umbilical and epigastric hernias may be present on abdominal exam. An umbilical hernia is the protrusion of abdominal contents into the umbilicus, causing an outpouching that is soft and easily reducible (Figure 9.6). It usually does not warrant treatment and usually resolves spontaneously in the first few years of life. Umbilical hernias are more commonly seen in African American infants, infants with congenital hypothyroidism, and infants with Beckwith–Wiedemann syndrome.[1] An epigastric hernia is a small, firm, palpable nodule seen between the umbilicus and the xiphoid process. It is midline in location, may be reducible, and is more easily visualized when an infant is bearing down or crying. It results from fat protruding through a small opening in the muscle. Surgical intervention is necessary for this type of hernia, as it rarely resolves on its own.[17]

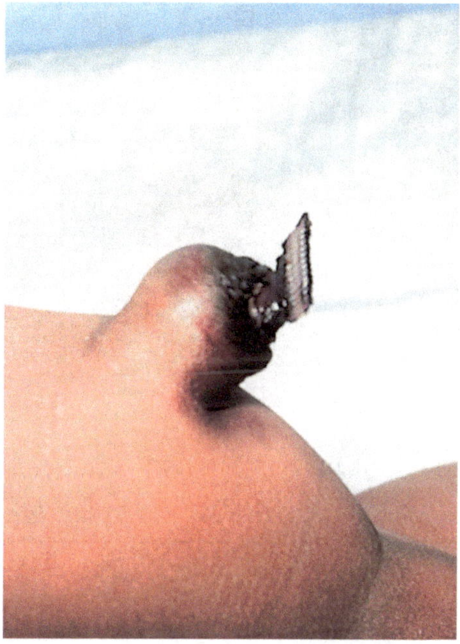

FIGURE 9.6 Umbilical hernia

Source: Zitelli BJ, McIntire SC, Nowalk AJ, Garrison J, and Davis HW. 2022. *Zitelli and Davis' Atlas of Pediatric Physical Diagnosis*, 8th ed. Zitelli BJ, McIntire SC, Nowalk AJ, and Garrison J, eds. Elsevier.

Abdominal-Wall Defects

Defects in formation of the abdominal wall may occur during embryonic life, resulting in abnormal externalization of the abdominal contents. Three such defects are omphalocele, gastroschisis, and exstrophy of the bladder. Both gastroschisis and omphalocele vary greatly in size, from smaller than a golf ball to so large that all the abdominal contents (including the liver) are externalized. An omphalocele is the herniation of abdominal contents into the umbilical cord (Figure 9.7). The hernia is contained in a translucent sac that is contiguous with the umbilical cord. The sac may rupture at or before delivery (Figure 9.8), so careful examination is necessary to distinguish between a ruptured omphalocele and gastroschisis. The incidence of omphalocele is 2 to 2.5 per 10,000 live births.[1] Omphaloceles are thought to result from failure of the bowel to reenter the abdominal cavity after its normal extrusion

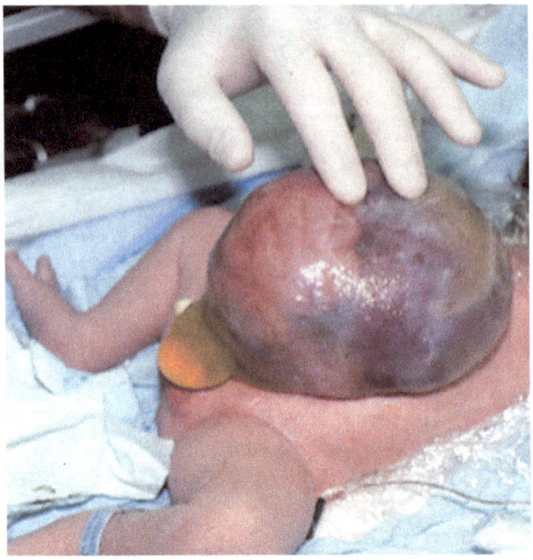

FIGURE 9.7 Omphalocele

Source: From Children's Mercy Hospital, Department of Surgery, Kansas, City, MO.

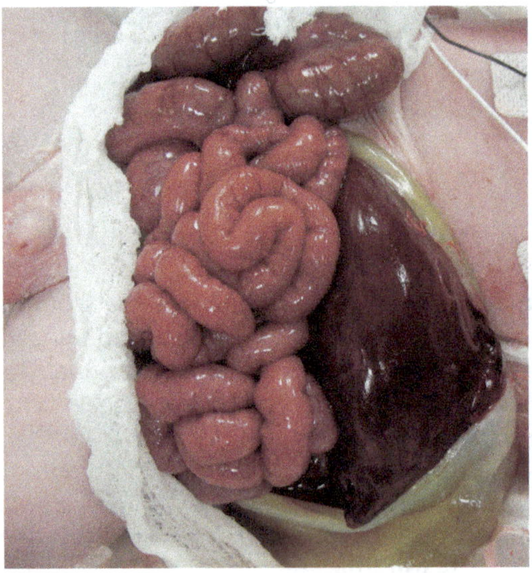

FIGURE 9.8 Ruptured omphalocele

Source: From Children's Mercy Hospital, Department of Surgery, Kansas City, MO.

into the cord between the 10th and 12th week of gestation.[16] Thus, any herniation of abdominal content into the umbilical cord past 12 weeks gestation is diagnostic for an omphalocele.[18]

Omphaloceles are associated with other structural abnormalities 55% to 58% of the time. They are associated with chromosomal abnormalities 10% to 30% of the time.[18] Omphaloceles are also frequently associated with Beckwith–Wiedemann syndrome and with trisomies 13, 18, and 21.[1,18,19] When the liver is involved, causes of omphalocele have been found to be less likely related to chromosomal abnormalities. The risk of concurrent genetic anomalies are highest with smaller defects, only including the small bowel, and when other structural anomalies are present, including midline defects, CNS anomalies, and clubfeet.[1]

Gastroschisis is a defect in the abdominal wall through which the viscera protrude. There is no sac covering this defect, and the umbilical cord is discrete from it. The gastroschisis is usually to the right of midline (Figure 9.9). The etiology of gastroschisis is suggested to be a failure in the normal attachment between the umbilical cord and umbilical ring in embryonic life. Other theories include vascular accident interfering with normal formation of abdominal musculature or failure of mesenchymal migration. The incidence of gastroschisis is approximately 1.5 per 10,000 live births. Associated defects occurring with gastroschisis occur at a rate much less than omphaloceles, with

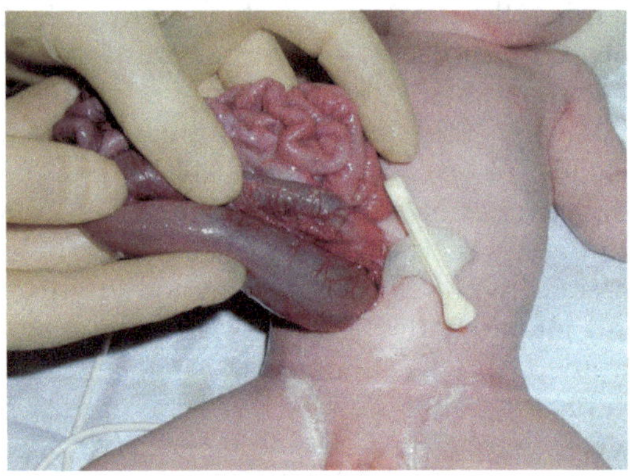

FIGURE 9.9 Gastroschisis defect to the right of the umbilicus with small bowel and colon involvement

Source: Polites SF and Nathan JD. 2021. *Pediatric Gastrointestinal and Liver Disease*, 6th ed. Wyllie R, Hyams JS, and Kay M, eds. Elsevier.

an incidence of approximately 5% to 20%. Most associated defects are intestinal atresias related to an ischemic insult or damage to the eviscerated bowel prior to birth.[1]

Exstrophy of the bladder is a rare defect. It is a malformation sequence resulting from lack of normal formation of the lower abdominal wall early in gestation. The posterior wall of the bladder is exposed, and urine drains into the abdomen. Exstrophy of the bladder is more common in males, and there may be associated urogenital abnormalities in both males and females.[20] This condition is discussed further in Chapter 10.

Perianal Abnormalities

When there is an imperforate anus present (Figure 9.10), often there is a fistula connecting the rectum to another organ allowing meconium to pass. The most common defect in males is a rectourethral fistula, or a connection between the urethra and rectum.[20] The most common defect in females is a rectovestibular fistula, where there is a third opening in the vestibule allowing meconium to pass.[20]

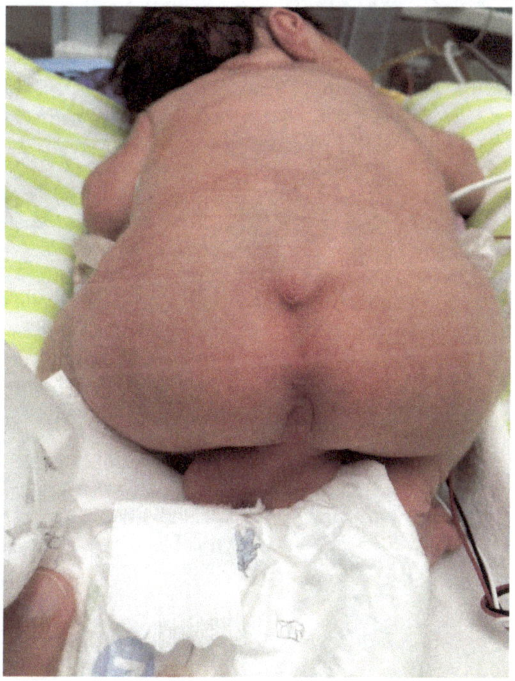

FIGURE 9.10 Imperforate anus

Source: From Children's Mercy Hospital, Department of Surgery, Kansas City, MO.

Femoral and Groin Abnormalities

An inguinal hernia is a defect in the muscle wall that allows the intestine to slip into the scrotum in males (Figure 9.11) and into the labia in females. The presence of a hernia is most easily evaluated when the infant is crying because intra-abdominal pressure increases. Inguinal hernias are more common in the preterm infant when compared to the term infant. The hernia should be soft and reducible into the body cavity without difficulty. Incarceration occurs when intestines become lodged in the inguinal canal. Presentation may include erythema, edema, and firmness at the site, along with nausea, vomiting, and abdominal pain.

Surgical repair is required for inguinal hernias, but in most cases, surgery is deferred to allow for growth of the infant. If incarcerated and unable to be reduced, surgery should not be deferred. Often incarceration will release once the infant is under general anesthesia, but if not, it is repaired surgically.[2]

SUMMARY

The examination of the abdomen involves observation, auscultation, and palpation.

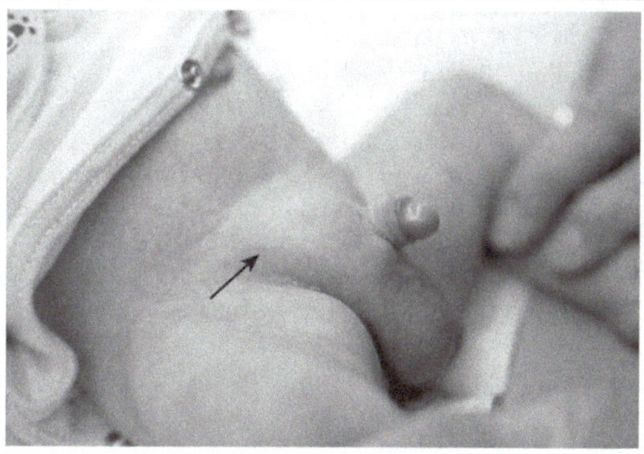

FIGURE 9.11 Inguinal hernia "bulge"

Source: Polites SF and Nathan JD. 2021. *Pediatric Gastrointestinal and Liver Disease*, 6th ed. Wyllie R, Hyams JS, and Kay M, eds. Elsevier.

Following a systematic routine and taking measures to ensure a quiet and cooperative infant will facilitate the exam. With practice, the examiner will learn to differentiate normal variations from abnormal findings, permitting timely intervention when abnormalities are found.

ADDITIONAL RESOURCES

SPRINGER PUBLISHING CONNECT™ | A robust set of resources designed to supplement this text is located at http://connect.springerpub.com/content/book/978-0-8261-4063-0. Qualifying instructors may request access by emailing textbook@springerpub.com.

REFERENCES

1. Dingeldein M. 2019. Selected gastrointestinal anomalies in the neonate. In *Fanaroff and Martin's Neonatal—Perinatal Medicine: Diseases of the Fetus and Infant*, 11th ed. Martin RJ, Fanaroff AA, and Walsh MC, eds. Elsevier, 1541–1570.
2. Amin R, and Oldham KT. 2021. Small and large bowel stenosis and atresias. In *Pediatric Gastrointestinal and Liver Disease*, 6th ed. Wyllie R, Hyams JS, and Kay M, eds. Elsevier, 588–592.
3. Spitzer AR. 2005. *Intensive Care of the Fetus and Neonate*, 2nd ed. Elsevier-Mosby.
4. Fletcher MA. 1998. *Physical Diagnosis in Neonatology*. Lippincott-Raven.
5. Cavaliere TA. 2019. Neonatal assessment. In *Golden Hours: Care of the Very Low Birth Weight Neonate*, 2nd ed. Bissinger RL, Annibale DJ, and Fanning BA, eds. The National Certification Corporation, 181–195.
6. Chiocca EM. 2015. *Advanced Pediatric Assessment*, 2nd ed. Springer Publishing Company, LLC.
7. Lissauer T, and Hansen A. 2020. Physical examination of the newborn. In *Fanaroff and Martin's Neonatal–Perinatal Medicine: Diseases of the Fetus and Infant*, 11th ed. Martin RJ, Fanaroff AA, and Walsh MC, eds. Elsevier, 440–457.
8. Gomella TL, Eyal FG, and Bany-Mohammed F. 2020. *Gomella's Neonatology: Management, Procedures, On-Call Problems, Diseases, and Drugs*, 8th ed. McGraw-Hill.
9. Muller A, Schurink M, Bos AF, et al. 2013. Clinical importance of a fixed bowel loop in the treatment of necrotizing enterocolitis. *Neonatology (Basel, Switzerland)* 105(1): 33–38. doi: 10.1159/000355064
10. Donlon CR, Furdon SA, and Clark DA. 2002. Look before you clamp: Delivery room examination of the umbilical cord. *Advances in Neonatal Care* 2(1): 19–26. doi: 10.1053/adnc.2002.31512
11. Thureen PJ, Deacon J, Hernandez J, and Hall D. 2004. *Assessment and Care of the Well Newborn*, 2nd ed. Elsevier Saunders.
12. Duderstadt K. 2019. *Pediatric Physical Examination: An Illustrated Handbook*, 3rd ed. Elsevier.
13. Alexander MM, and Brown MS. 1979. *Pediatric History Taking and Physical Diagnosis for Nurses*, 2nd ed. McGraw-Hill.
14. Bickley LS, Szilagyi PG, Hoffman RM, and Soriano RP. 2021. The abdomen. In *Bates' Guide to Physical Examination and History Taking*, 13th ed. Soriano RP, ed. Wolters Kluwer Health, 661–673.
15. Ball JW, Dains JE, Flynn JA, Solomon BS, and Stewart RW. 2022. *Seidel's Guide to Physical Examination: An Interprofessional Approach*. 10th ed. Elsevier.
16. De la Cruz DM, and Neu J. 2021. Disorders of the gastrointestinal tract. In *Avery's Neonatology: Pathophysiology & Management of the Newborn*, 7th ed. MacDonald MG, and Seshia MMK, eds. Wolters Kluwer, 546–563.
17. Walsh DS, Ponsky TA, and Bruns NE. 2017. *The SAGES Manual of Pediatric Minimally Invasive Surgery*. Springer International Publishing.
18. Melamed N, Kennedy A, and Glanc P. 2018. The fetal gastrointestinal tract and abdominal wall. In *Diagnostic Ultrasound*, 5th ed. Rumack CM, and Levin D, eds. Elsevier, 1304–1335.
19. Jones KL, del Campo M, and Jones MC. 2022. *Smith's Recognizable Patterns of Human Malformation*, 8th ed. Elsevier, Inc.
20. Rentea MR, and Levitt MA. 2019. Anorectal atresia and cloacal malformations. In *Holcomb and Ashcraft's Pediatric Surgery*, 7th ed. Holcomb GW, Murphy JP, St. Peter SD, and Gatti JM, eds. Elsevier, 577–598.

10 GENITOURINARY ASSESSMENT

Terri A. Cavaliere

A comprehensive newborn physical assessment includes an evaluation of the genitourinary (GU) system, which consists of kidneys and the urinary and reproductive tracts. These organs are closely related both anatomically and embryologically. This chapter focuses on examination of the GU system in the neonate using techniques of inspection, palpation, and percussion. Normal newborn characteristics and simple variations from normal are presented first, followed by a discussion of abnormalities and malformations.

HISTORY REVIEW

A newborn physical assessment begins with a review of prenatal history. Renal impairment or GU anomalies may be suggested by maternal, paternal, or family history of structural or functional anomalies, or abnormal findings on fetal ultrasounds (hydronephrosis, oligohydramnios).[1] Antenatal sonography often assists in diagnosis of disorders before birth or onset of symptoms in the newborn. Family history is an important consideration as certain GU anomalies have a genetic predisposition.[2,3] Parents of newborns with GU disorders should be questioned as to the occurrence of anomalies in family members. Genetic counseling may be appropriate in some instances.

Related Findings

Even without a documented history of oligohydramnios, physical signs of intrauterine compression in the newborn, such as flattened facies, malformed ears, and contraction deformities of the limbs (also known as *oligohydramnios (Potter) sequence*; Figure 10.1), suggest urogenital defects. Pulmonary hypoplasia, presenting as respiratory distress, may occur secondary to oligohydramnios or limited movement of the diaphragm caused by an intra-abdominal mass.[1,2]

There is a well-established correlation between GU anomalies and those of other systems. Careful evaluation of the GU system is warranted in newborns with other congenital anomalies such as myelomeningocele, complex congenital heart disease, and VACTERL association (**V**ertebral anomalies, **A**nal atresia, **C**ardiac abnormalities, **T**racheo **E**sophageal abnormalities, **R**enal abnormalities, and **L**imb anomalies).

The presence of oliguria or anuria may indicate underlying urologic disease. Ninety-eight percent of babies void in the first 30 hours of life, however it is not uncommon for the initial void at the time of delivery to go unnoticed. Lack of urine output in the first 48 hours of life in an *otherwise healthy* newborn should not be cause for alarm. However, diagnostic evaluation and/or intervention are necessary if there are any signs of illness or abnormalities (palpable bladder, abdominal mass, and renal disease) or if more than 48 hours pass without urination.[1] Anuria or oliguria after the first 48 hours of life can also be a sign of malformation or obstruction of the urinary tract.

Urine output is normally low during the first 2 days of life: full-term newborns may void one to four times, whereas a preterm newborn may void more frequently. The volume of urine production rises as intake

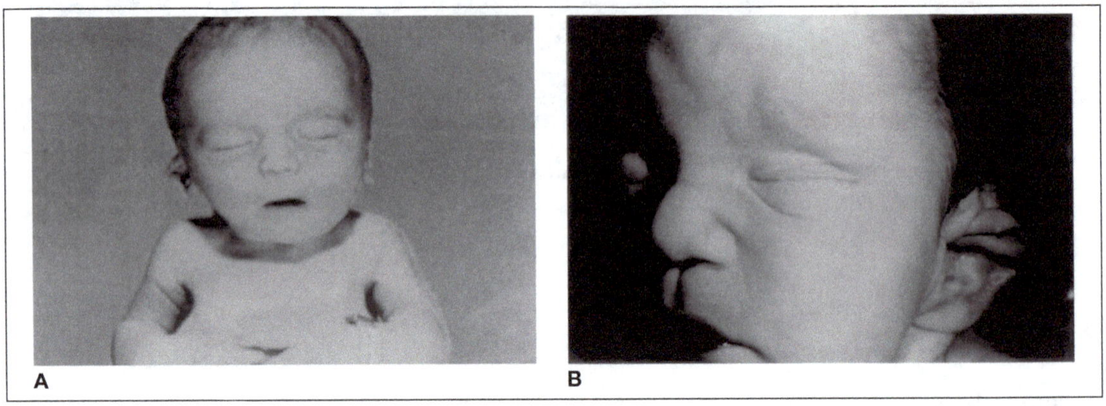

FIGURE 10.1 Compression effects of oligohydramnios, which may signal possible genitourinary or renal abnormalities. (A) Joint contractures, narrow thorax, malformed ear. (B) Typical facies; flattened nose, epicanthal fold, furrowed brow

Courtesy of J. Hernandez MD, The Children's Hospital, Denver, CO.

increases.[3] Documentation of adequate urinary output is important.

NORMAL PHYSICAL EXAMINATION

Abdomen

A comprehensive abdominal examination is described in Chapter 9. Those details pertinent to the GU system are presented here also. On inspection, the abdomen of a term newborn is rounded and symmetric, with smooth, opaque skin. A preterm newborn has a more protuberant abdomen because of immature muscle development, and the skin covering the abdomen may be thinner, with more prominent blood vessels.

The umbilical cord should be evaluated for appearance, length, diameter, number of vessels, and insertion site. At birth, the umbilical cord is gelatinous, bluish white in color, and contains three vessels: two arteries and one vein. There should be no exudate or discharge from the umbilicus. At term, the average cord length is 55 cm, with an average diameter of 2 cm. Cord length and appearance can provide clues to abnormalities. Abnormally short cords can indicate conditions such as fetal hypotonia, oligohydramnios, and uterine compression, while cords longer than 70 cm have higher risks for knotting, wrapping around fetal body parts, and/or prolapse.[4] Fetal distress, anomalies, and fetal demise may be seen when the cord is straight and untwisted.[4]

Palpation of the abdomen is easiest in the first 24 to 48 hours of life before air fills the entire gastrointestinal tract and before abdominal tone increases. All four quadrants should be examined to detect any masses. Palpation is best performed on a quiet newborn lying in a supine position with knees and hips maintained in flexion by the examiner's hand. Providing a gloved finger to evoke the sucking reflex may help to relax the abdominal musculature. The presence of a fussy, crying newborn or stool-filled intestines may make this portion of the examination somewhat difficult. If the examiner is unable to palpate the kidneys, the presence of *some* renal tissue is confirmed when the neonate voids.

The newborn's kidneys are in a lower position in the abdomen than they will be in later life. Normally, the inferior poles of both kidneys can be felt; the right kidney is usually lower than the left. Normal-sized kidneys, 4.5 to 5 cm in length in a term newborn, can be palpated in the flank areas above the level of the umbilicus.[5] They should be approximately equal in size and smooth to the touch. Ureters are not palpable under normal conditions. Enlarged kidneys are easy to detect; this finding should prompt further investigation.

Figure 10.2 illustrates one technique for palpating kidneys. The upper hand palpates the upper and lower quadrants, while the other hand supports the flank. The process is repeated on the opposite side. An alternate method is depicted in Figure 10.3. Place the fingers of one hand under the infant, with the thumb on the abdomen. To palpate the kidneys, compress the fingers against the thumb, the fingers support the flank while the thumb explores the area.[5]

The bladder can usually be palpated between the umbilicus and the symphysis pubis. Because the bladder wall is thin, this organ may be difficult to palpate. Percussion may be helpful to detect a full bladder over the symphysis pubis, or in differentiating between a urine-filled organ and a solid mass. A bladder containing urine will yield a tympanic sound, whereas a solid mass will invoke a dull sound.[6]

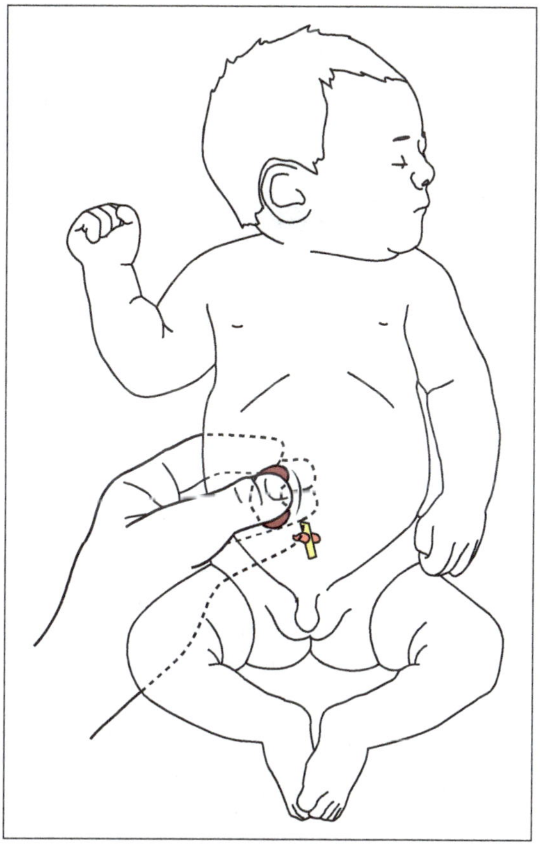

FIGURE 10.3 Alternate method for palpating the kidneys

Male Genitalia

Inspect the urogenital area with the male newborn in the supine position. Figure 10.4 depicts normal male genitalia. Gestational age has a great impact on the appearance of external genitalia. Figure 10.5 illustrates changes in external genitalia with advancing gestation. Rugae (wrinkles or creases) begin to form on the ventral surface of the scrotum at approximately 36 weeks gestation. At term, the scrotum is fully rugated and more deeply pigmented than the surrounding skin.

Palpate the scrotal sac and inguinal canal to locate the testes and detect any masses.

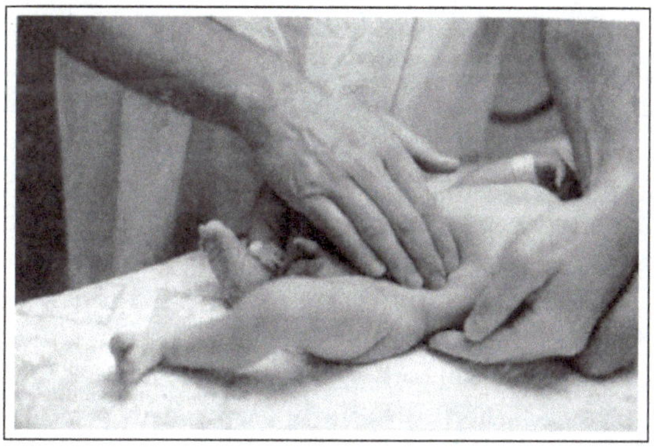

FIGURE 10.2 One technique for palpating the kidneys

Source: From Coen RW, and Koffler H. 1987. *Primary Care of the Newborn*. Boston, MA: Little, Brown, 30. Reprinted by permission.[18]

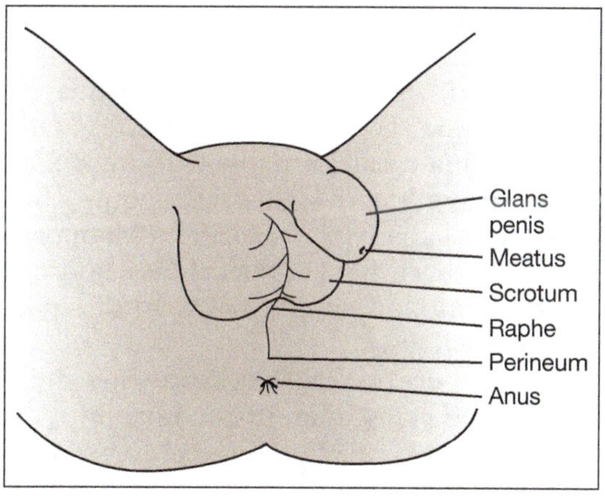

FIGURE 10.4 Normal newborn genitalia (male)

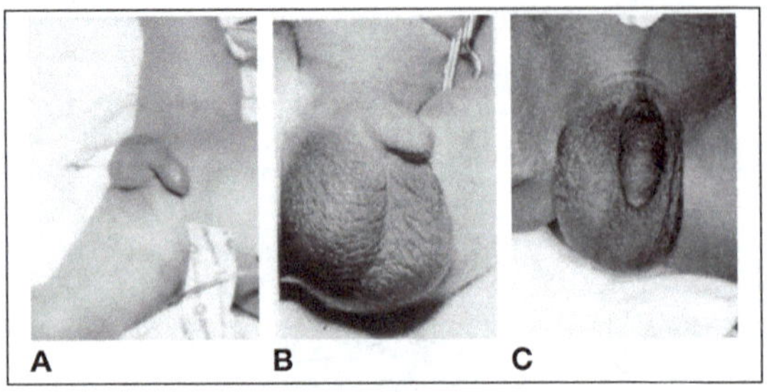

FIGURE 10.5 Appearance of genitalia in (A) preterm, (B) term, and (C) postterm male neonates

Source: Term infant is from Lepley CJ, Gardner SL, and Lubchenco LO. 1989. Initial nursery care. In *Handbook of Neonatal Intensive Care*, 2nd ed. Merenstein GB, and Gardner SL, eds. Philadelphia, PA: Mosby, 88. Reprinted by permission.[19]

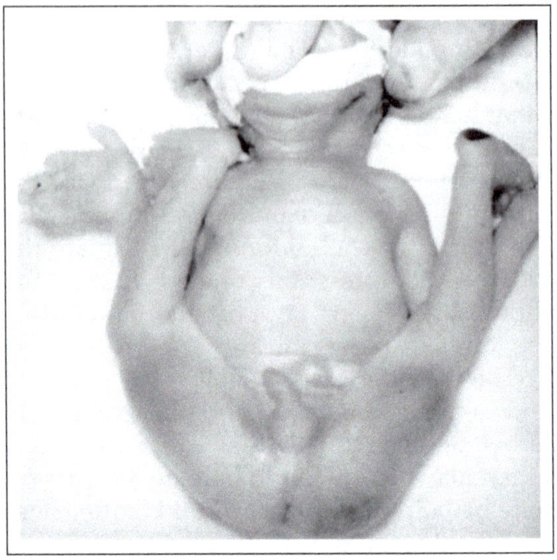

FIGURE 10.6 Genital bruising with breech presentation

Courtesy of Dr. David A. Clark, Albany, NY, Medical Center and Wyeth-Ayerst Laboratories, Philadelphia, PA.

Prior to 28 weeks gestation, the testes are abdominal organs; at 28 to 30 weeks, they begin to descend into the inguinal canal. By term, the testes should be well situated in the scrotum.[1,7] Normal testes are firm and smooth and comparatively equal in size. They are ovoid in shape, usually mobile, measuring approximately 8 to 14 mm at term.[8,9] The following technique is effective for detecting testes in the inguinal area: (a) Place the infant supine; (b) apply soap or oil to the skin and examiner's fingers; and (c) using gentle to firm pressure, slide two or three fingers along the inguinal canal toward the scrotum. It may be necessary to repeat this maneuver numerous times before testes can be felt.[9]

Newborn males may have edema of the genitalia because of transplacentally acquired maternal hormones. Trauma may occur during breech deliveries (Figure 10.6) or in very large babies causing ecchymosis, edema, or even hematomas. These findings are transient and should begin to dissipate after a few days.

The prepuce, or foreskin, covers the entire head of the penis in an uncircumcised male newborn. The function of the foreskin is to protect the urethral meatus from minor trauma.[9] Normally, the prepuce is tight, with a tiny orifice, but the opening is usually adequate to allow urination.[1] In newborns, the prepuce is adherent to the glans and cannot be retracted without disrupting its natural adherence to the surface of the glans. Therefore, forceful retraction should be avoided.[1] Physiologic phimosis, the inability to retract the foreskin, is normal in newborns and the foreskin generally becomes retractable during the first few years of life.[9]

Gentle traction is applied on the foreskin to visualize the urethral meatus at the central tip of the penis. The penis should be straight; erections are commonly seen in newborns. Observation and documentation of the force and direction of the urine stream while voiding is important. The urine stream should be forceful, straight, and continuous.

Penile length and width should be assessed. The average stretched length of the penis in a term newborn is 3.5 cm with a width of 0.9 to 3 cm, measured from the pubic bone to the tip of the glans (omitting excess foreskin).[2] Some newborns have a large deposit of adipose tissue overlying the pubic bone, giving the illusion of a small penis. In such cases, it is important to depress the fat pad while stretching the shaft for assessment of length. Comparative nomograms are available to enable the examiner to evaluate an abnormally sized penis.[7] There may be gestational and racial differences in the size of genitalia.[7] Male newborns with measurements that lie outside of the normal range should be compared to those of the same gestational age and racial background if such information is available. Figure 10.7 demonstrates a measurement technique for penile length. Penile width is measured midshaft on a stretched penis.

Female Genitalia

Female genitalia are best assessed with the newborn in the supine position. External female anatomy is illustrated in Figure 10.8; the labia majora are the outermost structures, extending from the mons pubis to the labial commissure. Medial to the labia majora are the labia minora, which join anteriorly to form the prepuce of the clitoris.

For the first 8 weeks of life, the term female newborn may have prominent labia, a large clitoris, and a urethral meatus that is difficult to visualize because of the influence of maternal estrogen. Maternal hormone exposure can stimulate a white, mucoid vaginal discharge and/or bleeding (pseudomenses).

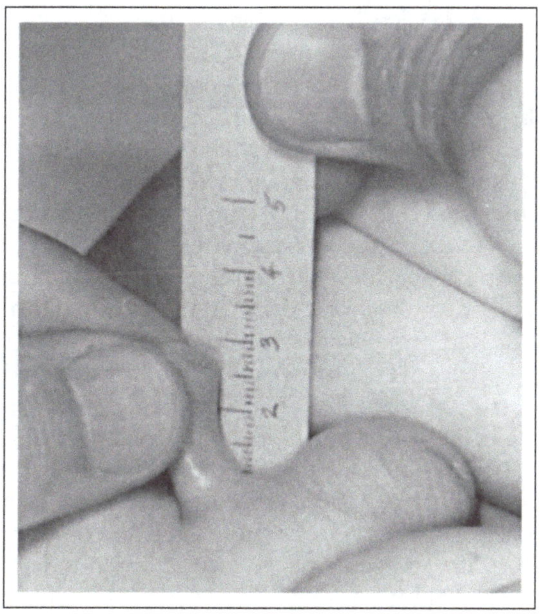

FIGURE 10.7 Technique for measuring penile length

Source: From Shulman RM, Palmert MR, and Wherrett DK. 2011. Disorders of sex development. In *Fanaroff and Martins Neonatal–Perinatal Medicine: Diseases of the Fetus and Infant*, 9th ed. Martin RJ, Fanaroff AA, and Walsh MC, eds. Philadelphia, PA: Mosby, 1592. Reprinted by permission.[20]

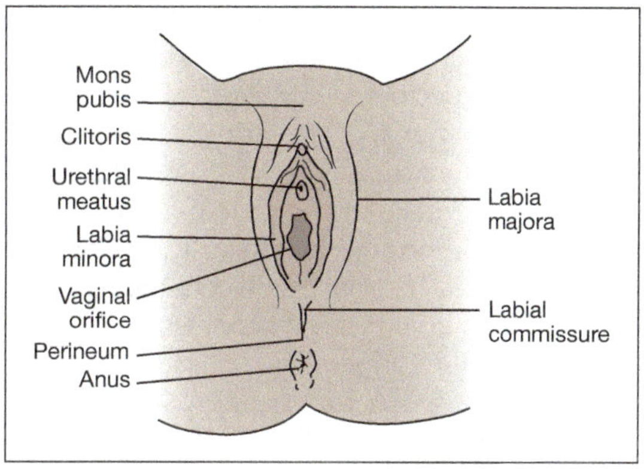

FIGURE 10.8 Normal newborn genitalia (female)

These findings may persist for up to 10 days. The genitalia of breech-positioned and large newborns may be edematous and ecchymotic for several days after delivery.[7] Gestational age influences the appearance of the female genitalia (Figure 10.9). In preterm females, the labia minora and clitoris are very prominent, and the labia majora are small because of a lack of adipose tissue. The labia majora are larger in more mature newborns; in term females, they usually cover the clitoris and labia minora. The urethral meatus should be just ventral to the vaginal opening. Deviation from this position may indicate a urogenital sinus or ambiguous genitalia.[10]

The labia and the inguinal and suprapubic areas are inspected and palpated to detect any masses, bulges, or swelling. The labia are then separated with gentle lateral and downward traction of the examiner's fingers. The clitoris is the uppermost structure, located at the junction of the labia minora. The normal clitoral width is 2 to 6 mm.[8]

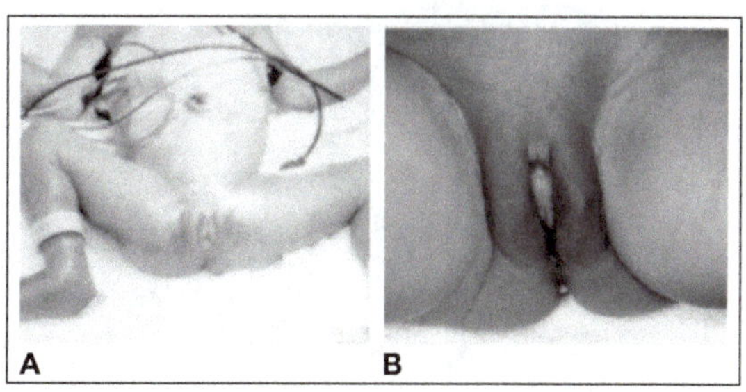

FIGURE 10.9 Appearance of genitalia in (**A**) preterm and (**B**) term female neonates

Directly below the clitoris and above the vaginal opening (3–4 mm slit) is the urethral meatus. The perineum is the area between the vaginal opening and the anus; it should be smooth, without dimpling or fistulas. Normally, in the term female, the perineum is as wide as a fingertip. Abnormal length of the perineum with abnormal spacing between the vaginal, urethral, and anal orifices is occasionally associated with GU anomalies.[10] The hymen is a thickened avascular membrane with a central orifice. A hymenal tag (Figure 10.10) is a common neonatal variation that usually disappears in a few weeks.[7]

ABNORMAL FINDINGS ON ABDOMINAL EXAMINATION

Abdominal Distention

Abdominal distention is a frequent finding in newborns because of poorly developed abdominal musculature. However, masses or, less commonly, ascites can be a cause of abdominal distention. Most palpable abdominal masses in newborns are of renal origin, and the most common causes are hydronephrosis and multicystic, dysplastic kidneys.[11] The urinary bladder is higher in the abdomen in the newborn than in the older infant, so bladder distention is a frequent cause of abdominal distention and the most common midline abdominal mass. Persistent bladder distention can signify structural urethral defects, bladder obstruction, or neuromuscular disease. Dilated, enlarged ureters caused by urinary tract obstruction can also present as abdominal masses. An abdominal mass is a cause for concern and warrants further investigation.

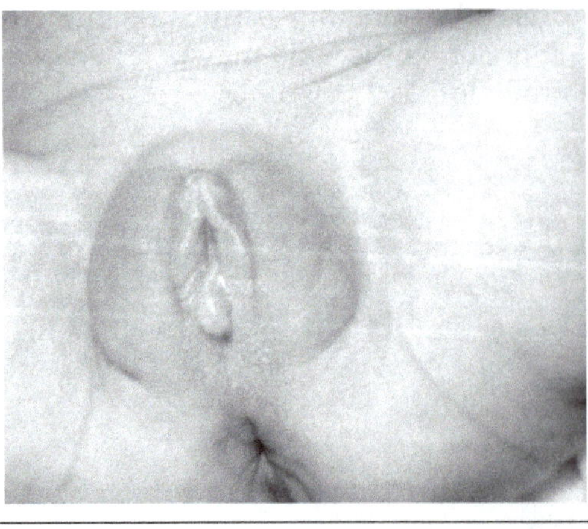

FIGURE 10.10 Hymenal tag in a neonate

Ascites refers to an intra-abdominal collection of fluid. Percussion reveals its presence. Lower urinary tract obstruction, particularly posterior urethral valves in the male, can be a cause of ascites. In these cases, ascitic fluid is composed of urine that has either escaped through a frank rupture in the collecting system or leaked through a renal calyx into the peritoneal cavity.[1]

Abdominal-Wall Defects

Eagle–Barrett syndrome (EBS), or triad syndrome, historically referred to as prune belly syndrome, is a congenital deficiency of the abdominal musculature that is readily apparent at birth (see Figure 9.5). The incidence of EBS is approximately one out of 35,000 to 50,000 births.[1] The characteristics of this syndrome are a large, flaccid, and wrinkled abdominal wall; undescended testes; and various GU malformations, such as hydroureter, hydronephrosis, and renal dysplasia. Occasionally, imperforate anus, intestinal malrotation, rib cage anomalies, cardiovascular abnormalities, and lower limb defects are also present. This syndrome is seen almost exclusively in males; reports of affected females are rare.

The spectrum of malformations called *exstrophy–epispadias complex (EEC)* involves defects of the urinary and genital tracts, musculoskeletal system, and sometimes the intestinal tract. *Exstrophy of the bladder* is a part of this spectrum. EEC is an uncommon condition, occurring in approximately one in 10,000 births, with a male predominance.[1] There is an absence of muscle and connective tissue in the anterior abdominal wall over the bladder caused by an embryologic defect, the incomplete closure of the inferior part of the abdominal wall. This presents as eversion and protrusion of the bladder through an abdominal-wall defect (Figure 10.11). The ureteral orifices can be identified on the exposed bladder surface. Complete exstrophy of the bladder is associated with epispadias in some male infants (Figure 10.12). In bladder exstrophy and epispadias, the upper urinary tract is usually normal, but renal agenesis, horseshoe kidneys, hydronephrosis, and other renal anomalies have been reported.

Cloacal exstrophy, the most severe defect, is more extensive and may include an omphalocele containing intestines, liver, and spleen (Figure 10.13).[1] Loops of cecum and terminal ileum may be seen dividing the exposed bladder into two sections. In males, the penis is small and divided in half, whereas females may present with a bifid clitoris and uterus and a duplicate or exstrophic vagina.[1]

A wide array of abnormalities involving the cardiac, gastrointestinal, renal, musculoskeletal, and neurologic systems is associated with cloacal exstrophy.[1]

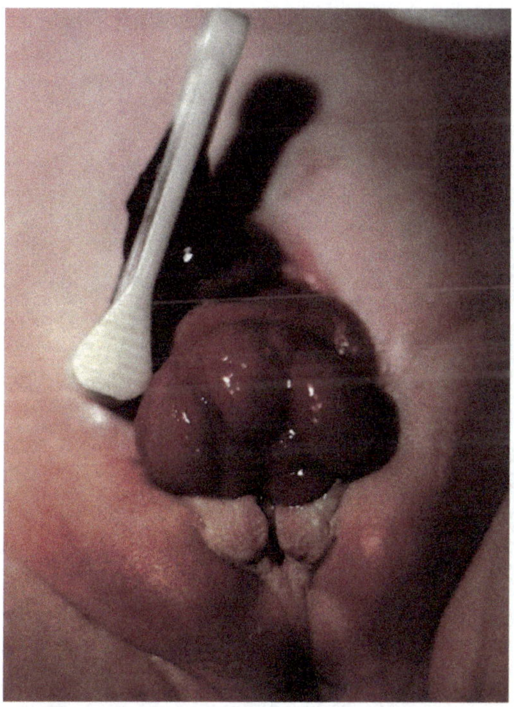

FIGURE 10.11 Exstrophy of the bladder

Source: Clark DA. 2000. *Atlas of Neonatology*. Philadelphia: Saunders, 201. Reprinted with permission.[22]

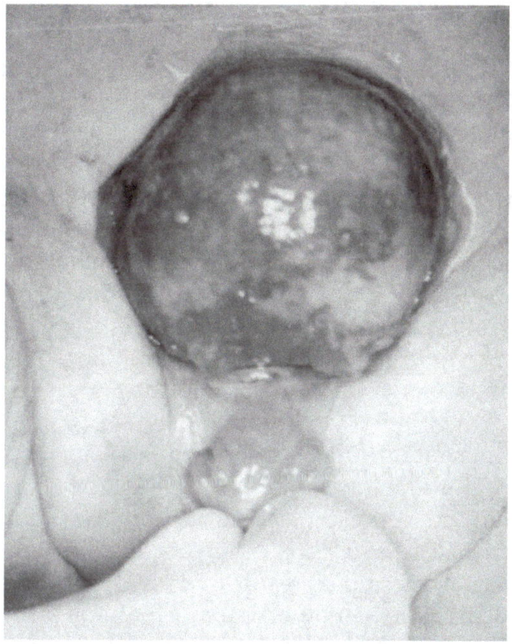

FIGURE 10.12 Exstrophy of the bladder with epispadias

Source: Kaplan GW, and McAleer IM. 2005. Structural abnormalities of the genitourinary tract. In *Neonatology. Pathophysiology and Management of the Newborn*, 6th ed. MacDonald MG, Mullett MD, and Seshia MMK, eds. Philadelphia: Lippincott Williams & Wilkins, 1077. Reprinted by permission.[23]

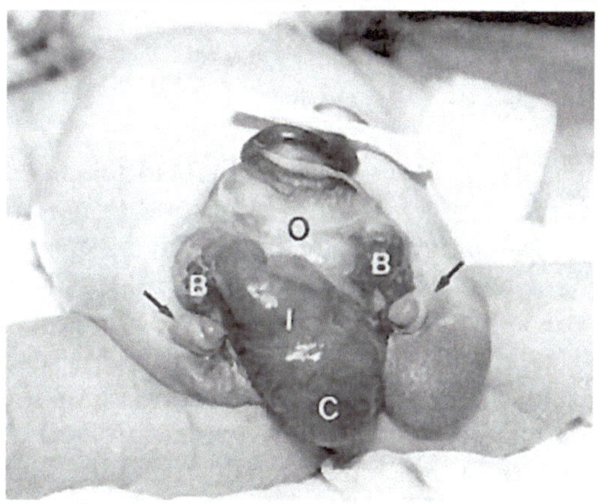

FIGURE 10.13 Newborn genetic male with cloacal exstrophy

Note: Separate bladder components **(B)**, associated omphalocele **(O)**, terminal ileum **(I)**, cecum **(C)**, and bifid penis *(arrows)*.

Source: From Zaontz MR, and Packer MG. 1997. Abnormalities of the external genitalia. *Pediatric Clinics of North America* 44(5): 1282. Reprinted by permission.[24]

Umbilical Cord Anomalies

A single umbilical artery (SUA) is found in 0.3% of newborns and can be identified on fetal ultrasound. It can be associated with an elevated risk of asymptomatic renal anomalies in 2% to 10% of cases. It is most often an isolated finding, therefore with absence of any other symptoms, additional diagnostic workup is no longer routinely recommended. When occurring as an isolated finding in an otherwise normal infant, other anomalies usually are not found, or if there are any renal anomalies, they are usually transient or mild.[4]

The urachus is an embryologic structure that connects the fetal bladder with the umbilicus. Postnatal patency of the urachal remnant can at times result in a clear discharge (urine) from an otherwise normal-appearing umbilical cord. The discharge of urine may be intermittent or minimal. A large, edematous umbilical cord that does not separate in the normal amount of time may be the only sign.[5] Urinary drainage from a urachal remnant can lead to umbilical granuloma, redness, or swelling below the umbilicus.

ABNORMALITIES OF THE MALE GENITALIA

The Penis

Aphallia (absence of a penis) and *diphallia* (duplicated penis) are rare conditions that require extensive reconstructive surgery. There are two types of duplications: bifid penis and true duplication. Bifid penis may occur in EEC and is characterized by separation of the corporal body of the penis into two halves, with a single urethral meatus at the base of the shafts. In true diphallia, there may be total duplication, with voiding and erectile function in individual shafts.[12]

Hypospadias is the abnormal location of the urethral meatus on the ventral surface of the penis. Hypospadias is a common abnormality, occurring in approximately 8.2/1,000 births, and results from the incomplete development of the anterior urethra.[9] Failure of the urethra to develop inhibits proper development of the prepuce. Most newborns with hypospadias also have a hooded or malformed prepuce (Figure 10.14).[9] It is important to locate the urethral meatus in a newborn with a malformed or hypoplastic prepuce and not simply to dismiss the malformation as a "natural circumcision."

Hypospadias can be classified into three categories based on meatal position: (a) Balanic (glanular) hypospadias exists when the urethral opening is ventrally situated at the base of the glans (Figure 10.15); (b) penile hypospadias occurs when the meatus is found between the glans and the scrotum (Figure 10.16); and (c) *penoscrotal hypospadias* (Figure 10.17) and *perineal hypospadias* are defined as the urethral opening at the penoscrotal junction and on the perineum, respectively. Isolated balanic (glanular) and penile hypospadias without other genital abnormalities or dysmorphic features are rarely associated with chromosomal or endocrine disorders or with problems of sexual differentiation. Newborns with penoscrotal or perineal hypospadias have a higher risk for these problems. In newborns with hypospadias and additional genital anomalies,

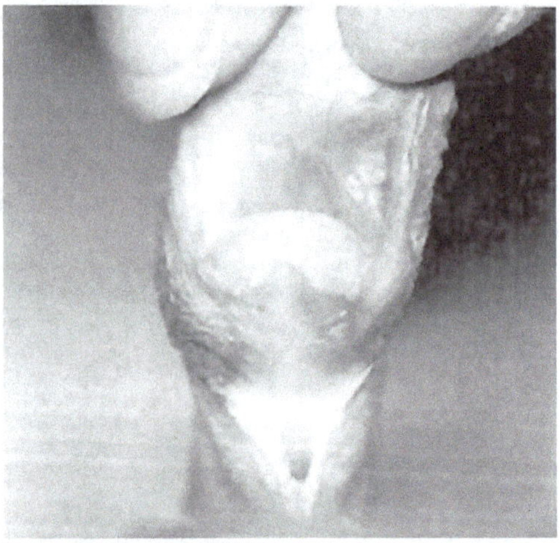

FIGURE 10.14 Distal hypospadias

Note: Dorsal hooded foreskin, flattened glans, and distal shaft meatus.

Source: From Zaontz MR, and Packer MG. 1997. Abnormalities of the external genitalia. *Pediatric Clinics of North America* 44(5): 1268. Reprinted by permission.[24]

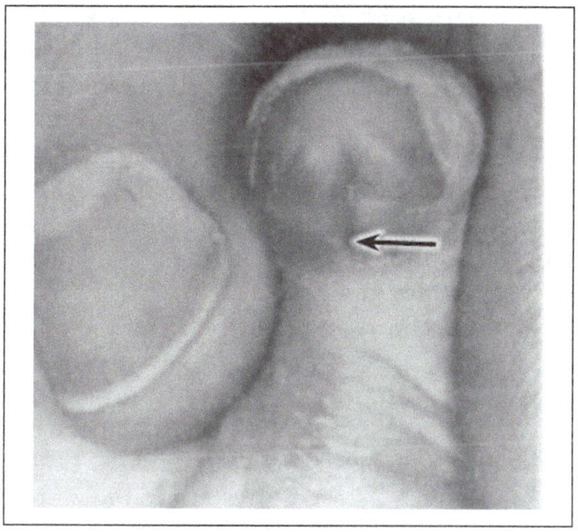

FIGURE 10.15 Balanic (or glanular) hypospadias

Notes: This is the most common form of hypospadias. The external urethral orifice is indicated by the arrow. There is a shallow pit at the usual site of the orifice. Note the moderate degree of chordee, causing the penis to curve ventrally.

Source: From Jolly H. 1968. *Diseases of Children*, 2nd ed. Oxford, UK: Blackwell Scientific Publications. Reprinted by permission via Copyright Clearance Center.[25]

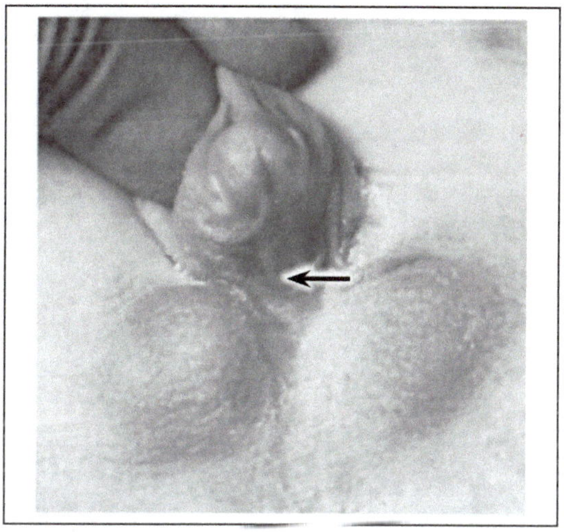

FIGURE 10.16 Penile hypospadias

Note: The penis is short and curved (chordee). The external urethral orifice (arrow) is near the penoscrotal junction.

Source: From Moore KL, and Persaud TVN. 1998. *Before We Are Born: Essentials of Embryology and Birth Defects*, 5th ed. Philadelphia, PA: Saunders, 320. Reprinted by permission.[26]

such as cryptorchidism or micropenis (both discussed later in this chapter), the risk for endocrine imbalance or problems with sexual differentiation rises.[9] Further investigation is warranted in these cases.

Chordee is a bend in the shaft of the penis, an aspect of penile development that occurs between the 16th and 20th week of gestation and may be seen in some normal premature newborns. In these newborns, chordee may resolve spontaneously within the first few months of life.[11] However, it is more common for chordee to be caused by fibrous tissue growth in an area of failed urethral development or by skin traction from skin deficiency as seen in hypospadias or epispadias.[1,12] Chordee may not be evident without the presence of an erection.[11] Ventral chordee frequently, but not always, accompanies hypospadias (see Figure 10.15).

A variant of hypospadias that can be identified only after circumcision is called *megameatus with intact prepuce*. In this type, there is a well-formed, complete foreskin; the hypospadias is hidden by the prepuce, and there is no chordee.[12]

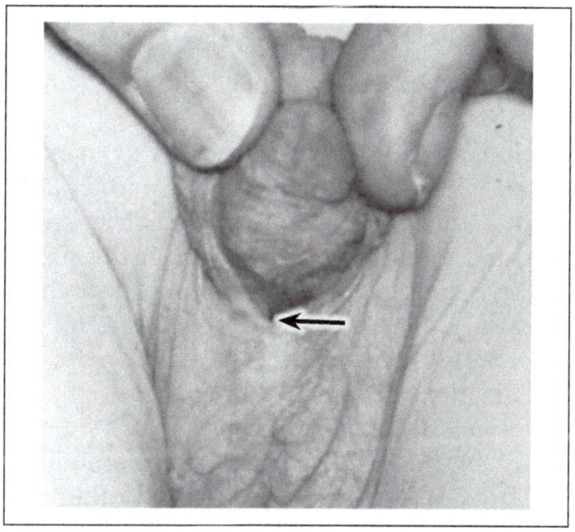

FIGURE 10.17 Penoscrotal hypospadias

Note: The external urethral orifice (arrow) is located at the penoscrotal junction.

Source: From Moore KL, and Persaud TVN. 1998. *Before We Are Born: Essentials of Embryology and Birth Defects*, 5th ed. Philadelphia, PA: Saunders, 320. Reprinted by permission.[26]

Epispadias, the location of the urethral meatus on the dorsal aspect of the penis, varies in severity from a glanular defect (Figure 10.18) to the complete version seen in exstrophy of the bladder (see Figure 10.12). Males with

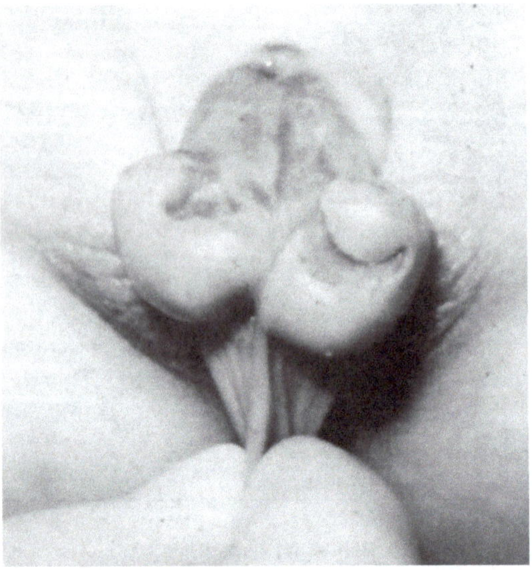

FIGURE 10.18 Epispadias

Source: Kaplan GW, and McAleer IM. 2005. Structural abnormalities of the genitourinary tract. In *Neonatology: Pathophysiology and Management of the Newborn*, 6th ed. MacDonald MG, Mullett MD, and Seshia MMK, eds. Philadelphia: Lippincott Williams & Wilkins, 1087. Reprinted by permission.[23]

epispadias have a dorsal chordee, while females have a bifid clitoris.[2]

Circumcision should be delayed in newborns with hypospadias or epispadias until after a consultation with a pediatric urologist; the foreskin may be used in the repair of these defects if a surgical repair is deemed necessary. Parents should be notified of the possibility of reconstructive surgery. Repair is generally performed after 6 months of age.[2]

Phimosis, which is generally physiologic in infants (see earlier in "Male Genitalia"), can become pathologic because of inflammation and scarring at the tip of the foreskin. Phimosis can occur due to forcefully retracting the foreskin.[12] Paraphimosis is a condition in which the foreskin has been retracted proximal to the glans penis and cannot be restored to its proper position because of swelling due to venous congestion.[12]

Hypospadias or epispadias can cause abnormalities in voiding.[12] In the male newborn, a weak urine stream, especially in the presence of a distended bladder, suggests the possibility of lower urinary tract obstruction (commonly, posterior urethral valves). A newborn with a spinal cord abnormality, such as a sacral tumor, spinal cord tethering, caudal regression syndrome, or myelomeningocele, can also have abnormalities in voiding as the result of a neurogenic bladder. In these newborns, lesions of the nervous system interrupt the conduction of impulses from the brain to the bladder, preventing normal micturition.

A *micropenis* is an abnormally short or thin penis that is more than 2.5 standard deviations below the mean of length and width for age using standard charts. Occasionally the penis appears small but, in reality, the measurement is within acceptable limits when stretched. This is termed an *inconspicuous penis*[12]; the measurement technique is illustrated in Figure 10.7. Evaluation and management of a newborn with a true micropenis frequently requires an endocrinologist and a geneticist[1] (see "Disorders of Sexual Development"). An acquired form of an inconspicuous penis is a phallus that becomes surrounded by the suprapubic fat pad after circumcision is performed.[12]

Priapism is a persistent, apparently painless, penile erection lasting less than 4 hours, typically resolving spontaneously. The most common cause is sickle cell disease. Other factors that may contribute to its development are polycythemia and birth trauma. Many cases of priapism are idiopathic.[12,8] In a neonate with a *webbed penis* (Figure 10.19), there is a normal urethra and scrotum. However, the scrotal skin extends onto the ventral surface of the shaft, obscuring the penoscrotal angle and making the penis appear short.[12]

Penile torsion is a rotational deformity of the shaft, most often counterclockwise (to the left). This deformity is not obvious until after a circumcision or foreskin retraction and may be an isolated finding or may accompany other penile abnormalities.[11]

The Scrotum

Cryptorchidism is the lack of a palpable testis/testes in the scrotum, referring to a testis or testes in an extra scrotal location.[10,13] Cryptorchidism is diagnosed by the inability to palpate one or both testes in the scrotal

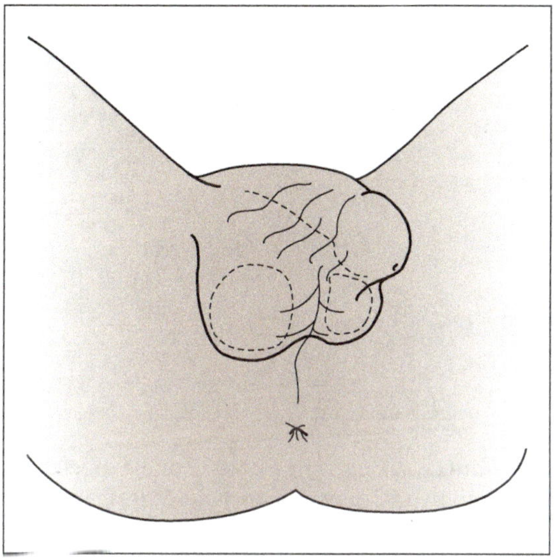

FIGURE 10.19 Webbed penis

Source: Adapted from Grumbach TA, and Bloom DA. 1997. Male genital tract. In *Surgery of Infants and Children: Scientific Principles and Practice*, Oldham KT, Colombani PM, and Foglia RP, eds. Philadelphia, PA: Lippincott-Raven, 1547. Reprinted by permission.[21]

sac. Cryptorchidism is seen in approximately 3.4% of term males, 30% of all preterm newborns, and nearly 100% in extremely preterm infants since testicular descent typically occurs at approximately 7 to 8 months of gestation.[10,13] A unilateral, undescended testis is more common than bilateral cryptorchidism. Bilateral cryptorchidism (anorchia) presents as an empty, hypoplastic scrotal sac.

A truly undescended testis is one that is interrupted in its usual path of descent, whereas an ectopic testis pursues an abnormal course of descent and may be found in a superficial inguinal pouch.[10,12] A retractile testis is a normally descended organ that recedes into the inguinal canal because of activity of the cremasteric muscle. Because this muscle is inactive in newborns, retractile testes do not occur in this age group.[20] Thus, an empty or a hypoplastic scrotal sac in a newborn, when detected by observation and palpation, indicates truly undescended testes, ectopic testes (outside the external inguinal ring), or anorchia (absence of testicular tissue).[13]

Most undescended testes (50%) will descend by 3 months of age. Spontaneous descent rarely occurs after 9 months of age.[10,13] Diagnosis of true cryptorchidism and subsequent surgical intervention, called *orchiopexy*, is important because of an associated risk for infertility and malignancy in the cryptorchid testis.[10,13] Retractile testes usually grow and develop normally.[10]

Cryptorchidism may be an isolated defect, or it may exist with other GU anomalies such as hypospadias or micropenis. Newborns with undescended testes and other abnormal features, such as micropenis, bifid scrotum, and hypospadias, should be evaluated for endocrine problems and gender ambiguity.[10,13]

Hydroceles and hernias commonly present as bulges or swellings in the groin or scrotum.[14] Both are the result of a patent processus vaginalis; however, they differ in several ways. A *hydrocele* (Figure 10.20) is generally a nontender, fluid-filled, scrotal mass overlying the testis and spermatic cord presenting as a scrotal swelling. This is caused by the passage of peritoneal fluid through the patent processus vaginalis into the scrotum or by the persistence of peritoneal fluid that has not been resorbed.[13,15] Upon examination, the entire circumference of the testis can be palpated. An actual or a potential indirect *inguinal hernia* (IH) may be associated with a hydrocele. Loops of intestine can herniate through the persistent processus vaginalis into the scrotum (Figure 10.21). The incidence of hernias is inversely proportional to gestational age and birth weight. Both positive family history and prematurity increase the incidence of IH in both males and females, although they present more often in males.[21] Other conditions associated with the development of an IH are hydrops fetalis, meconium peritonitis, urinary and chylous ascites, ambiguous genitalia, hypospadias, epispadias, cryptorchidism, cystic fibrosis, ventriculoperitoneal shunts, congenital hypothyroidism, and Beckwith–Wiedemann syndrome.[15] An examiner should be able to palpate a testis located in a soft hydrocele, but they may not be able to do so in the presence of a tense hydrocele. The presence of intestines in the scrotal sac renders the entire circumference of the testis impalpable.[7]

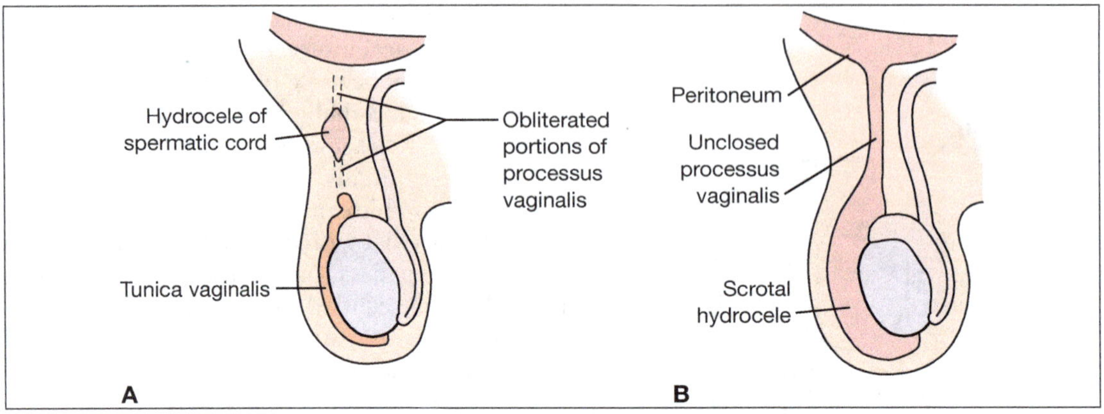

FIGURE 10.20 Hydrocele. (A) Large hydrocele that resulted from an unobliterated portion of the processus vaginalis. (B) Hydrocele of the testis and spermatic cord resulting from peritoneal fluid passing into an unclosed processus vaginalis

Source: From Moore KL, Persaud TVN, and Torchia MG. 2013. *The Developing Human: Clinically Oriented Embryology*, 9th ed. Philadelphia, PA: Saunders, 286. Reprinted by permission.[27]

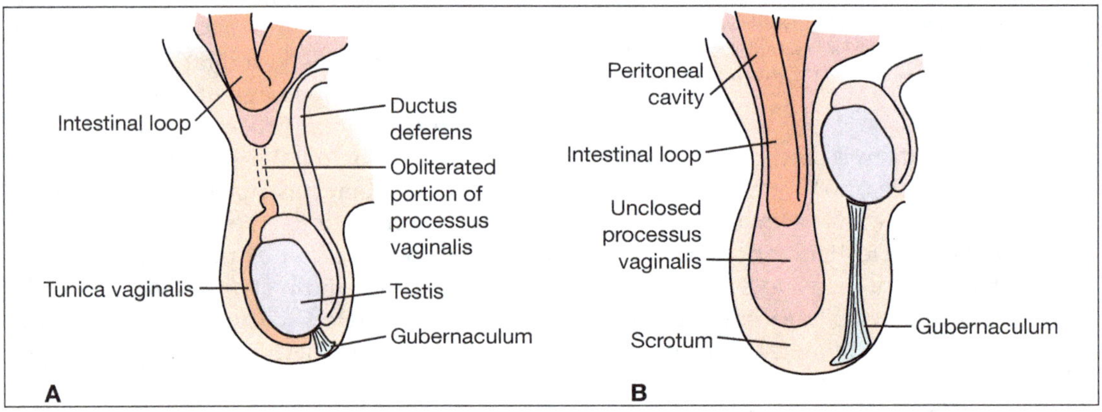

FIGURE 10.21 Inguinal hernia. (A) Incomplete congenital inguinal hernia resulting from persistence of the proximal part of the processus vaginalis. (B) Complete congenital inguinal hernia into the scrotum resulting from persistence of the processus vaginalis. Cryptorchidism, a commonly associated anomaly, is also illustrated

Source: From Moore KL, Persaud TVN, and Torchia MG. 2013. *The Developing Human: Clinically Oriented Embryology*, 9th ed. Philadelphia, PA: Saunders, 286. Reprinted by permission.[27]

A scrotal mass or swelling from a hydrocele may be further distinguished from swelling caused by a hernia because a hydrocele typically appears translucent on transillumination (Figure 10.22). However, hernias may also transilluminate because the bowel contains air.[15] Hernias are reducible, and hydroceles are not. To reduce a hernia, the examiner should grasp the most distal portion of the scrotum on the affected side with the fingers of one hand and apply firm, steady, upward pressure in the direction of the internal ring. The scrotal sac will decrease in size as the intestines return to the abdomen through the internal ring.[15]

Bowel incarceration, strangulation, and ischemic injury to the testes are potential complications of IH. Incarceration is the inability to easily reduce the hernia; in strangulation, the loop of the bowel becomes trapped, leading to ischemia and ultimate necrosis. Redness, pain, symptoms of intestinal obstruction, and difficulty in reduction are evidence of incarceration.

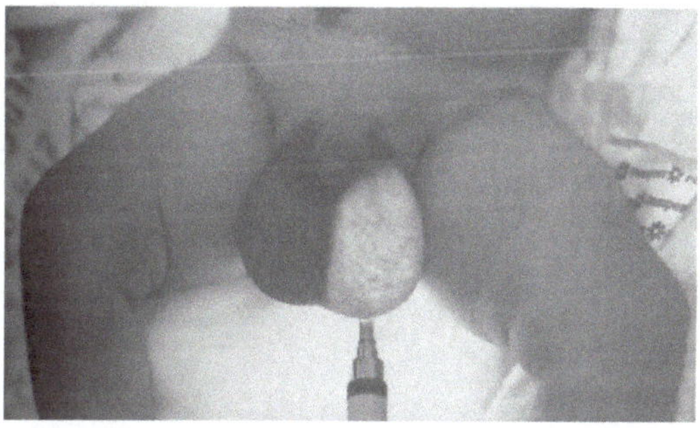

FIGURE 10.22 Transillumination of a scrotal hydrocele

Source: From Coen RW, and Koffler H. 1987. *Primary Care of the Newborn*. Boston, MA: Little, Brown, 33. Reprinted by permission.[18]

Most hydroceles resolve in the first year of life.[15]

Testicular torsion, or twisting of the testis on its spermatic cord, may occur prenatally and is usually unilateral. The neonate presents with a hard, swollen scrotum that is red to bluish red in color and does not transilluminate. This condition compromises blood supply to the testis; therefore, it requires urgent evaluation and possibly emergency management.[20] Ischemia of more than 4 to 6 hours duration usually results in irreversible damage and loss of the gonad.[20] With prenatal torsion, the duration of the torsion is unknown; by birth, irreversible ischemic damage to the testis may have occurred. Testicular torsion is painful in older children, but pain is not a universal finding in newborns.[9] Therefore, one should not be misled into discounting the possibility of testicular torsion in the case of a newborn male with a red, swollen scrotum that is not tender.

ABNORMALITIES OF THE FEMALE GENITALIA

There are several types of perineal masses found in newborn genetic females. *Periurethral cysts* are the most common, appearing as a whitish epithelial covering adjacent to the unaffected urethral meatus. An *imperforate hymen* is frequently identified as a white midline bulge symmetrically located between the labia. Hydrocolpos (distention of the vagina) and hydrometrocolpos (distention of the vagina and the uterus; Figure 10.23) are the result of either incomplete canalization of the vagina during gestation or an imperforate hymen.[16,17] These conditions present in the newborn as lower abdominal masses and frequently as urinary tract obstructions. The most common complication of hydrocolpos is compression of the bladder, leading to urinary retention and hydronephrosis, which can ultimately cause kidney damage. This can be prevented by drainage of the accumulated fluid.[2]

When the hymen is imperforate, it may bulge secondary to the accumulation of vaginal secretions, creating the appearance of a shiny, cystic mass between the labia.[17] IH occur less frequently in females than in males; they arise more frequently in extremely premature neonates than in those born closer to term. The uterus, fallopian tubes, and ovaries, as well as the bowel, may herniate. When IH does occur, it sometimes presents as a reducible swelling of the labia (Figure 10.24). If a gonad is palpable in the suprapubic region of a female, there may be concern over whether the neonate is a genetic female with an ovarian prolapse or a genetic male with a disorder of sexual differentiation (DSD). This is because only testes usually descend, not ovaries.[29]

Clitoromegaly has been defined as an 8- to 10-fold increase in the clitoral index (defined as

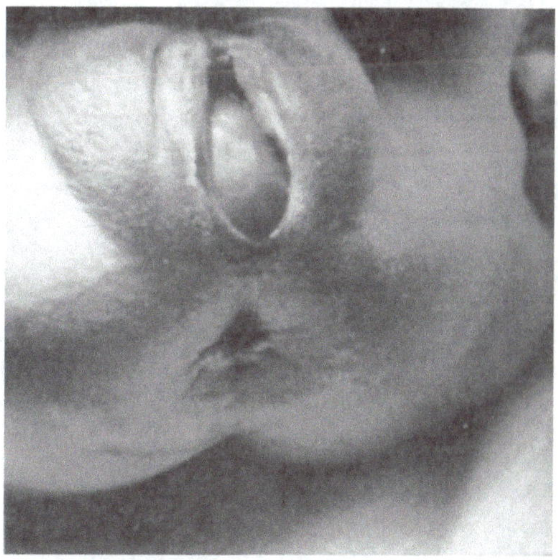

FIGURE 10.23 Hydrometrocolpos

Source: From Coen RW, and Koffler H. 1987. *Primary Care of the Newborn*. Boston, MA: Little, Brown, 90. Reprinted by permission.[18]

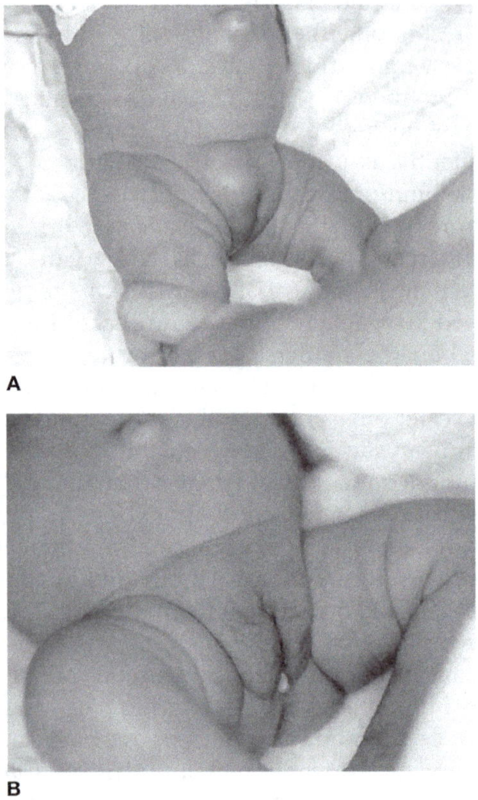

FIGURE 10.24 Inguinal hernias (A) before and (B) after reduction. Hymenal tag is apparent after reduction (B).

Source: From Fletcher M. 1998. *Physical Diagnosis in Neonatology*. Philadelphia: Lippincott-Raven, 388. Reprinted by permission.[8]

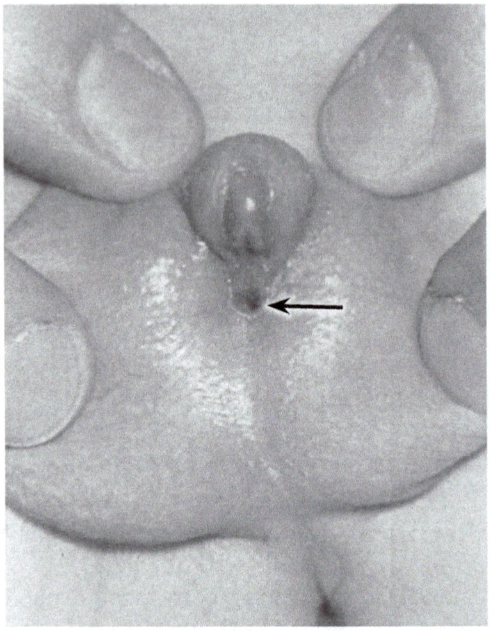

FIGURE 10.25 Newborn male infant (46, XY) with ambiguous genitalia

Note: Penoscrotal hypospadias (arrow). Testes are palpable in the scrotum.

Source: From Palmert MR, and Dahms WT. 2006. Abnormalities of sexual differentiation. In *Fanaroff and Martin's Neonatal–Perinatal Medicine: Diseases of the Fetus and Infant*, 8th ed. Martin RJ, Fanaroff AA, and Walsh MC, eds. Philadelphia, PA: Mosby, 1565. Reprinted by permission.[28]

width times length). Causes of clitoromegaly in the newborn include endocrine abnormalities (congenital adrenal hyperplasia), maternal factors (increased androgen production, drugs), and syndromes (Beckwith–Wiedemann, true hermaphroditism).[1,8] Typically the large appearing clitoris in premature neonates is due to a temporary deficiency of adipose tissue in the labia. As weight gain occurs, the clitoris becomes covered by the labia (see normal female genitalia, Figure 10.8).

Disorders of Sexual Development

The presence of (a) a phallic structure that is not discretely male or female, (b) an abnormally located urethral meatus, or (c) an inability to palpate one or both gonads in males is typically referred to as ambiguous gentalia (Figure 10.25).[10] One should suspect challenges with sexual differentiation in phenotypic males with bilateral impalpable testes, perineal hypospadias, or a unilateral undescended testis with hypospadias. Similarly, phenotypic females with clitoral hypertrophy, a palpable gonad, inseparably fused labia, or abnormal openings or dimpling on the perineum should also be evaluated (Figure 10.26).[1,10] The association of ambiguous genitalia with serious underlying endocrine disorders and the understandable distress of the parents require rapid identification and evaluation of these newborns. A multidisciplinary team consisting of an endocrinologist, a genetic specialist, a urologist,

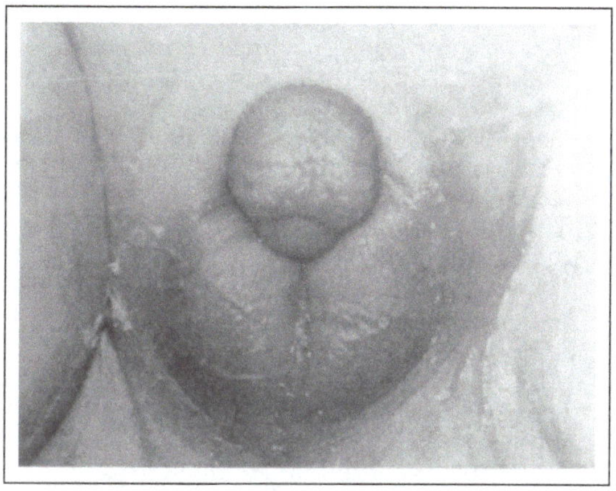

FIGURE 10.26 Newborn female with ambiguous genitalia: Clitoral enlargement and fusion of labia majora

Source: From Moore KL, and Persaud TVN. 1998. *Before We Are Born: Essentials of Embryology and Birth Defects*, 5th ed. Philadelphia, PA: Saunders, 307. Reprinted by permission.[26]

and a psychologist/social worker should be included on the neonatal/pediatric evaluation team. The newborn's parents should be involved in a discussion as to how they wish the baby will be referred to until the appropriate sex of the newborn is determined. Until this decision is made the newborn may be referred to as "baby" or "newborn."

SUMMARY

Evaluation of the GU tract in the newborn is important to ensure rapid detection and treatment of abnormalities. Too frequently, this examination is cursory, and abnormalities, both major and minor, go unnoticed. Identification of problems in the neonatal period may preserve organ function and prevent mortality and morbidity in the future.

ADDITIONAL RESOURCES

SPRINGER PUBLISHING CONNECT™ | A robust set of resources designed to supplement this text is located at http://connect.springerpub.com/content/book/978-0-8261-4063-0. Qualifying instructors may request access by emailing textbook@springerpub.com.

REFERENCES

1. Vogt BA, and Springel T. 2020. The kidney and urinary tract of the neonate. In *Neonatal–Perinatal Medicine: Diseases of the Fetus and Infant*, 11th ed. Martin RJ, Fanaroff AA, and Walsh MC, eds. Philadelphia, PA: Elsevier, 93, 1871–1895.
2. Murgerian PA, and Rowe CK. 2018. Developmental abnormalities of the genitourinary system. In *Avery's Diseases of the Newborn*, 10th ed. Gleason CA, and Juul SE, eds. Philadelphia, PA: Elsevier, 88, 1260–1273.
3. Bates CM, and Schwaderer AL. 2018. Clinical evaluation of renal and urinary tract disease. In *Avery's Diseases of the Newborn*, 10th ed. Gleason CA, and Juul SE, eds. Philadelphia, PA: Elsevier, 89, 1176–1181.
4. Nathan AT. 2020. The umbilicus. In *Nelson Textbook of Pediatrics*, 21st ed. Kleigman RM, Blum NJ, Shah SS, St. Geme JW, Tasker RC, and Wilson KM, eds. Philadelphia, PA: Elsevier, 125, 975–976.
5. Ngo KD, and Shah M. 2020. Gastrointestinal system. In *Comprehensive Neonatal Nursing Care*, 7th ed. Kenner C, Altimier LB, and Boykova MV, eds. New York, NY: Springer Publishing Company, 8, 179–210.
6. Parker LA. 2020. Genitourinary system. In *Comprehensive Neonatal Nursing Care*, 6th ed. Kenner C, Altimier LB, and Boykova MV, eds. New York, NY: Springer Publishing Company, 18, 449–480.
7. Cavaliere TA. 2020. Assessment of the newborn and infant. In *Comprehensive Neonatal Nursing Care*, 7th ed. Kenner C, Altimier LB, and Boykova MV, eds. New York, NY: Springer Publishing Company, 4, 65–104.
8. Fletcher M. 1998. *Physical Diagnosis in Neonatology*. Philadelphia, PA: Lippincott-Raven, 388.
9. Rozanski TA, and Bloom D. 1997. Male genital tract. In *Surgery of Infants and Children: Scientific Principles and Practice*, Oldham KT, Colombani PM, and Foglia RP, eds. Philadelphia, PA: Lippincott Williams & Wilkins, 1543–1558.
10. Sorbara JC, and Wherrett DK. 2020. Disorders of sex development. In *Neonatal–Perinatal Medicine: Diseases of the Fetus and Infant*, 11th ed. Martin RJ, Fanaroff AA, and Walsh MC, eds. Philadelphia, PA: Elsevier, 898, 1665–1705.
11. Elder JS. 2016. Renal dysgenesis: Dysplasia, hypoplasia, and cystic anomalies. In *Nelson Textbook of Pediatrics*, 20th ed. Kliegman RM, Stanton BMD, St. Geme J, and Schor N, eds. Philadelphia, PA: Elsevier, 2554–2556.

12. Elder JS. 2020. Abnormalities of the penis and urethra. In *Nelson Textbook of Pediatrics*, 21st ed. Kleigman RM, Blum NJ, Shah SS, St. Geme JW, Tasker RC, and Wilson KM, eds. Philadelphia, PA: Elsevier, 559, 2821–2826.
13. Elder JS. 2016. Disorders and anomalies of the scrotal contents. In *Nelson Textbook of Pediatrics*, 21st ed. Kleigman RM, Blum NJ, Shah SS, St. Geme JW, Tasker RC, and Wilson KM, eds. Philadelphia, PA: Elsevier, 560, 2827–2833.
14. Aiken JJ. 2020. Inguinal hernia. In *Nelson Textbook of Pediatrics*, 21st ed. Kleigman RM, Blum NJ, Shah SS, St. Geme JW, Tasker RC, and Wilson KM, eds. Philadelphia, PA: Elsevier, 373, 2064–2070.
15. Barthold JS, and Hagerty JA. 2016. Etiology, diagnosis and management of the undescended testes. In *Campbell–Walsh Urology*, 11th ed. Wein AJ, Kavoussi LR, Partin AW, and Peters CA, eds. Philadelphia, PA: Elsevier, 3430–3452.
16. Karfer M. 2016. Management of abnormalities of the genitalia in girls. In *Campbell–Walsh Urology*, 11th ed. Wein AJ, Kavoussi LR, Partin AW, and Peters CA, eds. Philadelphia, PA: Elsevier, 3453–3465.
17. Lee RS, and Borer JG. 2016. Perinatal urology. In *Campbell–Walsh Urology*, 11th ed. Wein AJ, Kavoussi LR, Partin AW, and Peters CA, eds. Philadelphia, PA: Elsevier, 2873, 2892.
18. Coen RW, and Koffler H. 1987. *Primary Care of the Newborn*. Boston, MA: Little, Brown, 30, 33, 90.
19. Lepley CJ, Gardner SL, and Lubchenco LO. 1989. Initial nursery care. In *Handbook of Neonatal Intensive Care*, 2nd ed. Merenstein GB, and Gardner SL, eds. Philadelphia, PA: Mosby, 88.
20. Shulman RM, Palmert MR, and Wherrett DK. 2011. Metabolic and endocrine disorders, Part 4: Disorders of sex development. In *Fanaroff and Martin's Neonatal–Perinatal Medicine: Diseases of the Fetus and Infant*, 9th ed. Martin RJ, Fanaroff AA, and Walsh MC, eds. Philadelphia, PA: Mosby, 1592.
21. Grumbach MM, and Conte FA. 1992. Disorders of sexual differentiation. In *William's Textbook of Endocrinology*, 8th ed. Wilson JD, and Foster DW, eds. Philadelphia, PA: Saunders, 331.
22. Clark DA. 2000. *Atlas of Neonatology*. Philadelphia, PA: Saunders, 201.
23. Kaplan GW, and McAleer IM. 2005. Structural abnormalities of the genitourinary tract. In *Neonatology: Pathophysiology and Management of the Newborn*, 6th ed. MacDonald MG, Mullett MD, and Seshia MMK, eds. Philadelphia, PA: Lippincott Williams & Wilkins, 1077.
24. Zaontz MR, and Packer MG. 1997. Abnormalities of the external genitalia. *Pediatric Clinics of North America* 44(5): 1268, 1282.
25. Jolly H. 1968. *Diseases of Children*, 2nd ed. Oxford, UK: Blackwell Scientific Publications.
26. Moore KL, and Persaud TVN. 1998. *Before We Are Born: Essentials of Embryology and Birth Defects*, 5th ed. Philadelphia, PA: Saunders, 307, 320.
27. Moore KL, Persaud TVN, and Torchia MG. 2020. *The Developing Human: Clinically Oriented Embryology*, 11th ed. Philadelphia, PA: Elsevier, 12, 223–262.
28. Palmert MR, and Dahms WT. 2006. Abnormalities of sexual differentiation. In *Fanaroff and Martin's Neonatal–Perinatal Medicine: Diseases of the Fetus and Infant*, 8th ed. Martin RJ, Fanaroff AA, and Walsh MC, eds. Philadelphia, PA: Mosby, 1565.
29. Laufer MR. 2022. *The Pediatric Physical Examination: General principles and standard measurements*. Chakrabarti A, ed. UpToDate. Retrieved from https://www-uptodate-com.proxy.library.stonybrook.edu/contents/congenital-anomalies-of-the-hymen-and-vagina

11 MUSCULOSKELETAL SYSTEM ASSESSMENT

Ellen P. Tappero

The musculoskeletal system of the body provides stability and mobility for all physical activity. It consists of the body's bones (Figure 11.1), joints, and their supporting and connecting tissues. In addition to allowing movement and providing structure, the musculoskeletal system protects vital organs (brain, spinal cord), stores minerals (calcium, phosphorus), and produces red blood cells and white blood cells. Careful scrutiny of the musculoskeletal system during the newborn's physical examination is imperative because (a) it is vital to the confirmation of musculoskeletal abnormalities detected on prenatal ultrasound such as spinal malformations, limb length discrepancies, and clubfoot deformities; and (b) the information recorded during the first examination forms the database for all future examinations, ordering of diagnostic tests, and development of management plans.

The bones of the newborn are soft because they are composed mostly of cartilage, which contains only a small amount of calcium. The process of ossification occurs rapidly during the first year of life. Compared with the skeleton of an adult or a child, the newborn's skeleton is flexible, and the joints are elastic. This elasticity is necessary to enable the infant to pass through the birth canal.

Unlike the bones of the skeletal system, the muscular system is almost completely formed at birth. Growth in the size of the muscle is caused by hypertrophy, rather than by hyperplasia of the cells.[1,2]

A thorough evaluation of the musculoskeletal system involves the techniques of inspection, palpation, and, on some occasions, listening. It includes an appraisal of the following:

1. Posture, position, and gross anomalies
2. Discomfort from bone or joint movement
3. Range of joint motion
4. Muscle size, symmetry, and strength
5. Configuration and motility of the back

Normal variations in shape, size, contour, or movement may be the result of position in utero or genetic factors. These normal variations should be distinguished from congenital anomalies and birth trauma. Early diagnosis of musculoskeletal disorders and early intervention often preempt the need for complex medical treatment and lead to more favorable outcomes.[3] Disorders that affect the musculoskeletal system may also originate from the neurologic system. An asymmetric Moro reflex, for example, may be caused by pain from a broken bone or a muscle injury, or it may be the result of a neurologic defect. Because there is some overlap between the musculoskeletal and neurologic examinations, assessment of muscle strength and motor activity are discussed with other neurologic assessments in Chapter 12.

PRENATAL HISTORY

Obtaining a comprehensive prenatal history is vital to the musculoskeletal assessment because the uterine environment is essential to the development of the fetus. Any event or condition that changes the intrauterine environment can alter fetal growth, movement, or position. Such prenatal factors as oligohydramnios, maternal uterine malformations, abnormal growth patterns, exposure to teratogenic agents, and breech presentation may

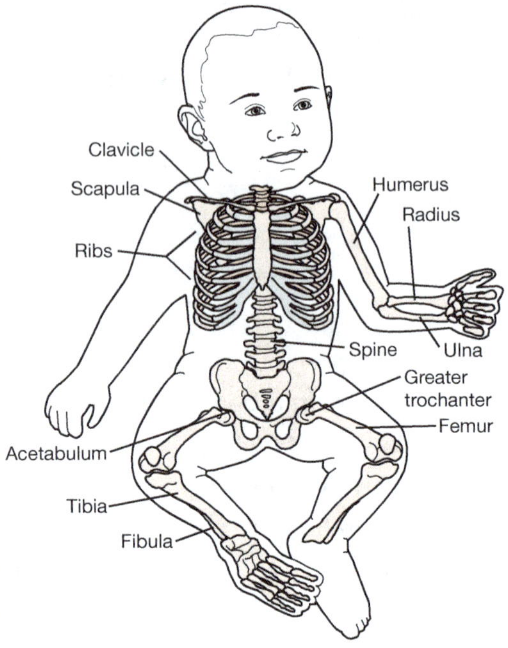

FIGURE 11.1 Infant's skeletal structure

adversely affect the development and maturation of the musculoskeletal system in utero. The perinatal history should be reviewed for possible birth trauma or neurologic insult. The examiner must note such factors as duration of labor, signs of fetal distress, and the type of delivery (vaginal or cesarean). These factors may have a bearing on conditions such as cerebral palsy, brachial plexus palsy (BPP), facial asymmetry, and torticollis. The birth order is also worth noting because there is a higher incidence of developmental dysplasia of the hip (DDH) in firstborn children.[4,5] An accurate gestational age assessment or estimated date of confinement from the obstetric record is necessary for accurate assessment of the infant's posture and muscle tone.

GENERAL SURVEY

Ideally, a thorough physical examination is completed within the first 24 hours after delivery. Because it is difficult to find a totally motionless, cooperative newborn, much of the musculoskeletal examination must be done while watching the newborn or while examining other systems. Nondisturbing maneuvers should be performed early in the examination and potentially distressing maneuvers near the end. For example, the head and neck should be palpated early, and the hips examined near the end. The examiner must compile all the information produced by the examination and record all findings concerning the musculoskeletal system in a systematic manner. See Table 11.1 for pertinent terms used for the musculoskeletal examination.

For examination, the newborn should be completely undressed and positioned initially on the back. The examination area should be well lit, warm, and free of drafts. A radiant warmer or other heat source is necessary to prevent loss of body heat. The practitioner should develop a routine for examining the newborn so that no part of the musculoskeletal system is overlooked. The examination routine varies from practitioner to practitioner but should be performed in a systematic head-to-toe manner. During assessment, the practitioner should consider general appearance and then proceed to specific areas.

Examination of the bony structures is important in a newborn examination because it is one of the first opportunities to assess intrauterine development. Deviations from normal may be the first indicator of a genetic abnormality or disease.[6]

Measurements are an important part of the musculoskeletal examination. The best instrument for measuring an infant's length, head circumference, and chest circumference is a narrow steel measuring tape or flexible plastic tape. However, most nurseries provide paper tapes, which may be less accurate. Folding the paper tape half-lengthwise may add strength and decrease slippage when measuring rounded contours like the head.

Measurements

Measurement of growth as reflected in increasing body weight and length along expected pathways and within certain limits is one of the most important indicators

TABLE 11.1: MUSCULOSKELETAL TERMINOLOGY

Use the following terms to accurately and consistently describe skeletal positions and muscle movements observed during the examination:	
Abduction	Moving a limb away from the midline of the body
Adduction	Moving a limb toward or past the midline of the body
Dorsiflexion	Flexing a limb toward the back, as in flexing the foot so that the forefoot is higher than the ankle
Everted	Turning a limb out and away from the midline of the body
Extension	Straightening a limb at a joint
Flexion	Bending a limb at a joint
Inverted	Turning a limb inward toward the midline of the body
Plantar flexion	Extending the foot so that the forefoot is lower than the ankle
Pronation	Turning the face down
Rotation (neck)	Turning the face to the side
Supination	Turning the face up
Valgus	Bending outward or twisting away from the midline of the body
Varus	Turning inward

of health in an infant.[6] Measurements taken soon after birth demand careful attention to detail because they will act as a baseline for subsequent assessments of growth and development. All measurements are plotted on a growth chart and correlated with gestational age (Chapter 4).

Weight

Infants should be weighed without clothing or diaper and at approximately the same time each day. Using an infant manual or electronic platform scale, put a protective cloth or paper liner in place, and then place the infant on the scale.[7] Weigh newborns in both pounds and ounces, and in grams. Newborn weight varies with gestational age, gender, ethnicity, and socioeconomic status. Average weight for a term newborn is 2,500 to 4,000 g (5 lb 8 oz–8 lb 13 oz).[1,7–9] All newborns initially lose weight, with a loss of 10% to 20% of birth weight considered acceptable. Variations in weight are a result of body water changes. Preterm infants lose more weight and regain birth weight slower than term infants. Weight gain usually begins within the first 2 weeks, with an average daily weight gain of 10 to 30 g/kg/day.[7,10] In general, infants double their birth weight by 4 to 5 months of age and triple their birth weight by 12 months of age.[7,8]

Length

The infant's length is a better indicator of body mass and long-term growth because it is not influenced by changes in body water content. The infant's recumbent length is measured from the heel to the crown (top of the head). The infant should be placed supine, with legs extended and the head flat. Make a mark on the bed to indicate the crown, and a mark at the heel of the infant. Measure the distance between those two marks. Direct measurement of the infant is difficult because of head molding and incomplete extension of the knees. An alternate method for measuring length, although less accurate, is to hold the zero point of the tape at the heel and to run the tape along the surface of the bed to the top of the head. Mark the spot on the tape with a finger, remove the tape, and read the measurement.[7,11] Infant length boards are available in some facilities and provide another accurate approach to obtaining length measurements.

The length of term newborns at birth is 46 to 56 cm (18–22 inches).[1,7] Average linear growth in preterm infants is 0.8 to 1 cm/week; in term infants, linear growth is 0.69 to 0.75 cm/week.[10] The average infant grows 10 cm (3 inches) in the first 3 months of life and length increases by 50% in the first year.[7,8]

Head Circumference

The head should be measured with a disposable tape measure around the occipital and parietal areas and over the frontal prominence, avoiding the ears. Intrauterine head growth is 0.5 to 0.8 cm/week and is an indicator of brain growth. The average findings in a term newborn are 33 to 35 cm (13–14 inches), with normal variations of 32.5 to 37.5 cm (12.5–14.5 inches).[1,7,9] The head circumference measurement can change markedly in the first few days of life because of molding of the head during delivery. Head circumference in preterm infants should be obtained weekly and plotted on a gestation-specific growth chart to be used as a reference for the future. Head circumference is correlated with long-term neurodevelopment.[9,10] Generally, the head circumference in centimeters is equal to one fourth of the body length in centimeters.[7,8]

Chest Circumference

Measurement of chest circumference is no longer a routine part of newborn physical examination in many hospitals. It can, however, be a useful measurement when compared with the head circumference if the examiner suspects a problem in the head or chest size. If it is measured, the chest circumference should be assessed at the nipple line during expiration. In term infants, the average chest circumference is approximately 2 cm smaller than the head circumference, with the average being 30.5 to 33 cm (12–13 inches).[1,7,11] The head circumference may exceed the chest circumference for the first 5 months of life. From the fifth month of life to 2 years of age, head and chest circumferences can be about the same.[7]

OBSERVATION

Observation, or inspection, should proceed from the general to the specific. General inspection includes observation for movement symmetry, size, shape, general alignment, position, and symmetry of different parts of the body. Soft tissues and muscles should be observed for swelling, muscle wasting, and symmetry.

In the extremities, asymmetry of length or circumference, constrictive bands, or length deformities should be noted. Unequal length or circumference has been associated with skeletal anomalies, tumors, and intra-abdominal neoplasms.[7,12]

The ratio of extremity length to body length is also observed. If a discrepancy is seen, measurements of thoracic length and extremities should be recorded. The gestational age of the newborn determines the normal values for these measurements. In the term newborn, the ratio of upper body length to the length of the lower body segment should not exceed 1.7:1.[13,14] If this ratio is too high, then the extremities are short; if the ratio is too small, then either the limbs are long, or the trunk is too short. This ratio is most useful in determining whether a small newborn is proportionate or has congenitally shortened lower extremities, as in achondroplasia (see later, Figures 11.39 and 11.40).[14,15]

Term newborns lie in a symmetric position with the limbs flexed and the legs partially abducted at the hips so that the soles of the feet may nearly touch each other (Figure 11.2). The head is slightly flexed and

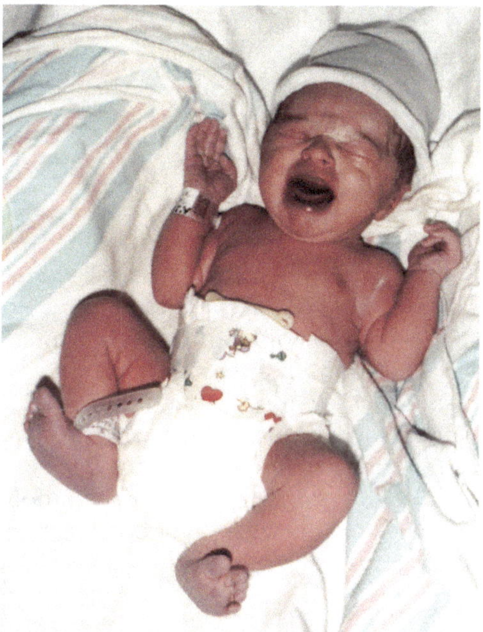

FIGURE 11.2 Posture of a term newborn

positioned in the midline or turned to one side. The resting position of the newborn is often that of the tonic neck reflex (see Figure 12.5). Spontaneous motor activity of flexion and extension, alternating between the arms and legs, is random and uncoordinated. The fingers are usually flexed in a fist, with the thumb under the fingers. Slight tremors may be seen in the arms and legs with vigorous crying during the first 48 hours of life. Any tremors noted after 4 days of age while the infant is at rest are considered abnormal and signal a neurologic problem.[6] The resting posture of the preterm infant is one of extension (Figure 11.3) and is discussed in Chapter 12.

The position and appearance of the extremities at birth can reflect intrauterine position. Because the lower extremities of the fetus have been folded on the abdomen, the newborn's lower extremities often appear externally rotated and bowed, with everted feet. The infant delivered in a breech presentation often has flexed, abducted hips and extended knees (Figures 11.4 and 11.5). These positional deformities can usually be corrected by

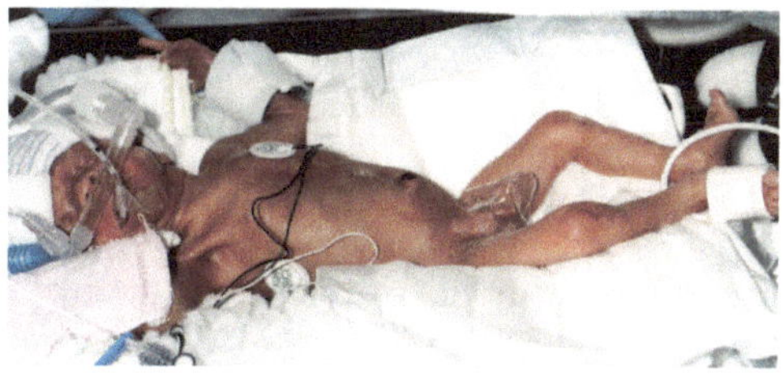

FIGURE 11.3 Posture of the preterm infant

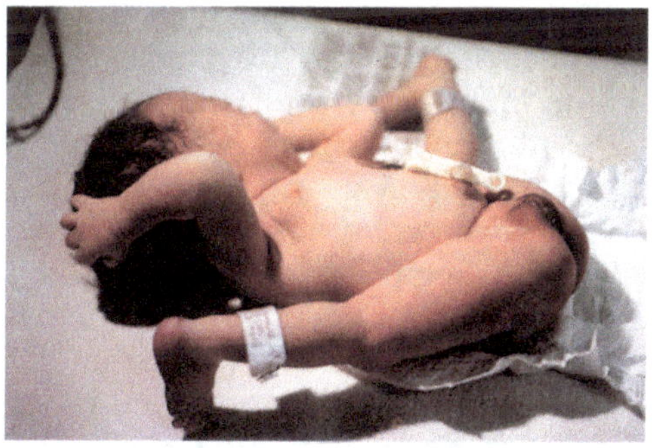

FIGURE 11.4 Breech presentation showing flexed, abducted hips and extended knees

Source: From Clark DA. 2000. *Atlas of Neonatology*. Philadelphia: Saunders, 9. Reprinted by permission.[16]

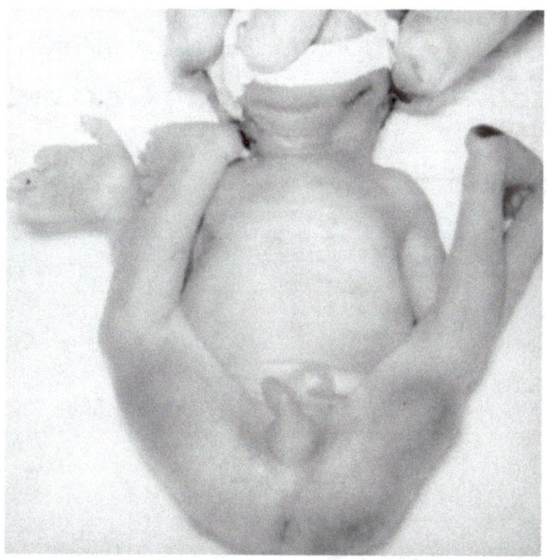

FIGURE 11.5 Abducted hips and perineal bruising with breech presentation

Source: Courtesy of Dr. David A. Clark, Albany Medical Center, Albany, NY, and Wyeth-Ayerst Laboratories, Philadelphia, PA.

passive joint manipulation and should not be confused with congenital malformations.

PALPATION

Palpation is the next important technique used in the examination of the newborn's musculoskeletal system. This technique, along with observation, is used on each extremity to identify component parts (e.g., the two bones in the forearm), function, and normal range of motion. Some aspects of this assessment are shared with the gestational age assessment. Muscular contour in the term infant is smooth, and despite lack of strength, the infant's muscles should feel firm and slightly resist pressure. If an infant feels limp, the condition should never be mistaken for a mere characteristic of immaturity. Further assessment is necessary to rule out a neurologic defect. When testing range of motion, note any asymmetry, tightness, or contractures. Range of motion of all joints is greatest in infancy, gradually lessening as the infant matures. As with posture and muscle tone, the range of joint motion varies with gestational age. It is not necessary to assess the exact number of degrees of range of motion, but only whether the range of movement is less than normal or significantly beyond normal findings. Never use excessive force to assess range of motion.

Neck

The neck is passively examined for rotation and for anterior and lateral flexion and extension. Rotation of 80° and lateral flexion of 40° to both the right and left sides are considered normal. In anterior flexion, the chin should touch or almost touch the chest, and on extension, the occipital part of the head should touch or almost touch the back of the neck. When there is asymmetric rotation or lateral flexion or when range of motion is limited, x-rays of the neck should be taken.

Upper Extremities

Examination of the upper extremities includes the bones of the shoulder girdle (the clavicle and scapula) as well as the humerus, elbow, forearm, and hand. Normal ranges for joint movements of the upper extremities are listed in Table 11.2. Asymmetry in range

TABLE 11.2: NORMAL NEONATAL RANGE OF MOTION IN THE UPPER EXTREMITIES

JOINT OR BONY UNIT	FLEXION	EXTENSION	EXTERNAL ABDUCTION	INTERNAL ROTATION	ROTATION
Shoulder	Close to 180°	>25°	Close to 180°	>45°	>80°
Elbow	145°	165° to 170°			
Forearm				Supination[a] >80°	Pronation[a] >80°
Wrist	75° to 80°	65° to 75°			
Digits	Able to clench	Full extension			
Metacarpophalangeal		0°			
Interphalangeal		0°–5° to 15°			

Note: [a]These maneuvers are done while the humerus is held immobile and the elbow is at 90°.

Source: From Scanlon JW, Nelson T, Grylack LJ, and Smith YF. 1979. *A System of Newborn Physical Examination*. Baltimore: University Park Press, 40. Reprinted by permission of the author.[13]

of motion may indicate weakness, paralysis, fractures, or infection. Failure to spontaneously move an extremity can indicate spinal cord injury or BPP.

Clavicles

The clavicles are inspected and palpated for size, contour, and crepitus (grating that can be felt or heard on movement of ends of a broken bone). A fractured clavicle should be suspected when there is a history of difficult delivery. It can also occur after an apparently normal labor and delivery and is thought to be secondary to forces of labor, maternal pelvic anatomy, and the position of the fetus in utero. Any irregularity in contour, shortening, tenderness, or crepitus on palpation and with passive movement can be a sign of a fractured clavicle.[17] An asymmetric Moro reflex (Chapter 12) may also be seen. If there is pain or discomfort with routine handling, the fracture can be treated by immobilization of the affected limb and shoulder with the elbow flexed 90 degrees. Immobilization is discontinued when a callus has formed at 8 to 10 days. A broken clavicle is one of the most common birth injuries in newborns occurring in 2 to 35 per 1,000 vaginal births. X-rays confirm the diagnosis of fracture.[3,17–19]

Humerus

Length and contour of each humerus should be noted. A fractured humerus should be suspected if there is a history of difficult delivery, one feels a mass caused by hematoma formation, or there are signs of pain during palpation. The Moro reflex on the affected side may be absent. After the clavicle, the humerus is the bone most often fractured during the birth process. X-rays confirm the diagnosis of fracture.[17,18]

Elbow, Forearm, and Wrist

The elbow, forearm, and wrist are examined for size, shape, and number of bones, as well as for range of joint motion. It is sometimes difficult to evaluate the elbow in infants because the normal neonate has a mild flexion contracture that does not disappear until a few weeks after birth. Wrist flexion varies with the infant's gestational age, with greater wrist flexion seen in the term than in the preterm infant.

Hand

The hand should be examined for shape, size, and posture while the fingers are examined for number, shape, and length. Inspection of palm creases should also be included. Although a single crease across the palm (Figure 11.6) is usually associated with Down syndrome (45%), it can also be a nonspecific finding in 4% of the population and is seen bilaterally in 1%.[9,19] However, a combination of short fingers, an incurved little finger, a low-set thumb, and a single palmar (simian) crease should lead the examiner to investigate the possibility of Down syndrome. In term infants, the distance from the tip of

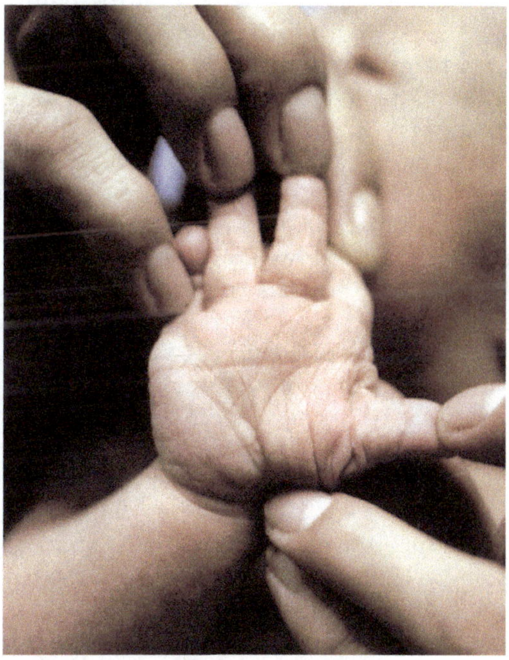

FIGURE 11.6 Single palmar crease (simian crease)

Source: From Clark DA. 2000. *Atlas of Neonatology*. Philadelphia: Saunders, 31. Reprinted by permission.[16]

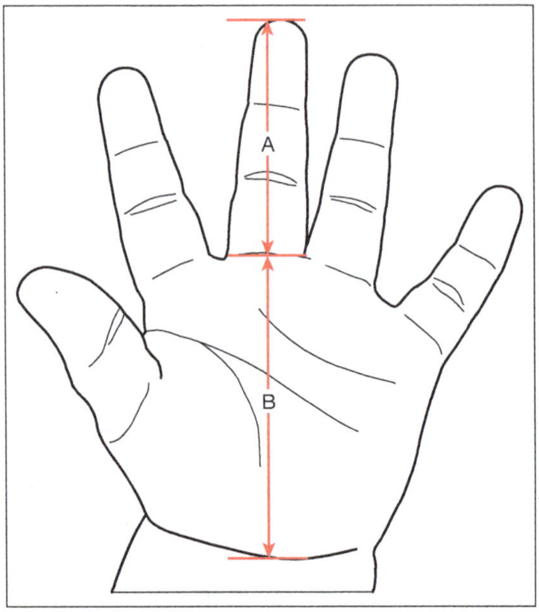

FIGURE 11.7 Landmarks used in measuring palm and finger length

Source: Adapted from Feingold M. 1994. Congenital malformations. In *Neonatology: Pathophysiology and Management of the Newborn*, 4th ed. Avery GB, Fletcher MA, and MacDonald MG, eds. Philadelphia, PA: Lippincott Williams & Wilkins, 761. Reprinted by permission.[20]

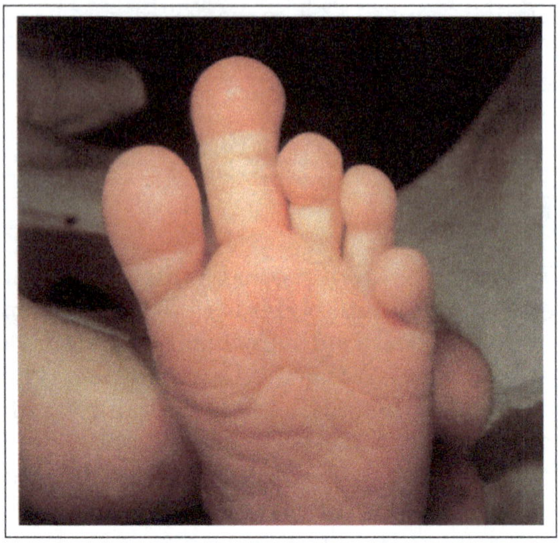

FIGURE 11.8 Macrodactyly

Source: From Clark DA. 2000. *Atlas of Neonatology.* Philadelphia: Saunders, 225. Reprinted by permission.[16]

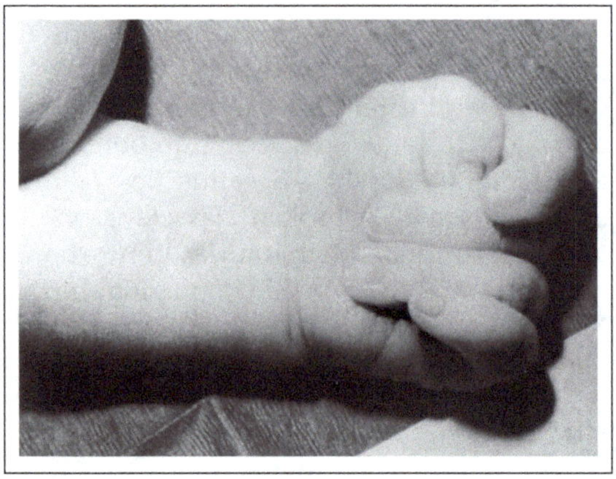

FIGURE 11.9 Finger position in an infant with trisomy 18

Courtesy of Eva Sujansky, MD, University of Colorado Health Sciences Center, Denver, CO.

the middle finger to the base of the palm is 6.75 ± 1.25 cm. Middle finger length to total hand length is usually 0.38 to 0.48:1 (Figure 11.7).[13,14] Macrodactyly, an abnormal enlargement of the finger or toe due to bone, blood vessel, nerve, and other soft-tissue enlargement, may be normal, or it may be a sign of neurofibromatosis, lymphedema, hemangioma, arterial vascular fistulas, fibrous dysplasia, or lipomas (Figure 11.8).[3] Flexed fingers with the index finger overlapping the third finger (Figure 11.9) should lead one to investigate the possibility of trisomy 18.[14] Puffy hands and feet in a newborn may appear as a result of lymphedema and are a characteristic finding of Turner and Noonan syndromes (Figure 11.10).[14,21]

Examine the nails for size and shape. The nails are usually smooth and soft and extend to the fingertips. They may be long in postterm infants or may be absent or spoon-shaped in the presence of some syndromes. Nails may appear hypoplastic if the infant's hands are edematous. A detailed discussion of nail examination is found in Chapter 5.

Spine

The back is examined with the newborn lying prone or held suspended with the examiner's hand under the chest. First inspect the spine from the base of the skull to the coccyx, noting any skin disruption, tufts of hair, soft or cystic masses, hemangiomas, a pilonidal dimple (Figure 11.11), cysts, or sinus tracts. Such pathologic conditions may be signs of a congenital spinal or neurologic anomaly.

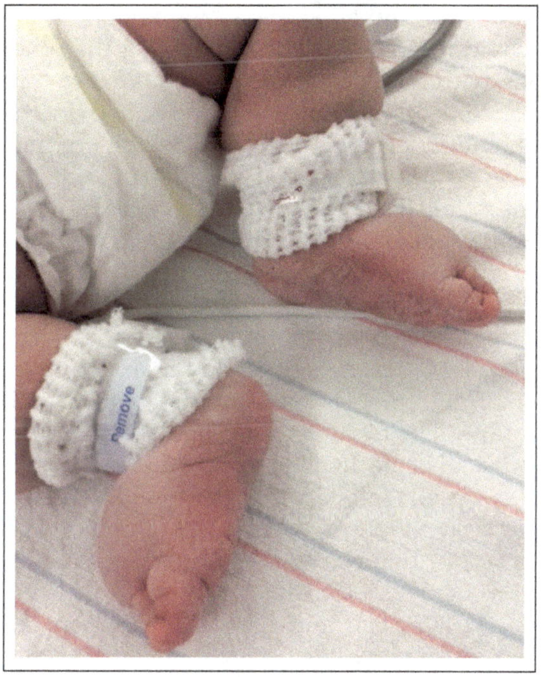

FIGURE 11.10 Turner syndrome

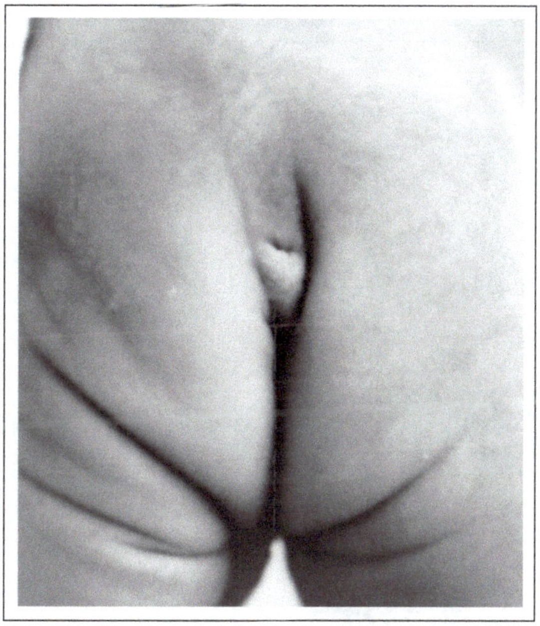

FIGURE 11.11 Pilonidal dimple

Source: Courtesy of Dr. David A. Clark, Albany Medical Center, Albany, NY.

The position of the scapulae should also be noted while the infant is in the prone position to rule out Sprengel deformity, a winged or elevated scapula.

The entire length of the spine should be palpated to determine the presence of dorsal spinal processes and any abnormal curvatures. Significant abnormalities, such as scoliosis (Figure 11.12), lordosis, and kyphosis, are easily observed. A lateral curvature, however, is usually secondary to in utero position. A convex curvature of the thoracic and lumbar spine will be apparent when the infant is in a sitting position (Figure 11.13). The lumbar and

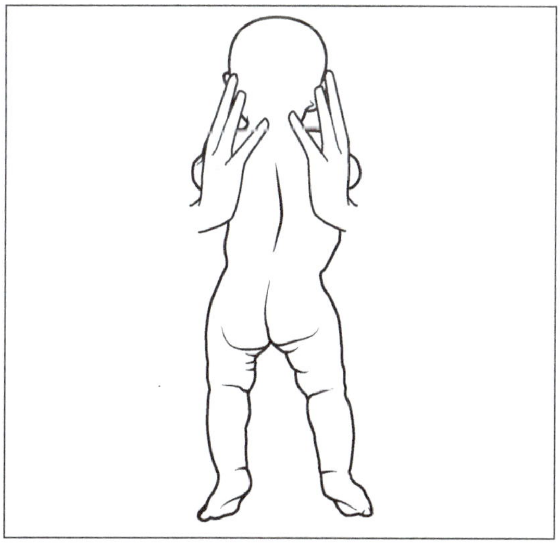

FIGURE 11.12 Scoliosis denotes spinal curvature convex to the right or left. When the baby is lifted by the axilla, the scoliosis is usually obvious

Source: Adapted from Milner RDG, and Herber SM. 1984. *Color Atlas of the Newborn*. Oradell, New Jersey: Medical Economics, 88. Reprinted by permission of Blackwell Science.[22]

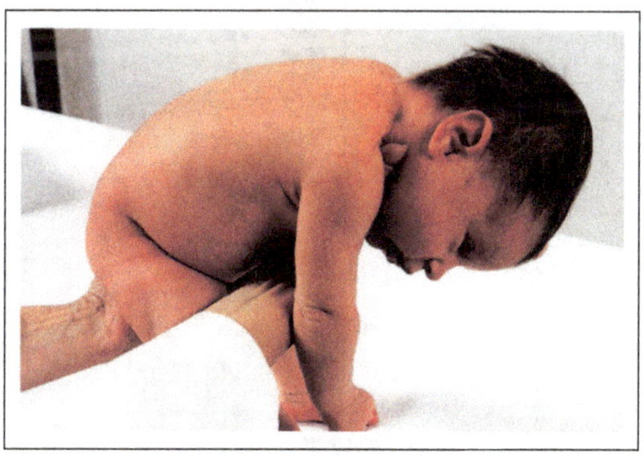

FIGURE 11.13 Convex curvature of the thoracic and lumbar spine

Source: From Jarvis C. 2012: *Physical Examination & Health Assessment*, 6th ed. Philadelphia, PA: Saunders, 600. Reprinted by permission.[23]

sacral curves that are seen in adults develop later, when the infant sits up and begins to stand (Figure 11.14).[11] Extension and lateral bending of the spine can be noted by passive flexion. Flexion and extension should be smooth and rhythmic, without muscle spasm. A neurologic evaluation is necessary to complete the examination of the spine. Techniques are explained in Chapter 12.

Lower Extremities

Examination of the lower extremities includes the hips, femurs, tibias, fibulas, knees, ankles, and feet. Normal ranges for joint movement in the lower extremities are listed in Table 11.3.

Hips

The hips of a newborn generally have a flexion contracture. When the pelvis is stabilized and the lumbar spine is flattened out by extending one leg flat and flexing the other leg with the knee to the chest, a flexion contracture of the hip can be detected in the extended leg. The degree of flexion contracture on the extended leg is the angle that is measured between the thigh and the horizontal plane of the bed or examining table.[7] Normal newborns have an approximately 20° to 30° flexion contracture that usually resolves by 4 to 6 months of age. The newborn hip is externally rotated in extension to 80° to 90°, and internal rotation has a limitation of 0° to 40°.[3,13] The stability of the hip must also be evaluated to rule out DDH. Asymmetry of skin folds in the gluteal and femoral regions is a sensitive but nonspecific indicator that suggests that the hip is abnormal (Figure 11.15).[4,7,13]

The Ortolani and Barlow maneuvers are the most reliable screening tests for evaluating hip stability (Figure 11.16). Although they are described as separate tests, in clinical practice, both maneuvers are done in a

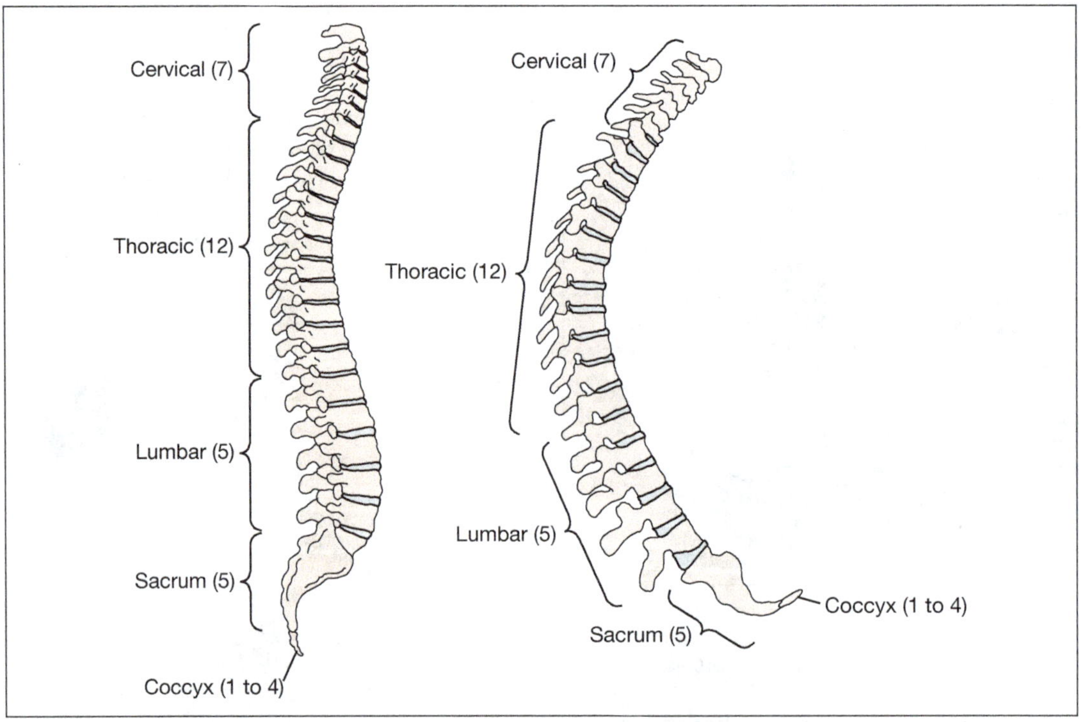

FIGURE 11.14 Spinal curves of the adult *(left)* and infant *(right)*

Source: From Alexander MM, and Brown MS. 1979. *Pediatric History Taking and Physical Diagnosis for Nurses*, 2nd ed. Philadelphia, PA: Mosby, 292. Reprinted by permission of the authors.[24]

TABLE 11.3: NORMAL NEONATAL RANGE OF MOTION IN THE LOWER EXTREMITIES

JOINT OR EXTREMITY	FLEXION	EXTENSION	ABDUCTION	ADDUCTION	INTERNAL ROTATION	ROTATION
Hip	145°		90°	10° to 20°	40°	80°
Knee	120° to 145°	90°				
Ankle	Dorsiflexion: Above resting position Plantar flexion: >10° from resting position					
Forefoot			≥10° to 15°	≥10° to 15°		
Hindfoot			Valgus ≥10°	Varus ≥5°		

Source: From Scanlon JW, Nelson T, Grylack LJ, and Smith YF. 1979. *A System of Newborn Physical Examination.* Baltimore, MD: University Park Press, 42. Reprinted by permission of the author.[13]

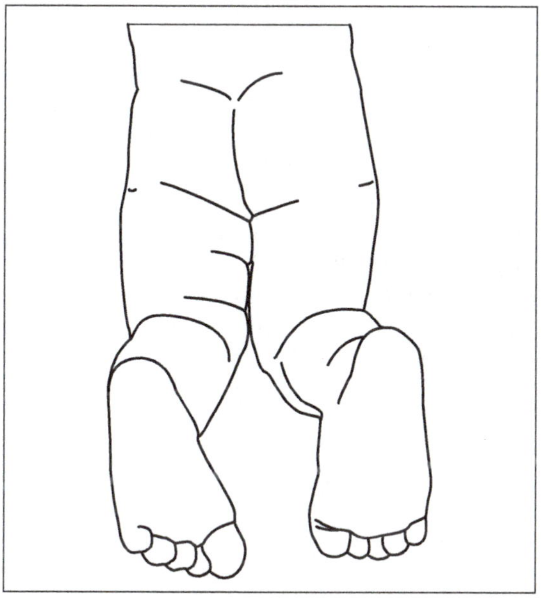

FIGURE 11.15 Asymmetric gluteal folds

sequence, not as separate examinations. The infant must be in a supine position and on a relatively firm surface. These are not forceful examinations; a forceful examination only makes the infant cry and yields unreliable results. A crying, kicking infant can generate enough muscle strength by tightening the adductors and hamstrings to create a false result.[9] The cooperation of the infant and the patience of the examiner affect the accuracy of the examination.

The Ortolani maneuver is a test of hip reduction. It produces the reduction of the dislocated femoral head into the acetabulum by abduction. A helpful tip is to remember that the O in Ortolani means that the hip is "out." The maneuver is used to place the hip back into a normal position. With the infant positioned supine, the practitioner flexes the infant's knee and hip, and then grasps the thigh with the thumb positioned along the inner thigh and the third or fourth finger placed over the greater trochanter laterally. While the examiner abducts the hip, the finger on the greater trochanter presses up against the head of the femur, and the hand presses the shaft of the femur toward the mattress. A positive Ortolani maneuver is produced when a palpable "clunk" is noted, indicating that the femoral head has slipped from a dislocated position into the acetabulum. Higher pitched clicks and snaps can be heard and felt but are not associated with hip pathology; they usually result from movement of tendons, ligaments, or fluid in the hip joint.[18,25,27]

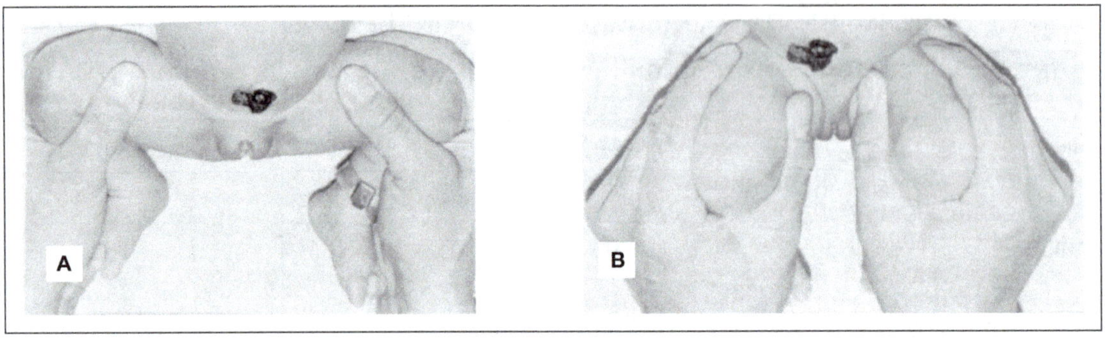

FIGURE 11.16 Ortolani and Barlow maneuvers. (A) Ortolani: The fingers are on the trochanter and the thumb grips the femur as shown. The femur is lifted forward as the thighs are abducted. If the femur head is dislocated, it can be felt to reduce. (B) Barlow: The thighs are adducted, and if the femur head dislocates, it will be both felt and seen as it suddenly jerks over the acetabulum

Source: From Robertson WW. 2005. Orthopedics. In *Neonatology: Pathophysiology and Management of the Newborn*, 6th ed. MacDonald MG, Seshia MMK, and Mullett MD, eds. Philadelphia: Lippincott Williams & Wilkins, 1429. Reprinted by permission.[26]

The Barlow maneuver determines whether the femoral head can be dislocated from the acetabulum and is the opposite of the Ortolani maneuver. The practitioner's hand position is the same as for the Ortolani maneuver, with the infant's hip and leg flexed. As the knee is brought to the center (adducted) from the abducted position, the practitioner's thumb pushes laterally on the upper inner thigh. A "clunk" indicates that the femoral head has slipped over the lateral edge of the acetabulum and demonstrates an unstable hip joint that is dislocatable. The amount of force needed to push the femoral head out of or into the acetabulum is minimal.

A variation of the Barlow maneuver is to stabilize the pelvis with one hand while using the other hand to try to move the thigh anteriorly and posteriorly (upward and downward) without flexing the hip. This maneuver enables the practitioner to determine whether the femoral head can be displaced posteriorly out of the acetabulum.

Legs

Palpate the legs to confirm the presence of the femur, tibia, and fibula. Fractures should be suspected when there is a history of difficult delivery or when palpation reveals irregularities in contour, crepitation, or masses resulting from hematoma formation.

Although birth trauma rarely causes a fracture of the femur (0.13/1,000 births), dislocation or avulsion of the femoral epiphysis can occur and should be suspected if there is pain on passive movement or little spontaneous movement of the leg.[17,18] Femoral length can be observed by testing for the Galeazzi (or Allis) sign. Keeping the feet flat on the bed and the femurs aligned, flex both of the infant's knees. With the tips of the big toes in the same horizontal plane, face the feet and observe the height of the knees.[7,11,25] It will be apparent if one knee is higher than the other, a positive sign. A discrepancy in knee height should lead one to investigate for DDH (Figure 11.17).[5,7,27] Twenty-four percent of

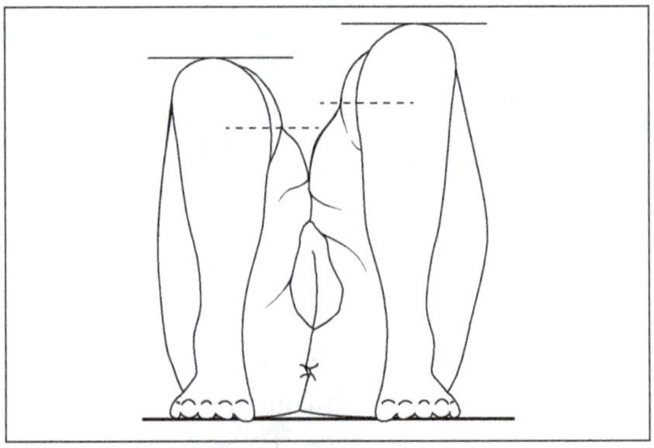

FIGURE 11.17 Allis sign

Source: Adapted from Alexander MM, and Brown MS. 1979. *Pediatric History Taking and Physical Diagnosis for Nurses*, 2nd ed. St. Louis, MO: Mosby-Year Book, 301. Reprinted by permission of the authors.[24]

patients with congenital constricting bands have leg length discrepancy.[12]

The lower extremities are examined for length and shape. Congenital limb deficiencies are easy to identify, and an x-ray will confirm the deficiency (Figures 11.18 and 11.19). The lower extremities of newborns frequently have mild bowing and internal rotation of the lower leg because of intrauterine environmental conditions and fetal positioning. The bowed appearance is usually a combined rotational deformity caused by external rotation of the hip and internal tibial torsion from in utero positioning.[3,18,25] With the infant supine, draw an imaginary line connecting the anterior superior iliac spine with the mid patella, and continue down to the foot. If the line falls medial to the big toe, external tibial torsion is present. If the line falls lateral to the second toe, internal tibial torsion (a slight varus curvature) is present (Figure 11.20). Internal tibial torsion is a common physiologic feature of almost all newborns and is the usual cause of intoeing in children from birth to 2 years of age. Because this is a physiologic rather than a pathologic condition, spontaneous recovery can be anticipated with normal growth and development.[3,18,25] Although lateral tibial

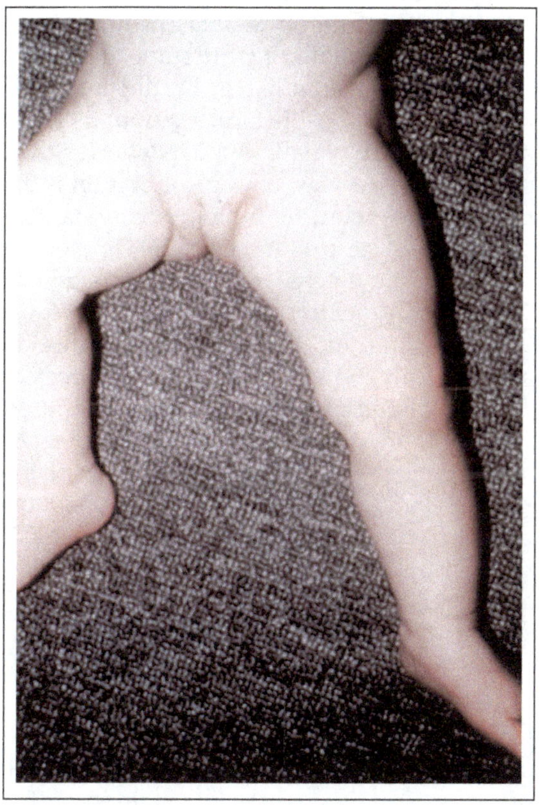

FIGURE 11.18 Infant with congenital limb deficiency of the leg

Courtesy of Mark Erickson, MD, Children's Hospital Colorado, Aurora, CO.

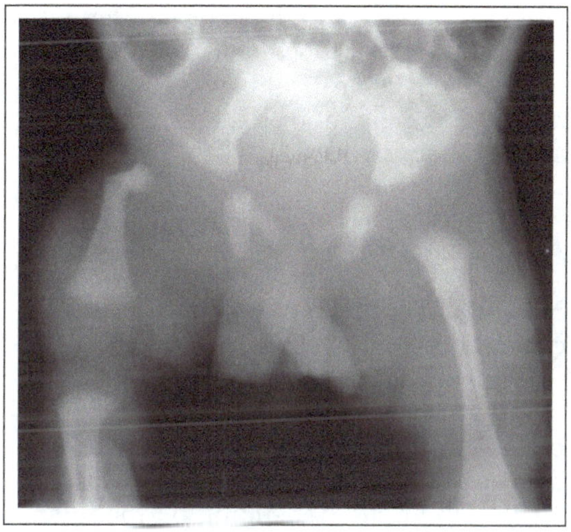

FIGURE 11.19 X-ray of congenital limb deficiency

Courtesy of Mark Erickson, MD, Children's Hospital Colorado, Aurora, CO.

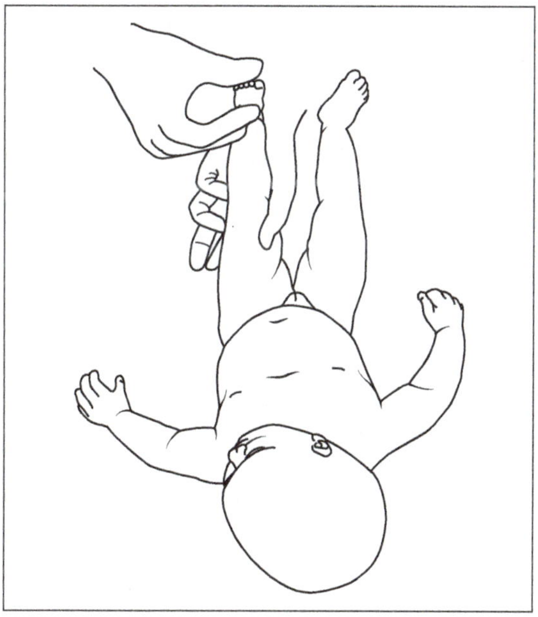

FIGURE 11.20 Examination for tibial torsion

bowing without a significant shortening of the extremity is considered normal in the newborn, anterior tibial bowing is an abnormal finding, and an orthopedic consultation should be sought.

Ankles and Feet

Examination of the ankles and feet includes observation of the resting position and stimulation for active motion. To stimulate for motion, stroke the sole as well as the dorsal, medial, and lateral sides of the foot. Passive motion of the ankle in dorsiflexion and plantar flexion varies, depending on the infant's position in utero. For example, ankle and forefoot adduction, a positional deformity, can be differentiated from congenital equinovarus (clubfoot) malformation by passively positioning the foot in the midline and dorsiflexing it. A clubfoot or other structurally abnormal foot and ankle will not have a full range of motion and will resist dorsiflexion.

The toes should be examined for number, position, and spacing between them. Overlapping toes in infancy are usually hereditary; conservative treatment measures for mild cases may involve only stretching or stabilizing the toe by taping it in the correct position.[28] The soles of the feet should be inspected as part of the gestational age assessment. Most newborns are flat-footed as the result of a plantar fat pad (a pad of fat in the longitudinal arch of the foot), which gradually disappears during the first year of life.

MUSCULOSKELETAL ANOMALIES

Congenital anomalies (birth defects) are structural or functional anomalies that occur during intrauterine life and are identifiable at birth. They are deviations from the norm. Most anomalies are isolated defects and not associated with other major anomalies. Musculoskeletal anomalies are seen in 10.25 to 14.15 per 10,000 newborns.[14] Congenital anomalies of the musculoskeletal system may be evident as the absence of a part, extra parts, or malformed or malfunctioning tissue. Congenital anomalies usually affect the infant's movement, muscle tone, or posture. It is not within the scope of this chapter to discuss all the musculoskeletal anomalies the practitioner may encounter. However, many of the common problems and other special conditions seen in neonates are included in this section.

Anomalies of the Neck

Klippel–Feil Syndrome

Klippel–Feil syndrome is a defect of the cervical vertebrae in which there is both a decrease in the number of vertebrae and a fusion of two or more vertebrae. It can be detected throughout life, but those diagnosed in the newborn period tend to have upper cervical spine involvement as opposed to lower cervical involvement. The condition varies in severity depending on the number of vertebrae that are fused. The cause is unknown, although current theories involve generalized fetal insult, in utero vascular insult, or neural tube abnormalities.[25] In some instances, the syndrome is familial, indicating a genetic transmission.[29] On physical examination, the neonate's neck usually appears shorter than normal, and decreased range of motion is the most frequent clinical finding. Rotational loss is usually more pronounced than is the loss of flexion and extension. The classic signs on physical examination of short neck, low posterior hairline, and limitation of neck motion are seen only in those more severely affected. The asymmetric motion may be confused with torticollis (see next section), but an x-ray of the neck will confirm the presence of the Klippel–Feil deformity. Other bony abnormalities, such as Sprengel deformity, congenital scoliosis, and congenital limb deficiencies, are associated with Klippel–Feil deformity.[25,29]

Torticollis

Congenital torticollis, or wry neck, is "a spasmodic, unilateral contraction of the neck muscles."[13] It is an injury sustained to the sternocleidomastoid muscle or to a cervical spine abnormality. It is thought to be the result of birth trauma, intrauterine malposition, muscle fibrosis, or venous abnormality in the muscle.[3,17,25] This anomaly is not usually seen in the immediate newborn period, but a hematoma may sometimes be palpated, or soft-tissue swelling may be noted over the involved sternocleidomastoid muscle shortly after birth. Torticollis usually appears as a firm, fibrous mass or tightness in the sternocleidomastoid muscle at approximately 2 weeks of age. The mass is 1 to 2 cm in diameter, hard, immobile, and felt in the midportion of the sternocleidomastoid muscle.[3,25] In infants with this condition, the head is tilted laterally toward the involved side, with the chin rotated away from the affected shoulder (Figure 11.21).[3,25] Infants with this anomaly should be further evaluated for associated conditions such as metatarsus adductus, hip dysplasia, and congenital anomalies of the cervical spine. If the mass is detected early, most neonates with congenital muscular torticollis can be treated with stretching exercises performed by the parents.[3,17,25,29] If the mass goes unnoticed, however, the torticollis may not be detected until there is plagiocephaly, or asymmetry of the face and skull development. If the torticollis persists or goes untreated, there is a flattening of the occiput on the opposite side and a flattening of the frontal bones on the side of the lesion.[17,25,29]

Spinal Deformities

Congenital Scoliosis

Scoliosis in the neonate may range from undetectable to very severe. It is not thought to be chromosomal or inherited, but rather an embryonic defect. It is a condition in which there is a lateral S- or C-shaped curvature of the spine that is usually associated with a rotational deformity of the spine and ribs. The structural basis for congenital scoliosis is a failure of vertebral formation, segmentation, or a variety of both. The failures can be in any area of the vertebral body (Figure 11.22). Failures of formation indicate the absence of a portion of the vertebra, such as a hemivertebra. Failure of segmentation is the absence of the normal separation between the vertebras. Females are affected more often than males, and their curvature is more likely to worsen. If the defect goes undetected, severe deformities can develop and affect neurologic function as well as cosmetic appearance.[5,25] Congenital scoliosis may occur as an isolated condition or with associated conditions. Upon diagnosis, the infant should also be evaluated for genitourinary tract anomalies (unilateral renal agenesis being the most common), occurring in

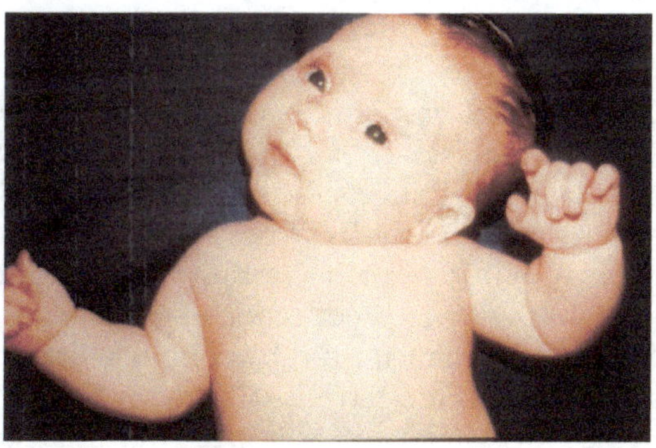

FIGURE 11.21 Torticollis

Courtesy of Mark Erickson, MD, Children's Hospital Colorado, Aurora, CO.

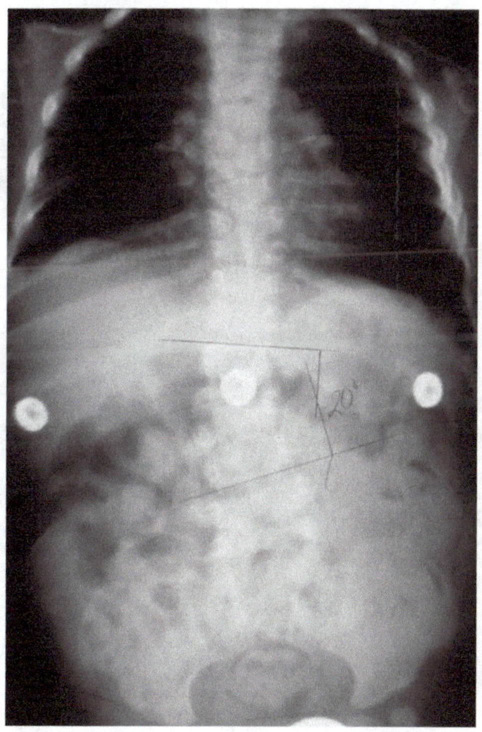

FIGURE 11.22 X-ray of congenital scoliosis

Courtesy of Mark Erickson, MD, Children's Hospital Colorado, Aurora, CO.

20% to 30% of infants, and cardiac anomalies, seen in 10% of infants with congenital vertebral anomalies.[25,30] Klippel–Feil syndrome, Sprengel deformity of the scapula, and **V**ertebral anomalies, **A**nal atresia, **C**ardiac abnormalities, **T**racheo **E**sophageal abnormalities, **R**enal abnormalities, and **L**imb anomalies (VACTERL) syndrome are also seen with congenital scoliosis.[25,29,30]

Myelomeningocele

Myelomeningocele is the most severe type of spina bifida. It is a congenital neural tube defect in which the bones of the spine do not completely form. The defect usually presents as a failure of closure at the caudal (tail) end of the vertebral column, permitting the meninges and sometimes the spinal cord to protrude into a saclike structure (Figure 11.23). Skin disruption is not always present; however, any soft mass noted over the spine or just off the midline must be examined closely to rule out myelomeningocele. Because the functional deficit of the lower extremities is linked to the level of involvement of the myelomeningocele, it is important to examine the muscle function of the lower extremities. Other congenital spinal cord or musculoskeletal defects that may also be seen with myelomeningocele include syringomyelia and hip dislocation.

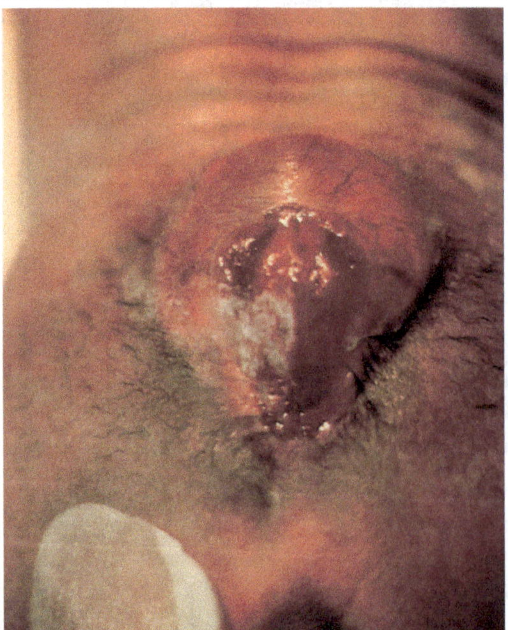

FIGURE 11.23 Myelomeningocele

Source: From Clark DA. 2000. *Atlas of Neonatology*. Philadelphia: Saunders, 131. Reprinted by permission.[16]

Upper Extremity Anomalies

Sprengel Deformity (Congenital Elevated Scapula)

Sprengel deformity is one of the more common congenital anomalies of the shoulder girdle. It is characterized by an abnormally small, elevated scapula.[25,31] The elevation may be unilateral or, in 10% to 30% of cases, bilateral.[31] The asymmetry of the shoulder seen with unilateral involvement makes diagnosis relatively easy. On examination, the scapula is noted to be hypoplastic, elevated, and malrotated so that, when palpated, the vertebral border lies superiorly and more horizontal than normal. The angle of the scapula may give the newborn the appearance of a webbed neck or a fullness at the base of the neck.[31] There is usually limitation of shoulder motion, particularly in abduction and forward flexion.[29,31] Internal and external shoulder rotation may be only slightly affected. Sprengel deformity appears to be a familial predisposition, and in 70% of cases another congenital abnormality is present such as congenital spinal problems, renal anomalies, torticollis, and Klippel–Feil syndrome.[19,25]

Cleidocranial Dysostosis

Cleidocranial dysostosis, also known as *cleidocranial dysplasia* or *mutational dysostosis*, is a rare defect that affects the growth of bones in all parts of the body. It can occur either spontaneously or be inherited as an autosomal dominant trait with no predilection of sex or ethnic group. It is characterized by complete or partial absence of the clavicles (Figure 11.24).[15,32,33] Symptoms vary and can range from mild to severe. Frequently, the chest is narrow; the shoulders are down sloping; and there is a high arched palate, frontal bossing, and a

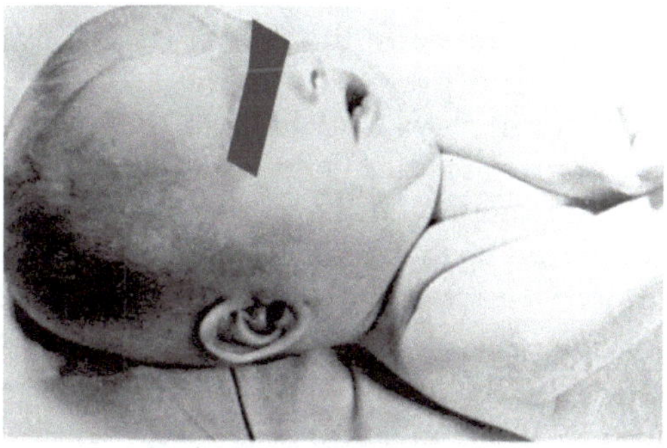

FIGURE 11.24 Cleidocranial dysostosis

Source: From Swaiman KF, and Wright FS. 1982. *The Practice of Pediatric Neurology*. Philadelphia, PA: Mosby, 441. Reprinted by permission.[33]

sloping forehead. It is usually caused by a mutation of the RUNX2 gene, located at chromosome 6p21. This gene encodes a protein necessary for the correct functioning of osteoblast cells, which regulate bone differentiation.[32] Bilateral absence of the clavicles, which occurs in 10% of cases, or segmental loss of the lateral or middle portion of the clavicles allows for excessive scapulothoracic motion where the newborn's shoulders touch in midline without discomfort.

Complete absence of the clavicle is usually accompanied by defective ossification of the cranium, large fontanels, and delayed closure of the sutures.[15,32] As the infant ages, there is a delay in the eruption and/or an absence of permanent teeth. Although the deformities may not be cosmetically pleasing, there is usually little functional disability. No treatment of the newborn is required, but genetic counseling is recommended for the parents.[32]

Brachial Plexus Palsy

BPP is one of the more common birth injuries detected on the newborn examination and the most frequent neurologic abnormality found in an otherwise healthy newborn, with an incidence of 0.9 to 5 per 1,000 live births.[18,34,35] BPP is a paralysis involving the muscles of the upper extremity that follows mechanical trauma to the spinal roots of the fifth cervical through the first thoracic nerves (the brachial plexus).[17] BPPs are associated with clavicle and humerus fractures as well as torticollis.[18,35] The incidence of BPP has not decreased over the last three decades, which may be partly due to an increase in population birth weights. However, the incidence of lower plexus lesions has decreased significantly with the decline in vaginal breech births.

Most cases of BPP are thought to be the result of prolonged and difficult labor involving traction and lateral flexion of the neck.[3,17,34] Brachial plexus injury has also been attributed to abnormal in utero forces on the posterior shoulder of the fetus as it passes over maternal bony prominences such as the sacral promontory. Increased in utero pressure and traction have also been proposed as the cause in an abnormal uterus such as a bicornuate or fibroid uterus.[17] Other perinatal risk factors include prolonged labor, large maternal body mass index, large-for-gestational-age fetuses, shoulder dystocia, and breech presentation.[3,18,34] BPP, therefore, is seen most often in large neonates, who, because of their size, are vulnerable to stretching injuries to the components of the brachial plexus.[17,31] Shoulder dystocia in vertex deliveries and difficult arm or head extraction in breech deliveries increases the risk for brachial plexus injuries.[17,18,31] A cesarean delivery does not protect against BPP as 10% of affected infants have a history of cesarean delivery.[3]

There are three types of BPP, each with a different clinical presentation, depending on the site of injury and extent of neural injury:

1. Upper lesion injuries are the most frequent type of brachial plexus injury and involve complete or partial paralysis of the shoulder muscles as a result of injury to cranial nerves 5 (CN V), 6 (CN VI), and occasionally 7 (CN VII). This type of palsy is known as *Erb palsy*, and the clinical presentation frequently is referred to as the *bad shoulder, good hand* scenario.[3,17] An infant with this type of upper arm paralysis holds the affected arm adducted and internally rotated, with extension at the elbow, pronation of the forearm, and flexion of the wrist (Figure 11.25). The grasp reflex remains

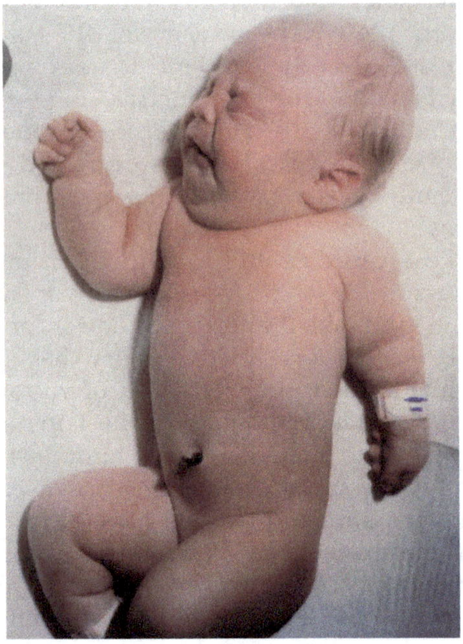

FIGURE 11.25 BPP (Erb palsy)

Source: From Clark DA. 2000. *Atlas of Neonatology*. Philadelphia: Saunders, 138. Reprinted by permission.[16]

intact, but the Moro reflex is absent on the affected side.

2. A second type, Klumpke palsy, is an example of a lower lesion injury presenting clinically as the *good shoulder, bad hand* scenario. This palsy involves cranial nerve 8 (CN VIII) and thoracic nerve 1 (T1), with complete or partial paralysis of the forearm and hand muscles. This lower arm paralysis is rare. When the lower plexus is involved, the shoulder is in a relatively normal position with the wrist and hand flaccid, having little or no control.
3. The third type of BPP, complete paralysis of the arm, involves injury to the plexus at all levels. It includes paralysis of the wrist and hand, in addition to shoulder and elbow dysfunction.[17,34] Because of the possibility of birth trauma as an etiology for the palsy, skeletal injury may coexist and should be ruled out radiographically.[3]

In cases of BPP in which the nerve roots are not disrupted, infants regain neurologic function within several days as the hemorrhage and edema in the area resolve. Gentle handling and protection of the arm for the first 7 to 10 days will help to avoid additional injury to the plexus. Initial treatment is aimed at preventing contractures of the shoulder, elbow, forearm, and hand during the observational recovery phase by gentle passive range-of-motion exercises. Although most infants gain significant functional improvement by 3 months of age, close examination usually reveals tightness of the shoulder on internal rotation, difficulties in supination of the forearm, and abduction of the shoulder.[3,17]

If improvement is not noted in the first few months, an electromyography and nerve conduction studies are performed to determine the extent of the damage. Secondary treatment involves nerve repair to restore neurologic function that has not occurred spontaneously. Infants with total plexus involvement require brachial plexus exploration and reconstruction if there is no return of biceps function at 3 months of age. If the arm remains flaccid at 2 to 3 months of age for infants with upper BPP, surgery is undertaken at 3 to 6 months of age.[18,34] In newborns with peripheral nerve disruption or nerve root disruption, early intervention with microsurgery is recommended. Approximately 20% of brachial plexus injuries require surgery, and 90% of these infants achieve useful function of muscle groups above the elbow.[17,34]

Erb palsy generally has a favorable prognosis and can be completely resolved in the first year of life if recovery begins within the first 4 weeks. However, if the muscle remains without reinnervation, the injury becomes irreversible at 18 to 24 months. Early management with close follow-up is recommended.[35]

Congenital Absence of the Radius (Radial Dysplasia)

Congenital absence of the radius is sometimes referred to as *radial dysplasia* and is easy to recognize. Clinically, the infant presents with the hand and wrist deviated 90° or more (Figure 11.26). The forearm is shortened, with bowing of the ulna. The thumb is usually

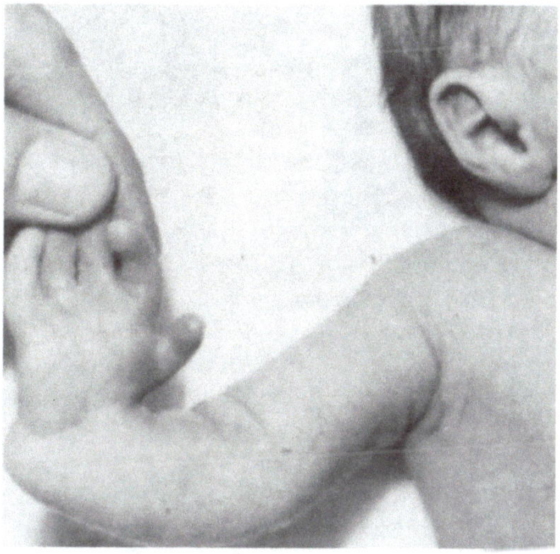

FIGURE 11.26 Congenital absence of the radius

Source: From Robertson WW. 2005. Orthopedics. In *Neonatology: Pathophysiology and Management of the Newborn*, 6th ed. MacDonald MG, Seshia MMK, and Mullett MD, eds. Philadelphia: Lippincott Williams & Wilkins, 1432. Reprinted by permission.[26]

absent or hypoplastic. There is marked limited movement of the hand, wrist, and forearm. It occurs in 1 of 30,000 to 1 of 100,000 live births and is seen in males more often than females.[25,31,36] Although radial hypoplasia alone may be inherited sporadically, infants presenting with this anomaly should be further evaluated for associations such as VACTERL, Fanconi anemia, and Holt–Oram syndrome.[31,36] Treatment comprises both operative and nonoperative options and is recommended for cosmetic and functional reasons.[25,31,36] A consultation with a pediatric hand surgeon is required.

Lower Extremity Anomalies

Developmental Dysplasia of the Hip

DDH is one of the most significant deformities of the newborn period and the most common neonatal hip disorder. It covers a spectrum of conditions that arise from abnormal development of the hip joint. These conditions range from minimal instability (in which the femoral head remains in the acetabulum) to irreducible dislocation (in which the femoral head loses contact completely with the acetabular capsule and is displaced over the fibrocartilaginous rim). DDH is thought to be caused by lack of acetabular depth, ligamentous laxity limited to the hip joint that is influenced by hormonal and genetic factors, and/or abnormal intrauterine positioning, as in intrauterine breech position.[4,25,37]

Approximately 30% to 50% of all DDH occurs in infants born after breech presentation.[2,36,37] Approximately 2.5 to 6.5 infants/1,000 live births develop hip dysplasia, but the true incidence of DDH can only be presumed because of disparities in the definition of the condition, the type of examinations used to detect hip abnormalities, the differing skill levels of examiners, and the populations being studied.[27] The overall incidence of DDH with evidence of clinically detectable hip instability has been reported to be as high as 1 of 100 newborns and with clinically and/or radiographic hip dislocation, 1 to 28 per 1,000 newborns.[2,25,37] Recent large ultrasound screening studies place the incidence of ultrasound detectable abnormalities leading to intervention at 5% to 7% of all newborns.[37] The etiology of DDH is unknown. However, both genetic and environmental influences play a role in the incidence of the condition. African and Asian infants have a very low incidence, whereas Native Americans and Eastern Europeans have an incidence reported as high as 25 to 50/1,000 live births.[27,38] These differences may be due less to genetic predisposition and more to child-rearing practices, such as swaddling, that keep the newborn's hips in adduction and extension.[38] Females are more prone to the condition than males, unilateral dislocation is twice as frequent as bilateral, and the left hip is affected twice as often as the right hip.[19,37,38] A family history revealing that a parent had a dislocated hip as a child or that an older sibling has hip dysplasia increases the risk for dislocated hip in the infant.[2,4,19] DDH is also more common in infants with other orthopedic conditions, such as torticollis, and in those with congenital foot deformities, such as clubfoot and metatarsus adductus.[25,38]

Early and routine screening for DDH is important because treatment prior to 6 months of age is easier and more effective while later detection has a higher risk for long-term disability. The clinical manifestations of DDH depend on the severity of the condition. Findings that should lead a practitioner to investigate further include (a) asymmetry of gluteal or thigh folds, (b) limb length discrepancy (Galeazzi/Allis sign), (c) positive Barlow maneuver (hip reduced but dislocatable), and (d) positive Ortolani sign (hip dislocated, but reducible).[36,39] Early diagnosis and treatment appropriate to the specific anomaly are important to create normal hip anatomy and function. There is no uniformly accepted method for diagnosis of DDH during the newborn period. Sixty percent to 80% of hip deformities identified in children by clinical examination resolve on their own without intervention.[5,39] The most effective diagnostic tool for screening hip joint problems during the first 6 months of life is ultrasonography. Ultrasounds should be completed on infants with high-risk factors, such as infants born in the breech position or those with positive Ortolani or Barlow maneuvers.[2,39] Universal newborn ultrasonographic screening is not recommended in North America because of the expense, inconvenience, inconsistency, and high false positive rates considering the overall incidence of the anomaly. Selective ultrasonographic screening is recommended to clarify suspicious findings on physical examination after 3 to 4 weeks of age or to detect clinically silent DDH in high-risk infants after 6 weeks of age and up to 6 months.[39] Radiographs of newborns with suspected DDH are of limited value because the femoral heads do not ossify until 4 to 6 months of age.[2,39]

Infants with a stable clinical hip examination but with abnormalities noted on ultrasonography can be followed without a brace. For infants with clinically unstable hips, when treatment is initiated early using abduction devices such as the Pavlik harness (Figure 11.27) and the von Rosen splint, there is a 95% success rate.[2,18,38] The longer the dislocation remains untreated, the greater the chance of problems in returning the femoral head to its normal position, and the less satisfactory the results. The hips of infants with normal examination should continue to be examined for signs of DDH at subsequent health visits. Normal findings at age 6 to 8 weeks do not definitively exclude DDH.

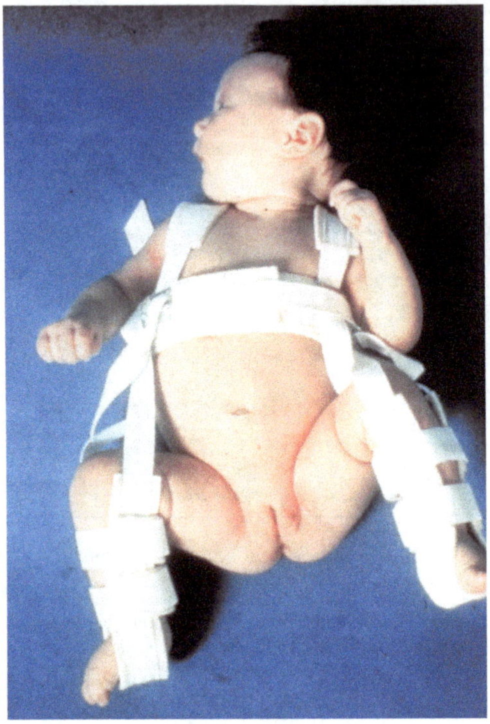

FIGURE 11.27 Pavlik harness

Source: Courtesy of Mark Erickson, MD, Children's Hospital Colorado, Aurora, CO.

Congenital Absence of the Tibia or Fibula

Although congenital absence of a long bone is unusual, when it does occur, the deformity is easily recognized. Tibia or fibula absence may be partial or complete. When a portion of the bone is present, the deformity is likely to be less severe. In the absence of the tibia, the clinical presentation is mild to marked shortening of the lower leg. The knee is unstable and has a flexion contracture. The foot may be normal or fixed in a mild to severe varus position.[40] In absence of the fibula, the clinical presentation is shortening of the involved leg, with bowing of the tibia anteriorly and medially (Figure 11.28). The foot deformity is often severe, with a valgus position.[18,41]

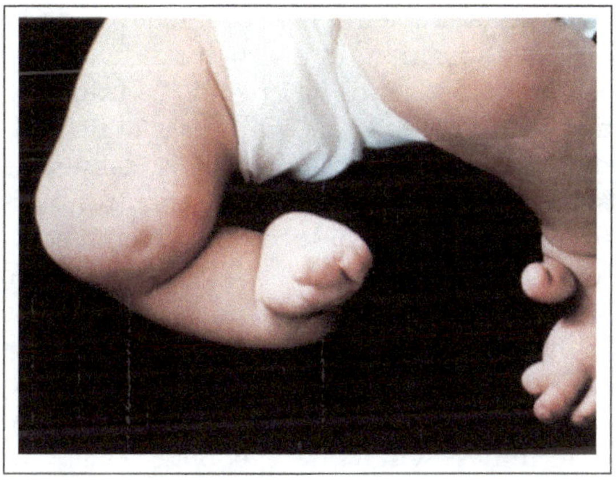

FIGURE 11.28 Congenital absence of the fibula

Courtesy of Mark Erickson, MD, Children's Hospital Colorado, Aurora, CO.

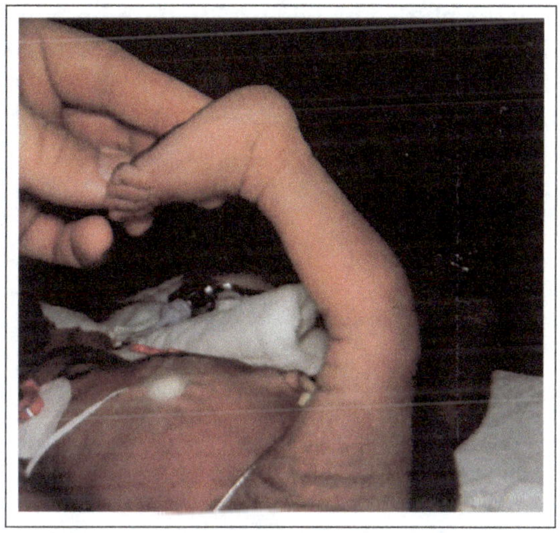

FIGURE 11.29 Genu recurvatum

Source: Form Clark DA. 2000. *Atlas of Neonatology*. Philadelphia: Saunders, 9. Reprinted by permission.[16]

Treatment depends upon the severity of the condition and focuses on the problems of foot deformity and leg length discrepancy. These deformities should be seen by an orthopedist early in the neonatal period. Many infants with congenital limb deficiencies frequently have other associated anomalies that represent an inherited syndrome. Because of the high potential for genetic transmission of the disorder, the parents should be offered genetic counseling.[40]

Genu Recurvatum

Genu recurvatum, a rare anomaly with an estimated incidence of one per 100,000 live births, is a congenital dislocation or hyperextension of the knee (Figure 11.29). It is thought to result from a frank breech position in utero (41% of otherwise normal newborns exhibiting this anomaly were breech). It can be the result of a prenatal developmental defect, a specific disease of the muscles or nerves of the leg, or a manifestation of generalized joint laxity, as seen in "floppy baby" syndrome. It can also be associated with oligohydramnios, anomalies of the elastic tissues, and fibrosis of the quadriceps muscle along with deficient hamstrings.[36,42] More common in females, genu recurvatum is usually seen bilaterally. Treatment for mild presentation of genu recurvatum includes physical therapy and progressive reduction of hyperextension through serial splinting. Other infants may require serial casting to hold the knee in flexion.[42] Genu recurvatum associated with dislocation of the knee requires surgery. A Pavlik harness, the mainstay of therapy for DDH, is typically not used to treat congenital knee dislocation unless it is associated with a hip dislocation. Typically, knee dislocation is treated before hip dysfunction. Because early treatment prevents further deformity or interference with normal function, an orthopedic consultation should be initiated early.

Metatarsus Adductus

The most common congenital foot anomaly, metatarsus adductus is a deformity of the forefoot in which the metatarsal bones deviate medially. The condition is typically a result of intrauterine positioning. Multiple gestation pregnancies and oligohydramnios, two conditions that decrease the intrauterine room available for fetal movement, predispose the newborn to metatarsus adductus.[7,11] It is associated with DDH in 10% to 20% of cases.[2,36] Other than the deviation, there are no pathologic changes in the structure of the foot. It occurs equally in both males and females and is seen bilaterally in approximately 50% of newborns who exhibit the anomaly.[36] Metatarsus adductus may be a positional (flexible) deformity with no bony abnormality involved or a structural (fixed) deformity (Figure 11.30). In a positional deformity, the forefoot is very mobile and can be easily abducted; the heel is likely to be in a neutral position. In a structural deformity, the arch appears to be greater than normal, and there may be a medial crease at its middle portion; the forefoot usually cannot be abducted beyond the midline (neutral position). In infants with severe structural anomaly, the heel (hindfoot) is in a valgus position. Approximately 85% of neonatal metatarsus adductus deformities resolve by 3 years of age and develop normal foot position and function without treatment.[11,36] Positional deformities will correct spontaneously or can be treated with stretching exercises. In a rigid foot, an orthopedic consultation is necessary for early treatment because manipulative stretching exercises and casting may be required. Surgery is indicated only when casting is unable to produce a flexible foot.[25,28]

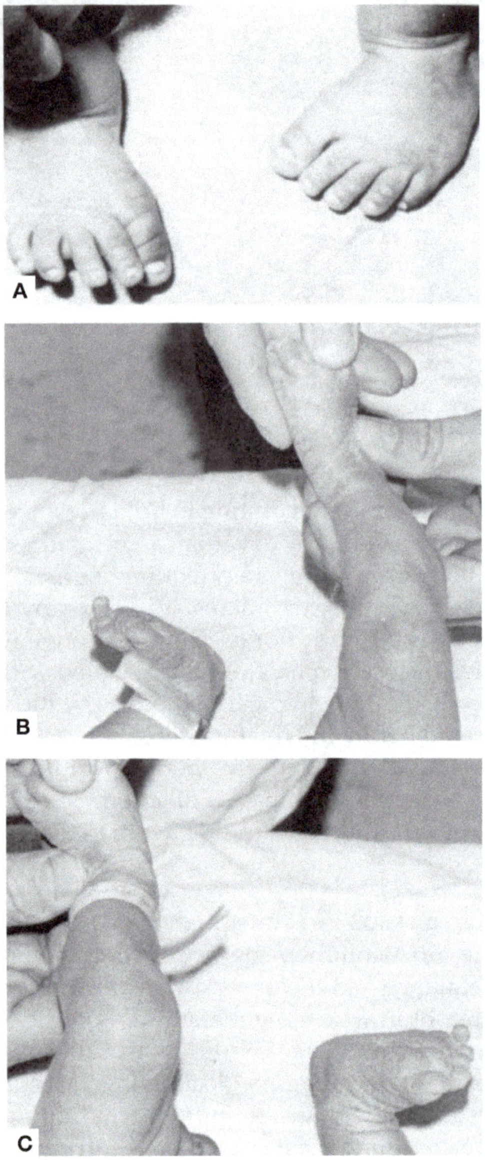

FIGURE 11.30 Metatarsus adductus. (A) Structural metatarsus adductus. (B) Structural metatarsus adductus. The forefoot does not abduct beyond neutral. (C) Positional metatarsus adductus. The forefoot abducts beyond the midline

Source: Robertson WW. 2005. Orthopedics. In *Neonatology: Pathophysiology and Management of the Newborn*, 6th ed. MacDonald MG, Seshia MMK, and Mullett MD, eds. Philadelphia: Lippincott Williams & Wilkins, 1434. Reprinted by permission.[26]

Clubfoot (Talipes Equinovarus)

Clubfoot (Figure 11.31) is a complex foot deformity in which the foot turns inward and downward and is readily apparent at birth. It is one of the most common congenital orthopedic anomalies, whose incidence varies with race and gender. In Caucasians, the birth frequency is approximately one per 1,000 live births, with males affected twice as often as females.[5,25,28] The highest incidence is seen in Polynesians at a rate of 6.8/1,000 births. Asian infants are the least likely to present with clubfoot, with it occurring at

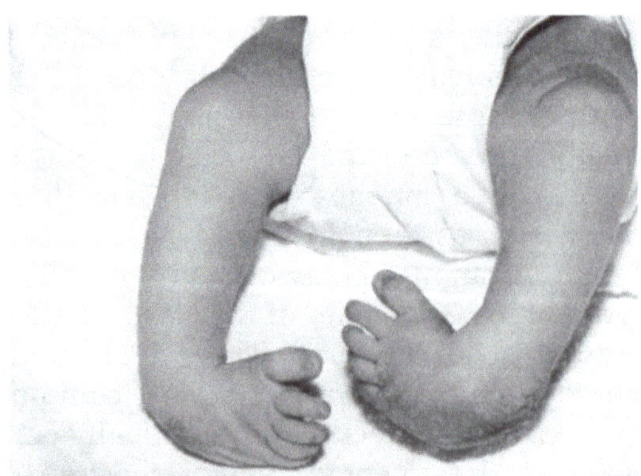

FIGURE 11.31 Clubfoot

Courtesy of Carol Trotter, St. John's Mercy Medical Center, St. Louis, MO.

a rate of 0.6/1,000 live births.[28] The cause of congenital clubfoot is unknown, but it is likely a combination of genetic and environmental factors. It may also be associated with chromosomal abnormalities or congenital syndromes. However, most cases are idiopathic and found in infants in whom there is no genetic or chromosomal abnormality and no other extrinsic cause can be found. Neural, muscular, and osseous abnormalities are other possible predisposing conditions. Within affected families, the probability is approximately 3% for siblings and 20% to 30% for the offspring of affected parents.[25,36]

Clinical presentation of the deformity is characterized by three primary components: (a) adduction of the forefoot (points medially) and accounts for approximately 95% of idiopathic cases, (b) pronounced varus of the heel, and (c) downward pointing of the foot and toes (equinus positioning). Clubfoot may be unilateral, but involvement is bilateral in about 50% of cases.[25,28] There are variations in the severity of clubfoot. Some are relatively flexible and correctable with conservative measures such as exercises and serial casting. Surgical correction is necessary for severe deformities or when nonoperative treatment methods are unsuccessful.[5,25] Treatment can often be started in the nursery. Clubfoot demonstrates excellent success rates in correction if recognized early and treated appropriately. An orthopedic consultation should be initiated as an early diagnosis facilitates an ideal long-term outcome.

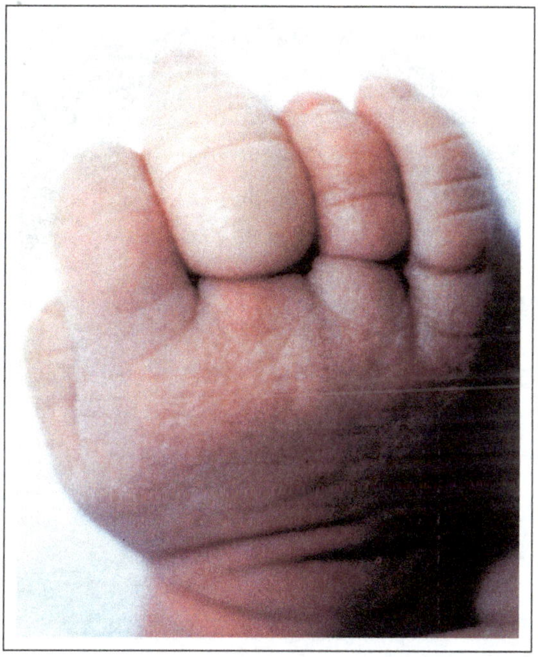

FIGURE 11.32 Congenital constricting bands (amniotic bands)

Source: From Clark DA. 2000. *Atlas of Neonatology*. Philadelphia: Saunders, 23. Reprinted by permission.[16]

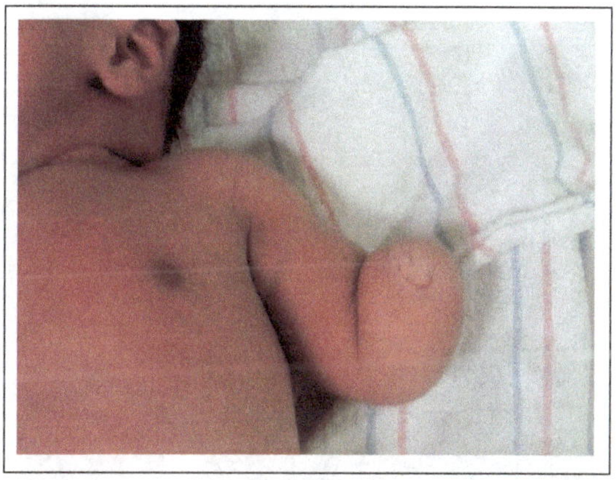

FIGURE 11.33 Congenital constricting bands (amniotic bands)

Conditions Affecting Upper and/or Lower Extremities

Congenital Constricting Bands

Constricting band syndrome (also know as amniotic band syndrome; amnion rupture sequence; amniotic deformity, adhesions, mutilations [ADAM] complex; and Streeter dysplasia) present as a band encircling the arms, legs, fingers, or toes. It can vary from mild, shallow indentations of the soft tissue to severe constrictions causing partial or complete amputation (Figures 11.32–11.35). Occasionally, craniofacial structures are affected, resulting in cleft lip, cleft palate, and other facial deformities.[31,43] No two cases of amniotic band syndrome are exactly alike, and the associated syndromes are highly variable. This deformity is estimated to occur in 1 per 1,000 to 1 per 15,000 live births, with the upper extremities more frequently involved than the lower extremities.[31,36,43] There are no gender or ethnic predispositions, and there

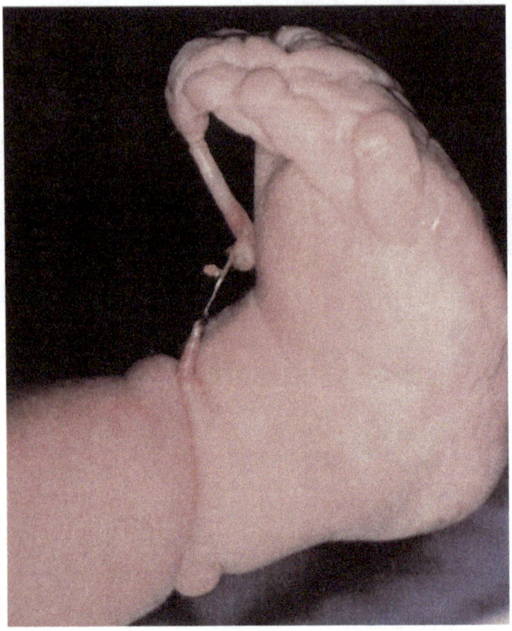

FIGURE 11.34 Congenital constricting bands (amniotic bands)

Source: From Clark DA. 2000. *Atlas of Neonatology*. Philadelphia: Saunders, 24. Reprinted by permission.[16]

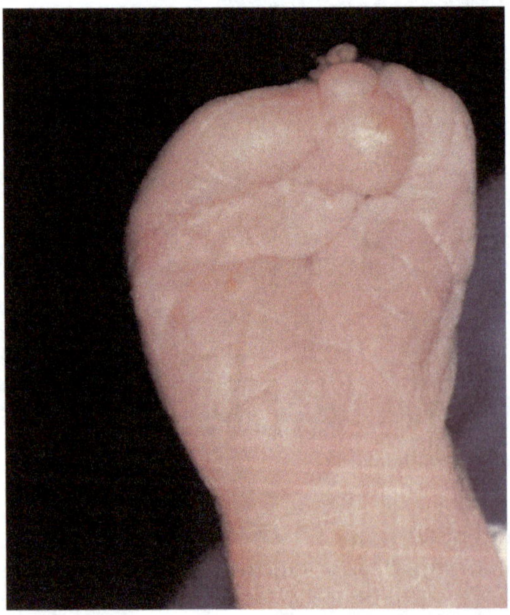

FIGURE 11.35 Amniotic bands resulting in finger amputation

Source: Clark DA. 2000. *Atlas of Neonatology*. Philadelphia: Saunders, 23. Reprinted by permission.[16]

is no known inheritance pattern. It is associated with other musculoskeletal deformations in 50% of cases; the most common being clubfoot.[36] The etiology is unknown, but the majority of evidence suggests that there is an abnormal attachment of the amnion to the fetus, because the amnion has either lost its integrity or ruptured and adhered to a fetal body part, causing compression or amputation.[19,36,43] Amniotic band syndrome can develop at any point during the first 20 weeks of pregnancy, but the most severe complications occur when it develops early in the first trimester. Treatment depends on the severity of the condition. Severe presentation of bands may need to be treated as an emergency, especially if there is evidence of vascular or lymphatic obstruction. Depending on the anatomical structure involved, consultation with a pediatric general surgeon, orthopedic surgeon, and/or craniofacial surgeon may be needed. Physical and occupational therapy are needed to ensure optimal use of affected fingers, toes, arms, and legs.[43]

Syndactyly

Congenital webbing of the fingers or toes—syndactyly—is one of the most common congenital anomalies of the upper extremities with an incidence of one per 2,000 to 3,000 live births (Figure 11.36).[36,44] While syndactyly is more common in the feet than the hands, it is more disabling in an upper extremity and accounts for 20% of congenital hand malformations. It occurs bilaterally in 50% of cases and is most often an isolated autosomal dominant inherited condition. This anomaly affects males twice as often as females and is 10 times more common among Caucasians than among infants of other races.[44] Syndactyly is caused by failure during the sixth to eighth week of gestation of the usual necrosis of skin that normally separates the fingers. Syndactyly is sporadic in most cases, with 10% to 40% familial and with variable penetrance. It can occur as an isolated anomaly or be associated with other congenital anomalies such as Apert and Streeter dysplasia.[14,25,44] The severity of involvement varies from minimal "bridging" between adjacent fingers and toes to complete webbing of the

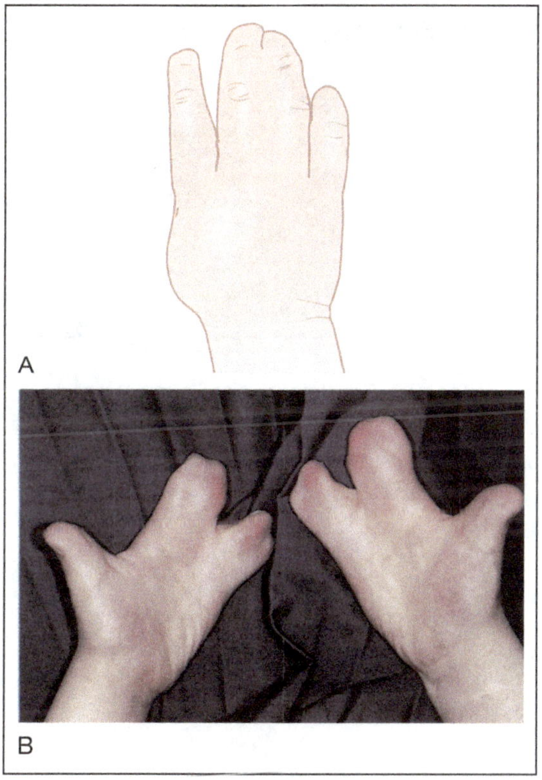

FIGURE 11.36 Two variations of syndactyly of the fingers

Source: Clark DA. 2000. *Atlas of Neonatology*. Philadelphia: Saunders, 222. Reprinted by permission.[16]

hand or foot. The more severe the syndactyly, the greater the likelihood of associated bony abnormalities. Syndactyly of the toes does not interfere with function but may be cosmetically undesired. Although surgical treatment is not required, it may be requested by the parents. Treatment for syndactyly of the fingers depends on the severity of the webbing and the presence or absence of bony abnormalities. When multiple fingers are involved, function may deteriorate as the fingers grow. Therefore, an early orthopedic consultation should be obtained, especially if the affected fingers are of unequal length, to determine if an operative approach is necessary.

Polydactyly

Extra digits—polydactyly—are common duplication abnormalities affecting both the hands and the feet (Figures 11.37 and 11.38), with an incidence of approximately 1.7 to 2 per 1,000 live births.[36,45] Postaxial (small finger, small toe) polydactyly has a variable racial incidence. It is seen more commonly in African American infants, with an incidence of 3.6 to 13.9 cases per 1,000 live births,

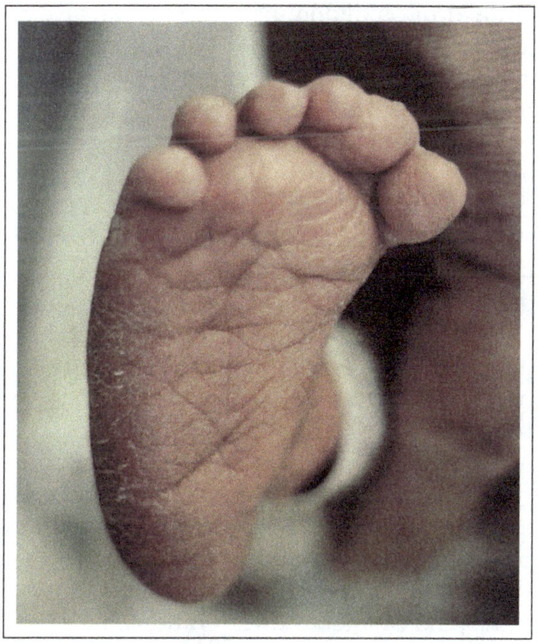

FIGURE 11.37 Polydactyly of the toes

Source: Clark DA. 2000. *Atlas of Neonatology*. Philadelphia: Saunders, 225. Reprinted by permission.[16]

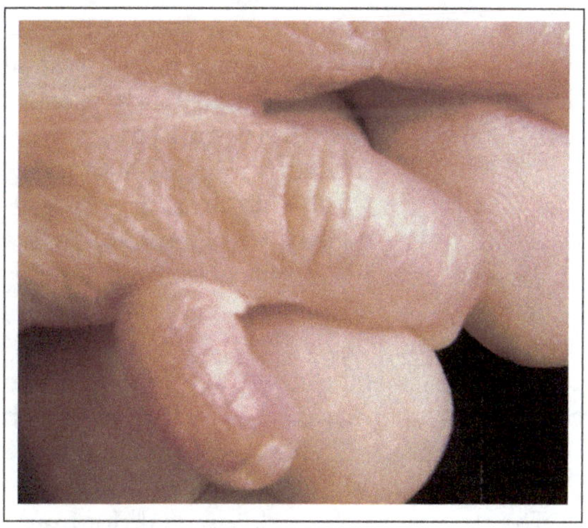

FIGURE 11.38 Polydactyly of the fingers

Source: Clark DA. 2000. *Atlas of Neonatology*. Philadelphia: Saunders, 222. Reprinted by permission.[16]

whereas the incidence in Caucasian infants is 0.3 to 1.3 per 1,000 live births. Polydactyly is bilateral in 50% of cases, and it affects males slightly more than females, hands more than feet, and left limbs more often than right.[14,45] It occurs more frequently in infants who have a positive family history.[41,45] Polydactyly can occur as an isolated anomaly or be inherited as an autosomal dominant trait. It can also be a manifestation of a multiple malformation syndrome such as trisomy 13, trisomy 21, or Meckel–Gruber syndrome.[14,41] Postaxial polydactyly in African Americans is almost always an isolated malformation. Postaxial polydactyly in Caucasians without a family history is infrequent and associated with chromosomal abnormalities, or other skeletal malformations.[31,36]

The most common type of polydactyly is a floppy digit or skin tag on either the radial or the ulnar side of the hand. Polydactyly may, however, involve the duplication of a normal-looking digit, giving the infant a functional six-fingered hand or a foot with six toes. Treatment depends on the extent of the anomaly. Consultation is needed so that therapeutic decisions can be based on functional and cosmetic considerations.

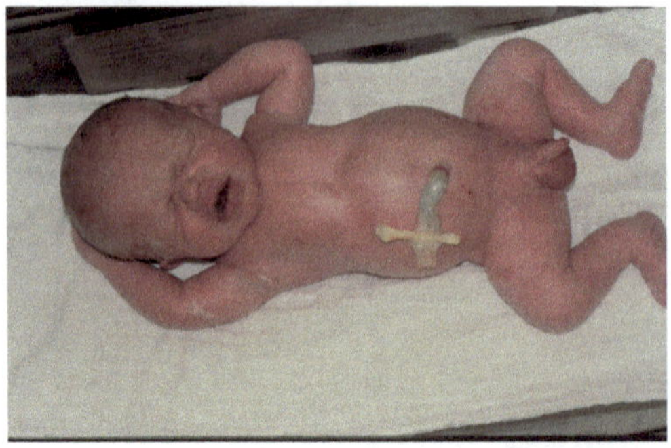

FIGURE 11.39 Achondroplasia: Flattened nasal bridge, frontal bossing, and shortened limbs

Source: Courtesy of L. Lilien, MD, Phoenix, AZ.

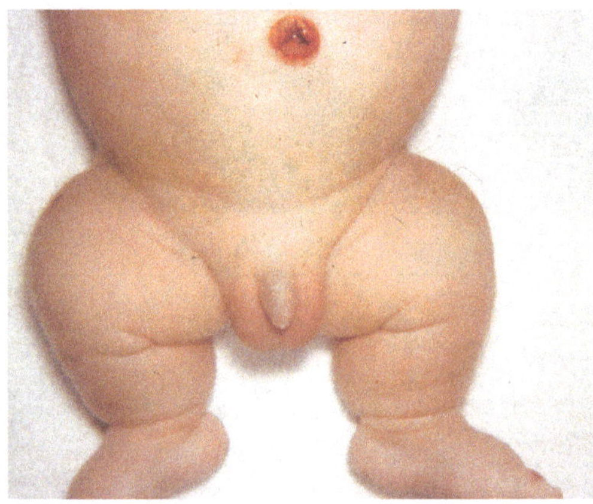

FIGURE 11.40 Achondroplastic dwarf: Short femurs and tibias

Source: From Clark DA. 2000. *Atlas of Neonatology*. Philadelphia: Saunders, 227.[16]

Skeletal Dysplasias: Achondroplasia

Skeletal dysplasias are a group of conditions associated with various abnormalities of the skeleton. These conditions are caused by disturbances of bone growth that begin in fetal development's early stages. Achondroplasia, a form of short-limbed dwarfism (Figures 11.39 and 11.40), is the most common form of nonlethal skeletal dysplasia with an incidence estimated to be 1 per 10,000 to 1 per 30,000 live births and affecting both males and females equally.[25,46] Achondroplasia occurs in all races with equal frequency. The estimated occurrence rate for this form of skeletal dysplasia in children of fathers over 50 years of age is much higher when compared to the frequency in the general population.[46]

The disorder has an autosomal dominant inheritance pattern with most cases appearing as spontaneous mutations. Approximately 80% of infants with achondroplasia have parents with normal stature. Heterozygous achondroplasia has not been shown to impact intelligence or life expectancy. Homozygous achondroplasia on the other hand is a lethal condition due to respiratory insufficiency caused by an underdeveloped rib cage and neurologic deficits secondary to cervicomedullary stenosis. Achondroplasia is caused by mutations in the gene for fibroblast growth factor receptor 3 (FGFR3) of chromosome 4. FGFR3 is responsible for providing instructions for making a protein that converts cartilage to bone. The mutations cause the FGFR3 protein to be overly active, which interferes with skeletal development and bone growth.[25,46,47] Infants with achondroplasia have short upper arms and thighs, limited range of motion at the elbows, an enlarged head with frontal bossing, midface hypoplasia, a depressed nasal bridge, and an average-sized torso with a protuberant abdomen. Hyperextensibility of the knees and hands is common. The hands are short and broad with the fingers exhibiting a three-pronged appearance (trident configuration) at birth due to an inability to oppose the third and fourth fingers. Infants usually lie with hips abducted, and lower legs have some degree of bowing (genu varum). In newborns, mild to moderate hypotonia is a typical finding and contributes to the delay of developmental motor milestones.[25,46]

Because most children with achondroplasia have delayed motor milestones, problems with persistent or recurrent middle ear infections, and bowing of the lower legs, treatment includes frequent monitoring and follow-up care. Although seen less often, infants may have serious health consequences related to hydrocephalus, craniocervical junction compression, upper airway obstruction, or thoracolumbar kyphosis. Anticipatory care should be directed at identifying infants who are at high risk and intervening to minimize risk of complications and prevent serious sequelae. Evaluations by genetic, orthopedic, and neurologic consultants are needed for best outcomes.[25,46,47]

SUMMARY

The examination of the musculoskeletal system provides a wealth of information about the overall development of the infant in utero, as well as the newborn's potential for normal development and function. Many of the common congenital anomalies of infancy are found in the musculoskeletal system. Although these abnormalities may not interfere with vital functions (as do those of the respiratory, cardiovascular, or other systems), they are a frequent cause of parental anxiety. The more accomplished the examiner becomes at performing the musculoskeletal examination, the easier it is to recognize deviations from normal, potential problems, and the need to initiate early interventions.

ADDITIONAL RESOURCES

SPRINGER PUBLISHING CONNECT™

A robust set of resources designed to supplement this text is located at http://connect.springerpub.com/content/book/978-0-8261-4063-0. Qualifying instructors may request access by emailing textbook@springerpub.com.

REFERENCES

1. Wheeler B. 2019. Health promotion of the newborn and family. In *Wong's Nursing Care of Infants and Children*, 11th ed. Hockenberry MJ, Wilson D, and Rodgers CC, eds. St. Louis, MO: Elsevier, 196–237.
2. Woiczik MR, McDaniel MG, and Butterfield RJ. 2019. Alterations of musculoskeletal function in children. In *Pathophysiology: The Biological Basis for Disease in Adults and Children*, 8th ed. McCance KL, and Huether SE, eds. St. Louis, MO: Elsevier, 1472–1495.
3. Liu RW, and Thompson GH. 2020. Musculoskeletal disorders in neonates. In *Neonatal—Perinatal Medicine: Diseases of the Fetus and Infant*, 11th ed. Martin RJ, Fanaroff AA, and Walsh MC, eds. Philadelphia, PA: Elsevier, 1980–1988.
4. American Academy of Orthopedic Surgeons. 2022. *Developmental Dislocation (Dysplasia) of the Hip (DDH)*. https://orthoinfo.aaos.org/en/diseases--conditions/developmental-dislocation-dysplasia-of-the-hip-ddh. Updated June 2022. Accessed October 2, 2022.
5. Butler KD. 2019. Disorders of musculoskeletal function: Developmental and metabolic disorders, activity, intolerance and fatigue. In *Porth's Pathophysiology*, 10th ed. Norris, TL, ed. Philadelphia, PA: Wolters Kluwer, 1378–1392.
6. Bickley LS, Szilagyi PG, Hoffman RM, and Soriano RP, eds. 2021. Children: Infancy through adolescence. In *Bates' Guide to Physical Examination and History Taking*, 13th ed. Philadelphia, PA: Wolters Kluwer, 943–992.
7. Ball JW, Dains JE, Flynn JA, Solomon BS, and Stewart RW, eds. 2023. *Seidel's Guide to Physical Examination*, 10th ed. St. Louis, MO: Elsevier, 110–132, 537–580.
8. Paris J, Ricardo A, and Reynolds D. 2019. Physical development in infancy and childhood. In *Child Growth and Development*. Open Textbook Library. Johnson A, ed. https://www.open.umn.edu/

opentextbooks/textbooks/750. Updated January 4, 2021. Accessed September 23, 2022.

9. Lissauer T, and Hansen A. 2020. Physical examination of the newborn. In *Neonatal—Perinatal Medicine: Diseases of the Fetus and Infant*, 11th ed. Martin RJ, Fanaroff AA, and Walsh MC, eds. Philadelphia, PA: Elsevier, 440–457.
10. Rao R, and Attarian S. 2020. Nutritional management. In *Neonatology: Management, Procedures, On-Call Problems, Diseases, and Drugs*, 8th ed. Gomella TL, Eyal FG, and Bany-Mohammed F, eds. New York, NY: McGraw-Hill, 125–165.
11. Jarvis C. 2019. *Physical Examination and Health Assessment*, 8th ed. St. Louis, MO: Elsevier, 139–160, 783–792.
12. Noonan KJ, and Halanski MA. 2021. Leg-length discrepancy. In *Lovell and Winter's Pediatric Orthopaedics*, 8th ed. Weinstein SL, Flynn JM, and Crawford HA, eds. Philadelphia, PA: Wolters Kluwer, 1296–1342.
13. Scanlon JW, Nelson T, Grylack LJ, and Smith YF. 1979. *A System of Newborn Physical Examination*. Baltimore, MD: University Park Press, 39–43, 50–51.
14. Mitchell AL. 2020. Congenital anomalies. In *Neonatal—Perinatal Medicine: Diseases of the Fetus and Infant*, 11th ed. Martin RJ, Fanaroff AA, and Walsh MC, eds. Philadelphia, PA: Elsevier, 489–513.
15. Sponseller PD, and MacKenzie WG. 2021. The skeletal dysplasias. In *Lovell and Winter's Pediatric Orthopaedics*, 8th ed. Weinstein SL, Flynn JM, and Crawford HA, eds. Philadelphia, PA: Wolters Kluwer, 214–258.
16. Clark DA. 2000. *Atlas of Neonatology*. Philadelphia, PA: Saunders, 9, 23, 24, 31, 131, 138, 222, 225, 227.
17. Prazad PA, Rajpal MN, Mangurten HH, and Puppala BL. 2020. Birth injuries. In *Neonatal—Perinatal Medicine: Diseases of the Fetus and Infant*, 11th ed. Martin RJ, Fanaroff AA, and Walsh MC, eds. Philadelphia, PA: Elsevier, 458–488.
18. White KK, Bouchard M, and Goldberg MJ. 2018. Common neonatal orthopedic conditions. In *Avery's Diseases of the Newborn*, 10th ed. Gleason CA, and Juul SE, eds. Philadelphia, PA: Elsevier, 1438–1449.
19. Balest AL, Riley MM, O'Donnell B, and Zarit JS. 2023. Neonatology. In *Zitelli and Davis Atlas of Pediatric Physical Diagnosis*, 8th ed. Zitelli BJ, McIntire SC, Nowalk AJ, and Garrison J, eds. Philadelphia, PA: Elsevier, 43–70.
20. Feingold M. 1994. Congenital malformations. In *Neonatology: Pathophysiology and Management of the Newborn*, 4th ed. Avery GB, Fletcher MA, and MacDonald MG, eds. Philadelphia, PA: Lippincott Williams & Wilkins, 761.
21. Haldeman-Englert CR, Saitta SC, and Zackai EH. 2018. Chromosome disorders. In *Avery's Diseases of the Newborn*, 10th ed. Gleason CA, and Juul SE, eds. Philadelphia, PA: Elsevier, 211–223.
22. Milner RDG, and Herber SM. 1984. *Color Atlas of the Newborn*. Oradell, NJ: Medical Economics, 88.
23. Jarvis C. 2012. *Physical Examination & Health Assessment*, 6th ed. Philadelphia, PA: Saunders, 600.
24. Alexander MM, and Brown MS. 1979. *Pediatric History Taking and Physical Diagnosis for Nurses*, 2nd ed. Philadelphia, PA: Mosby, 292.
25. McClincy MP, Olgun ZD, and Dede O. 2023. Orthopedics. In *Zitelli and Davis Atlas of Pediatric Physical Diagnosis*, 8th ed. Zitelli BJ, McIntire SC, Norwalk AJ, and Garrison J, eds. Philadelphia, PA: Wolters Kluwer, 766–849.
26. Robertson WW. 2005. Orthopedics. In *Neonatology: Pathophysiology and Management of the Newborn*, 6th ed. MacDonald MG, Seshia MMK, and Mullett MD, eds. Philadelphia, PA: Lippincott Williams & Wilkins, 1429.
27. Kim HKW, and Herring JA. 2022. Developmental dysplasia of the hip. In *Tachdjian's Pediatric Orthopaedics*, 6th ed. Herring J, ed. Philadelphia, PA: Elsevier, 422–526.
28. Mosca VS, and Bouchard M. 2021. The foot. In *Lovell and Winter's Pediatric Orthopaedics*, 8th ed. Weinstein SL, and Flynn JM, eds. Philadelphia, PA: Wolters Kluwer, 1342–1465.
29. El-Hawary R, and Pahys JM. 2021. The cervical spine. In *Lovell and Winter's Pediatric Orthopaedics*, 8th ed. Weinstein SL, and Flynn JM, eds. Philadelphia, PA: Wolters Kluwer, 820–884.
30. Abbasi D, and Shilt J. 2021. *Congenital scoliosis*. Orthobullets. http://www.orthobullets.com/spine/2060/congenital-scoliosis. Updated June 24, 2021. Accessed October 2, 2022.
31. Bauer AS, and Waters PM. 2021. The upper limb. In *Lovell and Winter's Pediatric Orthopaedics*, 8th ed. Weinstein SL, Flynn JM, and Crawford, HA, eds. Philadelphia, PA: Wolters Kluwer, 885–962.
32. National Center for Advancing Translational Sciences. 2021. *Cleidocranial Dysostosis*. Genetic and Rare Disease Information Center. https://rarediseases.info.nih.gov/diseases/6118/cleidocranial-dysplasia. Updated November 8, 2021. Accessed October 8, 2022.
33. Swainman KF, and Wright FS. 1982. *The Practice of Pediatric Neurology*. Philadelphia, PA: Mosby, 441.
34. Storment M. 2022. *Guidelines for Therapists: Treating Children with Brachial Plexus Injuries*. United Brachial Plexus Network. www.ubpn.org/resources/medical/pros/therapists/122-therapyguidelins. Updated 2022. Accessed October 8, 2022.
35. Basit H, Ali CDM, and Madhani NB. 2022. Erb palsy. In *StatPearls* [Internet]. Treasure Island, FL: StatPearls Publishing. https://www.ncbi.nlm.nih.gov/books/NBK513260/. Accessed September 23, 2022.
36. Son-Hing JP, and Thompson GH. 2020. Congenital anomalies of the upper and lower extremities and spine. In *Neonatal—Perinatal Medicine: Diseases of the Fetus and Infant*, 11th ed. Martin RJ, Fanaroff AA, and Walsh MC, eds. Philadelphia, PA: Elsevier, 1995–2015.
37. American Academy of Orthopaedic Surgeons. 2022. *Management of Developmental Dysplasia of the Hip in Infants Up to Six Months of Age*. https://www.aaos.org/globalassets/quality-and-practice-resources/pddh/ddh-auc_generalist-2022-reissue.pdf. Reissued August 22, 2022. Accessed September 28, 2022.

38. Weinstein SL. 2021. Developmental hip dysplasia and dislocation. In *Lovell and Winter's Pediatric Orthopaedics*, 8th ed. Weinstein SL, Flynn JM, and Crawford HA, eds. Philadelphia, PA: Wolters Kluwer, 963–1088.
39. Yang S, Zusman N, Lieberman E, and Goldstein RY. 2019. Developmental dysplasia of the hip. *Pediatrics* 143(1): e20181147. doi: 10.1542/peds.2018-1147
40. Bowen RE, Otsuka NY, and Doty SA. 2021. The child with a limb deficiency. In *Lovell and Winter's Pediatric Orthopaedics*, 8th ed. Weinstein SL, Flynn JM, and Crawford HA, eds. Philadelphia, PA: Wolters Kluwer, 1466–1536.
41. Mackenzie WG, and Thabet AM. 2020. Orthopedic and musculoskeletal problems. In *Neonatology: Management, Procedures, On-Call Problems, Diseases, and Drugs*, 8th ed. Gomella TL, Cunningham MD, and Eyal FG, eds. New York, NY: McGraw Hill, 1013–1021.
42. Iobst C, Jain V, and McCarthy JJ. 2021. The lower extremity. In *Lovell and Winter's Pediatric Orthopaedics*, 8th ed. Weinstein SL, Flynn JM, and Crawford HA, eds. Philadelphia, PA: Wolters Kluwer, 1223–1295.
43. Singh AP, and Gorla SR. 2022, January. Amniotic band syndrome. In *StatPearls* [Internet]. Treasure Island, FL: StatPearls Publishing. Updated June 9, 2022. https://www.ncbi.nlm.nih.gov/books/NBK545283. Accessed August 30, 2022.
44. Hinkley JR, and Fallahi AKM. 2022, January. Syndactyly. In *StatPearls* [Internet]. Treasure Island, FL: StatPearls Publishing. Updated September 18, 2022. https://www.ncbi.nlm.nih.gov/books/NBK557704. Accessed August 24, 2022.
45. Novick C. 2020. *Polydactyly of the foot*. Medscape. https://emedicine.medscape.com/article/1260255-overview. Updated October 9, 2020. Accessed October 12, 2022.
46. Parikh S. 2022. *Achondroplasia*. Medscape. https://www.emedicine.medscape.com/article/1258401-overview. Updated January 10, 2022. Accessed September 23, 2022.
47. Savarirayan R, Ireland P, Irving M, Thompson D, Alves I, Baratela, WAR, Betts J, Bober MB, Boero S, Briddell J, Campbell J, Campeau PM, Carl-Innig P, Cheung MS, Cobourne M, Cormier-Daire V, Deladure-Molla M, del Pino M, Elphick H, Fano V, Fauroux B, Gibbins J, Groves ML, Hagenäs L, Hannon T, Hoover-Fong J, Kaisermann M, Leiva-Gea A, Llerena J, Mackenzie W, Martin K, Mazzoleni F, McDonnell S, Costanza Meazzini M, Milerad J, Mohnike K, Mortier GR, Offiah A, Ozono K, Phillips JA, Powell S, Prasad Y, Raggio C, Rosselli P, Rossiter J, Selicorni A, Sessa M, Theroux M, Thomas M, Trespedi L, Tunkel D, Wallis C, Wright M, Yasui N, and Fredwell SO. 2022. International consensus statement on the diagnosis, multidisciplinary management and lifelong care of individuals with achondroplasia. *Nature Reviews Endocrinology* 18: 173–189. doi: 10.1038/s41574-021-00595-x

12 NEUROLOGIC ASSESSMENT

Bresney A. Fanning

The neurologic evaluation is a critical part of neonatal assessment and is comprised of history, physical examination and if appropriate, specialized studies. The neurologic examination is a detailed and organized exam and should guide diagnosis, management, and prognosis. A single examination may verify the presence of normal or abnormal neurologic responses. Serial follow-up of the abnormal neurologic examination is necessary to validate unusual findings and to document changes or improvements over time.

A common approach to assessment of neurologic status is through the systematic testing of specific functions of the nervous system, including the motor system, reflexes, sensory system, and cranial nerves. More formal neurologic assessments, designed as clinical and research tools, are available. The neurologic evaluation developed by Amiel-Tison is designed to evaluate neonates at term or corrected term age during the first year of life and emphasizes neuromotor function.[1] Prechtl also developed and validated a neurologic examination for the term neonate.[2] Another comprehensive neurologic examination was designed by Lilly and Victor Dubowitz and is applicable to both term and preterm neonates.[3] The Dubowitz examination places heavy emphasis on evaluation of movement, tone, and also includes some behavioral items evaluated on the Brazelton assessment, further discussed in Chapter 13.

HISTORY

The neurologic examination should be preceded by a thorough review of the history. This should include the maternal and family history for genetic or neurologic problems, maternal medications during pregnancy as well as anesthetic agents and medications administered during labor and at delivery, and any history of alcohol or illicit drug use. A detailed prenatal history should be obtained to note results of chromosome analysis, prenatal ultrasound findings, and tests of fetal well-being and maturity. Review the intrapartum course for abnormal presentation, prolonged labor, precipitous delivery, fetal distress, and difficult or operative extraction. Postnatal history should include Apgar scores, cord blood pH, presence of depression at birth, difficulties in transition, feeding ability, and gestational age. An accurate assessment of gestational age and the impact of maturation on the neurologic exam (refer to Chapter 4) is crucial.

OBSERVATION

After obtaining the history, the neonate should be carefully observed to determine behavioral state, posture, autonomic activity, facial symmetry, spontaneous movement, and more, prior to an intrusive assessment. In a critically ill neonate, requiring invasive monitoring and access, vigorous assessment and manipulation can skew the neurologic examination. During observation, the behavioral state should be assessed. The level of alertness will vary depending on gestational age, timing of last feeding, environment, and recent activity and is affected at some point with most central nervous system (CNS) disorders. In a stable sleep state, the infant should appear quiet and restful with minimal body and facial movement and decreased response to the environment. Abnormal findings would include restlessness, facial twitching or grimacing, and sensitivity to environmental factors. A neonate in the awake state should be alert, be able to focus on objects depending on gestational age, and be consolable. Abnormal findings include a low-level arousal or hyper-alert state and irritability with difficulty being consoled. Levels of alertness can be categorized as normal, stupor, and coma and are determined by the response to stimulation and the quantity and quality of movement.[4] A stuporous neonate may be described as sleepy or lethargic with diminished arousal response. For infants in deep stupor, arousal is absent, and the neonate appears to be sleeping. Neonates in coma have absence of arousal with low-level motor responses.

Prior to 28 weeks gestation, it is difficult to identify periods of wakefulness. Stimulation may result in eye opening and short periods of alertness. At approximately 28 weeks gestation, there is an increase in the level of alertness, and both stimulated and spontaneous alerting can be seen.[4] The premature neonate has longer sleep cycles than the term neonate. Sleep–wake cycles are more apparent by 32 weeks gestation, and stimulation is usually not necessary to arouse and alert the neonate.[4] By 36 weeks gestation, increased alertness can be readily observed.[4]

If the neonate is awake and crying, attention should be paid to the *quality of the cry, symmetry of movement*, and *facial expression*. A loud, lusty cry is typical in the term neonate. A weaker cry may be heard in the premature, depressed, or ill neonate. A high-pitched cry may be heard in infants with neurologic disturbances, metabolic abnormalities, neonatal abstinence syndrome, or infections such as meningitis. Self-regulation can be observed and noted as appropriate for gestational age.

Facial symmetry and extremity movement symmetry should be assessed in the active or crying infant during the observation period. Facial asymmetry or weakness may be evidence of a birth trauma, cranial nerve abnormality, intrauterine positioning, Bell's palsy, or neuromuscular junction disorders, such as myasthenia gravis and infantile botulism. Other etiologies for generalized facial weakness include posterior fossa hematoma, cerebral contusion, neonatal encephalopathy, and some congenital syndromes. Lack of movement of an extremity may indicate trauma and/or nerve damage.

The *quality of movements* should also be evaluated in the active neonate. Term neonates move their limbs smoothly. In the preterm neonate, tremors and jitteriness can be normally present. Jitteriness can also be benign in term neonates and is sometimes seen with vigorous crying. It may also be a sign of disorders such as hypoglycemia, hypocalcemia, drug withdrawal, and neonatal encephalopathy. Jitteriness must be distinguished from seizure activity (Table 12.1). Although the distinction can be subtle in the neonatal period, jitteriness is characterized by rapid alternating movements of equal amplitude in both directions. In contrast, the clonic movements seen during true seizures have a fast and slow component. Noise, touch, or other environmental stimuli can

TABLE 12.1: DISTINGUISHING SEIZURE ACTIVITY FROM JITTERINESS

CLINICAL FINDING	SEIZURE	JITTERINESS
Abnormal gaze or eye movements	Yes	No
Stimulus sensitive	No	Yes
Ceases with passive flexion	No	Yes
Autonomic changes	Yes	No
Predominant movement	Clonic jerking	Tremor

Source: Adapted from Volpe JJ. 2018. *Neurology of the Newborn*, 6th ed. Philadelphia, PA: Elsevier, 289. Reprinted by permission.[4]

elicit jitteriness, which can be stopped by flexing or holding the involved extremity. Seizures are generally not initiated by stimulation, nor can they be stopped by flexing or holding. In addition, jitteriness is not associated with any subtle signs of seizure activity, such as abnormal eye movements or autonomic changes.

The neonate's resting *posture* should be noted and its appropriateness for gestational age gauged. Typically, a term neonate lies with hips abducted and partially flexed and with knees flexed. The arms are usually adducted and flexed at the elbow (Figures 12.1). The hand is loosely fisted, and the thumb may lie in the palm or adjacent to the fingers. At 28 weeks gestational age, the newborn's arms and legs are extended, with little tone. From 28 to 40 weeks gestational age, tone increases in a caudocephalic direction, with increased tone in flexion observed first in the legs (around 32–34 weeks) and later in the arms (around 34–36 weeks). In the premature neonate, the adductor muscles are hypotonic; although flexion is seen as gestational age increases, the limbs are often flat against the bed surface. In this posture, the legs are abducted, and the lateral thigh rests against the surface of the bed. This position, often referred to as the *frog leg* position, is abnormal in neonates of more than 36 weeks gestation. Neonates of 32 weeks gestation or more who lie with their extremities completely extended are demonstrating depressed postural tone. Depressed postural tone in the arms is suggested by flaccid extension of the arms or by some degree of flexion at the elbow but with open palmar surfaces facing up at 36 weeks or greater. In addition, cortical thumb—a persistent tightly fisted hand in which the thumb is firmly enclosed by the fingers—may indicate neurologic

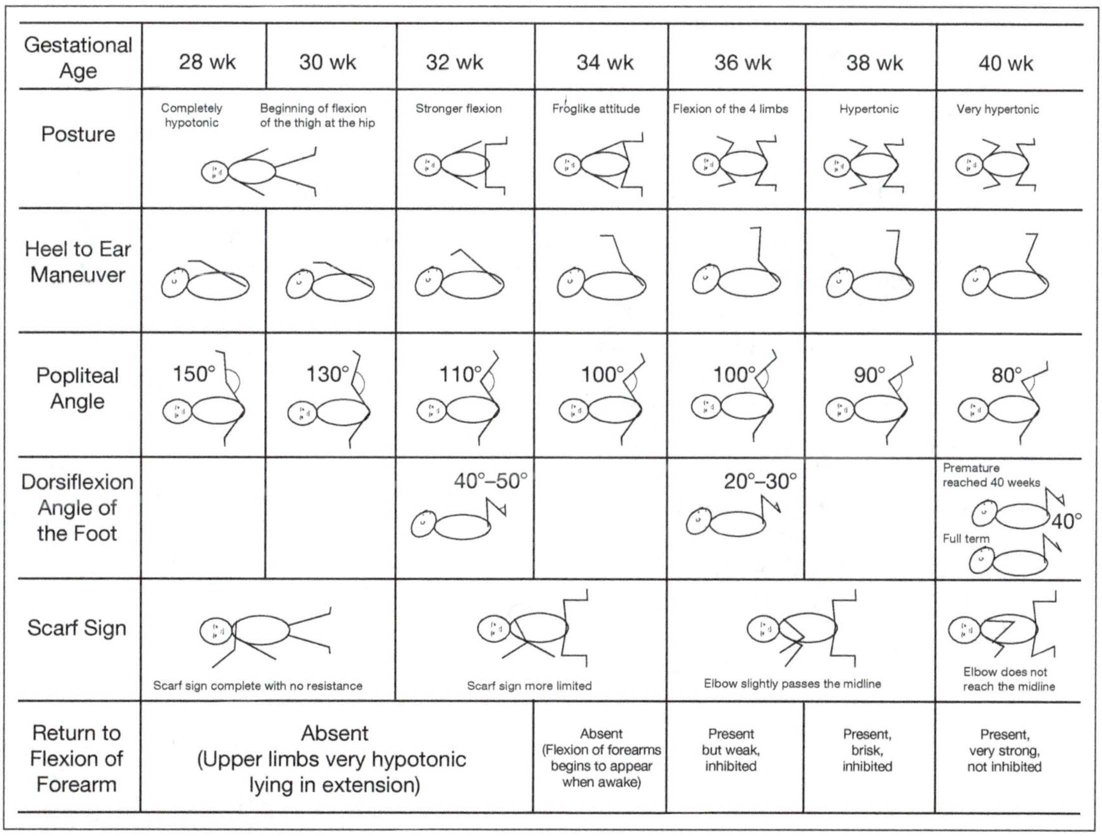

FIGURE 12.1 Posture and passive tone; tone increases with maturity, showing the ascending direction of tone

Source: From Amiel-Tison C. 1991. Examination of the newborn infant. In *Rudolph's Pediatrics*, 19th ed. Rudolph CD, et al., eds. New York: McGraw Hill, 178. Reprinted by permission.[5]

abnormality. When observation identifies any postural abnormality, it should be reconfirmed during the motor examination of tone and reflexes.

The autonomic system can reflect changes in neurologically compromised and injured neonates and, when able, should be observed in a quiet infant. Function of the segmental and peripheral centers of the autonomic nervous system is well established in the term neonate. This system has priority in maturation because it controls the activity of systems and organs essential for life. Vital signs, skin, and sphincters are areas that can be assessed. Observations of trends in temperature, perfusion, heart rate, blood pressure, respiratory rate, and pupillary response to light should be made.

In stressed or clinically ill neonates, the skin may be mottled, pale or cyanotic. Any skin abrasions, bruises, lacerations, or edema should be documented. This may point to evidence of birth trauma. A normal variant demonstrating autonomic vasomotor instability in the neonate is the harlequin sign (see Chapter 5). When the neonate is lying on their side, the dependent area becomes red, and the upper area appears pale in contrast (see Figure 5.2).

Certain types of *skin lesions* may be significant in specific neurologic abnormalities and should be noted for number, size, shape, color, and texture. Café au lait spots of 1.5 cm or larger or more than three in number may indicate the presence of neurofibromatosis, one of the more common autosomal dominant genetic disorders. Port-wine nevi involving both eyelids, with bilateral distribution or those that are unilateral but involve all three branches of the trigeminal nerve, are associated with a significantly higher incidence of eye and CNS abnormalities.[4] These lesions may indicate the presence of Sturge–Weber syndrome with underlying arteriovenous malformations. Glaucoma and leptomeningeal vessels in the brain can lead to seizures or other abnormalities. Areas of skin depigmentation should be noted because they can indicate the earliest manifestation of tuberous sclerosis, presenting as white, macular lesion(s), with irregular leaflike borders.

PHYSICAL EXAMINATION

Head and Spine

The examination of the head should include the size and shape. A head circumference provides valuable information in reference to intracranial volume. Head shape can affect the head circumference and should be considered. Head circumference is measured and plotted on a growth chart, and the percentile is determined based on gestational age. A neonate with a head circumference greater than the 90th percentile for gestational age yet weight and height below the 90th percentile may have hydrocephaly, macrocephaly, or hydranencephaly. The skull configuration in hydrocephalus is frequently globular. Posterior ballooning of the skull is seen with hydrocephalus caused by Dandy–Walker syndrome. When a large head circumference and percentile for gestational age are identified, transillumination of the skull can be helpful. In a dark room and after the examiner's eyes have adapted to the reduced light, a rubber-cuffed flashlight or other transillumination device is applied firmly to the skull (see Figure 1.3). A glow of more than 2 cm around the rubber cuff of the flashlight is abnormal and reflects fluid accumulation. Ultrasound, which is readily available in most hospitals, is the most common way to diagnose hydrocephalus in the newborn.

A head circumference of less than the third percentile for gestational age is considered microcephaly, and can be seen in chromosomal abnormalities, maternal drug and alcohol use, or intrauterine infections. **T**oxoplasmosis, **O**ther agents (including syphilis), **R**ubella, **C**ytomegalovirus, and **H**erpes simplex (TORCH) should be ruled out.

The fontanels and sutures should be evaluated by gentle palpation in the non-crying neonate (see Chapter 6) to determine size and to assess whether they are soft and flat or full and bulging. A full or bulging fontanel with widened sutures may indicate increased intracranial pressure and hydrocephalus. Widening of the sutures alone, with a normal anterior fontanel, may be caused by abnormal ossification seen with intrauterine growth restriction. Assessment for cephalohematoma, caput succedaneum, subgaleal hemorrhage, or any abnormalities in the scalp such as aplasia cutis congenita should be done at this time. The face should be examined for structural abnormalities, misplacement, or abnormalities of the ears. The presence of neck skinfolds, hair whorls, or poliosis should be documented.

Head shape can lead to suspicion of craniosynostosis, or premature closure of the cranial sutures (covered in Chapter 6 "Head, Eyes, Ears, Nose, Mouth, and Neck Assessment"). Although not a routine part of the newborn physical examination, auscultation of the skull for bruits may be of value when arteriovenous malformation or aneurysm is suspected. Flow disturbances resulting from interference with the normal laminar flow through vessels may cause vessel wall vibrations heard as systolic murmurs and referred to as *bruits*. Bruits may be heard in Sturge–Weber syndrome, usually accompanied by facial port-wine nevi; it is therefore important to listen for bruits in neonates with this skin lesion. Arteriovenous malformations may lead to unexplained high-output cardiac failure in neonates, and an examination for bruits may assist in making the diagnosis. Auscultation is carried out with the bell of the stethoscope placed over the temporal, frontal, and occipital areas.

Careful examination of the back and spine should be done, identifying any asymmetry, lesions or masses, dimples or pits, and hair tufts. A dimple on the spine should be differentiated from a sinus. A dimple is a common finding and rarely indicates an underlying problem. It is usually located just superior to the anal opening. A dermal sinus can occur anywhere along the midline of the back but is most frequently seen in the lumbar region. Although dimples generally have no clinical significance, sinuses may terminate in subcutaneous tissue, a cyst, or a fibrous band, or may be associated with spina bifida and extend into an open spinal cord.

To inspect the dimple or sinus, try to visualize the skin covering the end of the site. This may be difficult with deep sinuses. Probing the site with instruments is contraindicated; in the case of an open spine, direct trauma to spinal elements as well as possible introduction of bacteria into the defect could occur. Ultrasound of the involved area is preferred to assist in identifying any vertebral abnormalities and the relationship of the defect to the meninges and cord.

Evaluation of the Cranial Nerves

Olfactory—Cranial Nerve I

The neonate's sense of smell is rarely tested because disturbances in olfaction are rarely a feature of neurologic disease in the neonate. The sense of smell is present in neonates, and those of nursing mothers can discriminate between their mother's breast pad and that of another female.[4] Gross evaluation can be done using strong-smelling substances, such as anise, peppermint, or clove oil, and evaluating for sucking, grimacing, sniffing, or startle responses (Table 12.2). Abnormalities can be seen in infants with disturbances of porencephalic development such as holoprosencephaly.

Optic—Cranial Nerve II

Visual acuity, visual fields, and a funduscopic examination provide information on the function of the optic nerve. A term neonate's visual fixation is well developed, and some behavior associated with visual fixation can be detected by 32 weeks. The ability of the neonate's eyes to fix on an object and follow it over a 60-degree arc can be evaluated. The object may be the examiner's face, simple black-and-white pictures depicting facial features, or a ball held 10 to 12 inches from the neonate's eyes and moved from side to side. During the examination, occasional nystagmus (an involuntary rapid movement of the eyeball) may be seen in the neonate. Wandering or persistent nystagmus is abnormal and may indicate a neurologic abnormality. When a light is introduced into the periphery of the neonate's visual field, the head should turn toward the light. Tracking

TABLE 12.2: TESTING CRANIAL NERVE FUNCTION OF INFANTS

CRANIAL NERVE	FUNCTION
I	Smell
II, III, IV, and VI	Optical blink reflex—shine light in open eyes, note rapid closure
	Size, shape, equality of pupils
	Regards face or close object
	Eyes follow movement
V	Rooting reflex, sucking reflex
VII	Facial movements (e.g., wrinkling forehead and nasolabial folds) symmetric when crying or smiling
VIII	Loud noise yields Moro-like reflex or startle (until 4 months)
	Acoustic blink reflex—infant blinks in response to a loud hand clap 30 cm (12 inches) from head (avoid making air current)
	Eyes follow direction of sound
IX, X	Swallowing, gag reflex
XI	Head turns normally from side to side, shoulder height is equal
XII	Coordinated sucking and swallowing
	Pinch nose, infant's mouth will open and tongue rise in midline

Source: Adapted from Jarvis C. 2019. *Physical Examination & Health Assessment*, 8th ed. Philadelphia, PA: Saunders. Reprinted by permission.[6]

can be seen by 34 weeks, and by 37 weeks the infant should turn toward soft light. Response to light differs across gestational ages. By 26 weeks gestation, the infant should consistently blink when light is present, and by 32 weeks, light causes eye closure until the light disappears.

Funduscopic examination should be performed, and the character of veins and arteries, the macula, and the optic disk evaluated. A thorough examination of the optic disk requires pupil dilation.

Oculomotor, Trochlear, and Abducens—Cranial Nerves III, IV, and VI

These nerves supply the pupil and the extraocular muscles. Pupillary size and constriction in response to light are also evaluated. By approximately 30 weeks gestation, pupillary reaction to light is present[5] but is not consistent until 32 to 35 weeks. Pupillary abnormalities and possible etiologies are shown in Table 12.3. Presence of ptosis, proptosis, sustained nystagmus, or strabismus should be noted.

Movement of the eyes as the position of the head is turned should be evaluated. The "doll's eye" maneuver consists of gently rotating the head from side to side and evaluating for deviation of the eyes away from the direction of rotation—for example, in a normal response, when the head is turned to the right, the eyes deviate to the left (Figure 12.2). If the eyes remain in a fixed position regardless of head rotation, brainstem dysfunction may be present. If the eyes move in the same direction as the head is rotated, brainstem or oculomotor nerve dysfunction may be

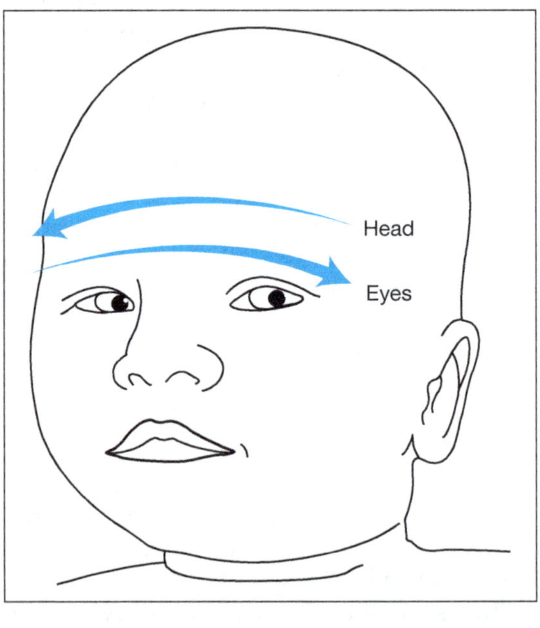

FIGURE 12.2 The "doll's eye" maneuver

TABLE 12.3: PUPILLARY ABNORMALITIES IN THE NEONATAL PERIOD

ETIOLOGY	PUPILLARY REACTIVITY
Bilateral increase in size	
HIE	Reactive early in course; unreactive later in course
IVH	Unreactive
Local anesthetic intoxication	Unreactive
Bilateral decrease in size	
HIE	Reactive
Unilateral decrease in size	
Horner syndrome	Reactive
Unilateral increase in size	
Subdural hematoma	Unreactive
Unilateral mass	Unreactive
Third nerve palsy	±Unreactive
HIE	±Unreactive

HIE, hypoxic-ischemic encephalopathy; IVH, intraventricular hemorrhage.

Source: Modified from Volpe JJ. 2018. *Neurology of the Newborn*, 6th ed. Philadelphia, PA: Elsevier, 207. Reprinted by permission.[4]

present. Complete ocular movement can be demonstrated with the doll's eye maneuver as early as 25 weeks gestational age.

Trigeminal—Cranial Nerve V

The trigeminal nerve supplies the jaw muscles and is responsible for the sensory innervation of the face. The three divisions of this nerve are mandibular, maxillary, and ophthalmic. If unilateral facial paralysis is present, damage to the motor component of this nerve may cause the jaw to deviate to the paralyzed side when the mouth is open. Strength of the masseter muscle is judged by placing a gloved finger in the neonate's mouth and evaluating the strength of the biting portion of the suck. The sensory component of this nerve can be estimated by response to touch (as in the rooting reflex) or by the response to gentle touching of the eyelashes with a piece of cotton. The corneal reflex can be tested by blowing air into the neonate's eye to elicit a blink or by gently touching the cornea with a small piece of cotton.

Facial—Cranial Nerve VII

The facial nerve controls facial expression. Facial symmetry is evaluated in the non-crying, undisturbed neonate and in the crying neonate. Severe injury to the facial nerve may result in marked facial weakness. If the entire nerve on one side of the face is damaged, the neonate will be unable to wrinkle his brow or close his eyes well with crying, and the mouth will appear to draw to the normal side. Nasolabial creases will also be asymmetric. Causes of facial weakness are listed in Box 12.1.

BOX 12.1: CAUSES OF FACIAL WEAKNESS IN THE NEONATAL PERIOD

Cerebral
Hypoxic-ischemic encephalopathy
Cerebral contusion

Nerve
Traumatic nerve damage
Hematoma in posterior fossa

Neuromuscular junction
Myasthenia gravis
Infantile botulism

Nuclear injury
Mobius syndrome
Hypoxic-ischemic encephalopathy

Muscle
Myotonic dystrophy
Muscular dystrophy
Facioscapulohumeral dystrophy
Myopathy
Mitochondrial disorder
Muscle hypoplasia

Source: Modified from Volpe JJ. 2018. *Neurology of the Newborn*, 6th ed. Philadelphia, PA: Elsevier, 210. Reprinted by permission.[4]

Auditory—Cranial Nerve VIII

The auditory component of cranial nerve VIII can be tested in the neonate by assessing response to a loud noise and can be elicited in neonates as young as 28 weeks gestation.[5] The response may be a blink or a Moro reflex. If the infant fails to respond to stimuli on repeat examinations, more accurate hearing tests (e.g., auditory evoked potentials) should be performed. The vestibular component is tested by rotating the neonate from side to side and eliciting the "doll's eye" movement.

Glossopharyngeal—Cranial Nerve IX

The glossopharyngeal nerve controls tongue movement. The nerve is assessed/evaluated by inspecting tongue movement, eliciting a gag reflex, and noting the position of the uvula. If weakness of the nerve is present, the uvula deviates to one side.

Vagus—Cranial Nerve X

The motor portion of the vagus nerve supplies the soft palate, pharynx, and larynx. Bilateral lesions of this nerve impair swallowing. Nerve function is evaluated by listening to the cry for abnormalities such as hoarseness, stridor, or aphonia. The ability to swallow indicates a functioning nerve.

Accessory—Cranial Nerve XI

Control of the sternocleidomastoid and the trapezius muscles originates with the accessory nerve. The neonate's head position should be evaluated when the head is turned from one side to the other. Paralysis of the sternocleidomastoid muscle is suggested by difficulty in turning the head to the affected side. Observations of shoulder height are made to evaluate the trapezius muscle function. When the upper fibers of the trapezius are paralyzed, the corresponding shoulder will be lower than the unaffected one.

Hypoglossal—Cranial Nerve XII

The hypoglossal nerve supplies the muscles of the tongue. Assess for atrophy or abnormal movements of the tongue, as well as the gag, suck, and swallow reflexes. A weak suck and delayed swallowing are present with damage to the nerve. Sucking requires function of cranial nerves V, VII, and XII; swallowing requires function of cranial nerves IX and X. Other causes of impaired suck and swallow are listed in Box 12.2.

MOTOR EXAMINATION

The motor examination should include evaluation of muscle tone and posture, motility and muscle power, and the tendon reflexes. All of these are affected by the neonate's gestational age and behavioral state. Most of

> **BOX 12.2: CAUSES OF IMPAIRED SUCK AND SWALLOW IN THE NEONATAL PERIOD**
>
> **Cerebral**
> Encephalopathy with bilateral cerebral involvement
>
> **Nuclear**
> Traumatic facial nerve damage
> Hypoxic-ischemic encephalopathy
> Möbius syndrome
> Werdnig–Hoffmann disease
> Arnold–Chiari malformation
>
> **Nerve**
> Hypoxic-ischemic encephalopathy
> Bilateral laryngeal paralysis
> Posterior fossa hematoma or mass
>
> **Neuromuscular junction**
> Myasthenia gravis
> Infantile botulism
>
> **Muscle**
> Myotonic dystrophy
> Muscular dystrophy
> Myopathies
> Facioscapulohumeral muscular dystrophy
>
> *Source*: Modified from Volpe JJ. 2018. *Neurology of the Newborn*, 6th ed. Philadelphia, PA: Elsevier, 210. Reprinted by permission.[4]

this examination should be done in the quiet alert stage.

Tone

Muscle tone examination involves evaluation of resting posture, passive tone, and active tone of the major muscle groups. Initial observation of posture can be valuable for the proper examination of tone (see Figure 12.1). Tone can be categorized as phasic and postural.

Phasic tone correlates with passive tone and deep-tendon reflexes. Multiple passive manipulation maneuvers can be done to evaluate tone. Resistance of the extremities to passive movements can be evaluated by the scarf sign (see Chapter 4), heel to ear, popliteal angle, and by arm and leg recoil. Tone develops in a caudal-rostral progression. Resistance is minimal at 28 weeks and increases with maturity.

Tendon reflexes are elicited by percussion with the examiner's finger or a small reflex hammer over the tendon of the designated muscle. In the term neonate, the pectoralis, biceps, brachioradialis, knee, adductor, and ankle jerks can be elicited. These are most active in the first 2 days after birth and when the neonate is alert. Tendon reflexes are less active in preterm neonates. The patellar or knee jerk reflex is most frequently demonstrated after birth. The knee jerk reflex is elicited by tapping the patellar tendon just below the patella while the examiner's hand supports the neonate's knee in a flexed position. The normal response is extension at the knee and visible contraction of the quadriceps.

Weak or absent tendon reflexes may be seen in neonates less than 28 weeks gestational age, in those with neonatal encephalopathy or sepsis, and in those with dysfunction of the motor unit (e.g., the motor neuron, peripheral nerve, muscle, and neuromuscular junction). Neonates with acute encephalopathy frequently have an absence of reflexes initially, but as the infant improves, tendon reflexes return, and then may become increased or exaggerated. Exaggerated deep-tendon reflexes are also seen in neonates with neonatal abstinence syndrome, selective serotonin reuptake inhibitor (SSRI) exposure, or nicotine exposure. Asymmetric deep-tendon reflexes may reflect either central or peripheral nervous system impairment.

Clonus is rapid movement of a particular joint brought about by sudden stretching of a tendon. Ankle clonus can be evaluated by holding the anterior portion of the neonate's foot with the hip and knee in flexion and dorsiflexing the forefoot. The response usually consists of several repetitive jerks (beats) of the foot or no movement at all. Symmetrical ankle clonus of 5 to 10 beats in the absence of other abnormal neurologic signs should be considered normal.[4] Clonus typically disappears by 3 months of age, and persistence of more than a few beats should be considered abnormal.

Postural tone is best tested by the traction response (or pull-to-sit maneuver; Figure 12.3) in an awake alert state. The traction response is tested by grasping the neonate's hands and pulling slowly from the supine to a sitting position. The normal-term neonate reinforces this maneuver by contracting the shoulder and arm muscles, followed by flexion of the neck. As the neonate is pulled to sit, the head leaves the bed almost immediately, lagging only minimally behind the body (see Figure 12.3). When the infant reaches the sitting position, the head remains erect momentarily and then falls forward.

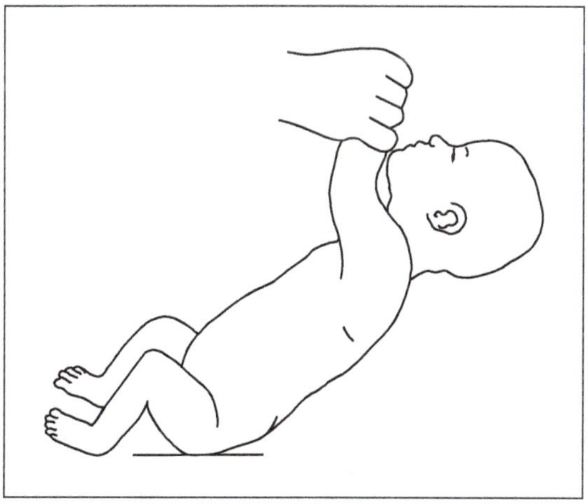

FIGURE 12.3 Normal traction response seen in the term neonate

During traction, flexion occurs in the elbows, knees, and ankles. In the term neonate, more than minimal head lag is abnormal and may indicate postural hypotonia (Figure 12.4).

Neck flexion in response to traction is absent in preterm neonates less than 33 weeks gestational age. Because normal postural tone requires the integrated functions of the entire CNS, hypotonia (indicating depressed postural tone) may result from disturbances in the CNS, the peripheral nervous system, or the skeletal muscles. When a large subgaleal hemorrhage or an extremely large caput is present, there may be more difficulty with the performance of neck righting in the pull-to-sit maneuver. It may be difficult to determine whether poor performance represents a mechanical problem caused by extra weight of the head or a neurologic problem related to birth trauma. When findings on the evaluation of other reflexes, tone, and activity are reassuring, the infant should be retested prior to discharge.

The motor examination may detect abnormalities in tone. *Hypotonia* is the most common tone abnormality observed in the neonatal neurologic examination. A focal injury to the cerebrum can result in contralateral hemiparesis involving the face and upper extremities more than the lower extremities. Injury to the parasagittal cerebral region (which may be caused by cerebral perfusion abnormalities) results in weakness of the upper limbs more than the lower limbs.

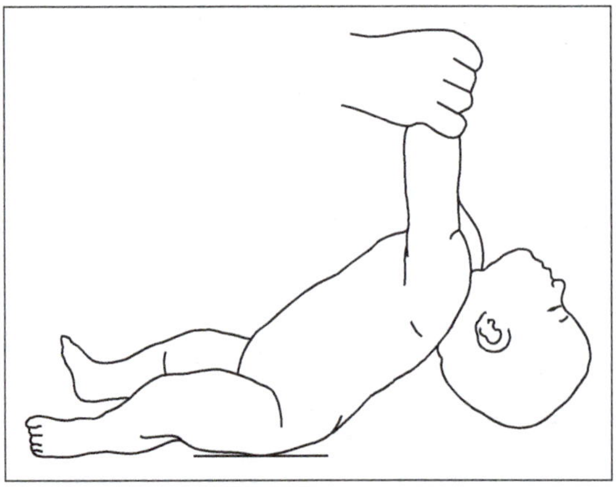

FIGURE 12.4 Traction response indicating hypotonia

If spinal cord injury occurs, it can result in flaccid weakness of the extremities; the face and cranial nerves are usually not affected. Neuromuscular junction diseases, such as myasthenia gravis and infantile botulism, cause generalized weakness and hypotonia. Disorders of the lower motor neurons (e.g., Werdnig–Hoffmann disease) cause flaccid weakness of the extremities with initial sparing of the face and cranial nerves. Fasciculation (spontaneous contraction of a group of fibers in a motor unit) can also be seen in Werdnig–Hoffmann disease and is best observed in the tongue. Inspection of the tongue reveals continuous and rapid twitching movements. Damage to nerve roots results in discrete patterns of focal weakness, the location of which depends on the root involved. One example is the unilateral loss of movement seen in the arm of a neonate with brachial plexus palsy.

Hypertonia is a less common finding in the neonatal period. If present, passive manipulation of the limbs often increases the tone. Hypertonia in the neonatal period may be associated with chronic injury (intrauterine) to the corticospinal tract or extrapyramidal system. Hypoxic-ischemic lesions are the most common cause of hypertonia.[4] Marked extensor hypertonia with arching of the back is sometimes seen with bacterial meningitis, severe neonatal encephalopathy, massive intraventricular hemorrhage (IVH), tetanus, and kernicterus. Table 12.4 lists patterns of abnormal muscle tone and their possible significance.

Muscle Power and Motility

Testing muscle strength is imprecise in the neonate because differentiating between hypotonia and muscle weakness is difficult. Strength of the upper extremities is gauged by using the pull-to-sit maneuver described previously and the grasp reflex. Strength of the lower extremities is evaluated by observing the infant's stepping reflex, readily elicited by 37 weeks gestational age, and gauging the neonate's ability to support its weight when the feet are against a flat surface if clinical status allows.

TABLE 12.4: PATTERNS OF ABNORMAL MUSCLE TONE IN THE NEONATE

ABNORMALITY	SIGNIFICANCE
Generalized increased or decreased tone	CNS insult or systemic illness
Increased arm flexor tone with increased leg extensor tone	Normal in crying neonate
	CNS irritability (e.g., hypoxic ischemic injury, hemorrhage, increased intracranial pressure)
Increased neck extensor tone more than neck flexor tone	Seen in crying neonates
	Hypoxic-ischemic injury
	Meningitis
	Increased intracranial pressure
Tight popliteal angle, increased as compared to leg tone	Intracranial hemorrhage
Asymmetric popliteal angles beyond 40 week	Hypertonia, hemiplegia

CNS, central nervous system.

Source: From Hill A. 1998. Development of tone and reflexes in the fetus and newborn. In *Fetal and Neonatal Physiology*, 2nd ed. Polin RA, and Fox WW, eds. Philadelphia, PA: Saunders, 2169. Reprinted by permission.[7]

Movement should be evaluated, and the presence of abnormal involuntary movements should be noted. At 28 to 32 weeks gestational age, slow twisting movements of the trunk and rapid, wide-amplitude movements of the limbs are seen. By 32 weeks gestational age, movements are more flexor and tend to occur in unison. At 36 weeks gestational age, active flexor movements of the lower extremities often occur in an alternating rather than a bilateral symmetric pattern. Term neonates' upper and lower extremities move in an alternating pattern. Typical of the neonatal period are mass movements that occur in response to environmental stimuli and discomfort. During the first few weeks of life, coarse tremors or brief trembling of the chin may occur normally, as may occasional uncoordinated movements. Abnormal movements include myotonia, fasciculations, jitteriness, and excessive startling. Myotonia is seen in myotonic dystrophy and is described by sustained contraction of a muscle group. Fasciculations are a feature associated with lower motor neuron disease. Fasciculations are more frequently observed in the tongue or fingers.

ASSESSMENT OF DEVELOPMENTAL REFLEXES

Developmental reflexes are sometimes referred to as *primary* or *primitive* reflexes because they do not require functional brain above the diencephalon. Although there are many developmental reflexes, assessment includes those normally present in the newborn. Development of reflexes with maturation from 28 to 40 weeks gestation is shown in Table 12.5.

Sucking Reflex

The sucking reflex is normally present at birth, even in the premature neonate, although it is weaker with decreasing gestational age. The stimulus consists of touching or gently stroking the lips. In response, the neonate's mouth opens, and sucking movements begin. The examiner's gloved finger can be introduced into the mouth to evaluate strength and coordination of the suck.

Rooting Reflex

To evaluate the rooting reflex, stroke the cheek and corner of the neonate's mouth. The infant's head should turn toward the stimulus, and the mouth should open. The rooting reflex starts at 28 weeks gestational age with full response by 32 weeks gestational age.[8]

Palmar Grasp

Stimulating the palmar surface of the neonate's hand with a finger should cause a grasp of the finger. Attempts to withdraw the finger should lead to a tightened grasp.

TABLE 12.5: DEVELOPMENT OF REFLEXES WITH MATURITY FROM 28 TO 40 WEEKS GESTATION

GESTATIONAL AGE (WEEKS)	28	30	32	34	36	38	40	DISAPPEARANCE (MONTHS)
Sucking	Weak and not synchronized with swallowing		Stronger and better synchronized with swallowing		Excellent			12
Grasp	Weak		Well established			Excellent		2 to 3
Response to traction	Absent		Begins to appear	Strong enough to lift part of the body weight		Strong enough to lift full body weight		
Moro reflex	Weak, may be obtained inconsistently and incomplete		Well established → → →					5 to 6
Crossed extension	Flexion and extension without purpose or pattern		Good extension; no tendency to adduction		Tendency to adduction but imperfect	Complete response with • Extension • Adduction • Fanning of the toes		
Stepping	—	—	Begins tiptoeing with good support on the sole and a righting reaction of the legs for a few seconds		Well established; fast tiptoeing	• A premature infant who has reached 40 weeks gestation; walks in a toe–heel progression or on tiptoes • A term newborn of 40 weeks gestation; walks in a heel–toe progression on the whole sole of the foot		3 to 4

Source: Adapted from Volpe JJ. 2018. *Neurology of the Newborn*, 5th ed. Philadelphia, PA: Elsevier, 203–205[4]; and Gardner SL, et al. 2021. *Neonatal Intensive Care and Interprofessional Approach*, 9th ed. St. Louis, MO: Elsevier, 338[9]; Kliegman, RM. 2020. *Nelson's Textbook of Pediatrics*, 21st ed. Philadelphia, PA: Elsevier, 3060[8]; Zenel JA. 2011. Chapter 44. Examination of the Newborn Infant. In: *Rudolph's Pediatrics*, Rudolph CD, Rudolph AM, Lister GE, First LR, and Gershon AA, eds. McGraw Hill[11].

When the palmar grasp is tested with both hands, the term neonate can be lifted off the bed for a few seconds. If palmar grasp is weak or absent in a term neonate, cerebral, local nerve, or muscle injury may be present.

Tonic Neck Reflex

To elicit the tonic neck reflex, place the neonate in the supine position and turn his or her head to one side. The neonate should extend the upper extremity on the side toward which the head is turned and flex the upper extremity on the opposite side (Figure 12.5). This is sometimes called the *fencing position*. If the response cannot be obtained or if even slight turning of the head consistently produces a marked tonic neck reflex, this may indicate concern for an abnormality.

Moro Reflex

The Moro reflex is a response to the sensation of loss of support. The most effective and reproducible method of stimulating this reflex is to hold the neonate in the supine position with the head several centimeters off the bed. Next, withdraw the hand supporting the head, and the infant's head will fall back into the examiner's hand. The infant's first response is a spreading movement in which the arms are extended and abducted, and the hands are opened (Figure 12.6). That response is followed by inward movement and some flexion of the arms, with closing of the fists. An audible cry may accompany this reflex in neonates older than 32 weeks of gestation. Premature neonates have incomplete responses, with abduction of the arms, but without flexion, adduction, or cry. Complete absence of the reflex is abnormal and may occur in depressed neonates. Asymmetry of movements may indicate a localized neurologic defect, such as brachial plexus injury or fractured clavicle.

A loud noise or bumping the side of the incubator or crib often produces a Moro-like response. This is usually a startle reflex—consisting of flexion of the extremities and palmar grasping—but not a complete Moro.

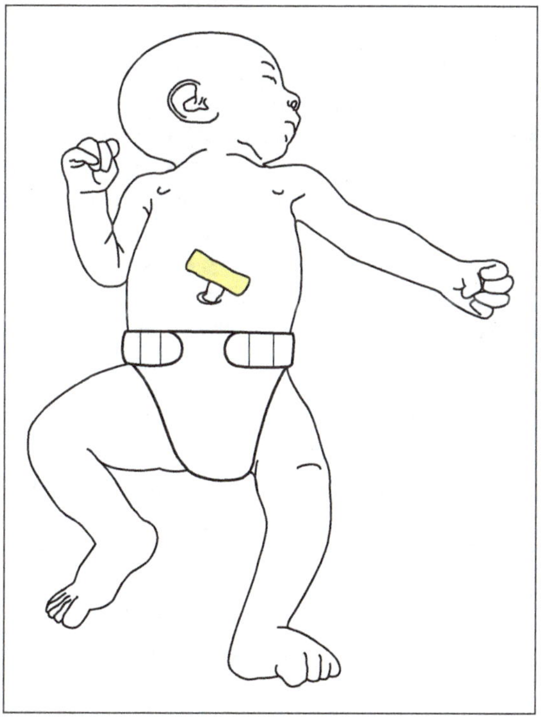

FIGURE 12.5 The tonic neck reflex

Stepping Reflex

When the neonate is held upright and the soles of the feet are allowed to touch a flat

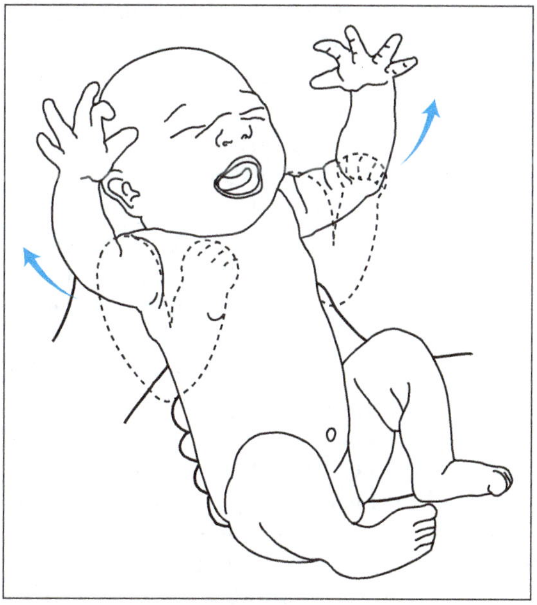

FIGURE 12.6 The moro reflex

surface, alternating stepping movements can be observed. Stepping is more active 72 hours after birth.

Babinski Reflex

The response to stimulation of the sole of the foot is usually plantar flexion. In the neonatal period, the Babinski reflex is positive if extension or flexion of the toes occurs. Consistent absence of any response is abnormal and may indicate central depression or abnormal spinal innervation.[8] In children older than 18 months, an abnormal response is extension or fanning of the toes; either response indicates upper motor neuron abnormalities.

Spinal Reflexes

The truncal incurvation reflex is tested with the neonate in ventral suspension, with the anterior chest wall in the palm of the examiner's hand. Firm pressure with the thumb or a cotton swab is applied parallel to the spine in the thoracic area. A positive response is flexion of the pelvis toward the side of the stimulus. The anocutaneous reflex, or "anal wink," is tested by evaluating the response to cutaneous stimulation of the perianal skin. The normal response is contraction of the external sphincter.

ASSESSMENT OF SENSORY FUNCTION

The peripheral sensory system functions include touch and pain. By 28 weeks gestational age, the infant can distinguish between touch and pain, resulting in different behavior responses.[4] The withdrawal reflex is stimulated to evaluate peripheral sensory function. Touching the sole of the foot with a pin provokes flexion of the stimulated limb and extension of the contralateral limb. Response is present in most neonates of 28 weeks gestational age and older. In neonates, extension of the contralateral limb varies, and sometimes flexion of both limbs is seen. Habituation is a normal neonatal response. This assessment is rarely performed as part of a routine neurologic examination but may be performed in cases such as spinal cord injury (to detect sensory level), peripheral lesions such as brachial plexus injuries, and infants with myelomeningocele or lesions of the cerebral hemispheres.

ABNORMALITIES

Neonatal Encephalopathy

Neurologic examination plays a significant role in the assessment of the depressed newborn. Neonatal encephalopathy results from an insult to the fetus or newborn causing a lack of oxygen and perfusion. It is associated with tissue hypoxia and acidosis. The biochemical definition of asphyxia is acidosis, hypoxia, and hypercapnia. Neonatal encephalopathy is a condition characterized by recognizable clinical, biochemical, and pathologic features. The spectrum of hypoxic-ischemic encephalopathy (HIE) can be divided into categories. *Mild encephalopathy* is associated with irritability, jitteriness, and hyper alertness. *Moderate encephalopathy* is characterized by lethargy, hypotonia, a decrease in spontaneous movements, and seizures. *Severe encephalopathy* is characterized by coma, flaccidity, disturbed brainstem function, and seizures. Infants at risk for encephalopathy include those with a low-cord pH, those with an Apgar score of less than 6 at 5 minutes of age, and those who need extended resuscitation continuing for 10 minutes. Early recognition is important in the infant at risk for HIE. A complete, early neurologic examination should be done on any infant identified at risk. Abnormal findings will guide the management of these infants including the use of total body cooling. Total body cooling initiation is time sensitive and can improve outcomes when used appropriately, so early and complete neurologic evaluation of the infant at risk is vital.[8]

The evolution of severe encephalopathy without intervention has been studied and is somewhat predictable.[4] From birth to 12 hours of age, the neonate with severe encephalopathy usually demonstrates stupor or coma, periodic breathing, minimal movement, and seizures. Pupillary and oculomotor responses are intact. By 12 to 24 hours, the neonate's level of consciousness appears to improve, but this apparent improvement is accompanied by apneic spells, weakness, jitteriness, and severe seizures. Between 24 and 72 hours of age, the neonate's level of consciousness deteriorates, and stupor and coma may be associated with respiratory arrest. Pupils become fixed and dilated, and doll's eye response is lost. Those neonates who survive 72 hours or longer usually demonstrate improvement in level of consciousness over days to weeks, but hypotonia and weakness are common. Disturbances in suck, swallow, gag, and tongue movements may impair the ability to feed.

Specific patterns of limb weakness reflect the area of brain injury resulting from asphyxia. In term neonates, injury occurs predominantly to the parasagittal areas, zones between the cerebral arteries that are most affected by changes in blood flow and oxygenation. Weakness of the shoulder girdle and proximal upper extremities results from injury to this area of the brain. Focal ischemic injury in the middle cerebral artery also presents frequently in the term neonate and is demonstrated by hemiparesis. In the premature neonate, decreased arterial blood flow affects the periventricular (PV) area and results in PV leukomalacia. Damage to the PV area results in weakness in the lower extremities with increased risk of developing cerebral palsy.[4]

Intrauterine Drug Exposure

Drugs that are unbound to protein will cross the placenta easily and affect the developing fetal brain. These effects depend on the type of drug, the gestational timing of the exposure, the duration of exposure, and use of multiple drugs. Drugs that have been prescribed to pregnant women have generally been studied and the effects on the fetus are known. Illicit drugs and alcohol have less known information on the effects to the developing fetus. Illicit drugs may have compounding effects on the fetus, not only disrupting blood flow, but also nutrition. Evidence has supported that both licit and illicit drug exposure of the fetus can have both short-term and long-term effects that can vary and affect the structure and function. Table 12.6 provides a review of specific drugs and their effects on the developing nervous system (see Chapter 16).

Neuromuscular Disorders

A variety of conditions affecting the peripheral nervous system, resulting in weakness, define neuromuscular disorders. They are generally organized according to the anatomical level affected. Diagnosis may be difficult, and careful history collections and physical examination is vital. The hallmark clinical findings associated with neuromuscular disorders in the neonate are hypotonia and weakness, often with an alert appearance. Assessment should be systematic and include both physical and neurologic aspects. Examination is directed toward evaluation of the muscle size, tone, tendon reflexes and strength, neonatal reflexes, cranial nerve abnormalities, sensory response, muscle fasciculation, and muscle fatiguing. Multiple factors should be considered, including gestational age.

Arthrogryposis is a neuromuscular disorder characterized by fixed position and limitation of limb movement. Atrophic muscles and decreased tendon reflexes are usually present. Limitation of fetal movement from any condition can lead to arthrogryposis, for example, conditions affecting the brain, anterior horn cells, nerves, neuromuscular junctions, or muscles. Neurogenic causes are the most common and include brain malformations, chromosomal defects, genetic syndromes, and destructive lesions of the CNS.[4] Other disorders include spinal muscular atrophy (SMA), transient or congenital myasthenia gravis, congenital myotonic dystrophy, and congenital muscular dystrophies. Early identification allows for early interventions with lesion-specific care.

TABLE 12.6: INTRAUTERINE DRUG EXPOSURE AND ASSOCIATED ABNORMALITIES

DRUG	CNS ABNORMALITY/ NEURODEVELOPMENTAL SEQUELAE	EXAM FINDINGS
Antiepileptic drugs (increased risk in older drugs—valproate, phenytoin, phenobarb—compared to newer drugs—topiramate, lamotrigine, levetiracetam, and gabapentin)	– CNS malformations (microencephaly, anencephaly, myelomeningocele, and hydrocephalus) – Hemorrhage (skin, liver, intracranial, GI, and thorax) – Neonatal abstinence – Cognitive delay	– Withdrawal (occurring ~7 days)—jitteriness, overactivity, abnormal sleeping pattern, inconsolability, hyperreflexia, and disturbed sucking. Worsen over the first several weeks and can persist for months.
Anticoagulants (warfarin)	– CNS malformations (microcephaly, hydrocephalus, atrophy, and Dandy–Walker syndrome) – Hemorrhage – Intellectual disability/ language difficulties	– Seizures – Spasticity
SSRIs	– Neonatal abstinence	– Tremors, shaking, agitation, spasm, hyper- or hypotonia, sleep disturbances, high-pitched cry, tachypnea, myoclonus, and GI disturbances
Opioids	– Microcephaly – Strabismus – Growth restriction – Neonatal abstinence – Language delays	– Withdrawal symptoms—irritability, hypertonia, seizures, tremors, GI disturbances, respiratory distress, fever, and sweating, sneezing
Stimulants (cocaine/ methamphetamines)	– CNS malformations (microcephaly, encephalocele, disorders of neuronal migration, and disorders of porencephalic development) – Cerebral infarction and IVH – Neonatal abstinence – Attention problems – Impacts on cognition, language, and behavior – Increased risk of SIDS	– Depressed interactive behavior – Poor state regulation – Altered sleep-wake patterns – Agitation – Hypertonicity/hyperreflexia – Tremors – Seizures
Sedatives (benzodiazepines)	– Unknown	– Neonatal withdrawal (jitteriness, irritability, hyperactivity, and hypertonicity) – Floppy infant syndrome (hypotonia, CNS depression, hypothermia, and poor suck)

(continued)

TABLE 12.6: INTRAUTERINE DRUG EXPOSURE AND ASSOCIATED ABNORMALITIES (*continued*)

DRUG	CNS ABNORMALITY/ NEURODEVELOPMENTAL SEQUELAE	EXAM FINDINGS
Marijuana	– Neurobehavioral difficulties – Issues with executive function – Language and attention problems	– Increased arousal – Dysregulation – Irritability – Disorganized cry – Altered sleep patterns
Alcohol	– CNS malformation (microcephaly, disorders of neural tube formation) – FAS – ARBDs – ARND – ND-PAE – Neonatal abstinence – Cognitive deficit or delays – Language and attention problems – Behavior problems – Motor and visual deficits	– Withdraw symptoms – Distinct facial features

ARBDs, alcohol-related birth defects; ARND, alcohol-related neurodevelopmental disorder; CNS, central nervous system; FAS, fetal alcohol syndrome; GI, gastrointestinal; IVH, intraventricular hemorrhage; ND-PAE, neurobehavioral disorder associated with prenatal alcohol exposure; SSRI, selective serotonin reuptake inhibitor; SIDS, sudden infant death syndrome.

Source: Adapted from Dodson WE. 1989. Deleterious effects of drugs on the developing nervous system. *Clinics in Perinatology* 16(2): 340–343, 348–353[12]. Volpe JJ. 2018. *Neurology of the Newborn*, 6th ed. Philadelphia, PA: Elsevier, 1149–1189.[4]

Spinal Cord Injuries

Injuries to the spinal cord are usually seen following deliveries that overstretch the vertebral axis or over-rotate the body in relation to the head. Risk factors include breech vaginal extraction, external cephalic version, vascular insults, asphyxia, forceps, difficult extraction, prematurity, and vertebral anomalies. Clinical manifestations depend upon the level and severity of the injury. Acute lesions include edema and hemorrhaging in the epidural and intraspinal spaces and can be followed by chronic changes to the cord perfusion. Acute lesions are associated with stretching, laceration, disruption, or transection. Transection injuries are irreversible. Partial or complete recovery is possible with injuries caused by compression or ischemia.

The level of spinal cord injury determines the presentation. Following spinal cord injury, a state of shock and difficulty initiating respiration are common. Lesions above C3 or C4 paralyze the diaphragm. Lower cervical and upper thoracic cord lesions result in flaccidity of the legs and portions of the arms. Lack of perceptible response to pinprick can be demonstrated below the level of spinal cord injury.[4] The site of injury determines the outcomes.

Defects in Closure of the Anterior Neural Tube

Anencephaly

Anencephaly is the result of defective closure of the anterior neural tube. The defect in the skull begins at the vertex and may extend to the foramen magnum. Dermal covering is absent; hemorrhagic and fibrotic cerebral tissue lies exposed to view. The cranium is underdeveloped, resulting in shallow orbits and protruding eyes. The most common variety of anencephaly involves the forebrain and variable amounts of the upper brainstem. Associated abnormalities (e.g., adrenal hypoplasia and lung defects) are frequently seen.

Encephalocele

Encephalocele is a restricted disorder of neural development involving closure of the anterior neural tube. There is a protrusion of meninges and sometimes cerebral tissue, which is covered by skin. The skull defect that allows protrusion is called cranium bifidum.

Occasionally, cranium bifidum may be present without protrusion of meninges or fluid and instead appears as a small, tissue-covered opening on the skull. Noticeable tufts of normal hair may surround the defect. Encephaloceles most often occur in the midline of the occipital bone, but they may also occur in the parietal, temporal, or a frontal nasopharyngeal area. They sometimes appear to be protruding from the eye socket.

Severity of clinical findings is related to the location, size, and contents of the sac. Encephaloceles may vary from tiny protrusions to massive protrusions the size of the skull. The sac may contain cerebrospinal fluid (CSF), meninges, and cerebral tissue. Severe deficits occur if brain tissue and part of the ventricular system are trapped in the defect. Encephaloceles are often complicated by hydrocephalus and absence of the corpus callosum. Microcephaly, spasticity, seizures, weakness, and cortical blindness are associated with structural defects of the occipital lobe. Skull x-rays are valuable in identifying the defect in the skull (the bifid cranium). Transillumination and ultrasound can be useful in identifying the extent of brain tissue in the sac.

Defects in Closure of the Posterior Neural Tube

Spina bifida, meningocele, and myelomeningocele are defects arising from abnormal closure of the posterior neural tube (Figure 12.7).

Spina Bifida Occulta

A malformation caused by non- or incomplete closure of the posterior portion of the vertebrae, spina bifida is the mildest form of neural tube defects. It occurs most often in the lower lumbar and lumbosacral area and is covered with skin. The meninges and spinal cord are normal. The presence of tufts of hair, lipomas, sinus, or other abnormalities along the spine may indicate the presence of underlying defects.

Meningocele

This lesion is associated with a disruption in secondary neurulation and is a closed neural tube defect. Typically, these lesions involve more than one vertebra. In this defect, the meninges and CSF protrude and are covered by skin, the spinal roots and nerves are normal, and neurologic deficits are unusual. Long-term complications can include cord tethering.

Myelomeningocele

Myelomeningoceles are the most common form of open neural tube defects and occur due to malformations in the closure of the posterior neuropore prior to 26 days gestational age. These lesions are associated with bilateral broadening of the vertebrae or absence of the vertebral arches. In this type of lesion, the meninges, spinal roots, and nerves protrude. Remnants of the spinal cord are fused, and the neural tube is exposed on the dorsal portion of the mass. Most of these lesions occur in the lumbar spine. Abnormalities in neurologic function depend on the level of the lesion (Table 12.7). Generally, the higher the defect is on the spine, the greater the degree of impairment. Thoracic-level defects may be associated with marked abnormalities in spinal curvature and defects of the hips and lower extremities. Attention should be paid to examination of the motor, sensory, and sphincter functions, and the reflexes.

Hydrocephalus is a frequent finding associated with myelomeningocele. The status of head size and its percentile for gestational

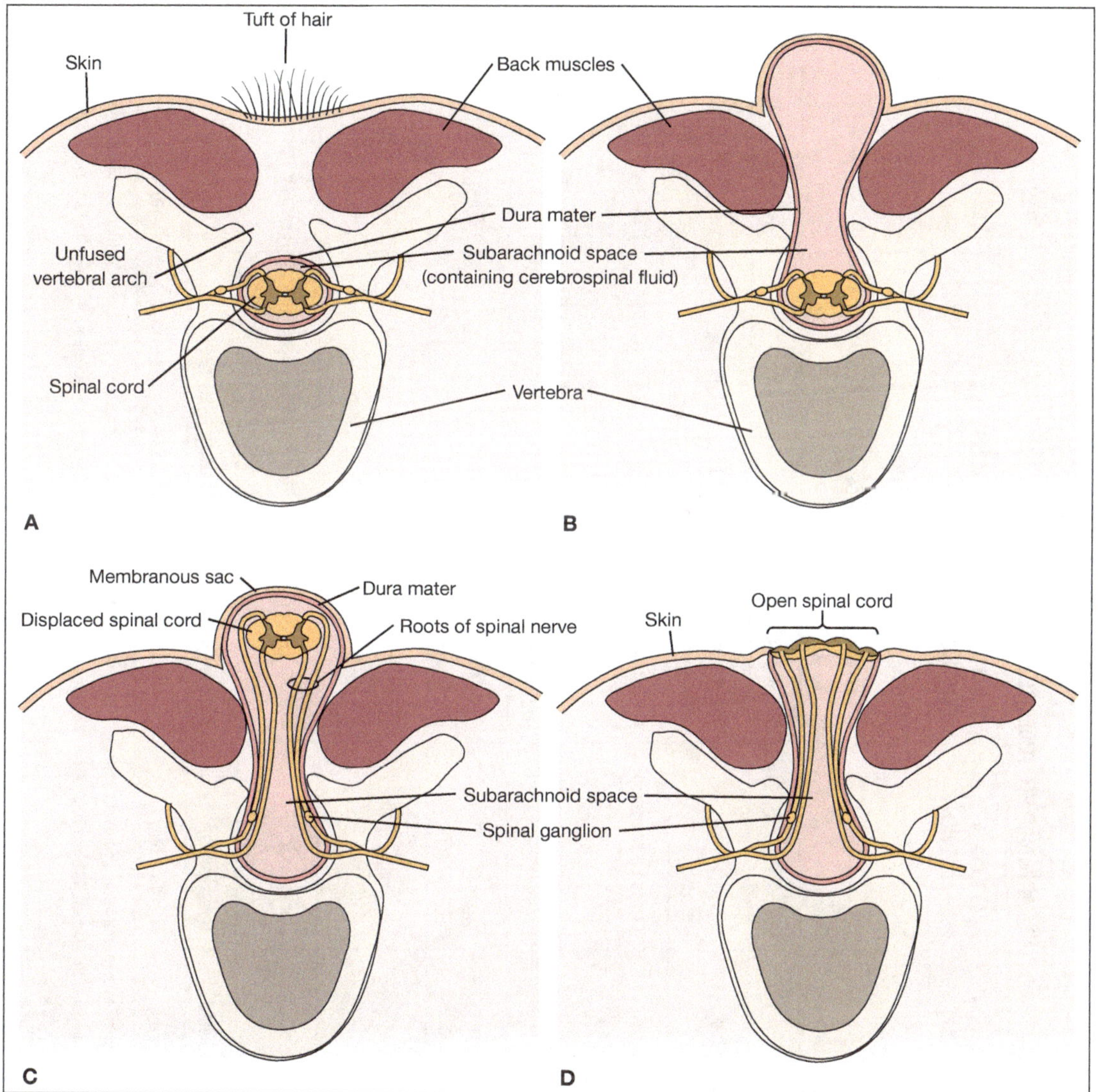

FIGURE 12.7 Types of spina bifida and the commonly associated malformations of the nervous system commonly associated with them. The diagrammatic sketches illustrate various types of spina bifida and the associated defects of the vertebral arches (one or more), spinal cord, and meninges. (A) Spina bifida occulta. Observe the unfused vertebral arch. (B) Spina bifida with meningocele. (C) Spina bifida with meningomyelocele. (D) Spina bifida with myeloschisis. The defects illustrated in B to D are referred to collectively as spina bifida cystica because of the cyst-like sac or cyst associated with them

Source: From Moore KL, Persaud TVN, and Torchia MG. 2019. *The Developing Human: Clinically Oriented Embryology*, 11th ed. Philadelphia, PA: Saunders, 357–394. Reprinted by permission.[13]

age, fontanel pressure, and width of sutures should be determined initially and periodically. Transillumination of the head following admission can be useful; serial brain ultrasounds are indicated.

Chiari malformation (inferior displacement of the medulla and fourth ventricle into the upper cervical canal and elongation and thinning of the upper medulla and lower pons) is an abnormality associated with myelomeningoceles. Inferior displacement of the lower cerebellum through the foramen magnum into the lower cervical canal is also a feature. Hydrocephalus is thought

TABLE 12.7: MYELOMENINGOCELE AND SENSORY, MOTOR, SPHINCTER, AND REFLEX FUNCTION

LESION	INNERVATION	CUTANEOUS SENSATION	MOTOR FUNCTION	WORKING MUSCLES	SPHINCTER	REFLEX
Cervical/ thoracic	Variable	Variable	None	None	None	—
Thoracolumbar	T12	Lower abdomen	None	None	None	—
	L1	Groin	Weak hip flexion	Iliopsoas	None	—
	L2	Anterior upper thigh	Strong hip flexion	Iliopsoas and sartorius	None	—
Lumbar	L3	Anterior distal knee and thigh	Knee extension	Quadriceps	None	Patellar
	L4	Medial leg	Knee flexion, hip adduction	Medial hamstrings	None	Patellar
Lumbosacral	L5	Lateral leg, medial knee and foot	Foot dorsiflexion and eversion	Anterior tibial	None	Ankle jerk
	S1	Sole of foot	Foot plantar flexion	Gastrocnemius, soleus, and posterior tibial	None	Ankle jerk
Sacral	S2	Posterior leg and thigh	Toe flexion	Flexor hallucis	Bladder and rectum	Anal wink
	S3	Middle of buttock	Toe flexion	Flexor hallucis	Bladder and rectum	Anal wink
	S4	Medial buttock	Toe flexion	Flexor hallucis	Bladder and rectum	Anal wink

Note: To assess the degree of dysfunction and level of lesion, evaluate the neonate with myelomeningocele for the presence of cutaneous sensation, motor function, working muscles, sphincter control, and reflexes.

Source: Adapted from Volpe JJ. 2018. *Neurology of the Newborn*, 6th ed. Philadelphia, PA: Elsevier, 14[4]; and Noetzel M. 1989. Myelomeningocele: Current concepts of management. *Clinics in Perinatology* 16(2): 318. Reprinted by permission.[14]

to result from aqueductal stenosis and blockage of the CSF outflow from the fourth ventricle. Neurologic, neurosurgical, urologic, and orthopedic consultations are commonly required for these patients.

INTRACRANIAL HEMORRHAGE

Primary Subarachnoid Hemorrhage

A common type of neonatal intracranial hemorrhage, primary subarachnoid hemorrhage may occur in both term and preterm neonates but is more common in the former. Bleeding occurs from vessels within the subarachnoid space and is usually most predominately located over the surface of the cerebral hemispheres (Figure 12.8). Hemorrhages are typically small due to venous bleeding. Etiology is thought to be related to trauma or hypoxia. Complications are rare.

Minor hemorrhages may go undetected because the neonate will generally be asymptomatic. Moderate degrees of hemorrhage may result in seizure activity in a neonate who otherwise appears well. One or more seizures can occur, but the neonate is stable between them.

Rarely, a massive subarachnoid hemorrhage may occur followed by rapid clinical deterioration and death. These neonates usually have histories of severe perinatal asphyxia and some degree of trauma. In those neonates surviving a major hemorrhage in the subarachnoid area, the development of hydrocephalus is possible. Hydrocephalus occurs with major subarachnoid hemorrhages because of decreased spinal fluid absorption by the inflamed arachnoid villi, resulting in adhesions in the subarachnoid space or around the outflow of the fourth ventricle.

Subdural Hemorrhage

Subdural hemorrhages occur below the dura and above the arachnoid meninges. These hemorrhages are caused by (a) rupture of

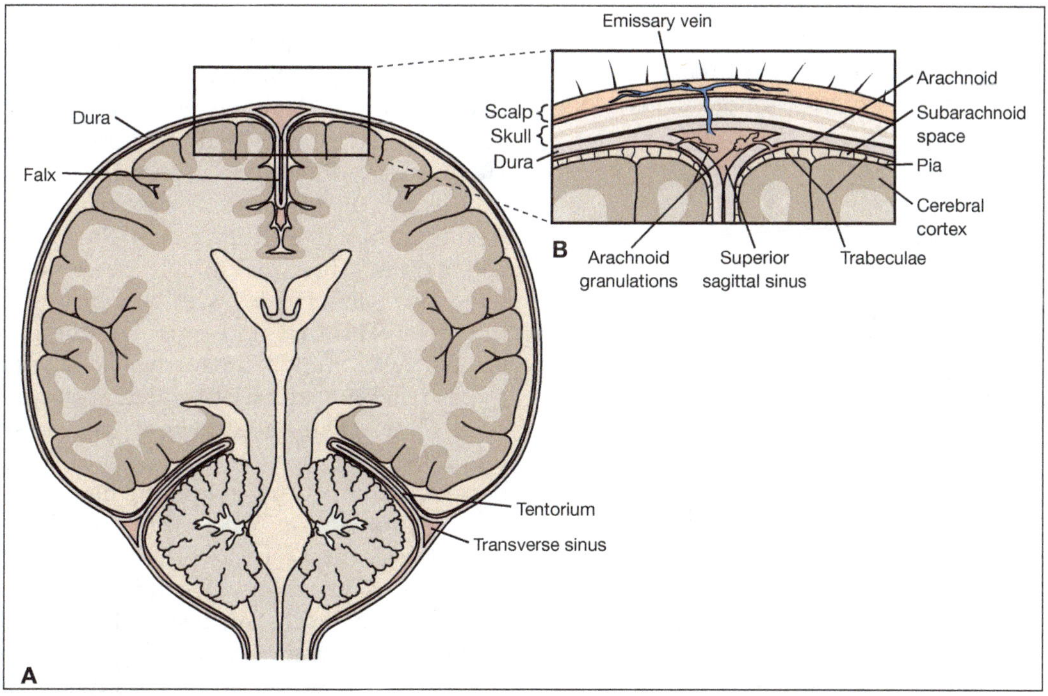

FIGURE 12.8 The brain and its coverings

Source: From Waxman SG. 2000. *Correlative Neuroanatomy*, 24th ed. New York, NY: Lange Medical Books/McGraw-Hill, 155. Reprinted by permission.[15]

the tentorium, (b) occipital diastasis, (c) falx lacerations, and (d) rupture of superficial cerebral veins.[4] Subdural hemorrhages are the least common type of intracranial hemorrhage, but risk increases with difficult deliveries with trauma. The dura mater is a fibrous tissue with two layers: an outer periosteal layer and an inner meningeal layer. These layers separate in areas to form sinuses into which major veins drain. One of the layers of separation is called the falx cerebri. The falx divides the cerebral hemispheres. The superior and inferior sagittal sinus and the vein of Galen lie close to the falx. Another area of the dura called the *tentorium* separates the cerebral hemispheres from the cerebellum. The straight sinus, vein of Galen, and transverse sinus lie near the tentorium.

Tentorial laceration is the most lethal and may result in rupture of the vein of Galen, straight sinus, or transverse sinus (Figure 12.9). Clots extend into the posterior fossa and, if large, cause compression of the brain. When the neonate has a large hemorrhage in this area, neurologic disturbances will be present from birth, with signs of midbrain–upper pons compression such as stupor, coma, lateral deviation of the eyes that does not change with the doll's eye maneuver, and unequal pupils with abnormal response to light. *Opisthotonos* may also be present. When bradycardia is seen, it generally indicates severe compression from a massive hemorrhage.

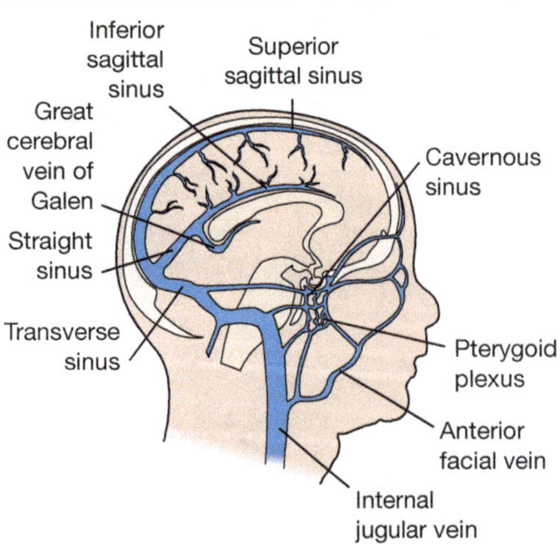

FIGURE 12.9 Major cranial veins and dural sinuses

Source: From Volpe JJ. 2018. *Neurology of the Newborn*, 6th ed. Philadelphia, PA: Elsevier, 1116. Reprinted by permission.[4]

Occipital osteodiastasis hemorrhages are caused by separation of the cartilaginous joint between the squamous and lateral portions of the occipital bone. This can lead to tearing of the dura and the occipital sinuses with massive bleeding below the tentorium. The same clinical features as described for tentorial laceration occur. Smaller degrees of hemorrhage and hematoma formation in the posterior fossa lead to a different clinical evolution of signs. Initially, the neonate may have no abnormal neurologic signs. These signs begin to develop over hours or days as continued seepage of blood and gradual enlargement of the hematoma occur. Clinical signs of increased intracranial pressure ensue, followed by signs of disturbance of the brainstem, including respiratory depression, apnea, oculomotor abnormalities, and facial paresis. Seizures are also commonly seen.

When *falx laceration* has occurred with bleeding from the superior sagittal sinus, hematoma development in the cerebral fissure occurs. Marked neurologic signs develop only when the clot has extended infratentorially, and then the clinical signs are those described for tentorial laceration.

Rupture of the superficial cerebral veins results in blood collecting over the cerebral convexities. Three neurologic presentations have been associated with hemorrhage in this area. The first and most common that occurs with minor hemorrhages is either hyperirritability and a hyperalert appearance or no clinical signs at all. The second presentation includes signs of focal cerebral disturbances. Seizures are common; hemiparesis with eye deviation to the side opposite the hemiparesis can occur. The doll's eye maneuver remains normal because this is a cerebral lesion, not a brainstem lesion. Dysfunction of the third cranial nerve, the oculomotor, on the side of the hematoma results in a poorly reactive or nonreactive pupil on the side of the lesion. The third presentation is secondary to chronic subdural effusion. The neonate has few or no clinical signs in the neonatal period but presents months later with an enlarging head.

Periventricular–Intraventricular Hemorrhage

PV–IVH is the most common intracranial hemorrhage seen in the premature neonate.[4] The incidence of IVH increases with decreasing gestational age. Correlation with gestational age is related to the site of bleeding, the subependymal germinal matrix. In this area of the brain, there is a matrix of poorly supported, thin-walled capillaries located near the caudate nucleus at or slightly posterior to the foramen of Monro. Autoregulation of cerebral blood flow does not occur in sick, premature neonates.[4] This lack of autoregulation renders the vessels of the subependymal germinal matrix vulnerable to blood flow alterations. Hemorrhage can result after a period of increased blood flow, decreased blood flow, increased central venous pressure, or with coagulation abnormalities. Ninety percent of IVHs are identified using ultrasound by 72 hours of age. At a gestational age of 28 weeks, the vessels in this area begin to involute, and involution continues so that the subependymal germinal matrix is no longer present by term gestation. Rarely, IVH is seen in the term neonate. The common site of IVH in term neonates is the choroid plexus within the ventricle. Trauma, infection, and hypoxic events are thought to be the pathogenic mechanisms.[4]

Hemorrhage that starts in the PV germinal matrix can be localized in this area, or may rupture into the ventricular system and, if large enough, cause distention of the lateral ventricles. Adjacent cerebral tissue can also be damaged by hemorrhage in the germinal matrix, resulting in a parenchymal clot or infarction.

Large IVHs have a high incidence of associated hydrocephalus. Most often, hydrocephalus occurs because of inflammation of the arachnoid villi, which absorbs CSF. With hemorrhage, they become inflamed or scarred from blood and particulate matter in the CSF. Obstruction to absorption of CSF then occurs.

Three clinical presentations have been described and are thought to be related to severity of hemorrhage. A catastrophic course is the least common but most dramatic presentation. Stupor progresses to coma, shallow respirations progress to apnea, generalized seizures occur, pupils become fixed and nonreactive to light, the doll's eye maneuver is abnormal, the eyes are fixed to vestibular stimulation, and marked hypotonia is present. A falling hematocrit, hypotension, bradycardia, metabolic acidosis, and a bulging anterior fontanel are also accompanying findings.[4]

A less dramatic course has been described in which the neonate presents with signs of a progressively decreasing level of consciousness, hypotonia, lethargy, subtle eye movement abnormalities, and partial response to the doll's eye maneuver.[4] Deterioration occurs over many hours, with periods of apparent stabilization followed by recurrence of abnormal signs. This progression of neurologic symptoms with periods of apparent stabilization may be seen over several days.

The third type of presentation is a clinically silent course in which a screening ultrasound detects the hemorrhage.

EXTRACRANIAL HEMORRHAGE

A caput succedaneum is caused by trauma to the scalp and results in hemorrhage and edema superficial to the periosteum and not confined by suture lines. The edema is soft and pitting. Subgaleal hemorrhage is associated with vaginal delivery and instrumentation. Cephalopelvic disproportion, prolonged labor, and tetanic contractions are also contributory factors.[4] They usually resolve within a few days without intervention.

A cephalohematoma is below the periosteum and confined by the cranial sutures. The periosteum of the cranial bone limits the potential space available for blood to expand. Cephalohematoma is associated with instrument-assisted deliveries, trauma, oligohydramnios, preterm premature rupture of membranes (PPROM), and head compression in utero. Findings include a firm collection of blood that is confined by suture lines. It may increase in size after delivery. It can be associated with a linear skull fracture in up to 25% of cases.[9] Cephalohematoma may contribute to jaundice but is rarely of clinical significance from a neurologic standpoint (see Figures 6.7 and 6.8). Most resolve over a few weeks to several months.

A *subgaleal hemorrhage* is located between the scalp (galea) and the cranial periosteum. The potential space for blood to accumulate extends from the orbital ridges to the nape.[4] A major portion of the neonate's blood volume can potentially be contained in this space, leading to severe hypovolemic shock, anemia, and death (see Figures 6.7 and 6.9). Clinical signs for early identification are an expanding boggy scalp, pallor, prolonged capillary refill, tachycardia, decreased responsiveness and spontaneous activity, a falling hematocrit, and signs of frank or impending shock. Seizure activity may be a late sign. Risk factors include vacuum extraction and vitamin K deficiency. Incidence of severe subgaleal hemorrhage has decreased due to limitations on the number of vacuum or forceps attempts at operative vaginal deliveries by the American College of Obstetricians and Gynecologists.[16]

MENINGITIS

Neonatal meningitis is of major clinical importance and can be associated with infection from bacteria, viruses, and fungi. Clinical features of bacterial meningitis present in two clinical syndromes: early onset and late onset. Early onset disease is often indistinguishable from those of neonatal sepsis, including temperature instability, irritability, poor feeding, and vomiting. Late onset disease may present with more obvious neurologic signs such as fever, abnormal feeding, lethargy, seizures, and extensor rigidity.[4] The fontanel may be full, and nuchal rigidity may be present.[9]

Findings in neonates with fungal meningitis are similar to those with bacterial meningitis. Other findings include acute respiratory failure, abdominal distention, and macular erythematous rash.[4]

The major infectious agents related to congenital viral infections of the CNS are termed TORCH syndrome.

CMV is among the most common congenital infections that can present asymptomatically or may present with microcephaly, petechiae, purpura, and jaundice on physical examination.[17] Other symptoms include seizures, cerebral calcifications, and encephalitis. Disturbances of neuronal migration such as polymicrogyria have also been documented. Hearing loss and neurodevelopmental deficits have been commonly described.

SEIZURES

Seizures are the most frequent sign of an underlying neurologic disorder.[5] Due to the preponderance of excitatory neurotransmitter influence as well as immature inhibitory systems, neonates are susceptible to seizures, and for this reason the risk of seizures is higher during the neonatal period than any other period in life. Clinical recognition of seizures in the neonate is not reliable, and suspicion should be confirmed by video electroencephalography (vEEG). Seizures can be electroclinical or electrographic. Electroclinical seizures can be characterized by their appearance pattern (Table 12.8). The most common etiology of seizures results from cerebral insult from hypoxic ischemic encephalopathy. Other causes include vascular insults, infections, brain malformations, metabolic derangements such as hypoglycemia or hypocalcemia, inborn errors of metabolism, epilepsy syndromes, or neonatal abstinence. In some cases, seizures have a familial basis. When seizure activity is identified, rapid evaluation of the cause and prompt treatment should follow.

TABLE 12.8: NEONATAL SEIZURES

SEIZURE TYPE	CHARACTERISTICS
Subtle	Seen in term and preterm infants; apneic spells; tonic horizontal eye deviation, jerking, sustained eye opening, eyelid blinking or fluttering; sucking, drooling, oral buccal movement; swimming, pedaling, and rowing movements
Generalized tonic	Primarily seen in preterm infants; characterized by tonic extension of all limbs or by tonic flexion of arms and extension of legs
Multifocal clonic	Seen primarily in term infants; clonic movement migrating from limb to limb in a sporadic pattern (e.g., right leg, then left arm)
Focal clonic	Seen more commonly in term than in preterm infants; well-localized clonic jerking in a conscious state
Myoclonic	Seen in both term and premature infants; synchronous jerks of flexion, single or multiple, affecting upper more than lower limbs

Source: Adapted from Volpe JJ. 2018. *Neurology of the Newborn*, 6th ed. Philadelphia, PA: Elsevier, 286–287.[4]

SUMMARY

A careful early neurologic assessment of the newborn is necessary for early intervention and optimal management. Serial examinations should be performed when a neonate is identified to be at risk or has abnormal findings. Gestational age should be considered throughout all aspects of the exam.

ADDITIONAL RESOURCES

SPRINGER PUBLISHING CONNECT™

A robust set of resources designed to supplement this text is located at http://connect.springerpub.com/content/book/978-0-8261-4063-0. Qualifying instructors may request access by emailing textbook@springerpub.com.

REFERENCES

1. Amiel-Tison C. 1986. *A Neurologic Assessment During the First Year of Life*. Oxford, UK: Oxford University Press, 7.
2. Prechtl H, and Beintema D. 1991. *The Neurological Examination of the Full-Term Newborn Infant*, 2nd ed. London, UK: Cambridge University Press, 3.
3. Dubowitz L, Dubowitz V, and Mercuri E. 2007. *The Neurological Assessment of the Preterm and Full-Term Newborn Infant*. London, UK: Heinemann, 9–11.
4. Volpe JJ. 2018. *Neurology of the Newborn*, 6th ed. Philadelphia, PA: Elsevier, 6–16, 108, 191–221, 275–321, 325–424, 593–698, 878, 1116, 1149–1190.
5. Amiel-Tison C. 1991. Examination of the newborn infant. In *Rudolph's Pediatrics*, 19th ed. Rudolph, AM, Rudolph CD, and Hoffman JI, eds. New York, NY: McGraw-Hill, 178–179.
6. Jarvis C. 2019. *Physical Examination & Health Assessment*, 8th ed. Philadelphia, PA: Saunders, 651.
7. Hill A. 1998. Development of tone and reflexes in the fetus and newborn. In *Fetal and Neonatal Physiology*, 2nd ed. Polin RA, and Fox WW, eds. Philadelphia, PA: Saunders, 2169.
8. Verklan MT, Walden M, and Forest S. 2021. *Core Curriculum for Neonatal Intensive Care Nursing*, 6th ed. St. Louise, MO: Elsevier, 99–130.
9. Gardner SL, Carter BS, Enzman-Hines MI, and Niermeyer S, eds. 2021. *Merenstein & Gardner's Handbook of Neonatal Intensive Care and Interprofessional Approach*, 9th ed. St. Louis, MO: Elsevier, 338.
10. Kliegman, RM. 2020. *Nelson's Textbook of Pediatrics*. 21st ed. Philadelphia, PA: Elsevier, 3060.
11. Zenel JA. 2011. Chapter 44. Examination of the Newborn Infant. In: *Rudolph's Pediatrics*, Rudolph CD, Rudolph AM, Lister GE, First LR, and Gershon AA, eds. McGraw Hill.
12. Dodson WE. 1989. Deleterious effects of drugs on the developing nervous system. *Clinics in Perinatology* 16(2): 340–343, 348–353.

13. Moore KL, Persaud TVN, and Torchia MG. 2020. *The Developing Human: Clinically Oriented Embryology*, 11th ed. Philadelphia, PA: Saunders, 357–394.
14. Noetzel M. 1989. Myelomeningocele: Current concepts of management. *Clinics in Perinatology* 16(2): 318.
15. Waxman SG. 2000. *Correlative Neuroanatomy*, 24th ed. New York, NY: Lange Medical Books/McGraw-Hill, 155.
16. American College of Obstetricians and Gynecologists. 2015. *Operative Vaginal Delivery: ACOG Practice Bulletin Number 154*. Washington, DC: American College of Obstetricians and Gynecologists.
17. Ku LC, Boggess KA, and Cohen-Wolkowiez M. 2015. Bacterial meningitis in the infant. *Clinics in Perinatology* 42(1): 29–45.
18. Swanson EC, and Schleiss MR. 2013. Congenital cytomegalovirus infection: New prospects for prevention and therapy. *Pediatric Clinics of North America* 60(2): 1–14.

13 BEHAVIORAL ASSESSMENT

Dorothy Vittner and Jacqueline M. McGrath

The newborn infant has truly amazing capabilities. Science supporting an increased understanding of the infant's capabilities and interactive behaviors has led to evolved awareness over the past 35 years. Born at term or preterm, the infant has a unique repertoire of behaviors that caregivers can observe to better understand what the infant is trying to accomplish. The infant's behaviors are a window for understanding the infant's developing brain. Assessing the infant's neurologic status and neurobehavioral patterns requires evaluating how the infant responds and interacts with others in context of their environment. The environmental context cannot be ignored and must be considered in every interaction with a newborn.

There is growing evidence that the premature infant and the developing brain are influenced by the environment especially during the vulnerable window of time when the infant is cared for in the NICU.[1] Although survival rates of extremely premature infants are steadily improving, the incidence of later developmental disabilities for these infants remains high.[2–5] It has been optimistically yet incorrectly proposed that healthy preterm infants without major complications will eventually catch up developmentally to full-term infants.[6] Rather, research suggests that as preterm infants mature, they remain increasingly disadvantaged on many neurodevelopmental outcomes.[7–11] Evidence also suggests racial and ethnic disparities influence preterm health outcomes accentuating the influence of the social determinants of health.[12,13] The United States Centers for Disease Control and Prevention (CDC) reports in 2021 that the rate of preterm births among African American females (14.8%) was approximately 50% higher than the rate of preterm births among White or Hispanic females.[14]

The womb is a dynamic, sensory-rich environment meant to prepare the infant for interaction after full-term birth. The neonate delivered early *experiences a very different sensory environment* in the task-driven, high-tech world of the NICU. To best respond to an infant as caregivers or parents, we must first understand the unique behavioral strategies the infant uses to cope with the intensive care nursery experience. At this point in development, the preterm infant's neurobiologic expectations are quite different from what they actually experience in the NICU. This mismatch in neurobiologic sensory expectations often leads to early life stress, and in the context of the developing brain is important to long-term developmental outcomes.[15]

Behavioral assessment provides information about the infant's neurobehavioral functioning and allows caregivers to design individualized, developmental guided plans of care for hospitalized infants. Evidence suggests that appropriate, individualized developmental care of preterm infants decreases the length of hospitalization.[15] A meta-analysis of individualized developmental assessment and care demonstrated a statistically significant impact on the requirement for supplemental oxygen and on neurodevelopmental outcome at 9 and 12 months, but not at 2 years.[16] Evidence suggests enhancement of developmental outcomes after discharge, when the infant's behavioral and physiologic cues were supported in the NICU.[16] McAnulty et al. reported individualized developmental care had enhanced neuropsychological and electrophysiological effects into school age, which were evaluated at 8 years corrected age.[17] Effectiveness of interventions are influenced by the environment; evidence for improving preterm outcomes was found with the Newborn Individualized Developmental Care Assessment Program (NIDCAP) intervention.[18] There is growing evidence for interventions included in developmentally supportive care. What is more difficult to sort out are the cumulative effects of this type of care on infant and family outcomes.[6,18]

On-separation between the infant–parent is imperative. Infants need parental contact for optimal physiologic and emotional development, and parents need meaningful relationships with their infants to establish their identities as parents.[19,20] Evidence suggests social determinants of health, underpinned by biological factors, can predict decreased synchrony in the mother–infant dyad which in turn influence infant short- and long-term health and well-being.[21]

Parental touch, particularly during skin-to-skin contact (SSC), has been shown to reduce some adverse consequences of prematurity.[22–24] This physical proximity allows for a continuously interactive environment known to enhance infant physiologic stability and affective closeness between parent and infant.[25–27]

Parents and professionals have long searched for early accurate indicators of competence, developmental delay, or disability in infants. Neurodevelopment is dynamic, influenced by relationships, the environment, and genetic predispositions. Despite advances in care for preterm infants, it remains difficult to predict adverse neurodevelopmental outcomes accurately.[7,11] Untimely and/or inappropriate predictions sometimes have caused both infants and families more harm than benefit.[15] Each approach to assessing the newborn represents the need to determine early which infants are progressing according to expected developmental milestones and which will benefit from therapeutic interventions and follow-up. The infant's developmental trajectory is influenced by evolving relationships. Parents are the infant's ideal nurturer and coregulator, enhancing the infant's competence and ability to build trust within the relationship.[15,28] Parents and infants benefit from the parents' awareness and responsiveness to the infant's behavioral capabilities and temperament. Parental ability to interpret the infant's behavioral cues has been shown to strengthen parent–infant interaction during the first year of life.[17,19,21] When parents have the skills to interpret their infant's cues and respond appropriately, the infant is better able to self-regulate and respond appropriately to the physical and social environment.[15,29] Providing infants with this foundation for trusting interactions increases their self-regulatory efforts and ability to respond to new situations.

The assessment of neurobehavioral functioning complements and elaborates on the neurologic assessment as described in Chapter 12. To differentiate, the neurologic examination assesses the function of the central nervous system and includes assessment of muscles and reflexes within the context of the infant's state of consciousness, whereas the behavioral examination relies on describing the infant's observable behavior in response to different stimuli. This behavior pattern is a reflection of the infant's underlying neurologic status and current level of functioning. A critical window of brain growth and differentiation occurs between 24- and 40-weeks postmenstrual age (PMA). How the caregiver interacts with the infant during this critical window influences brain development and function.[15]

Newborn behavioral assessments must be understood in the context that all human experiences have psychological, biological, and organic contexts that dynamically influence each other in connection with the physical and social environment. Another important consideration in the foundation for presenting the assessment findings is the acknowledgment that developmental behavior and function are not determined solely by the circumstances at birth. The human brain demonstrates a fascinating capacity to adapt and adjust to difficulties and conditions. Moreover, a child's development is a complex, dynamic process with many influences that occur over time in addition to the structural and functional changes within the infant's central nervous system.

The process of infant behavioral assessment has shifted to embrace a range of competencies building on strengths, rather than deficiencies. The recognition of the infant's functional competence led to the integration of the infant's regulatory efforts (or the infant's capacity to cope with his or her experiences) and the infant's interactive competencies, to be viewed within a social context.[29] The focus is on individual differences and what influences those differences. The evolving conceptualization of these differences affect the caregiver's behavior in addition to the infant's developmental trajectory. A priority for health professionals is to offer helpful and accurate information that can facilitate parent–infant attachment. Assessment of the infant's environment and of family and social interaction must also be included to fully assess the capacities and needs of infants who may be considered at risk during the perinatal period.[30] Ideally, the assessment should be repeated at different time intervals to determine the infant's current level of behavioral functioning while identifying strengths and vulnerabilities. Repeating the assessment provides the family with more information about how to best interpret their infant's unique set of cues and behaviors.

APPROACH TO BEHAVIORAL ASSESSMENT

Identifying conditions of risk, describing behavior patterns, and evaluating developmental functions are all important aspects of the neurobehavioral assessment. Credible evaluation relies primarily on the examiner's astute, accurate observational skills. The examiner must observe the infant's ability to organize, recognize signs of disorganization or stress, and modify the interaction based on the infant's behavioral response.

It is important to follow the basic principles of physical examination when assessing the infant's behavior. Perinatal history will provide important information on factors that will affect the infant's ability to interact with the environment. Repeated and prolonged stress influences the infant's behavioral patterns.[31] Factors such as time elapsed since birth, type of labor and delivery, as well as drugs used during pregnancy and delivery by the mother must be considered. Gestational age as well as postnatal age and medical status will also have a significant impact on both the behavioral findings and the infant's ability to participate actively in the examination. An infant with respiratory distress will exhibit different behaviors than one who is not in distress. Caregiving and activity provided before the examination must also be considered since they could exhaust the infant. Research with preterm infants has demonstrated that the sequence of care and the clustering of caregiving interventions can affect the infant's responsiveness and capabilities.[30,31]

The physical and social environment are important considerations that may affect the outcome of the examination. A warm, calm, quiet, and softly lit room provides the best environment in which to observe the infant's responses to stimuli and ability to regulate state. Performing the examination in the presence of the infant's parents or caregivers provides a valuable opportunity for the parent to better understand the infant's behavior and competencies.[32] Other supports that might be needed for some infants to perform at their best include the use of swaddling and containment. These postural supports encourage a tucked, neutral posture that decreases stress for the infant. In addition, the use of rest periods allows the infant to regain energy and focus during the examination. Another strategy to reduce the effects of the sensory environment is to reduce sounds and activity in the infant's immediate environment and thereby decrease stressful stimuli for the infant allowing the infant to focus on the interaction at hand. Premature and high-risk infants are easily stressed. There is often little leeway for the physiologically compromised infant to become overstressed. The infant who surpasses autonomic regulation thresholds may experience behaviors such as desaturations or bradycardia. When these occur, breaks can help, but sometimes the exam needs to be discontinued and considered for another time.

The infant's state of consciousness is another important consideration.[29] An infant's state depends on a variety of factors, such as time of last feeding, recent events (e.g., blood tests or circumcision), and the infant's individual sleep–wake cycle. It is important to be aware of these other factors and consider them in relationship to scheduling and performance of the infant during the examination. The response to stimuli and behavioral cues will vary according to the infant's state. Preterm infants exhibit subtle behaviors that are more difficult to identify than term infants. The examiner needs to be flexible to obtain the most valid outcomes and conclusions. It is important to remember while caring for these vulnerable infants that there is only a small window of leeway for state organization; infants can quickly go from being actively engaged in the interaction to being disorganized and stressed to the point of fatigue or withdrawal. Thus, caregivers are always balancing the need for assessing the infant's competence with the knowledge that the NICU sensory experiences may be impinging on the infant's ability to demonstrate appropriate behavioral responses.

In many intensive care nurseries and follow-up clinics, neurobehavioral assessment is an essential part of the comprehensive care of the high-risk newborn. Evaluating behavior is a useful concept because it facilitates understanding the infant's ability to cope with their experiences.[33] Evaluation also helps to provide an understanding of the infant's interactional capacities, including alerting and orienting to caregivers' faces and objects in the environment. Case studies providing examples of behavioral assessment of three different infants (well newborn, well preterm infant, and sick preterm infant) are found at the end of this chapter with the descriptions of the instruments that can be used for behavioral assessment. These examples demonstrate the need for the examiner to have a comprehensive understanding of infant behavior and the proper training to assess neurobehavioral functioning. This understanding is necessary for developing a rapport with the infant and administering a developmental assessment that elicits meaningful results.

Behavioral assessment is intended to identify an infant's current level of balance and smooth, integrated functioning. In other words, it is designed to identify in what situations and with what supports the infant exhibits its organized behavior. It is also the purpose of the assessment to describe the threshold of disorganization indicated in the infant's behaviors of coping and avoidance. The degree and types of stress and intensity of anxiety and frustration the infant experiences can be indicators of the degree of energy the infant has available. The behavioral assessment must also determine whether there is any leeway in the infant's responses. For example, if the infant can tolerate being moved from the examiner's shoulder (where he is flexed, tucked, and resting calmly) to the lap without an onslaught of disorganized behaviors (such as extended arms and hands, grimaces, fussiness, and irregular breathing), then the infant is demonstrating organization, even if working hard to achieve that organization. If disorganization is unavoidable, even when sensitive handling is provided, the infant's behaviors are demonstrating that more facilitation is needed before, during, and even after caregiving, with minimal activity during handling.

It is the intent of the behavioral assessment to describe the degree of competence and organization in the infant's behavioral repertoire, as well as when and how behaviors reflect disorganization or stressful responses. Are there changes in color, breathing, or movement patterns as the infant is moved? Or can the infant be moved from one place to another with minimal adjustments and limited cost to behavioral subsystems? What strategies does the caregiver need to employ to help the infant function smoothly? Behavioral assessment provides data that can answer all of these questions. The next several sections outline parameters often included in a behavioral assessment. It is important to note that not all parameters are included in all behavioral assessments.

Use of some parameters is dependent on the status of the infant. At times, a chosen assessment tool may bring each parameter used together in a meaningful way. For reliable administration, a thorough understanding of the elements of the assessment are needed. Once each parameter is discussed, then several different behavioral assessments are described with how they might be best used in the clinical setting.

IDENTIFYING STATES OF CONSCIOUSNESS

State refers to the level of consciousness exhibited by the infant (Table 13.1). State is determined by the level of arousal and ability to respond to stimuli. The infant's behavior, function, and response to the environment will depend upon which baseline state he is in, ranging from deep sleep to vigorous crying. Healthy infants can use their state to exert control over environmental input, but this ability may be limited in the preterm or sick infant. Often the preterm infant is awake with eyes closed; this can be mistaken for sleep. Premature and critically ill infants often have difficulty achieving the entire range of states, for example, a defined state of deep sleep or robust crying. Behavioral assessment begins with evaluating the infant's ability to control state, move smoothly from one state to another, and maintain alertness.[34]

TABLE 13.1: NEONATAL BEHAVIORAL STATES

STATE	CHARACTERISTICS
Deep sleep	No eye movements No activity Regular breathing
Light sleep	Low levels of activity Rapid eye movement possible
Drowsiness	Variable activity levels Dull, heavy-lidded eyes that open and close
Quiet alert	Wide, bright eyes Attention focused on stimulus
Active alert	Increased motor activity Periods of fussiness Irregular respirations
Crying	Increased motor activity Color changes

State is determined by observing an infant's level of arousal and accompanying behaviors or cues. Several scoring systems have been developed for identifying infant states. Brazelton's system is the most widely used and easiest to follow, particularly for the term infant.[79] For the preterm infant, more definitive state definitions may be useful, such as those developed by Als, Holditch-Davis, and Anderson.[15,35,36] The Anderson Behavioral State Scale (ABSS) has been used often in nursing research because it is easily learned and provides interrater reliability.[35] The ABSS was devised specifically for use with preterm infants. The underlying theoretical framework for this state scale is different from that of other scales. Most other state scales are nominal in nature: the coding is a categorical representation of clusters of behavioral states.[35] These state scales, then, have been designed to capture the *qualitatively* different aspect of behavioral clusters. The ABSS was designed with consideration for the linear relationships among the states, heart rate, and energy consumption. Thus, the differences are *quantitative* or ordinal in nature.[35] The ABSS is particularly useful for preterm infants because it breaks down the typical five or six behavioral states into 12 states. This delineation more closely captures behavioral states exhibited by preterm infants because differentiating sleep–wake states is more difficult in preterm infants. For example, the ABSS has four measures of sleep, five measures of awake, and three measures of crying, allowing a more sensitive indication of infant behavioral state.

Interobserver reliability with the ABSS has been easier to establish than with other scales. ABSS scores range from 1 to 12. The infant's sleep is categorized within scores of 1 to 4; the behavior observed with the infant's eyes closed (sleep) is used to differentiate the actual score itself. Scores of 1 or 2 are quiet sleep states and represent no body movement; these are considered optimal for recovery and/or growth because of decreased energy expenditures. Scores of 3 or 4 are more active sleep states, with beginning awareness of the environment. Apnea due to disorganized breathing is most likely to be seen in state 3 or 4. Drowsiness with eyes open and closed at times is a score of 5. Scores of 6 or 7 are alert states considered optimal for perception, interaction, and learning. Increasing activity with a degree of alertness are scores of 8 or 9. Scores of 10 to 12 represent increasing levels of agitation and crying. The examiner assigns a state based on ease of identification (the infant clearly exhibits that state). This may be more difficult in preterm or ill infants, whose states may be more fleeting.[32,34,37]

Sleep States

Deep sleep is characterized by closed eyes with no eye movements, regular breathing, and no spontaneous activity. There is a delayed response to external stimuli and then only a brief arousal, followed by a return to deep sleep. Isolated sucking movements or startles may be noted. Preterm infants may demonstrate a difference between very deep sleep, still sleep, and deep sleep with startles or muscle twitching.[37,38]

Light sleep consists of low levels of activity, with greater variability in response to external stimuli. (Figures 13.1 to 13.9 show progression of an infant through states of light sleep to crying, demonstrating time-out signals with visual stimuli). Rapid eye movement may be observed. Preterm infants may exhibit irregular respirations. Infants in light sleep may startle or make brief fussing or crying noises. Parents may need support in delaying response to these brief episodes during the light-sleep phase. Active sleep and lower-level alert states are seen more often in preterm infants than in term infants, who spend more time in deep sleep and quiet alert states.[38]

Transitional State

Drowsiness is the transitional state between sleep and awake. Drowsiness is characterized by a variable activity level, with smooth movements and occasional mild startles (Figure 13.2). The eyes open and close and appear dull and heavy lidded. The infant will react to stimuli, but the response is often delayed, and the infant may startle easily. From the drowsy state, the infant may either return to a sleep state or move to a more alert state. Caregivers may arouse an infant into a quiet alert state by providing an auditory or visual stimulus. Nonnutritive sucking has also been found to be effective in calming and bringing an infant to an alert state.[38]

Awake States

Quiet alert refers to the state in which the infant interacts most with the environment by exhibiting a brightening and widening of the eyes and an alert appearance (Figure 13.3). Attention is focused on available stimuli, whether visual or auditory (Figure 13.4). A minimal amount of motor activity is noted, and respirations are regular. This state provides the greatest opportunity for infant interaction with caregivers. Term newborns commonly experience a period of quiet alertness in the first few hours after birth, providing an opportunity for parents to interact with their infant.

Preterm infants may have difficulty maintaining a quiet alert state for long. Alert periods may be brief and fleeting. The infant may become "*hyperalert*," with an inability to decrease or end fixation on a stimulus (Figure 13.5). Preterm infants may also appear awake and alert but be unable to involve themselves in interaction.[37,38] During these periods, they are often noted to use gaze aversion to manage the overwhelming stimuli in the nursery environment.[38]

The *active alert* state is characterized by increased motor activity, with heightened sensitivity to stimuli. The infant may have periods of fussiness, yet is consolable. Although open, the eyes are less bright and attentive than in the quiet alert state. Respirations are

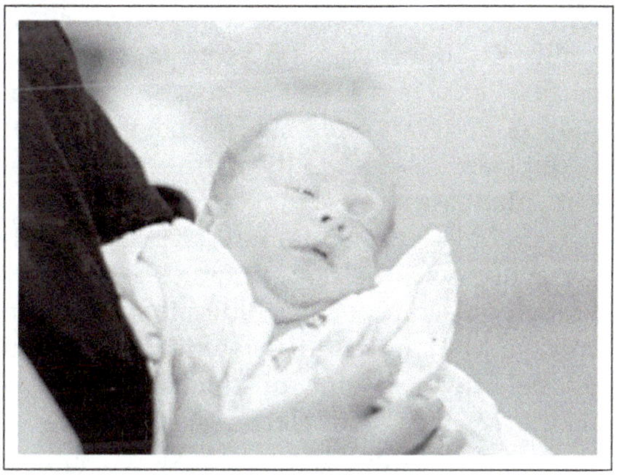

FIGURE 13.1 Light sleep

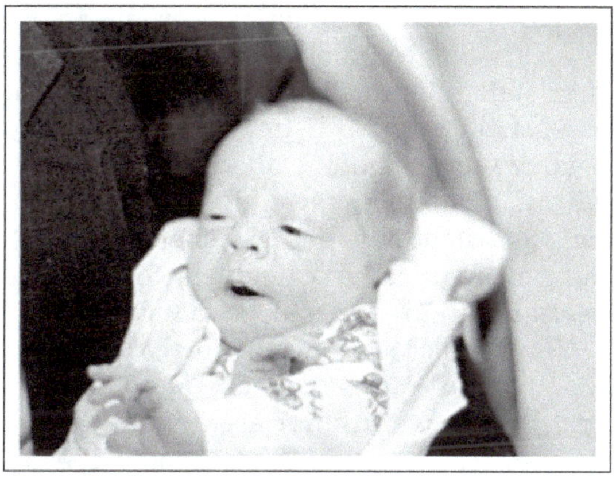

FIGURE 13.2 Drowsy

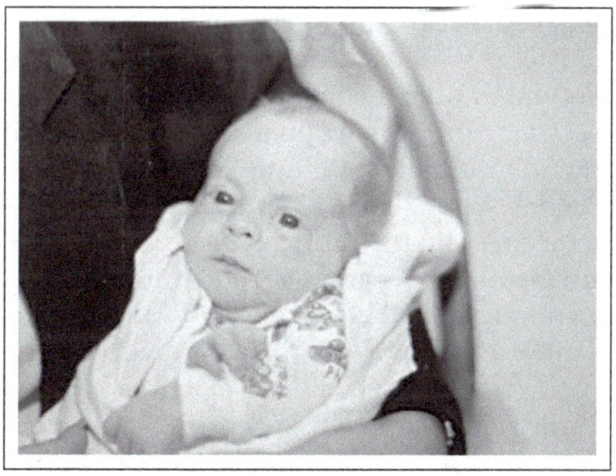

FIGURE 13.3 Quiet alert

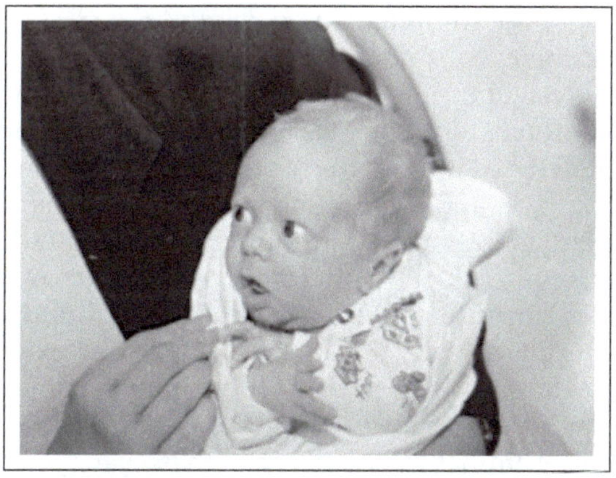

FIGURE 13.4 Signs of attentiveness

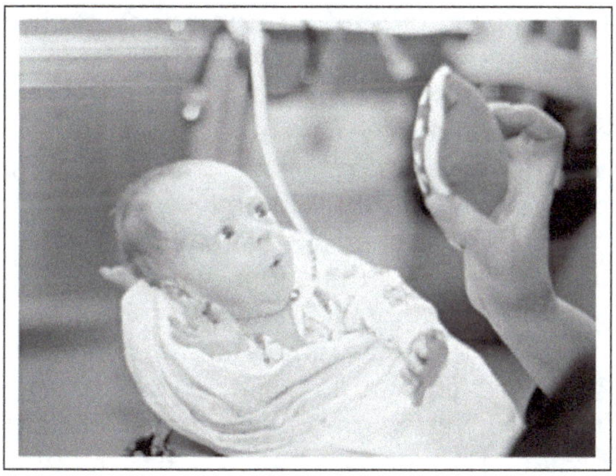

FIGURE 13.5 Hyperalert response to stimulus

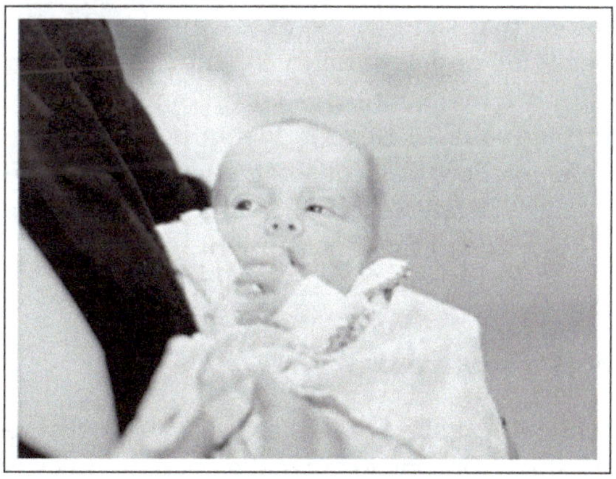

FIGURE 13.6 Self-consoling behavior; hand-to-mouth movements

irregular. The term infant may be able to use self-consoling techniques to return to a quiet alert state (Figure 13.6). The preterm infant will usually become distressed and unable to organize. Interventions such as waiting for the infant to settle, swaddling, containing, and reducing other environmental stimuli can be provided by caregivers to help the infant return to a quiet alert state.[37]

Crying is accompanied by increased motor activity and color changes. The infant is very responsive to unpleasant stimuli, both internal and external. Some infants console themselves and return to a lower state level, whereas others need help from caregivers such as facilitation with swaddling or holding. Preterm infants may exhibit a weak cry, or their cry is not audible due to intubation. Even without an audible cry, infants may demonstrate color changes, alterations in motor activity, or other signs of stress, such as a crying face, apnea, vomiting, or decreased oxygen saturation.[34,38] During crying, the infant may also extend and straighten his extremities, then lie still, remaining extended without the capacity to return to a neutral, flexed posture. As energy is lost, the infant becomes flaccid and appears depleted. The question the examiner must ask when these behaviors are observed is, "What does it take from the environment or caregiver to settle and help the infant recover and return to a modulated, interactive state?" Awareness of the infant's behavior and the ability of the caregiver to support the infant are core components of individualized, developmentally supportive care practices that conserve energy and facilitate the infant's ability to interact with the caregiver and the environment.

Maintenance of State

Although behavioral states can be distinguished from one another, the infant makes frequent transitions among them, changing from one state to another several times during the examination. The term infant should display smooth transitions between behavioral states and move from sleep to drowsy to wakefulness instead of moving from sleep to agitation with robust crying. Excessive lethargy or irritability is abnormal. The preterm or neurologically impaired infant may exhibit sudden changes between sleep and awake states, but abrupt state changes in the seemingly healthy term infant are a cause for concern.[38]

The ability to maintain an alert state with interaction varies among infants. Some have difficulty becoming alert initially and then struggle to maintain this state for any length of time. The infant may need facilitation from a caregiver to sustain alertness. Other infants have trouble filtering out noxious stimuli and progress rapidly to active alert or crying, becoming disorganized. Swaddling or a quiet, darkened environment may help these infants remain alert and focus on a single stimulus.

The examiner should acknowledge the amount of time the infant spends in the quiet alert state or focusing on a stimulus and reinforce the infant's attempts to build positive trusting interactions. Infants who have difficulty remaining alert can be frustrating for caregivers and parents. The examiner may spend time with parents exploring opportunities to support the infant to maintain an interactive alert state. The examiner should consider the situation and ask, "When does the infant look most comfortable?" or "What supports are necessary for the infant to be successful or comfortable?" The examiner then incorporates these individualized strategies, such as postural support, appropriate for this infant into the interaction with the infant.

Preterm infants have brief periods of alertness and may have difficulty maintaining this state. Brazelton describes the "cost of attention" as the amount of energy the infant must expend to maintain an interaction.[15] This cost of attention varies, depending on the health and maturity of the infant. Premature or sick infants show fatigue or stress sooner than do healthy term infants.[29] The caregiver's supportive responsiveness to the infant's distress is imperative to building trusting relationships.

Signs of stress or fatigue may include color changes, irregular respirations, apnea, changes in tone, irritability or lethargy, and vomiting. The infant may change states rapidly from crying to sleep or may become hyperalert. The examiner must be able to recognize these signs of stress and fatigue and support the infant or discontinue the examination when appropriate. After the infant has rested, the examiner may begin again. The cost to the infant or the amount of energy expended during the examination should be noted.[31,37] The preterm or ill infant may require completion of the examination in pieces, which is not optimal; yet completion in one time period may be too much for vulnerable infants.

ORGANIZATION

Organization reflects the infant's ability to integrate physiologic and behavioral systems in response to the environment without disruption in state or physiologic functions.[15,38] Physiologic functions include such parameters as heart rate, respiratory rate, oxygen consumption, and digestion. The behavioral system includes state (attention and self-regulation) and motor activity (tone, movements, and posture).

The organized, robust infant maintains stable vital signs, smooth state transitions, and even movements when interacting with the environment. The infant is able to self-console or be consoled easily and can habituate to or block out overwhelming stimuli. The disorganized infant will react to the environment with sudden state changes and will exhibit frantic, jittery movements, color changes, and irregular respirations. Some infants will respond with hypotonia. The ability to maintain organization depends on the infant's maturity level and overall well-being. Individual temperament may also play a role in organizational ability.

In evaluating organization of motor behavior, the examiner assesses the infant's movement patterns, energy level, and tone. Hand-to-mouth maneuvers to self-console are purposeful movements achieved by the mature, well-organized infant (see Figure 13.6). When a cloth is placed over the face of a term neonate, the infant will attempt to remove it by arching, rooting, and swiping at the cloth covering the eyes/face. As during most assessments of behavioral maturity, the preterm infant may have a diffused or delayed response.

Infants who are easily overwhelmed will benefit from care designed to enhance their organizational ability to cope and self-regulate. Clustering care to allow for uninterrupted restorative sleep, arousing the infant slowly, and introducing one stimulus at a time are all interventions that support the infant in being more successful or competent. However, it is important to consider those caregiving tasks that are clustered together and their overall effect on the infant; there is always a cost-benefit ratio to consider.[15,31] Providing postural support to encourage the infant to stretch and squirm to help steady breathing yet return to a neutral, tucked posture is essential for the infant to develop productive coping mechanisms. Being aware of and modifying sensory input is important so as not to increase stress for the high-risk infant. Some infants, however, can tolerate help in modulating their behavior during the examination. Quietly speaking to the infant in a way that provides comfort while interacting can also be a supportive strategy or intervention to obtain a comprehensive impression of the infant's strengths and vulnerabilities.

RECOGNIZING THE SENSORY THRESHOLD

Sensory threshold refers to the level of tolerance for stimuli within which the infant can respond appropriately. After reaching or exceeding this threshold, the infant becomes overstimulated and exhibits signs of stress and fatigue (Box 13.1). Preterm and neurologically impaired infants may have low thresholds compared to healthy term newborns. What would normally be considered routine care (e.g., talking to the infant during feeding) may be overstimulating to an infant with a low sensory threshold. These infants might do better when presented with a single stimulus or modified, muted sensory inputs such as providing a comforting quiet voice or briefly catching the infant with eye contact.

BOX 13.1: SIGNS OF OVERSTIMULATION (TIME-OUT)

Gaze aversion
Frowning
Sneezing
Yawning
Hiccuping
Vomiting
Mottled skin
Irregular respirations
Apnea
Increased oxygen requirement
Heart rate changes
Finger splaying
Arching
Stiffening
Fussing, crying

The mature newborn can regulate physiologic and emotional response to various stimuli. It is the infant's way of learning to control the effects of the surrounding environment. Evaluating infant responses to the environment allows the examiner to design an individualized plan of care that is unique to that infant.[39] Knowledge of infant responses also facilitates parent competence and involvement in infant care which can be defined as parent engagement.[10,24] Infants who are easily overwhelmed may require more frequent breaks during caregiving to adapt and regulate responses.

Observing Behavioral Cues

An infant's behavior indicates physical, psychological, and social needs. Caregivers who are responsive to these cues develop reciprocal relationships with the newborn. Responding to an infant's behavioral cues also reinforces behavioral organization.[21,27,30] This reciprocity helps to build trust, which is an essential component of emotional development and a key component in the foundation of secure attachment.[30] The infant relies on individualization, responsiveness, and respectfulness, which should be integrated into each interaction.[15,38]

Signs of approach (or attention) indicate the infant is ready to interact with the caregiver or the environment. Approach behaviors include an alert, focused gaze; regular breathing; and dilated pupils. The infant may also exhibit grasping, sucking, or hand-to-mouth movements (Box 13.2; see Figure 13.6).[38]

Avoidance behaviors (time-out signals) indicate the infant is becoming tired, overstimulated, or stressed and needs a break from the stimulus or interaction. Avoidance behaviors include averting the gaze, frowning, sneezing, yawning, vomiting, and hiccupping. The infant may also display finger splaying, arching, stiffening, or crying (Figures 13.7–13.9; see Box 13.1). Color changes, apnea, irregular breathing, and decreased oxygen saturation may also indicate the infant's need for time-out.[34,38] A state change may be an avoidance behavior, as demonstrated by the infant who withdraws or shuts down entirely by falling asleep during repeated or prolonged painful procedures. It is important to remember that while some infants may muster up the energy to protest a noxious stimulus, they seldom have the autonomic stability to sustain the response. Healthcare professionals must use these cues in planning routine care if they are to best support the infant and decrease energy consumption.[31,40]

HABITUATION

The infant's ability to decrease a response to a repeated stimulus is referred to as *habituation.*

BOX 13.2: SIGNS OF APPROACH (ATTENTION)

Quiet, alert state
Focused gaze
Dilated pupils
Regular respirations
Regular heart rate
Rhythmic sucking
Reaching or grasping
Hand-to-mouth movements

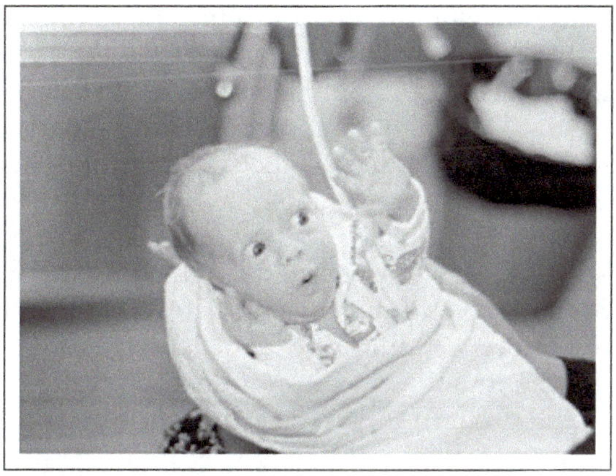

FIGURE 13.7 Sign of overstimulation in response to stimulus

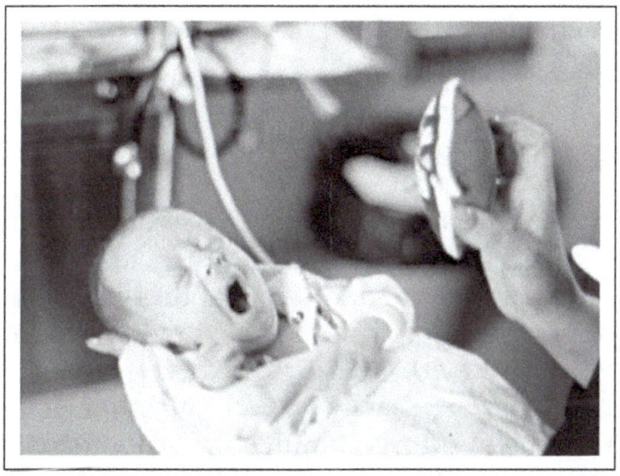

FIGURE 13.8 Sign of overstimulation in response to stimulus

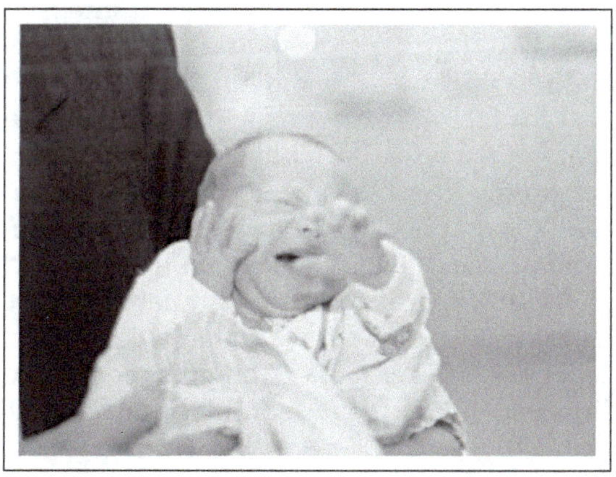

FIGURE 13.9 Crying as a response to continued stimulus

When a stimulus is repeated, the infant's initial response will gradually disappear. Habituation provides a defense mechanism for shutting out overwhelming or disturbing stimuli. For example, healthcare providers often habituate to the noxious noise of the NICU.

Habituation is best assessed when the infant is asleep or in a drowsy alert state.[29,38] The stimulus can involve the visual, auditory, or tactile senses. Visual habituation can be easily assessed by shining a light briefly onto the infant's closed eyes during sleep from 10 to 12 inches away. Repeat the stimulus every 5 seconds to a maximum of 10 times or until the infant ceases to respond (whichever comes first). Note the presence of startles, facial grimaces, blinking, and respiratory changes. If habituation occurs, responses will become delayed and eventually disappear. Infants who are able to habituate successfully to protect their sleep usually do so within five to nine flashes.

The infant's ability to habituate to an auditory stimulus can be tested in the same manner, using an object that makes a noise (e.g., a bell or rattle). Hold the object 10 to 15 inches from the baby and shake the object for about 1 second. Responses may include startles, squirming movements, facial grimaces, and respiratory changes. The following stimuli should be provided when the infant stops responding. Note the infant's ability to decrease her or his responses as the stimulus is repeated or if the infant continues to respond longer than 45 to 60 seconds, indicating he or she may need facilitation from the examiner to stop. As they do with visual habituation, most term infants decrease their reaction after five to nine repetitions.

Habituation to tactile stimulation can be determined by pressing the sole of the foot with a smooth object. Repeat the stimulus every 5 seconds. The infant may begin with a generalized body response, pulling both feet away. The response will gradually decrease to only the involved foot or will disappear altogether.

The ability to habituate varies among infants. Some (including those who are preterm) have difficulty tuning out noxious stimuli.[41] They are easily distracted and then become irritable and disorganized, displaying signs of stress and fatigue. The premature infant's brain development is strongly influenced by random frequent sensory stimulation. Their inability to cope with environmental sights and sounds may make interactions and feeding difficult. These infants may need to be fed in a quiet, darkened room or presented with one stimulus at a time during their quiet, alert state. Work with parents to reinforce identification of and response to their infant's behavior. This can facilitate a positive relationship between the infant and the family, supporting parental competence.

RESPONSE TO STIMULI

Visual Stimuli

The newborn has the ability to focus on and react to a variety of stimuli in the environment. The examiner should observe and record the infant's response to visual and auditory stimuli. For optimal evaluation, responses should be assessed with the infant in the quiet, alert state.

Two tests for visual response can be performed with the newborn. The first is a response to light. When a light is directed toward the infant's eyes, an appropriate response is a grimace and closure of the eyelids. This response will lessen with habituation. The second test evaluates the ability to fixate on an object and track it. Term infants are able to fixate briefly on an object (e.g., a face or a red ball). The newborn's visual field is fairly narrow, with the ability to focus on objects at a distance of about 10 to 12 inches. Objects closer or farther away will be ignored because newborns have decreased visual acuity that improves with maturation. The term newborn is able to follow or track an object horizontally about 60° and vertically about 30°, often with some head movement.[29,42]

The pupillary reflex develops at approximately 30 weeks PMA. Without this reflex, premature infants have a limited ability to maintain protective lid tightening and therefore should be protected from bright lights and visual stimulation.[43] As the pupillary reflex matures, preterm infants beyond 30 weeks PMA age demonstrate both response to light and ability to focus on simple patterns.[43,44] Preterm infants may take longer to focus on an object, as they have less visual acuity than term newborns, which accounts for this variability in response. It is important to continue monitoring light levels, protecting the infant's eyes from direct bright light. In the preterm infant, closed eyelids provide less protection from bright lights than they do in more mature term infants. Behavior responses to visual stimuli should be evaluated for signs of stress and fatigue.[38,42] An eye examination for the preterm infant may be a noxious procedure for which the infant may need supportive interventions to manage.

Auditory Stimuli

When in the alert state, newborns will respond to an auditory stimulus with brightening of the eyes and face and turning of the head in search of the sound. A rattle, bell, or voice will work well as an auditory stimulus. Keep in mind that a newborn may tune out a noxious auditory stimulus. With the baby's head in midline, initiate the stimulus 6 to 12 inches away from one ear, out of visual range. The infant should open their eyes and turn their head toward the sound; continue by alternating the stimulus on each side with sounds of varying rhythm and intensity based on the infant's responses.

Preterm infants begin to orient (look at and focus) to a soft sound source by approximately 28 weeks PMA, but often demonstrate sensitivity to obtrusive sounds and physiologic instability in the presence of random loud sounds.[45] The use of a soft voice and rhythmic cyclical auditory stimulation can be introduced based on the infant's behavioral response.[38] Careful attention must be paid to limiting environmental sounds because it has the ability to interfere with the responses to the behavioral examination. White and associates provide design guidelines for limiting sound in the NICU.[46]

EVALUATING CONSOLABILITY

Infants' abilities to quiet when in a crying state vary. The well-organized infant demonstrates observable activities to self-console during the examination. These include bringing the hands to the mouth; sucking on the fist or tongue; and using environmental stimuli (visual or auditory), such as a soft human voice, to self-console (see Figure 13.6).[25] Infants who make limited attempts or who show decreased ability to self-console may be more irritable or sensitive to stimuli.[25,46]

Most infants will respond to consoling attempts by caregivers. Irritable infants may be easily disturbed by stimuli from the environment and may be slower to respond (or may not respond at all) to attempts to console them. The examiner should try interventions that can lead to consoling the infant, such as talking softly, providing hand containment, or placing a hand over the infant's stomach, flexing the extremities near the trunk to prevent startle activity, holding, rocking, or offering nonnutritive sucking. Decreasing such environmental stimuli as light, sound, and sudden movement may also be helpful.[42] A common mistake is trying several interventions at the same time (e.g., rocking, talking softly, *and* offering a pacifier).[42,47] A combination of activities may overstimulate some infants. Therefore, limit the interventions to one at a time before using them as a group. If one intervention fails, try a different one and note which interventions work for this infant so they can be used again.

IDENTIFYING TEMPERAMENT

Infant temperament has been defined as the infant's behavioral style—how the infant behaves in relationship to the environment and caregiving interaction.[48] The developing relationship between infant and parent is affected by how the child's temperament is exhibited and perceived. The infant is neurobiologically connected to the parents. When there is synchrony within this dyad, there is said to be "goodness of fit." When synchrony is lacking, the infant is perceived as difficult and/or demanding by the mother/father (primary caregiver), and the asynchrony of the relationship predisposes the infant to long-term negative outcomes. Parents' perceptions of infant temperament are important and should be considered as individualized plans of care are created. Parents' perceptions and beliefs about the attributes of the infant affect how parents care for their infant and the symbiotic relationship that will support the infant's cognitive development. Thus, infant temperament has been measured by asking parents about their infants. How do they perceive the infant? Is the infant calm or demanding? How easily is the infant consoled or is the infant inconsolable? Understanding these dimensions can help the parent acquire realistic expectations for the child's behavior and perceive that he or she can meet them. Consider using reflective strategies, such as journaling or talking about the interaction with the infant, to support the parents in exploring their perceptions and better understanding their infant's behavior.[49]

As stated earlier, *temperament* refers to the way an individual interacts with the environment. Chess and Thomas describe nine behaviors that define variations in temperament.[50] A description of each behavior follows:

- *Activity level* refers to motor activity such as playing, dressing, eating, crawling, and walking. Sleep–wake cycles and their durations are also used in scoring activity level. Some infants are very active, with short sleep cycles; others are less robust.
- *Rhythmicity* refers to the regularity of functions such as hunger, sleep–wake patterns, and elimination.
- *Approach* or *withdrawal* describes the individual's reaction to a new stimulus such as food, a new toy, or a new person. Approach responses are positive; withdrawal responses are negative reactions to the new situation.
- *Adaptability* is the individual's response to new situations once the initial response has passed. Adaptability examines the

ability to adjust to the new situation or environment.

- *Threshold of responsiveness* refers to the amount of stimulation required to generate a response, either positive or negative.
- *Quality of mood* describes the overall mood of the individual or the amount of pleasant, friendly, happy behavior versus unpleasant, unfriendly, or fussy behavior.
- *Intensity of reaction* is the level of energy in a response, whether positive or negative.
- *Distractibility* is the ability of extraneous stimuli to interfere with the individual's current behavior.
- *Attention span* or *persistence* refers to the length of time an individual will pursue a specific activity, especially when obstacles interfere with it.

Based on these behaviors, three categories of temperament can be defined and frequently identified in the newborn:

1. The "easy" baby demonstrates regularity, positive approaches to new situations, adaptability to change, and an overall positive mood.
2. The "difficult" baby has an irregular schedule; trouble adapting to new situations; a low threshold for stimuli; and intense, often negative moods.
3. The "slow-to-warm" infant is characterized by mild intensity, positive or negative moods, and slow adaptation to new situations and people. These infants need repeated, slow exposure to a situation before they will respond positively.

Understanding and supporting an infant to best optimize temperament for interaction with the environment can help parents create an environment that will maximize their child's positive characteristics and minimize frustration.[47] Parents of a slow-to-warm child can allow extra time to adapt to new situations. The infant with a low sensory threshold may be easier to care for if activity is limited to a stimulus or two at a time.

TERM NEWBORN BEHAVIORAL ASSESSMENT

The best-known tool for behavioral assessment of the term infant is the Neonatal Behavioral Assessment Scale (NBAS) developed by Brazelton.[48] The tool was designed for use with healthy newborns born between 36 and 44 weeks gestation. A complete behavioral assessment using the NBAS takes about 30 minutes and is best administered by a trained examiner. However, even limited aspects of the examination performed by an untrained examiner can be used to provide helpful information about the infant's neurobehavioral status.[29,51] There are several studies in which the NBAS has been done in the presence of families to encourage them to see the vast capabilities of their infant.[29,51] The NBAS assesses the newborn's response to 28 behavioral items, each scored on a 9-point scale, and 18 elicited responses, each scored on a 4-point continuum. These items provide information about the newborn's ability to respond and adapt to his environment. Such items as reflexes, state regulation, orientation to visual and auditory stimuli, habituation, motor performance, and interaction with caregivers are assessed. The examination is usually done in one sitting, and items are most often presented in the same order to all infants.

The focus of the NBAS is assessment of the infant and intervention with the family.[51] The parents and examiner work together, using a nonjudgmental approach, to observe and understand the unique behaviors of the infant. Specific items selected from the NBAS by the examiner create opportunities to emphasize the infant's capabilities and to facilitate reciprocal interaction between parents and their infant. The model assumes that the parents and newborn are dynamically inseparable and that the family and infant require individualized attention. The examiner selects the behaviors and interactions with the infant that will have the most positive impact on establishing a parental–infant bond. During the examination, the examiner identifies infant strengths and builds on these successful strategies the infant is demonstrating and can also identify the infant's efforts to comfort and self-console. The examiner facilitates/guides parents to be most responsive to their infant. Anticipated areas of concern are addressed, and parents are encouraged to understand and communicate with their infant in ways that promote understanding of individual behavioral needs and communications. It is important to point out for parents when their infant is positively interacting with them and strategies they can use to support their infant. This can be an important opportunity to increase attachment between the infant and their parents.

The NBAS focuses on motor responses and maturity, interactive skills, visual and auditory orientation, management of sleep–wake cycles, and physiologic integrity and reflexes.[29,51] Self-quieting activity is highlighted, and parents learn how their infant can calm himself by bringing hands to mouth, sucking, looking, and changing position. If a baby cannot self-console, the nurse points out cues that signal stress or disorganization. Parents can then be aware of when their infant is stressed and modulate their reactions. Parents can be shown how to watch for stress cues and how to intervene without either overwhelming the infant with too much stimulation or failing to offer enough intervention to soothe.

The examination is structured with a preferred order of presentation of items. The infant's state plays a major role in the evaluation; therefore, observing the state of consciousness becomes the starting point. This sample evaluation using the NBAS describes some of the major responses of a healthy term newborn, but space does not permit description of the entire examination.

Initially, the examiner evaluates state of consciousness by observing respirations, eye movements, startles, and body movements. A specific scoring system is utilized to describe the initial state and the predominant states throughout the examination. The range and variety of state changes are noted. Once state is observed, habituation is evaluated. Habituation is the degree to which the nervous system reduces or inhibits responsiveness to a repeated stimulus until shutdown. Typically, the examination begins with the infant asleep or in a drowsy state. A flashlight is passed across the sleeping infant's closed eyes up to 10 times, and the degree of response and response decrement are noted. The assessment is repeated with a rattle and then a bell to note the infant's ability to shut out sound after repeated presentations. A typical response would be a startle or dramatic movement to the first stimulus, followed by decreasing responses to each of the remaining nine presentations of the stimulus. A range of responses is possible, but overall, one would like to see the infant react strongly at first and then show a reduction of responses over time. Next, the supine sleeping infant is uncovered slowly and the response to this change is noted. One may see no change, postural changes, color or breathing changes, or state changes. Next, a series of reflexes is evaluated with the infant still in a supine position. First, the reflexes of the hands and feet are evaluated, including plantar grasp, Babinski, heel prick, ankle clonus, passive tone in legs and arms, rooting response, sucking reflex, and glabella reflex. Each item is presented in a specific pattern with a watchful eye for change and variable responses.

Because the infant is supine, the examiner gently undresses the infant prior to assessing the palmar grasp and pull-to-sit reflexes. The infant is then picked up with his or her head facing away from the examiner, and standing and stepping reflexes are tested. The infant is then placed prone on the bed to evaluate the crawling reflex. Next, the infant is picked up to evaluate truncal incurvation. The infant is placed prone over the examiner's hand and raised in the air, and the examiner skillfully strokes along the right and left of the spine to evaluate for hip swing. The infant is then moved through space in a brisk manner, initially in an upright position, then in the horizontal position, and tonic deviation of head and eyes and nystagmus are assessed by eliciting the infant's vestibular reaction and neurobiologic capacities. These maneuvers also allow for observation of the degree and type of balance, and differentiation between relative extensor and flexor tone and posture. The infant is then held close to the examiner's body to evaluate cuddliness. A cloth is placed over the baby's eyes to evaluate attempts to remove it by swiping with the arms in a defensive movement pattern. Tonic neck reflex and Moro reflex are then tested.

By this time in the examination, the examiner can begin to define what is necessary to help this infant stay in a calm, alert state. When the infant is alert, the social interactive package can be administered. To set the stage for administration of these items, evaluate state, check room temperature and lighting, and have a comfortable chair available. Gently move the infant to the examiner's lap, providing postural support. Ideally, this change will not disrupt the alertness that has been achieved by the infant. The examiner then presents a red ball, a rattle, and the examiner's face alone, voice alone, and the two together. The responses evaluated are the degree of visual fixation, gazing, and any avoidance reactions, such as turning away, or nonresponsiveness. In addition, the examiner may see the degree of recognition of voice and sound in the infant's turning with head and/or eyes to "see" the sound off to the side of each ear.

Throughout the administration of these items, the examiner is vigilant in watching for state changes (e.g., change in the quality of alertness, becoming fussy, or crying). All state changes (if they last at least 15 seconds each) are recorded. The lability of crying and alertness are scored along with irritability. The degree of excitation and ease in consoling the infant are important (self-quieting and consolability). As crying or fussiness develops, the examiner does not immediately stop the cry, but gives the infant a chance to self-quiet, then offers a specific sequence of supports to see what level of support quiets the infant. The examiner watches for any attempts or strategies used by the infant to self-organize and quiet himself or herself (such as hands to mouth, bracing a foot, or sucking). The buildup to a full, intense cry state becomes important so the examiner can see the degree of self-quieting, as well as what it takes to calm the infant. If, at any time, any physiologic instability is observed, the examiner terminates the examination.

Throughout the examination, the examiner is scoring the infant's best performance. The examination moves from presentation of simple to more vigorous stimuli. A typical term newborn may show a variety of responses, from smooth responses that appear to come steadily and without cost or effort to vigorous activity levels with intense upset, demonstrating a need to be comforted. Some infants are more difficult to comfort than others. They may need specific levels of stimulation to elicit their ability to use the comforting resources available to them. A typical infant encompasses a wide range, and these responses can fall within normal limits.

Case Assessment of a Full-Term Infant

Newborn JF is a healthy 3-day-old newborn. Her mother, HF, had recovered from her delivery and was eager to get to know her baby but had been told that babies do not see well for the first few weeks. HF had many questions when the nurse came in to discuss JF with her. The nurse noted that JF's mother had already learned several things about her: how she liked to suck on her fist, what made her cry, and even how to calm her successfully. When the nurse pointed out JF's alertness and explained that JF could see her mother even at this early stage, HF seemed skeptical. The nurse suggested that because JF was awake now, HF should hold her in front of her and move her face out of JF's vision, call her name, and talk to her. As soon as JF heard her mother's voice, her eyes shifted in the direction of her mother's face. Encouraged to keep talking, HF was extremely pleased as JF continued to look and search until she found her mother's face and voice. As JF gazed at her mother, the nurse pointed out that if she kept JF's face within 10 to 12 inches of her own face, JF could focus and look (Figure 13.10). HF and JF sat gazing at each other, enthralled, for several minutes. After a few minutes, her nurse, who had remained quiet while letting them get to know each other, explained that JF could indeed see and even hear and look

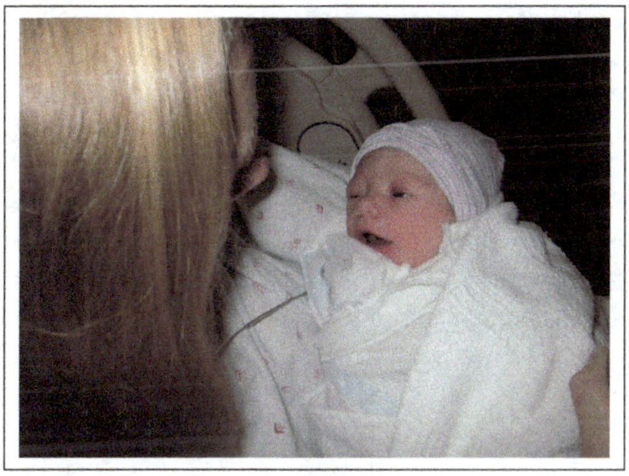

FIGURE 13.10 JF gazes at her mother's face

for her mother's voice and face. She suggested that this be a game they could play. HF was amazed and proud at the same time, marveling at her baby's capacity to interact at such an early age (Figure 13.11).

PRETERM INFANT BEHAVIOR ASSESSMENT

Als and associates developed an instrument for assessing the neurobehavioral development of the preterm infant. Their assessment of preterm infant behavior (APIB) examines the interplay of behaviors within five behavioral parameters (subsystems): *autonomic*, which refers to physiologically related changes such as pulse, respiration, skin color, and visceral responses; state, or state of consciousness on the continuum of sleep to wakefulness up to robust crying; *motor*, which assesses tone, posture, and movement patterns; *attention/interaction*, or the ability to attend and respond to the environment; and *self-regulatory*, the infants' efforts to cope with their experiences along with their ability to maintain state and self-console.[42,47] These parameters can be used to assess a preterm infant's current level of functioning as well as their ability to cope with the physical and social environment. It is important to note that the APIB is a dynamic, interactive examination that is provided by an examiner who is mindful of an infant's breathing/autonomic stability, and thus, the infant is facilitated to exhibit best performance. Once an infant's coping ability and organization are assessed, an individualized plan of care that is unique to the infant can be developed.[42,47]

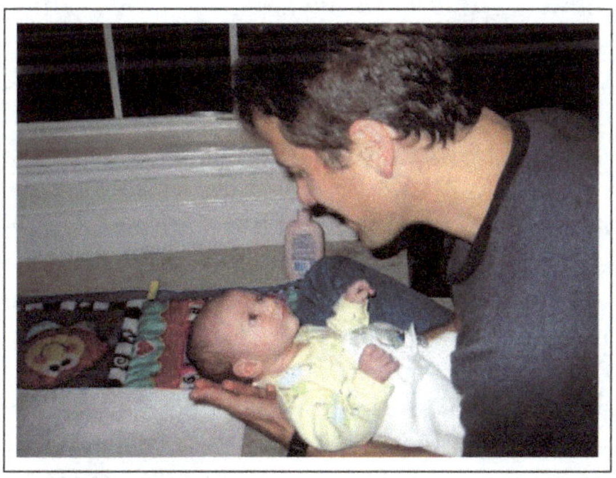

FIGURE 13.11 JF gazes at her father's face in full alert state

The assessment seeks to describe the unique way in which each infant interacts, copes with, and integrates experience from their environment. The interplay of behaviors is evaluated along with the degree of organization rather than maturation of the central nervous system as the focus; in this model, the preterm infant is seen as being in continuous interaction with the environment. The degree of facilitation by the examiner is also integrated into the scoring.

The APIB assessment is intended to identify an infant's current level of balanced and smooth integrated functioning (competence). In other words, identifying in which situations and with what supports the infant appears to function smoothly and is relaxed and comfortable and that enable the caretaker to promote modulated, organized behavior. The purpose of this assessment is to enable the examiner to describe the threshold of disorganization indicated in the infant's behaviors of defense and avoidance. The degree and kind of stress and intensity of frustration or defense that the infant experiences can be indicators of the degree of energy the infant has available. The assessment will show whether there is any leeway in the infant's responses. For example, can the infant tolerate being turned over to supine from prone (where he is flexed, tucked, and resting calmly) without demonstrating disorganized behaviors such as extended arms and hands, grimaces, and fussiness, or does the infant lose energy and become depleted with vestibular input of changing positions? What is the relationship between the infant's breathing and movement patterns? Does the infant stretch and squirm in an attempt to steady his or her breathing? Does the infant pause in breathing as he stretches and squirms? If the infant cannot display organized behavior when being handled sensitively, the infant may require greater facilitation before, during, and after caregiving interactions. As with the NBAS, training is required to become proficient at administering the APIB examination. However, an awareness of various behavior dynamics will increase the untrained examiner's ability to assess the infant's well-being and provide appropriate interventions.

Case Assessment of a Healthy Preterm Infant

Assessing the organizational function of a healthy preterm newborn follows much the same approach as examining the term infant, yet responses may be quite different. In the following example, LK represents a healthy, preterm newborn of an appropriate weight for gestational age when the infant was delivered at 33 weeks gestational age and who is now 36 weeks PMA. The infant is doing well with minimal respiratory support, is breastfed every 2 to 4 hours, and is bedded in a bassinet.

As the examiner begins the evaluation of this infant, she is positioned supine and loosely swaddled to support flexed, midline postures. Her hips and legs are tucked in close. One of the infant's hands is placed on top of her face, and the other arm is extended along the side of her body. LK is breathing regularly and has stable oxygen saturation levels. Her face is pink, and she is in a deep sleep. Her nicely flexed body position, regular breathing, and good color indicate organized sleep. The examination begins by assessing the habituation responses by passing a flashlight across the infant's eyes, which yields an intense startle at the first shine, followed by brief squirming and a return to sleep. The second and third flashes trigger a slightly delayed but less intense response. The fourth flash yields a cycle of activity starting with the startle, and then all arms and legs extend, followed by a brief stoppage and then a recycling of less intense movements. The next flash yields a facial movement only, and then stillness. LK's breathing is regular, but her face is now pale around her eyes and nose. The next two flashes produce no response. Thus, LK had some difficulty inhibiting the motor arousal with one cycle of response but was able to eventually settle and sustain sleep and shut out the remaining light stimuli. Using a rattle as an auditory sound stimulus, the examiner repeats a similar sequence of 10 trials. The first response shows a brief movement, with subsequent responses subsiding, and eventually LK successfully inhibits her motor response. The second auditory stimulus of a bell produces no response, and she remains asleep. This means that the sequence can end because she has shut down successfully. These are appropriate habituation responses for a healthy, preterm newborn.

The next part of the assessment evaluates movement, posture, and tone. The examiner begins by placing LK on her back. As she is touched, her color changes across her face, her hands become blue, and her trunk appears mottled. She makes jerky arm and leg movements in all directions; she awakens and squirms. The examiner places her hand on the soles of LK's feet and contains them, allowing the leg movements to slow, which softens the arm movements. As the examiner bends over the infant and talks quietly, her eyes open and the infant also quiets and fixates on the examiner's face.

Now that LK is calmer and is able to use motor inhibition to quiet her state and movement pattern, the examiner touches the sole of the infant's foot and begins a series of reflexive tests. As LK's feet are touched, she once again becomes active with uncontrolled activity of arms, legs, and trunk, resulting in prolonged tremors. The infant also begins breathing irregularly, and her color changes, so that face and body appear very pale then get quite red. She does not fuss or cry, but the examiner's tactile stimulation has aroused the motor system beyond the infant's capacity to regain any control on her own. As LK is placed on her abdomen, she squirms and attempts to regain control. By pressing her feet against the bottom wall of the bassinet and putting her hands to her face, the infant inhibits the squirming and motor movements. Her color and breathing once again come under control.

The examiner loosely wraps LK with her arms out of the blankets and lifts her to assess social skills. The examiner places LK on her lap with her face about 12 inches away from the infant. LK opens her eyes wide and actively avoids looking at the examiner, turning her gaze away. The examiner speaks softly and now keeps her face unavailable and out of LK's visual field. LK seems to relax, and her hands open and close rhythmically, her face softens, her mouth begins to purse, and eventually the infant turns her head in the direction of the voice. As LK continues to focus, looking and staying alert, her arms, hands, and head lift toward the examiner in a generalized movement of approach. At this approach's height, she yawns and sneezes, then settles into a drowsy state. Then the examiner presents the rattle to LK and sees a different response. She startles, frowns, and her face becomes pale. The examiner presents the sound again, but more softly, and the infant turns her head and eyes to the left, in the direction of the sound. LK appears more relaxed and with great effort shifts her eyes to search in the direction of the rattle. Even though her movements remain smooth, she becomes paler and frowns again, indicating the cost of this maneuver to her nervous system.

These responses indicate that although LK can process and respond to the stimulus, it is very taxing for her. Being held wrapped in a blanket and being placed on the examiner's lap helps LK respond more competently. She shows her ability to be selective, choosing the animate social voice of the examiner to turn to and avoiding the more difficult inanimate auditory stimulus of the rattle. LK's responses give the overall impression of a well-organized, healthy preterm newborn. LK can communicate within a wide range of behaviors in which she can function smoothly without stressing her overall well-being. Her sleep is stable, and her ability to process both visual and auditory stimuli indicates that she can handle stimuli without becoming upset or irritable. With the onset of a stimulus that is too loud, LK's autonomic system is taxed, and she becomes pale, but the assistance of being wrapped and supportiveness on the examiner's lap, along with a slower presentation of the stimulus, afford LK an opportunity to smoothly regulate her motor and autonomic systems. LK is able to avoid overwhelming input with some degree of specificity by rejecting taxing and costly stimulation.

If LK is provided with a supportive environment, several developmental achievements can be predicted for the next 2 to 3 months. First, her intense sensitivity to activity will lessen, and her autonomic nervous system will mature to a degree so that sleep and wakefulness will become more regular. LK can open her eyes and interact with her caregivers yet is easily taxed and moves past her threshold for stimulation as she closes her eyes and withdraws from the interaction. She demonstrates the capacity for consistent modulation of the ability to self-regulate as seen with her alertness and interactivity when the stimulation is appropriate. The facilitation and timing of the stimulus by the examiner are pivotal to eliciting the infant's best performance. As LK's organization increases, the examiner should see arousal of her motor system after tactile stimulation lessens. LK has demonstrated that she can modulate her arousal when the examiner provides containment (putting her hands on the infant's feet, wrapping her, and letting her press her feet against a surface). LK has also shown that her movements become smoother when motor arousal is diminished. Additional signs of motor organization include the ability to bring fingers to mouth and to fold hands under chin and keep them together. The infant is also demonstrating the ability to make a transition from one state to another without becoming upset. Figures 13.12 to 13.18 show LK in an organized state and a disorganized state, with some instances of infant cues.

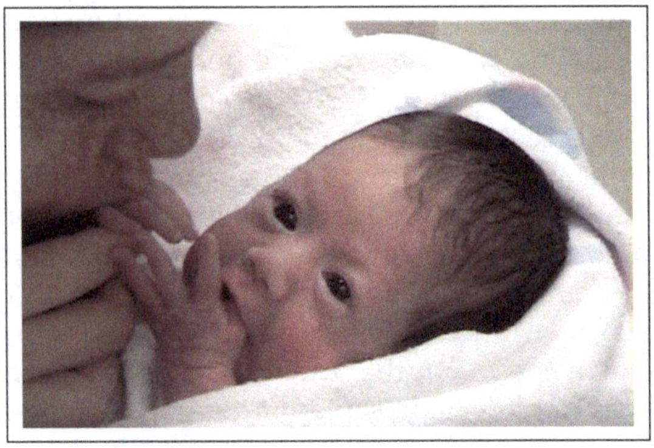

FIGURE 13.12 Containment helps the preterm infant to stay organized

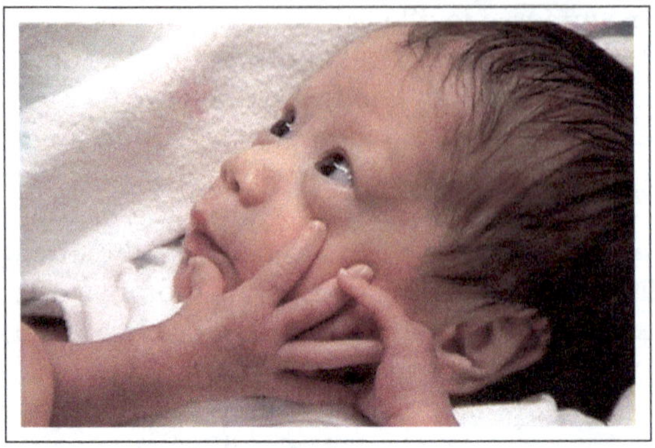

FIGURE 13.13 Alert state

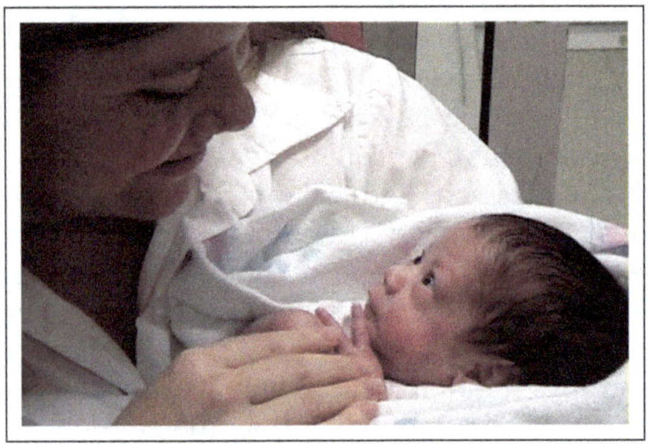

FIGURE 13.14 Organized preterm infant

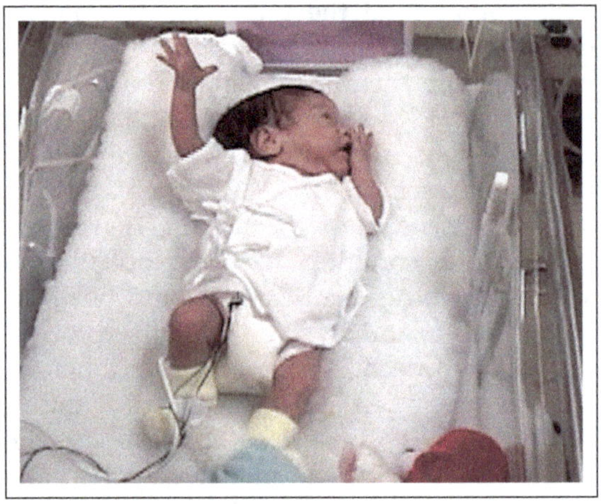

FIGURE 13.15 Disorganized preterm infant

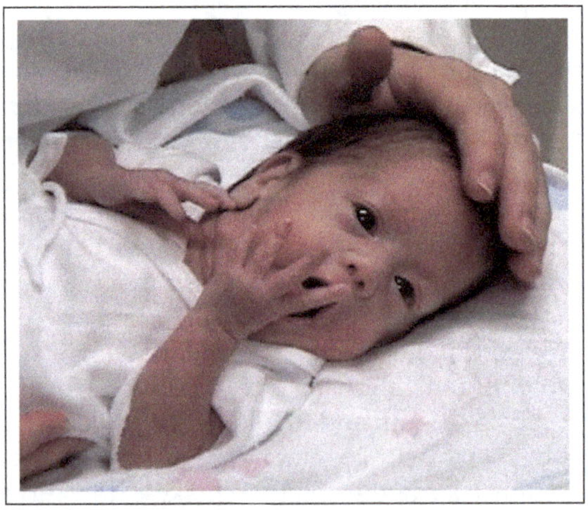

FIGURE 13.16 Disorganized preterm infant

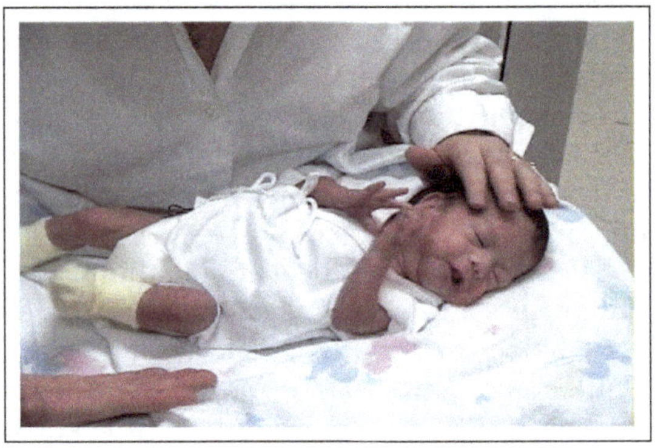

FIGURE 13.17 Disorganized preterm infant unable to cope with outside stimulation

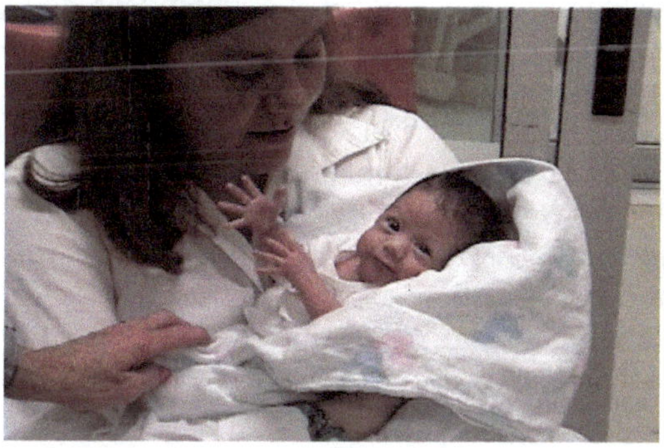

FIGURE 13.18 Preterm infant signals it is time for a pause

Case Assessments of Immature Preterm Infants

Some infants can show a range of immature or overly sensitive responses to interactions and environmental stimuli. At one extreme of the continuum of preterm functioning is MJ, a hyperreactive infant who reacts to all stimuli, lacking any ability to shut them out and protect himself. MJ appears to be "at the mercy of the stimuli," and his autonomic system pays a severe cost in terms of stress.[52,53] He overreacts to sound or to being touched with a series of startles and limb extensions, followed by uncontrollable flailing, arching, and squirming. Soon MJ is in a challenging cycle that goes on until he either stops breathing or drops his oxygen saturation level or heart rate. This is costly to him because it uses energy and delays his ability to consolidate the regulation of his motor and state systems.[38,46] MJ's high reactivity interferes with his growth and may lead to failure to thrive.

Unlike MJ, the hyperreactive preterm infant JL is a lethargic, withdrawn, or depleted infant who lies still and does not respond to stimuli.[42,47] This preterm newborn appears to want to preserve his fragile autonomic regulation. Because JL is past his thresholds and is depleted, he has little energy for interaction. His behavioral responses will be subtle and difficult to interpret as you attempt to interact with him. The challenge for JL is that this pattern of withdrawal does not facilitate his ability to develop or activate new pathways to take in new information. Therefore, he develops a rigid pattern of minimal range of behavioral responses. Autonomic behaviors, such as heart rate and oxygen saturation levels, will often fluctuate. This infant's presentation is very concerning, and his developmental trajectory is guarded.

Some premature infants exhibit a combination of these two types of response patterns, demonstrating an overreactive range of sensitivity at times and later becoming unavailable if overwhelmed by the constant sensory stimuli within the environment. In some disorganized infants, the pattern of protest takes the form of resistant squirms, turning away, pushing away, and avoidance behaviors while being held. These behaviors can be channeled into a more modulated level of interaction if the caregiver slowly introduces caregiving activities, allowing the infant time to ease into them.[47] For example, the caregiver can pause to allow the infant the opportunity to steady his or her breathing or regain energy during an interaction.

An appropriate behavioral assessment describes the infant's abilities to utilize intervention support and delineates the types of facilitation necessary to ensure smooth functioning. As the infant is supported to actively participate in the interaction despite a taxing sensory environment, the caregiver can articulate the infant's neurobehavioral agenda and emerging competence. Recognizing the infant's efforts to cope with stress and regain modulation leads to the infant's evolving behavioral agenda.[38,47]

The ability to understand and reveal the infant's full range of responses becomes essential when parents of a newborn infant begin to read behaviors as meaningful communications. The nurse's role is to help parents become attuned to the infant's responses and to facilitate their developing relationship. If parents can interpret the behaviors and understand the infant's messages, they can use strategies, such as reciprocity, to enhance the infant's competence. When parents and caregivers can support the infant based on behavioral cues, the infant is more successful and competent and can improve overall level of functioning while caregivers continue to develop their understanding of the infant's unique individuality as further maturation develops.

OTHER EMERGING INFANT ASSESSMENT TOOLS

There are several other infant assessment tools available. Previously a systematic review completed by Noble and Boyd found 27 different infant assessment instruments available in the literature for use in the newborn period (up to 4 months corrected age).[54] However, they chose only eight assessment instruments to include in their review—those that had good reliability in prediction, discrimination, and evaluation of change.[54] The Brazelton and APIB as described earlier were among those chosen. Other instruments found to be of high quality included the Test of Infant Motor Performance (TIMP),[52] the NICU Network Neurobehavioral Scale (NNNS),[34] Prechtl's Assessment of General Movements (GMs),[53] Neurobehavioral Assessment of the Preterm Infant (NAPI),[55] Dubowitz neurologic assessment of the preterm and full-term infant (Dubowitz),[56] and Neuromotor Behavioral Assessment (NMBA).[57] The GMs and Dubowitz are well known and described as primarily neurologic system assessments rather than behavioral assessments and as such are discussed elsewhere in this text. Each of the others is appraised in the following with some of the unique examination characteristics, psychometric properties, and clinical utility that might be of interest to those considering use of these assessments. These descriptions are not exhaustive but are considered an introduction to the different options available for discriminating infant behaviors.

Each of the instruments chosen in the review was found to have adequate content validity;[54] however, the TIMP created by Campbell was found to be suitable to be used as an outcome measure. This could be important if the instrument is being used to demonstrate effectiveness of previously delivered interventions. The TIMP is a standardized instrument for assessing neuromotor development in infants between 34 weeks PMA and 4 months postterm.[58] The TIMP includes 13 observation and 28 elicited items. The TIMP is an age-sensitive measure of motor performance that can differentiate for high and low risk of poor infant motor outcomes and has excellent psychometric properties.[56] Reliable administration of the TIMP requires extensive training. Primarily, physical or occupational therapists become reliable in the scoring when used for prediction or outcome measures. The NAPI has some similarities to the TIMP; however, it was developed only for use with preterm infants, whereas the TIMP can be used across infant groups. This makes the TIMP useful for comparison across populations.[58] The NAPI was designed to measure the progression of neurobehavioral performance in the preterm infant 32 weeks PMA to term.[52] Training to administer the NAPI is extensive but not as formalized as with some of the other assessment tools. The NMBA has less utility since its scoring is only reliable from 30 to 36 weeks PMA and was developed to identify preterm infants at risk for developmental delays. It is interesting that no formal training is required for the NMBA, not the extensive training required for other instruments. Only the TIMP and the NAPI have published preterm norms, and these two instruments may be better suited for clinical utility than other well-designed infant assessments available.

There has been a surge in the literature over the past few years, addressing the many components and complexities of infant neurobehavioral assessments, especially with the NNNS. This assessment has been utilized in research as well as within clinical settings and was designed to measure the infant's biobehavioral organizations as a valid biomarker for detecting at-risk infants, with the ability to predict developmental outcomes.[34,59,60] The NNNS examines both neurologic integrity as well as behavioral functioning and scores a full range of infant neurobehavioral performance that was intended to have broad applicability.[34] The standardized nature of the NNNS does not embody optimal performance criteria as a foundational principle and uses the integrity of the infant's innate organization to identify neurobehavioral patterns as an objective format. During the NNNS, the order of the items administered is more structured, and the emphasis to bring out the "best" in the infant is less apparent. The administration of the NNNS is completed in about 20 to 30 minutes and is scored easily by an experienced examiner. The examination is primarily state dependent and follows a relatively invariant sequence. This does not mean that the examiner disregards the infant's behavior and simply completes the maneuvers to the infant's detriment. The examiner is expected to read the infant's states and behaviors to develop a rapport with the infant that ensures the infant's active participation. Measurable antecedents of later developmental outcomes can be detected with neonatal neurobehavior using the NNNS.[60,61] The NNNS assessment is a valid, predictive biomarker for articulating high-risk infant neurobehavioral functioning. The infants' neurobehavioral patterns revealed by the NNNS, particularly presence of increased excitability, arousal, hypertonicity, and stress behaviors associated with lower quality of movement scores, orientation, and self-regulation, have been shown to be predictive of adverse outcomes.[61] The NNNS can be used with high-risk infants 34 to 44 weeks PMA and is easily administered in the NICU. It is imperative to acknowledge the concept of behavioral regulation, which is considered to be reflective of the infant's level of higher functioning and may be missed with routine neurological examinations.[34] The NNNS is a valuable tool available to nurses and other healthcare professionals who work with preterm infants to provide a strategy for obtaining accurate information about the infant's strengths and vulnerabilities.[60,61] Ideally, a behavioral assessment is completed prior to the infant's hospital discharge and incorporates the findings into the infant's medical discharge exam to identify infants most at risk for developmental delays to facilitate appropriate early-intervention services.

SUMMARY

An infant's behavioral patterns may be subtle and difficult to elicit and interpret, yet observing behavior is an integral part of a comprehensive newborn examination. The behavioral assessment allows the examiner an opportunity to evaluate aspects of the infant's neurologic status and helps establish guidelines for an individualized developmental plan of care for both term and preterm infants. Behavioral assessments can also be used to encourage parents to identify and respond to their newborn's behavioral cues and signals. Behavioral assessment provides an opportunity to consider the infant as a whole individual—an approach that enhances infant competencies and supports the infant–parent relationship.

ADDITIONAL RESOURCES

SPRINGER PUBLISHING CONNECT™

A robust set of resources designed to supplement this text is located at http://connect.springerpub.com/content/book/978-0-8261-4063-0. Qualifying instructors may request access by emailing textbook@springerpub.com.

REFERENCES

1. Romberg J, Wilke M, Allgaier C, Nägele T, Engel C, Poets C, and Franz A. 2022. MRI-based brain volumes of preterm infants at term: A systematic review and meta-analysis. *Archives of Disease in Childhood. Fetal and Neonatal Edition* 107(5): 520–526. doi: 10.1136/archdischild-2021-322846
2. Hodel A, Senich K, Jokinen C, Sasaon O, Morris A, and Thomas K. 2017. Early executive function differences in infants born moderate to late preterm. *Early Human Development* 113: 23–30. doi: 10.1016/j.earlhumdev.2017.07.007
3. Spittle A, and Treyvaud K. 2016. The role of early developmental intervention to influence neurobehavioral outcomes of children born preterm.

Seminars in Perinatology 40: 542–548. doi: 10.1053/j.semperi.2016.09.006

4. Loeb D, Imgrund C, Lee J, and Barlow S. 2020. Language, motor, and cognitive outcomes of toddlers who were born preterm. *American Journal of Speech-Language Pathology* 29(2): 625–637. doi: 10.1044/2019_AJSLP-19-00049
5. McGowan E, Hofheimer J, O'Shea T, Kilbride H, Carte, B, Check J, Helderman J, Nea C, Pastyrnak S, Smith L, Camerota M, Dansereau L, Della Grotta S, and Lester B. 2022. Analysis of neonatal neurobehavior and developmental outcomes among preterm infants. *Journal American Medical Association* 5(7): e2222249. doi: 10.1001/jamanetworkopen.2022.22249
6. O'Reilly H, Johnson S, Ni Y, Wolke D, and Marlow N. 2020. Neuropsychological outcomes at 19 years of age following extreme preterm birth. *Pediatrics* 145(2): e20192087. doi: 10.1542/peds.2019-2087
7. Chan E, Leong P, Malouf R, and Quigley M. 2016. Long-term cognitive and school outcomes of late preterm and early term births: A systematic review. *Child: Care, Health & Development* 42(3): 297–312. doi: 10.1111/cch.12320
8. Allotey J, Zamora J, Cheong-See F, Kalidindi M, Arroyo-Manzano D, Asztalos E, … Thangaratinam S. 2018. Cognitive, motor, behavioural and academic performances of children born preterm: A meta-analysis and systematic review involving 64 061children. *International Journal of Obstetrics and Gynaecology* 125: 16–25. doi: 10.1111/1471-0528.14832
9. Zhao T, Mishra V, Jeon T, Ouyang M, Peng Q, Chalak L, Wisnowski J, Heyne R, Rollins N, Shu N, and Huang H. 2019. Structural network maturation of the preterm human brain. *NeuroImage* 185: 699–710. doi: 10.1016/j.neuroimage.2018.06.047
10. Linsell L, Johnson S, Wolke D, Morris J, Kurinczuk J, and Marlow N. 2019. Trajectories of behavior, attention, social and emotional problems from childhood to early adulthood following extremely preterm birth: A prospective cohort study. *European Child Adolescent Psychiatry* 28(4): 531–542. doi: 10.1007/s00787-018-1219-8
11. Duncan A, and Matthews M. 2018. Neurodevelopmental outcomes in early childhood. *Clinics in Perinatology* 45(3): 377–392. doi: 10.1016/j.clp.2018.05.001
12. Anderson J, Rogers E, Baer R, Oltman S, Paynter R, Partridge J, Rand L, Jelliffe-Pawlowski L, and Steurer M. 2018. Racial and ethnic disparities in preterm infant mortality and severe morbidity: A population-based study. *Neonatology* 113(1): 44–54. doi: 10.1159/000480536
13. Beck A, Edwards E, Horbar J, Howell E, McCormick M, and Pursley D. 2020. The color of health: How racism, segregation, and inequality affect the health and well-being of preterm infants and their families. *Pediatric Research* 87(2): 227–234. doi: 10.1038/s41390-019-0513-6
14. CDC. Premature birth. 2022. Retrieved from https://www.cdc.gov/reproductivehealth/features/premature-birth/index.html
15. Als H, Duffy FH, McAnulty GB, Rivkin MJ, Vajapeyam S, Mulkern RV, Warfield SK, Huppi PS, Butler SC, Conneman N, Fischer C, and Eichenwald EC. 2004. Early experience alters brain function and structure. *Pediatrics* 113(4): 846–857.
16. Ohlsson A, and Jacobs S. 2013. NIDCAP: A systematic review and meta-analysis. *Pediatrics* 131(3): 881–893.
17. McAnulty G, Duffy F, Kosta S, Weisenfeld N, Warfield S, Butler S, Alidoos M, Bernstein J, Robertson R, Zurakowski D, and Als H. 2013. School-age effects of the newborn individualized developmental care and assessment program for preterm infants with intrauterine growth restriction: Preliminary findings. *BMC Pediatrics* 13: 25. doi: 10.1186/1471-2431-13-25
18. Aita M, De Clifford Faugère G, Lavallée A, Feeley N, Stremler R, Rioux É, and Proulx M. 2021. Effectiveness of interventions on early neurodevelopment of preterm infants: A systematic review and meta-analysis. *BMC Pediatrics* 21(1): 210. doi: 10.1186/s12887-021-02559-6
19. Roque A, Lasiuk G, Radünz V, and Hegadoren K. 2017. Scoping review of the mental health of parents of infants in the NICU. *Journal of Obstetric, Gynecologic, and Neonatal Nursing: JOGNN* 46(4): 576–587. doi: 10.1016/j.jogn.2017.02.005
20. Cheong J, Burnett A, Treyvaud K, and Spittle A. 2020. Early environment and long-term outcomes of preterm infants. *Journal of Neural Transmission (Vienna, Austria: 1996)* 127(1): 1–8. doi: 10.1007/s00702-019-02121-w
21. Golds L, Gillespie-Smith K, Nimbley E, and MacBeth A. 2022. What factors influence dyadic synchrony? A systematic review of the literature on predictors of mother–infant dyadic processes of shared behavior and affect. *Infant Mental Health Journal* 43(5): 808–830. doi: 10.1002/imhj.22011
22. Kostandy R, and Ludington-Hoe S. 2019. The evolution and the science of kangaroo mother care (skin-to-skin contact). *Birth Defects Research* 111(15): 1032–1043. doi: 10.1002/bdr2.1565
23. Linnér A, Westrup B, Lode-Kolz K, Klemming S, Lillieskold S, Markhus Pike H, Morgan B, Bergman N, Rettedal S, and Jonas W. 2020. Immediate parent–infant skin-to-skin study (IPISTOSS): Study protocol of a randomised controlled trial on very preterm infants cared for in skin-to-skin contact immediately after birth and potential physiological, epigenetic, psychological and neurodevelopmental consequences. *Brittish Medical Journal Open* 10(7): e038938. doi: 10.1136/bmjopen-2020-038938
24. Vittner D, Butle S, Smith K, Makris N, Brownel, E, Samra H, and McGrath J. 2019. Parent engagement correlates with parent and preterm infant oxytocin release during skin-to-skin contact. *Advances in Neonatal Care* 19(1): 73–79. doi: 10.1097/ANC.0000000000000558
25. Shattnawi K, and Al-Ali N. 2019. The effect of short duration skin to skin contact on premature infants'

physiological and behavioral outcomes: A quasi-experimental study. *Journal Pediatric Nursing* 46: e24–e28. doi: 10.1016/j.pedn.2019.02.005
26. Akbari E, Binnoon-Erez N, Rodrigues M, Ricci A, Schneider J, Madigan S, and Jenkins J. 2018. Kangaroo mother care and infant biopsychosocial outcomes in the first year: A meta-analysis. *Early Human Development* 122: 22–31. doi: 10.1016/j.earlhumdev.2018.05.004
27. Vittner D, McGrath J, Robinson J, Lawhon G, Cusson R, Eisenfeld L, Walsh S, Young E, and Cong X. 2018. Increases in oxytocin from skin-to-skin contact enhances development of parent–infant relationships. *Biological Research for Nursing* 20(1): 54–62. doi: 10.1177/1099800417735633
28. Feldman R. 2015. Sensitive periods in human social development: New insights from research on oxytocin, synchrony and high-risk parenting. *Development and Psychopathology* 27: 369–395. doi: 10.1017/S0954579415000048
29. Brazelton TB, and Nugent JK. 2011. *The Neonatal Behavioral Assessment Scale (Clinics in Developmental Medicine, No. 190)*, 4th ed. London, UK: MacKeith Press.
30. Vohr B. 2019. The importance of parent presence and involvement in the single-family room and open-bay NICU. *Acta Paediatrica (Oslo, Norway: 1992)* 108(6): 986–988. doi: 10.1111/apa.14783
31. Cong X, Wu J, Vittner D, Xu W, Hussain N, Galvin S, Fitzsimons M, McGrath J, and Henderson W. 2017. The impact of cumulative pain/stress on neurobehavioral development of preterm infants in the NICU. *Early Human Development* 108: 9–16. doi: 10.1016/j.earlhumdev.2017.03.003
32. Sannino P, Giannì ML, De Bon G, Fontana C, Picciolini O, Plevani L, Fumagalli M, Consonni D, and Mosca F. 2016. Support to mothers of premature babies using NIDCAP methods: A non-randomized controlled trial. *Early Human Development* 95: 15–20.
33. Macho P. 2017. Individualized developmental care in the NICU: A concept analysis. *Advances in Neonatal Care* 17(3): 162–174. doi: 10.1097/ANC.0000000000000374
34. Lester BM, and Tronick EZ. 2005. *NICU Network Neurobehavioral Scale (NNNS) Manual*. Baltimore, MD: Brookes.
35. Anderson CJ. 1981. Enhancing reciprocity between mother and neonate. *Nursing Research* 30(2): 89–93.
36. Holditch-Davis D, and Blackburn ST. 2014. Neurobehavioral development. In *Comprehensive Neonatal Nursing Care*, 5th ed. Kenner C, and Lott JW, eds. New York: Springer Publishing Company, 689–721.
37. Park J. 2020. Sleep promotion for preterm infants in the NICU. *Nursing for Women's Health* 24(1): 24–35. doi: 10.1016/j.nwh.2019.11.004
38. Als H, Lester BM, Tronick EZ, and Brazelton TB. 1982. Manual for the assessment of preterm infant's behavior. In *Theory and Research in Behavioral Pediatrics*, Fitzgerald HE, Lester BM, and Yogman MW, eds. New York, NY: Plenum Press, 65–132.
39. Vittner D, DeMeo S, Vallely J, Parker M, Baxter A, and McGrath J. 2022. Factors that influence NICU health care professionals decision making to implement family-centered care. *Advances in Neonatal Care* 22(1): 87–94. doi: 10.1097/ANC.0000000000000846
40. McPherson C, Miller S, El-Dib M, Massaro A, and Inder T. 2020. The influence of pain, agitation, and their management on the immature brain. *Pediatric Research* 88(2): 168–175. doi: 10.1038/s41390-019-0744-6
41. Malak R, Fechner B, Sikorska D, Rosołek M, Mojs E, Samborski W, and Baum E. 2021. Application of the neonatal behavioral assessment scale to evaluate the neurobehavior of preterm neonates. *Brain Sciences* 11(10): 1285. doi: 10.3390/brainsci11101285
42. Als H, Lester BM, Tronick EZ, and Brazelton TB. 1982. Assessment of preterm infant behavior (APIB). In *Theory and Research in Behavioral Pediatrics*, Fitzgerald HE, and Yogman M, eds. New York, NY: Plenum Press, vol. 1, 63–133.
43. Burstein O, Zevin Z, and Geva R. 2021. Preterm birth and the development of visual attention during the first 2 years of life: A systematic review and meta-analysis. *JAMA Network Open* 4(3): e213687. doi: 10.1001/jamanetworkopen.2021.3687
44. Gorski P, Lewkowicz D, and Huntington L. 1987. Advances in neonatal and infant behavioral assessment: Toward a comprehensive evaluation of early patterns of development. *Journal of Developmental and Behavioral Pediatrics* 8(1): 39–50.
45. Carlier M, and Harmony T. 2020. Development of auditory sensory memory in preterm infants. *Early Human Development* 145: 105045. doi: 10.1016/j.earlhumdev.2020.105045
46. White R, and Consensus Committee on Recommended Design Standards for Advanced Neonatal Care. 2020. Recommended standards for newborn ICU design, 9th edition. *Journal of Perinatology: Official Journal of the California Perinatal Association* 40(Suppl 1): 2–4. doi: 10.1038/s41372-020-0766-2
47. Als H. 2022. *Manual for the Naturalistic Observation of Newborn Behavior: Preterm and Full Term Infants*. Boston, MA: The Children's Hospital, 1–16.
48. Brazelton TB, and Nugent JK. 1995. *Neonatal Behavioral Assessment Scale*, 3rd ed. London, UK: Mac Keith Press.
49. Shea S, Jester J, Huth-Bocks A, Weatherston D, Muzik M, Rosenblum K, and Michigan Collaborative for Infant Mental Health Research. 2020. Infant mental health home visiting therapists' reflective supervision self-efficacy in community practice settings. *Infant Mental Health Journal* 41(2): 191–205. doi: 10.1002/imhj.21834
50. Chess S, and Thomas A. 1992. Dynamics of individual behavioral development. In *Developmental and Behavioral Pediatrics*, 2nd ed. Levine MD, Carey WB, and Croker AC, eds. Philadelphia, PA: Saunders, 84–94.
51. Barlow J, Herath N, Bartram Torrance C, Bennett C, and Wei Y. 2018. The neonatal behavioral assessment scale (NBAS) and newborn behavioral

observations (NBO) system for supporting caregivers and improving outcomes in caregivers and their infants. *The Cochrane Database of Systematic Reviews* 3(3): CD011754. doi: 10.1002/14651858.CD011754.pub2

52. Campbell SK, and Hedeker D. 2001. Validity of the test of infant motor performance for discriminating among infants with varying risk for poor motor outcome. *Journal of Pediatrics* 139(4): 546–551.
53. Einspieler C, and Prechtl, HRF. 2005. Prechtl's assessment of general movements: A diagnostic tool for the functional assessment of the young nervous system. *Mental Retardation and Developmental Disability Research Reviews* 11(1): 61–67.
54. Noble Y, and Boyd R. 2012. Neonatal assessments for the preterm infant up to 4 months corrected age: A systematic review. *Developmental Medicine and Child Neurology* 54(2): 129–139. doi: 10.1111/j.1469-8749.2010.03903.x
55. Korner AF, and Constantinou JC. 2001. The neurobehavioral assessment of the preterm infant: Reliability and developmental and clinical validity. In *Biobehavioral Assessment of the Infant*, Singer LT, and Zeskine PS, eds. New York, NY: Guilford Press.
56. Dubowitz L, Ricciw D, and Merceri E. 2005. The Dubowitz neurological examination of the full-term newborn. *Mental Retardation and Developmental Disability Research Reviews* 11(1): 52–60.
57. Carmichael K, Burns Y, Gray P, and O'Callaghan M. 1997. Neuromotor behavioral assessment of preterm infants at risk for impaired development. *Australian Journal of Physiotherapy* 43(2): 101–107.
58. Campbell SK. 2005. The test of infant motor performance. In: *Test User's Manual Version 2.0*. Chicago, IL: Infant Motor Performance Scales.
59. Lester BM, Tronick EZ, LaGasse L, Seifer R, Bauer CR, Shankaran S, Bada HS, Wright LL, Smeriglio VL, Lu J, Finnegan LP, and Maza PL. 2002. The maternal lifestyle study: Effects of substance exposure during pregnancy on neurodevelopmental outcome in 1-month-old infants. *Pediatrics* 110(6): 1182–1192.
60. McGowan E, Hofheimer J, O'Shea T, Carter B, Helderman J, Neal C, Pastyrnak S, Smith L, Soliman A, Dansereau L, Della Grotta S, and Lester B. 2020. Sociodemographic and medical influences on neurobehavioral patterns in preterm infants: A multicenter study. *Early Human Development* 142: 104954. doi: 10.1016/j.earlhumdev.2020.104954
61. McGowan E, Hofheimer J, O'Shea T, Kilbride H, Carter B, Check J, Helderman J, Neal C, Pastyrnak S, Smith L, Camerota M, Dansereau L, Della Grotta S, and Leste B. 2022. Analysis of neonatal neurobehavior and developmental outcomes among preterm infants. *JAMA Network Open* 5(7): e2222249. doi: 10.1001/jamanetworkopen.2022.22249

14 ASSESSMENT OF THE INFANT WITH DYSMORPHIC FEATURES

Susan R. Meier and Erin Mestas

Most infants are born healthy, and the first clinical assessment usually reveals no physical abnormality. However, birth defects remain one of the leading causes of infant mortality in the United States. Every 4½ minutes a baby in the United States is born with a birth defect, and as of 2017, one in five infant deaths was attributed to a congenital abnormality.[1]

About 15% of all newborn babies will have at least one minor malformation (e.g., one that does not interfere with normal functioning), and these often go unnoticed. However, their presence should prompt the practitioner to look for a major malformation, as newborns with one or more minor malformations are more likely to have a major malformation (e.g., causes dysfunction or requires surgical correction). If there is one minor malformation, the incidence of an associated major anomaly is 3%; this increases to 11% in the presence of two minor malformations and to as high as 90% with the presence of three minor anomalies.[2] Fifty to 60% of human congenital anomalies are of unknown etiology, and approximately one third are caused by genetic factors. As high as 10% of birth defects are the result of environmental agents, viruses, or drugs.[3] An ever-growing number of malformation syndromes have been delineated using standard karyotype as well as newer genomic technologies including microarray, fluorescence in situ hybridization, gene sequencing, methylation tests, and polymerase chain reaction-based techniques.[3]

The identification of dysmorphic features during the initial physical examination is a crucial first step in the continuum of care for affected infants. A thorough, systematic approach by a skilled examiner can yield important findings and direct the healthcare team in providing timely and appropriate care for the infant, as well as resources for parents.

MATERNAL AND FAMILY HISTORIES

A complete maternal medical, gynecologic, and obstetric history should be constructed when evaluating the infant with dysmorphic features. A history of adverse pregnancy outcomes, including multiple miscarriages and stillbirths, can be an important risk factor. Maternal age should be documented because chromosomal anomalies, such as trisomy 21, occur more frequently with advancing maternal age. Pregnancies complicated by medical conditions, such as diabetes mellitus or hypertension, increase the possibility for fetal physical deformities. Prenatal exposure to teratogens, including medications, infections, chemicals, and illicit drugs, must be documented because certain agents cause specific structural abnormalities and functional diseases to be exhibited in the fetus. Critical periods of fetal development, dosage, and duration of exposure to the teratogen, and genotype of the embryo must also be taken into consideration.[2] Results of prenatal testing, including multiple marker serum screening, maternal serum alpha-fetoprotein testing, chorionic villus sampling, and amniocentesis, should be recorded to identify an increased risk or a confirmed diagnosis of fetal disorders such as neural tube defects and trisomies. In addition, cell-free DNA testing, also known as noninvasive prenatal testing, examines cell-free fetal DNA in the mother's circulation and can detect most aneuploidies and sex chromosome differences. Cell-free DNA testing is a screening test and is not diagnostic and should not be treated as such.[4]

A comprehensive maternal and paternal family history is also helpful. Many congenital anomalies and medical conditions can be inherited and place an infant at risk for the disorder. Some of these conditions include spina bifida; hydrocephalus; muscular dystrophy; cleft lip; cleft palate; congenital heart defects; polydactyly; clubfoot; congenital hip dislocation; deafness; blindness; childhood cataracts; cystic fibrosis; dwarfism; polycystic kidney disease; and stomach, bowel, or kidney defects.

There are also genetic disorders that occur more commonly within particular ethnic groups. Descendants of Ashkenazi Jewish or French-Canadian ancestors may have an increased risk for Tay–Sachs disease, an often fatal disorder marked by degeneration of brain tissue and the maculae of the retinas. Infants of African ancestry are at an increased risk for inheriting sickle cell disease, a serious condition of red blood cells that are distorted in shape and tend to clump together and occlude blood vessels. Thalassemia, a group of hemolytic anemias, is more prevalent in Mediterranean and Asian populations.

If one or both parents are of Jewish, French Canadian, African, Mediterranean, or Asian descent or if a medical condition occurs repeatedly in one of the partner's families, the couple may consider genetic testing prior to conceiving a child. If either partner is a carrier for a specific inheritable condition, the significance of the results can then be discussed with the couple's healthcare provider.

PHYSICAL EXAMINATION

The newborn infant should have a thorough physical examination within 24 hours of birth. This first examination may reveal more abnormalities than any subsequent routine examination done. First, the family, maternal, pregnancy, and perinatal histories are reviewed. The examination is performed in an area that is warm and quiet with good lighting. A systematic approach should be used. Although the exact examination sequence is not important, a consistent approach ensures that all aspects are evaluated. Assessment of gestational age should be included. Knowledge of gestational age can be important in interpreting physical findings, especially in infants noted to have intrauterine growth restriction (IUGR). Each body part should be examined with emphasis on size, shape, color, position, spacing, and symmetry.

Appearance and Posture

An inspection is made for deformations and obvious malformations. An abnormal facial appearance or other abnormalities in appearance can indicate a syndrome. The newborn's posture at rest usually reflects intrauterine position, sometimes called the *position of comfort*.

Skin

The skin is inspected for abnormalities. Areas of abnormal pigmentation, congenital nevi, hemangiomas, macular stains, or other unusual lesions should be noted.

Head

The shape and size of the head are inspected. The presence of abnormal hair, lacerations, abrasions or contusions, scalp defects, unusual lesions, or protuberances should be noted. An asymmetric skull that persists for longer than 2 to 3 days after birth or a palpable ridge along a suture line is abnormal and suggests craniosynostosis. Although it occurs in normal infants, craniotabes can be a pathologic finding with syphilis and rickets.

A large anterior fontanel may be associated with congenital hypothyroidism, osteogenesis imperfecta, IUGR, Down syndrome, achondroplasia, or other skeletal anomalies.[5]

Neck

The neck is assessed for masses, decreased mobility, and abnormalities. Cystic hygroma, the most common lymphatic malformation in newborns, typically presents as a painless mass superior to the clavicle that transilluminates. Redundant skin in the neck may be a feature of some genetic syndromes. Examples include Turner syndrome, in which the neck appears webbed due to redundant skin along the posterolateral line, and Down syndrome, with excess skin posteriorly at the base of the neck.

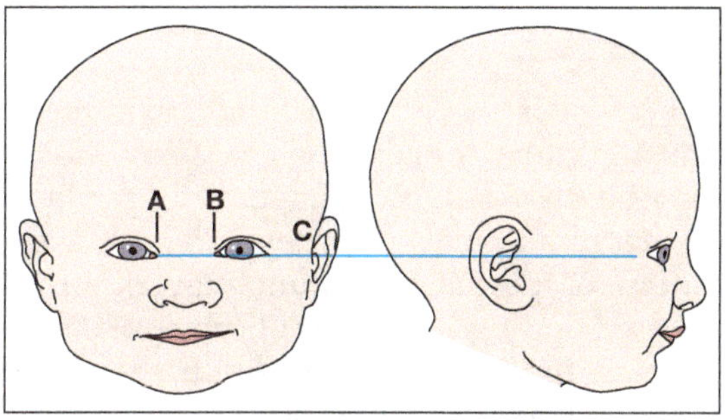

FIGURE 14.1 Ear placement

Source: From Halderman-Englert CR, Saitta SC, and Zackai EH. 2012. Evaluation of the dysmorphic infant. In *Avery's Diseases of the Newborn*, 9th ed. Gleason CA, and Devaskar SU, eds. Philadelphia, PA: Saunders, 189. Reprinted by permission.

Face

The face is examined for symmetry. Facial palsies and asymmetric crying facies are most obvious when the newborn is crying and may go unnoticed in the sleeping or quiet infant. Asymmetric crying facies are the result of hypoplasia or congenital absence of the depressor anguli muscle. Only the muscles controlling movement of one side of the mouth are affected, causing asymmetry of the face with crying. However, the muscles controlling movement of the upper face are normal; so, when the infant cries, the forehead wrinkles and both eyes close normally. Asymmetric crying facies have been associated with other anomalies, particularly those of the cardiovascular system.[6] Facial palsy may also be secondary to nerve compression during delivery, which can occur from a forceps-assisted delivery.

Eyes

If spacing appears abnormal, the distance between eyes can be measured and compared to standard values (see Figure 5.15). This part of the examination is especially important if other dysmorphic features that suggest a syndrome are present. The presence of epicanthal folds may be indicative of a syndrome, or based on ethnicity, a normal finding. The sclerae should be clear and white. If the sclerae appear deep blue, osteogenesis imperfecta should be considered. Glaucoma is manifested by a large cloudy cornea. Defects in the iris, such as coloboma, should be noted. Cataracts or retinoblastomas will present as a white pupil when the red reflex is assessed.

Ears

The ears are in normal position when the helix is intersected by a horizontal line drawn from the outer canthus of the eye perpendicular to the vertical axis of the head (Figure 14.1).[7] If the helix falls below this line, the ears are low set. An ear is posteriorly rotated if its vertical axis deviates more than 10 degrees from the vertical axis of the head. Malformations of the external ear are often associated with syndromes of multiple congenital anomalies that include renal malformations. The abnormalities may also indicate additional anomalies of the middle and inner ear associated with hearing loss.

Nose and Mouth

A depressed nasal bridge or an extremely thin or unusually broad nose may occur in some malformation syndromes. Clefts of the soft or hard palate are visible to inspection. Palpation may be needed to detect a submucosal cleft. Macroglossia, or enlargement of the tongue, can be seen with Beckwith–Wiedemann syndrome.

Chest

The chest is examined for size, symmetry, and structure. A malformed or small thorax may be the result of pulmonary hypoplasia or neuromuscular disorders. Pectus excavatum or pectus carinatum may occur as isolated findings or as part of congenital syndromes. Breast size and position should be noted, because widely spaced nipples occur with some genetic syndromes.

Abdomen

Asymmetry caused by congenital anomalies or masses may first be appreciated by observation. Abnormal, absent, or misplaced kidneys are assessed by using deep palpation (see Figures 10.2 and 10.3). Most abdominal masses in newborns are renal in origin.[8] A single umbilical artery is present in .05% to 5% of neonates, occurring more frequently in small-for-gestational-age (SGA) infants, premature infants, and twins.[9,10] Several large studies suggest that single umbilical artery is associated with increased risk for malformations, placental abnormalities, IUGR, and perinatal death.[11]

Genitalia

The genitalia are inspected immediately after birth to identify any potential abnormalities and the infant's sex (discussed in more detail in Chapter 10).

Females

The labia minora should be separated to detect whether the hymen, which normally has some opening, is imperforate. Enlargement of the uterus resulting from an imperforate hymen may be detected as a low midline abdominal mass.

Males

Hypospadias, ventral location of the meatus on the penis, is relatively common. The meatus may be located anywhere from the proximal glans to the perineum, with more severe cases having a more proximal meatus. Infants with perineal or scrotal hypospadias and those with hypospadias of any location accompanied by nonpalpable testes should be evaluated for disorders of sexual development (DSD) including congenital adrenal hyperplasia (CAH). Epispadias, dorsal location of the meatus, is uncommon and usually associated with bladder exstrophy.

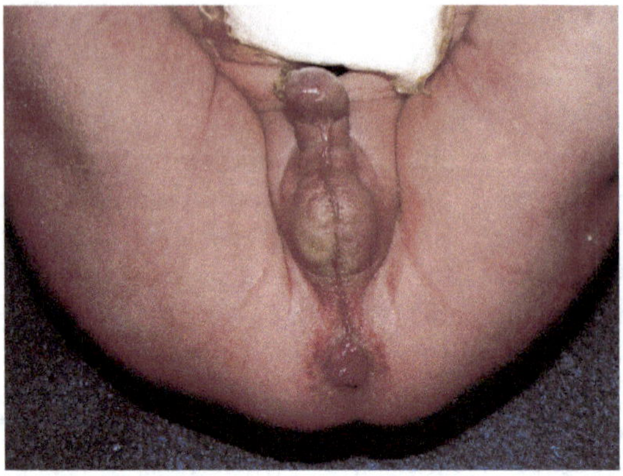

FIGURE 14.2 Cryptorchidism

Courtesy of Presbyterian/St. Luke's Medical Center, Denver, CO.

Ambiguous Genitalia

Ambiguous genitalia is considered a DSD and includes an enlarged clitoris, fused labial folds, and palpable gonads in a phenotypic female; and bifid scrotum, severe hypospadias, micropenis, and cryptorchidism (undescended testes; Figure 14.2) in a phenotypic male. DSDs are defined as congenital conditions characterized by atypical development of chromosomal, gonadal, or anatomic sex. Infants with ambiguous genitalia should be evaluated promptly for potential CAH as there is a risk for insufficient cortisol levels and an adrenal crisis. Further diagnosis and management should include pediatric specialists, such as an endocrinologist with expertise in DSD.[12]

Anus

The anus and rectum should be checked carefully for patency, position, and size. On

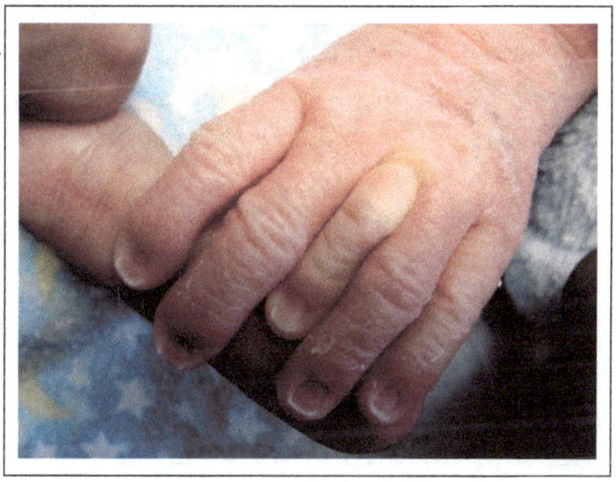

FIGURE 14.3 Polydactyly of the fingers

Courtesy of Presbyterian/St. Luke's Medical Center, Denver, CO.

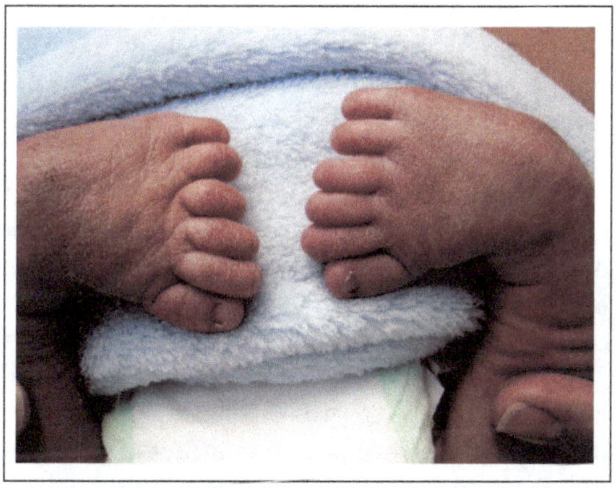

FIGURE 14.4 Polydactyly of the toes

Courtesy of Presbyterian/St. Luke's Medical Center, Denver, CO.

occasion, large fistulas are mistaken for a normal anus, but if one checks carefully, it will be noted that a fistula will be either anterior or posterior to the usual location of a normal anus.

Extremities

The extremities are examined for deformities and movement. The hands and feet are inspected for syndactyly (fusion of digits) and polydactyly (extra digits; Figures 14.3 and 14.4). Syndactyly and polydactyly can be normal variants in a newborn with an otherwise normal examination, may be associated with a strong family history, or may be associated with various syndromes. The presence of a single palmar crease, or simian crease, should be noted. A single palmar crease occurs in 5% to 10% of the normal population and is common in newborns with trisomy 21. Talipes equinovarus (clubfoot; Figure 14.5) is more common in males. The foot is turned downward and inward, and the sole is directed medially. If position can be corrected with gentle force, it will resolve spontaneously. If not, orthopedic treatment and follow-up are necessary. The hips should be examined to detect developmental dysplasia of the hip.[13]

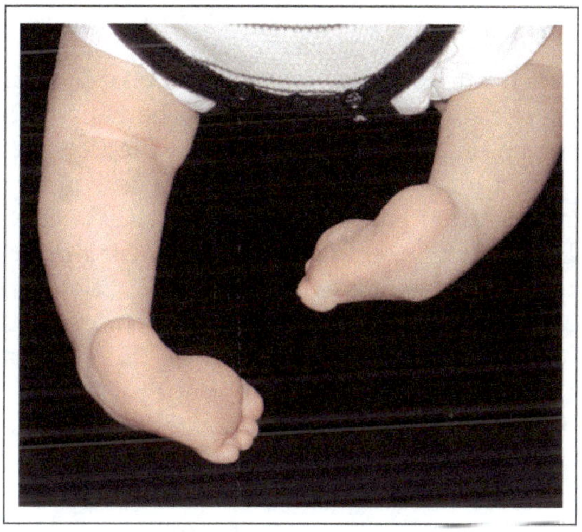

FIGURE 14.5 Clubfoot

Trunk and Spine

A tuft of hair, discoloration, or hemangioma in the sacrococcygeal area may suggest an underlying vertebral anomaly. Soft-tissue masses along the spine that are covered with normal skin may be lipomas or myelomeningoceles. A dimple without a visible base may indicate the presence of a pilonidal sinus or tract to the spinal cord.

In infants with one or more external malformations, a search should also be made for internal malformations, with surveillance that includes an echocardiogram, a renal ultrasound, and a cranial ultrasound. Chromosomal analysis should be completed in infants who have more than one major or multiple minor anomalies or dysmorphic features.

SHARING FINDINGS WITH PARENTS

When an anomaly is identified on physical examination, the infant should be shown to the parents as soon as possible. The physical finding may have been identified antenatally by ultrasound or may not have been expected. Either way, a spectrum of emotional responses from the parents is to be anticipated. Common responses of parents include fear, guilt, intense grief, anger, denial, frustration, and a sense of isolation. It is important to be sensitive to what the parents may be feeling. The defect should be shown to the parents and a factual description given, avoiding opinions or guesses. Care should be taken to ensure the use of person-first language in all discussions. Genetic counseling should be provided to help parents answer any questions regarding the prognosis for the child and genetic risks for future pregnancies. Medical geneticists and genetic counselors have extensive knowledge of genetic disorders and congenital anomalies and are trained to provide families with psychological and emotional support. However, even a healthcare professional with a basic knowledge of genetics and Mendelian inheritance can be helpful when discussing the physical findings with the parents and can provide answers to broad questions. Efforts should be made to connect parents with local resources, support networks, or other families experiencing a similar diagnosis as soon as is reasonable.

GENETICS

The nucleus of the human cell contains chromosomes, structures that include DNA and transmit genetic information during cell division and human development. Each human being has 46 chromosomes—22 pairs of autosomes and a pair of sex chromosomes (XX or XY) that determine gender. The chromosomes contain genes, the biologic units of inheritance. Genes control the physical, biochemical, and physiologic traits passed along to children from their parents. Genetic abnormalities are divided into three categories. Those that[14]

- Influence gene dosage (chromosomal abnormalities such as trisomies)
- Involve mutations in the genes themselves (over 6,000 rare single-gene disorders)
- Create a vulnerability to developmental errors that are then influenced by environmental factors (multifactorial inheritance disorders such as isolated malformations or schizophrenia)

The gene mutations that cause greater than 6,000 individually rare disorders can be further classified into four categories: autosomal dominant, autosomal recessive, X-linked, and mitochondrial mutations. Each individual receives two sets of chromosomes, one from each parent. Each pair of chromosomes contains a pair of genes, or alleles, that normally work together. A mutant gene is one that has altered in such a way that it can produce an abnormal trait.

Diseases caused by autosomal dominant genes are rare. A single mutant gene is dominant if it masks the effect of its paired gene and causes an obvious abnormality. The risk of the single mutant gene being passed on is 50%, but autosomal dominant disorders have a wide range of expression and will present in varying degrees between affected individuals due to influences of the normal paired gene as well as the genetic and environmental background of the individual. Examples of autosomal dominant disorders are retinoblastoma and neurofibromatosis.

Autosomal recessive disorders are also rare, although the number of carriers for these diseases can be high. These disorders are inherited from parents who both have the same recessive mutant gene. In most cases, both parents of an affected individual are heterozygous carriers of the disease yet have a normal phenotype. Typically, one-fourth of their offspring will be normal heterozygotes, one-half will be normal carrier heterozygotes, and one-fourth will be homozygotes who have the disease. An example of an autosomal recessive disease is cystic fibrosis.[15]

Genes located on the sex chromosomes cause X-linked disorders. The Y chromosome does not appear to carry any disease-causing genes. X-linked dominant traits are rare, but X-linked recessive diseases occur more commonly. A single copy of a mutant gene on the X chromosome will be expressed in the male because he has no unaffected partner gene. His daughters will all be carriers because they will receive his X gene, and his sons will all be unaffected because they receive his Y gene. Because females receive an X chromosome from each parent, they can be homozygous normal, homozygous for the X-linked disease, or heterozygous. Fifty percent of male offspring of X-linked recessive women will be affected, and 50% of her daughters will be carriers. Examples of X-linked disorders are Turner syndrome and Fragile X syndrome.[2]

Mitochondrial mutation disorders result from insufficient energy production in critical tissues. Most of these disorders present after the child is born, usually with visual loss, seizures, encephalopathy, progressive myopathy, or diabetes. The human egg is the source of mitochondria for all offspring and is therefore inherited only from the mother. Males with disorders caused by mitochondrial mutations have no risk of passing along the disorder to their offspring. Females, however, have a risk that approaches 100%. Female offspring of affected women will inherit some abnormal mitochondria, but may not manifest the disease.[14]

PROBLEMS IN MORPHOGENESIS

Abnormal morphogenesis may manifest in a variety of ways at the macroscopic and microscopic levels.[16] Anomaly is defined as a significant morphological or anatomic variation in the phenotype from the standard reference population.[16] A congenital anomaly is a structural defect, present at birth, a deviation from normal. Every structural defect represents an inborn error in morphogenesis (dysmorphogenesis). Based on the clinical implication, anomalies are classified as major and minor. Minor anomalies are unusual morphologic features that have no serious medical or cosmetic consequences to the patient. Almost any minor defect may occasionally be found as an unusual feature in a particular family. Minor external anomalies are most common in areas of complex and variable features, such as the face, ears, hands, and feet. Major anomalies have significant adverse implications in functional, anatomical, psychological, social, or cosmetic well-being.[16] Clinical diagnosis cannot usually be made based on a single defect. A specific diagnosis most often depends on recognition of an overall pattern of anomalies. Single minor anomalies occur in approximately 14% of neonates; 90% of infants with three or more minor anomalies also have one or more major anomalies, requiring significant surgical or cosmetic intervention.[3] Of the 3% born with clinically significant anomalies, multiple major anomalies are found in .7%, and most of these infants die.[3] Therefore, recognition of both minor and major anomalies is equally important.

Based on the developmental process involved in their formation, patterns of anomalies can be classified into four categories: malformation, deformation, disruption, and dysplasia. A malformation results from an abnormal morphogenesis (dysmorphogenesis) of the underlying tissue, which is attributed to a genetic or teratogenic factor. Malformations arise from intrinsic defects in genes that specify a series of developmental steps.[3] Often, but not always, a malformation in one part of the body is associated with malformations elsewhere. Examples of malformations are congenital heart defects or neural tube defects. Malformations occur in all gradations, the manifestations ranging from nearly normal to more severe.

Deformation is an alteration in form, shape, and/or position of a normally formed body part by biomechanical forces that distort the normally developing structure.[3,6] It usually occurs in the fetal period, not in embryogenesis, and is a secondary defect. Congenital hip dislocation and clubfoot are examples of deformations that can be caused by intrauterine constraint. Most deformations apparent at birth either resolve spontaneously or can be treated using external fixation devices to correctly position the affected part. Deformations may or may not be reversible.[16]

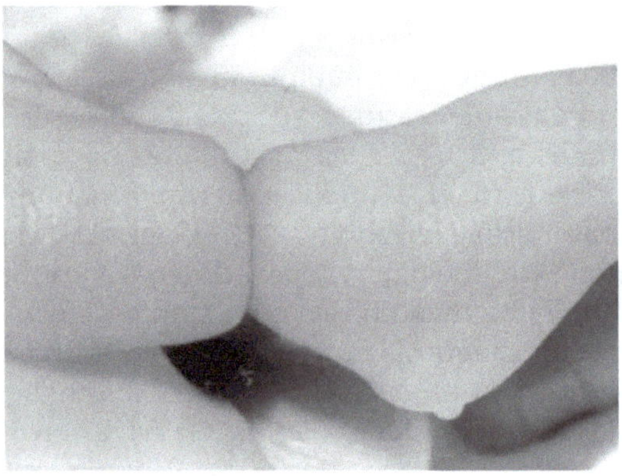

FIGURE 14.6 Constriction defect from amniotic band

Courtesy of J. Hernandez, MD, The Children's Hospital, Denver, CO.

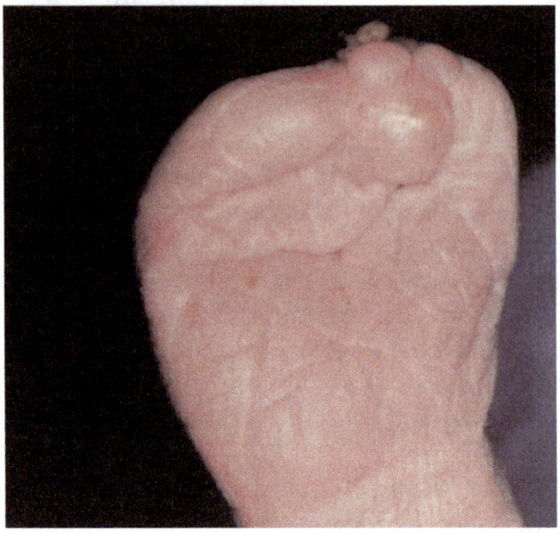

FIGURE 14.7 Amniotic bands resulting in finger amputation

Source: From Clark DA. 2000. *Atlas of Neonatology*. Philadelphia, PA: Saunders, 23. Reprinted by permission.

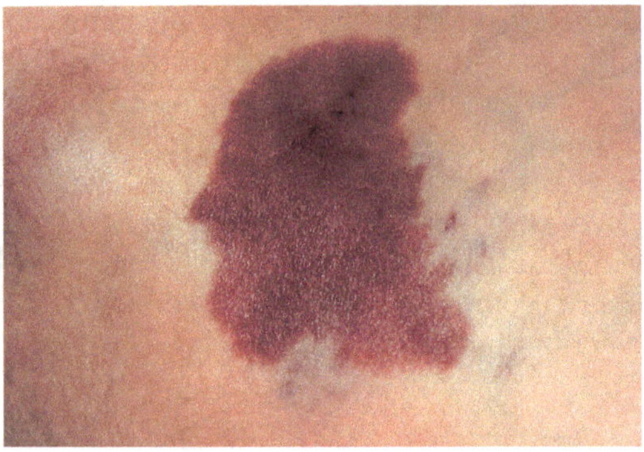

FIGURE 14.8 Hemangioma

Disruptions result from an extrinsic insult or destruction of originally normal fetal tissue.[16] This may cause the developmental arrest of the adjacent tissues, thereby leading to a secondary malformation. The process characteristically affects several tissue types in a specific anatomical region, and the phenotypic abnormalities may cross multiple embryonic cell lines.[16] Such disruptions may be vascular, infectious, or mechanical in origin. One example of this is disruption of normally developing tissues by amniotic bands (Figures 14.6 and 14.7).[3] Disruptions are more difficult to treat than deformations because they involve actual loss of normal tissue.

Dysplasia is a primary defect involving abnormal organization or differentiation of cells into tissue that results in clinically apparent structural or physiological changes.[3,16] Dysplasia can be triggered by genetic factors, teratogen exposure, or metabolic disorders. This can be localized, for example, a hemangioma (Figure 14.8), or generalized, such as achondroplasia (dysplasia of skeletal tissue). Dysplasias are usually not correctable, and the affected individual experiences the clinical effects of the underlying cell or tissue abnormality for life. However, in the case of hemangiomas interfering with vital functions, treatment is available (see Chapter 5, Skin Assessment).[10] Dysplasia may be associated with malformations.[16] Malformations and dysplasia are primary events in embryogenesis; disruptions and deformations occur secondarily. The concepts of malformation, deformation, disruption, and dysplasia are useful clinically to assist in recognition, diagnosis, and treatment of congenital anomalies. However, given the constellation of congenital anomalies, a neonate may present with combinations of these patterns of anomalies. The occurrence of congenital anomalies can further be divided into several categories: syndromes, sequences, associations, and teratogens.

SYNDROMES

A syndrome is a collection of anomalies involving more than one developmental region or organ system or a pattern of multiple anomalies thought to be pathogenetically related.[17] The anomalies can be malformations, deformations, disruptions, or dysplasia. Chromosomal syndromes are usually diagnosed in the neonatal period. The most common of these are trisomy 21, trisomy 18, trisomy 13, and 45, X. With the advent of the human genome project, more information is now available regarding chromosome structure. Once thought to be associations, DiGeorge; Beckwith–Wiedemann; and **C**oloboma, **H**eart defect, choannal **A**tresia, growth **R**etardation, **G**enital anomalies, **E**ar abnormalities (CHARGE) have now been found to have chromosomal abnormalities as an underlying etiology and are more correctly categorized as syndromes.[18]

Trisomy 21 (Down Syndrome)

The incidence of trisomy 21 is one per 660 to one per 1,000 live births, making it the most common pattern of malformation.[16] Down syndrome can usually be diagnosed at birth or soon after by its dysmorphic features, which produce a distinctive phenotype. Principal features include hypotonia, poor or absent Moro reflex, hyperextensibility of joints, excess skin at the nape of the neck, flat facial profile (Figure 14.9), low-set ears, slanted palpebral fissures, and single transverse palmar (simian) creases (Figure 14.10). Associated anomalies include congenital heart defects (30%–40%); increased incidence of duodenal atresia, esophageal atresia, and imperforate anus; and significant hearing loss (90%). Most of the features of trisomy 21 can occur as isolated features in normal infants. It is the combination of features forming a recognizable pattern that permits early diagnosis.[19]

Trisomy 18 (Edwards Syndrome)

The incidence of trisomy 18 is approximately one in 6,000 live births.[20] There is a 4:1 preponderance of females to males. The Edwards syndrome phenotype is as distinct as Down syndrome, but because it is less common, it is less likely to be recognized clinically. Trisomy 18 syndrome (Figure 14.11) is usually lethal, with 50% mortality within the first several weeks of life, predominantly due to an 85% incidence of congenital heart disease.[20] Common causes of death in trisomy 18 include central apnea or end-organ dysfunction, such as pulmonary hypertension or heart failure. Prognosis for this diagnosis has been regarded as poor, with studies citing up to a nearly 97% 1-year mortality rate; infants that do survive have severe mental deficiencies.[20] However, with changing guidelines and new literature showing increased survival in recent years with palliative cardiac surgery, postoperative mortality rates range between 12% and 15% with a roughly 50% complication rate, and those who survive to hospital discharge have an average survival of 16.2 years.[20] Physical findings include prenatal and postnatal growth deficiency, micrognathia, overlapping digits, complex congenital heart disease, low-set ears, rocker-bottom clubfeet, and generalized hypertonicity. Associated anomalies include tracheoesophageal fistula or esophageal atresia, hemivertebrae, omphalocele, myelomeningocele, and radial dysplasia.[14]

Trisomy 13 (Patau Syndrome)

The incidence of trisomy 13 is approximately one per 10,000 live births.[14] The prognosis for infants with trisomy 13 (Figure 14.12) is poor, and 80% of untreated affected infants do not survive past the first month.[21] Nearly all of the remaining affected infants die during infancy or early childhood, although some have longer survival. This malformation pattern is quite distinguishable and clinically recognizable. Physical findings include oral facial clefts, microphthalmia or absence of the eyes, low-set ears, rocker-bottom feet, moderate microcephaly, polydactyly, scalp cutis aplasia, and congenital heart disease. Associated anomalies include cleft lip and palate, cystic kidneys, holoprosencephaly, and other severe central nervous system

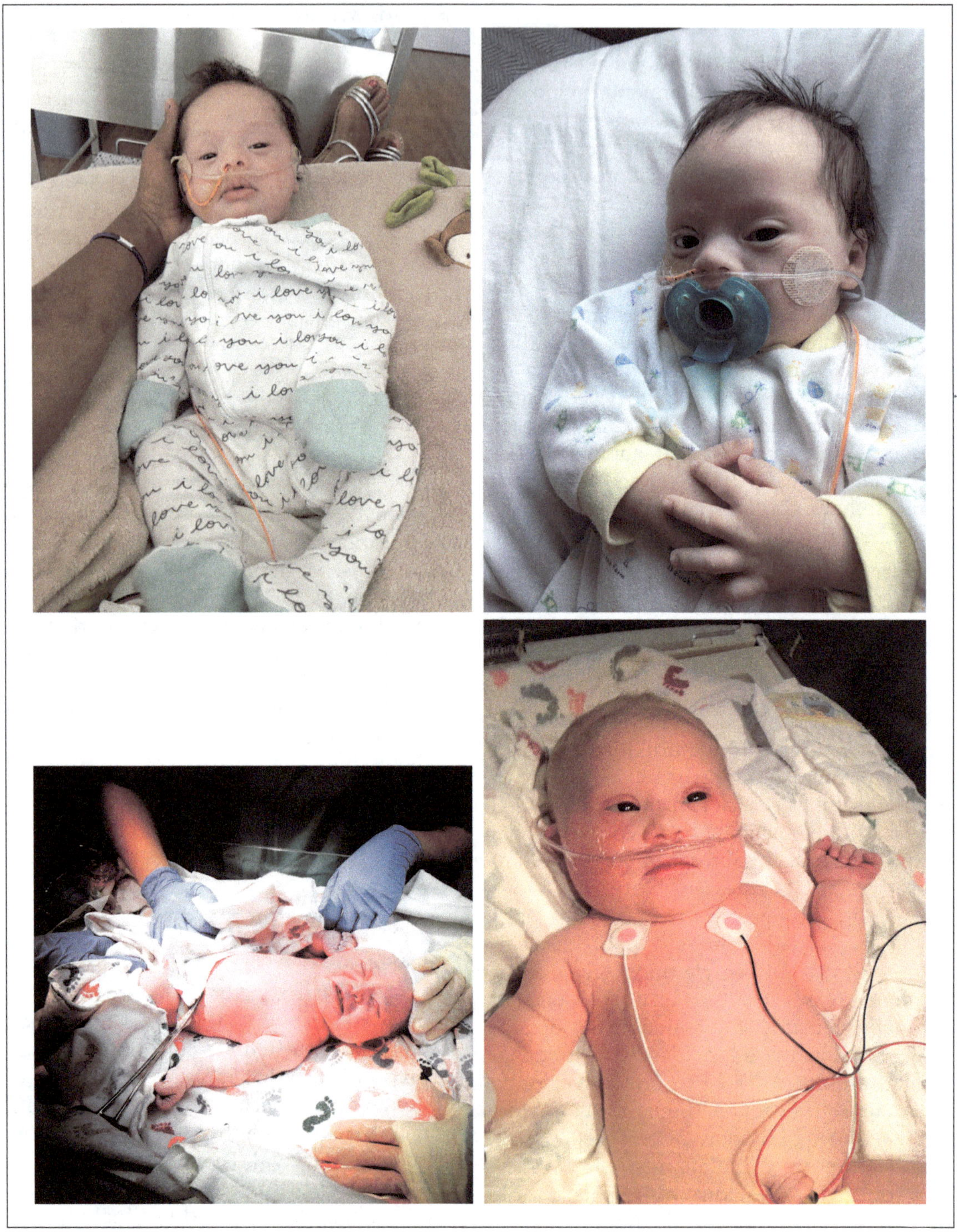

FIGURE 14.9 Trisomy 21 (Down syndrome)

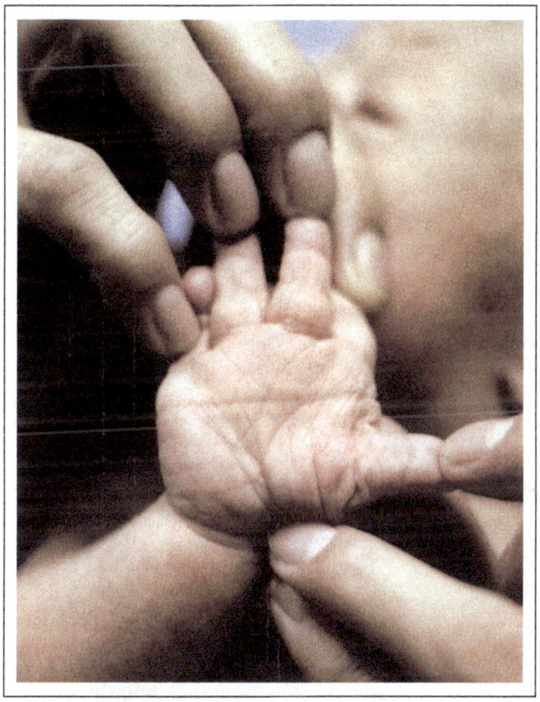

FIGURE 14.10 Single palmar crease

Source: From Clark DA. 2000. *Atlas of Neonatology*. Philadelphia: Saunders, 31. Reprinted by permission.

(CNS) malformations. The identification of multiple midline defects is an indicator to consider trisomy 13.[14]

45, X (Turner Syndrome)

The incidence of monosomy X or Turner syndrome is one in 2,500 live-born females.[14] Ninety-five percent of conceptions are miscarried or stillborn. The 45, X syndrome (Figure 14.13) is usually compatible with survival if the fetus reaches term gestation. Turner syndrome is the most common sex chromosomal abnormality in females.[22] Females with Turner syndrome can often be identified at birth or before puberty by their distinctive phenotypic characteristics. Physical findings include small stature, short neck with webbing, lymphedema of the hands and feet, frontal prominence, low posterior hairline, and broad chest with widely spaced nipples. Associated anomalies include congenital heart defects, structural kidney defects, and gonadal dysgenesis.[14]

DiGeorge Syndrome

DiGeorge syndrome is a chromosomal deletion of 22q11.2 characterized by structural or functional defects of the thymus, conotruncal heart defects, hypoparathyroidism, and secondary hypocalcemia.[23] 22q11DS is the most common microdeletion syndrome in humans. However, population-based estimates of the incidence and prevalence of 22q11DS differ. Most studies reported a prevalence of one in every 4,000 newborns.[23] Signs vary from patient to patient. Physical findings of DiGeorge syndrome include cardiac anomalies, usually conotruncal in nature, such as truncus arteriosus or aortic arch anomalies (approximately 75%), cleft palate (approximately 70%), immunodeficiency

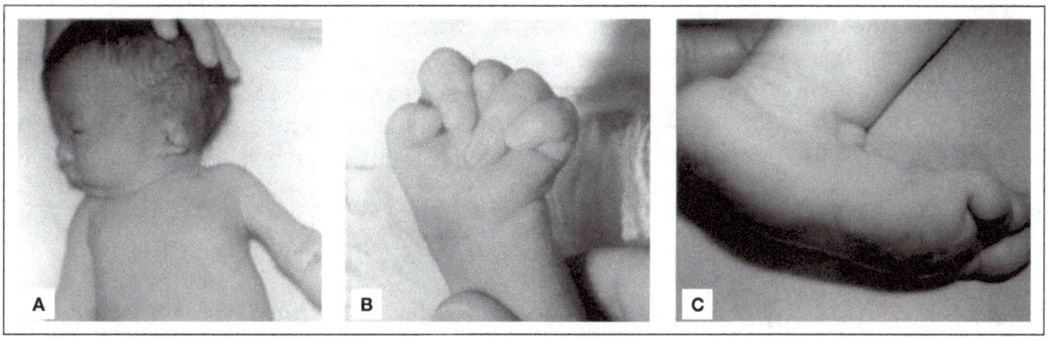

FIGURE 14.11 Trisomy 18 (**A**) prominent occiput; short sternum; micrognathia; malformed, low-set ears. (**B**) Overlapping fingers. (**C**) Rocker-bottom feet

Courtesy of J. Hernandez, MD, The Children's Hospital, Denver, Colorado.

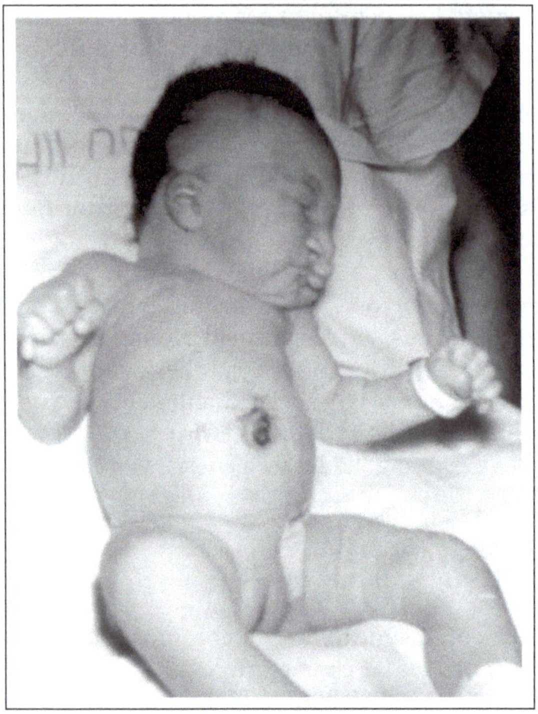

FIGURE 14.12 Trisomy 13

Courtesy of J. Hernandez, MD, The Children's Hospital, Denver, CO.

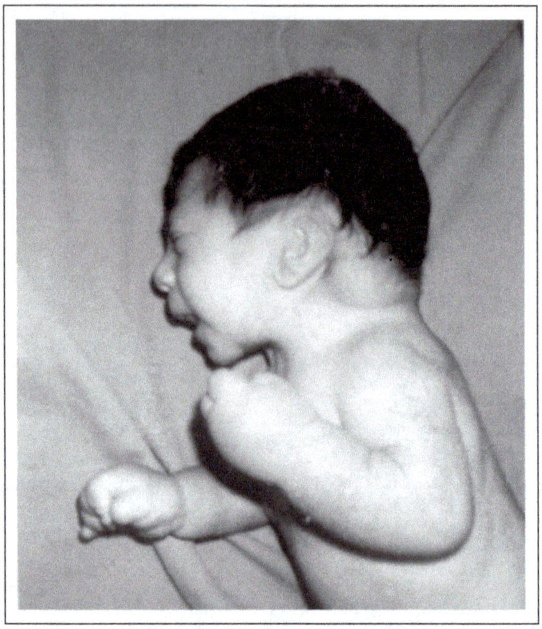

FIGURE 14.13 Turner syndrome lymphedema (hands), webbed neck, low posterior hair line, low-set ears

Courtesy of J. Hernandez, MD, The Children's Hospital, Denver, CO.

due to thymic hypoplasia (approximately 75%), and craniofacial features that include microcephaly, abnormally shaped ears, prominent nasal root with bulbous nasal tip, and hooded eyelids.[14] However, some neonates have no identifying craniofacial features. Associated findings include renal anomalies, hearing loss, significant feeding problems, and hyperextensibility of hands and fingers. Hypocalcemia is a prominent laboratory finding secondary to absence or hypoplasia of the parathyroid glands and thymus. Etiology has been associated with prenatal exposure to alcohol and isotretinoin (Accutane). There is significant neonatal morbidity and mortality associated with the cardiac defects, immunodeficiency, and seizures related to hypocalcemia.[24]

Beckwith–Wiedemann Syndrome

Beckwith–Wiedemann syndrome is caused by a mutation or deletion within the chromosome 11p15.5 region.[25] An estimated one in 13,700 newborns are affected.[25] Beckwith–Wiedemann syndrome is usually identifiable at birth because the infant will be large for gestational age, and have refractory hypoglycemia, a large tongue, creases on the earlobe, and an omphalocele. Hyperplasia of a limb or one side of the face or trunk may be present at birth. Classified as an overgrowth syndrome, affected infants are considerably larger than normal (macrosomia) and continue to grow and gain weight at an unusual rate during childhood. Associated anomalies include renal malformations and cardiomyopathy. Polyhydramnios and a high incidence of prematurity are also common historical findings. Early diagnosis and aggressive treatment of hypoglycemia may prevent mental deficits.[25]

CHARGE Syndrome

CHARGE syndrome is an acronym for **C**oloboma, **H**eart anomaly, choanal **A**tresia, **R**estricted growth and development, **G**enital anomalies, **E**ar anomalies and/or deafness caused by mutations on the chromodomain helicase DNA binding protein 7 (CHD7) gene located on chromosome 8q1.[26] Not all features need be present for a diagnosis to be made, and the extent of involvement of each system is widely variable.[17] CHARGE syndrome is diagnosable when three or four major criteria or two major and three minor criteria are present. The occurrence of CHARGE syndrome is one per 12,000 live births.[26] CHARGE syndrome often presents as a medical emergency because of the presence of choanal atresia, serious heart defects, and swallowing difficulties. Associated anomalies include cleft lip and palate as well as unilateral facial palsies. Most patients have some degree of mental deficiency or CNS defect and visual or auditory anomalies that further compromise cognitive function.

SEQUENCES

A sequence is a pattern of multiple anomalies derived from a single known or presumed structural defect or mechanical factor followed by a cascade of secondary effects.[8] The most common nonchromosomal deformation or disruption sequences diagnosed in the neonatal period are oligohydramnios (Potter) sequence, amniotic band sequence, arthrogryposis, and Pierre Robin sequence.[8]

Oligohydramnios (Potter) Sequence

The incidence of oligohydramnios (Potter) sequence is one of 3,000 to one of 9,000 live births.[15] Almost all of these infants die in the neonatal period due to pulmonary hypoplasia. Oligohydramnios sequence is caused by severe oligohydramnios (Figure 14.14). Renal agenesis, polycystic kidneys, urinary tract obstruction, or chronic leakage of amniotic fluid may be the cause of oligohydramnios. This results in intrauterine constraint of the fetus and pulmonary hypoplasia. Physical findings include refractory respiratory distress, frequently with concomitant pneumothoraces, clubfeet, hyperextensible fingers, large ears, low inner eye folds, and a beak nose. Anuria is typically present in the newborn. Associated anomalies include congenital heart defects, Eagle–Barrett syndrome (prune belly syndrome [absent abdominal musculature, urinary tract abnormalities, and cryptorchidism]), esophageal and duodenal atresias, imperforate anus, and Pierre Robin sequence.

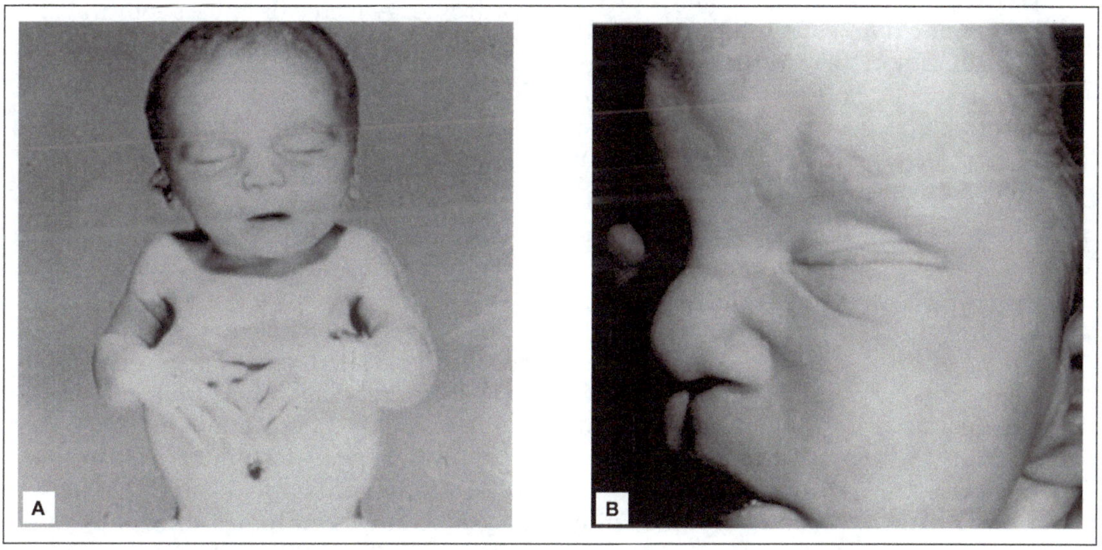

FIGURE 14.14 Constraint deformities (A) secondary to oligohydramnios (Potter) sequence: Narrow, flared thorax, folded ear. (B) Typical potter facies: Flattened nose, ear anomalies, furrowed brow

Courtesy of J. Hernandez, MD, The Children's Hospital, Denver, CO.

Diagnosis is usually confirmed by renal ultrasound and autopsy findings of urinary tract abnormalities.[27]

Amniotic Band Sequence

Amniotic band sequence is a collection of fetal disruptions that results from in utero entrapment of fetal parts by fibrous bands. The cause of amniotic band sequence is unclear; the extrinsic model suggests a sequence mechanism of disruption of the amnion that leads to the entanglement of fetal structures by mesodermic bands.[28] The incidence of amniotic band sequence is approximately one in 10,000 to one in 15,000 live births.[28] Early amnion rupture occurs, and small bands of amnion encircle developing structures, usually limbs, leading to constrictions, intrauterine amputations, and/or umbilical cord constriction (see Figures 14.6 and 14.7). In addition, deformational defects occur secondary to decreased fetal movement, the result of tethering of a limb by an amniotic band. The decreased fetal movement may result in scoliosis or foot deformities. No two affected fetuses will have the exact same features, and there is no single feature that consistently occurs. Anomalies of the extremities include congenital partial or irregular amputations, constriction rings, and distal swellings. Craniofacial anomalies can include microcephaly, encephaloceles, and facial clefts. Examination of the placenta and membranes is diagnostic.[28]

Arthrogryposis (Multiple Joint Fixations)

Arthrogryposis occurs in approximately one of 8,000 live births.[14] Physical findings include joint contractures, extensions, and dislocations. Joint contractures can be secondary to intrinsic factors affecting the fetus such as early onset of neurologic, muscle, and joint problems or to extrinsic factors such as fetal crowding and constraint. Neurologic abnormality is the most common cause of arthrogryposis. Non-joint-related anomalies may indicate that the arthrogryposis is part of a multiple defect syndrome. Affected infants should also be assessed for scoliosis (Figures 14.15 and 14.16) and hip dislocation.

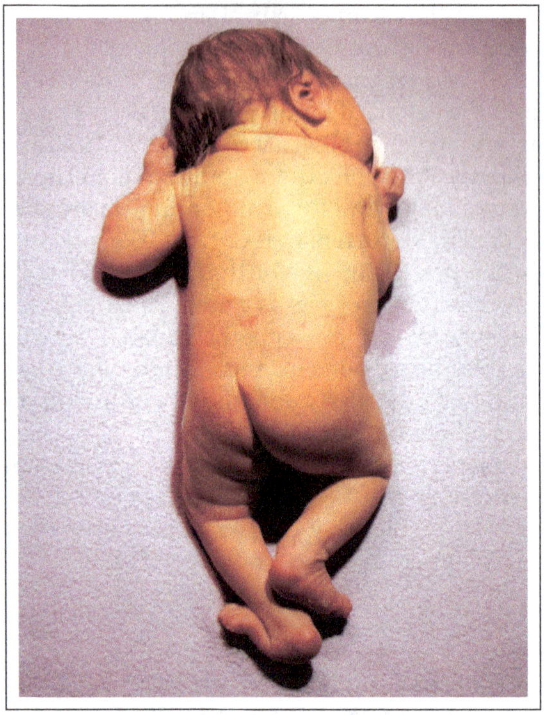

FIGURE 14.15 Scoliosis

Courtesy of Presbyterian/St. Luke's Medical Center, Denver, CO.

Pierre Robin Sequence

Pierre Robin sequence occurs in approximately one of 8,500 live births.[14] The initiating defect of this sequence is severe hypoplasia of the mandible, causing the tongue to be posteriorly located, resulting in severe upper airway obstruction and cleft palate. Physical findings include micrognathia, cleft palate, and low-set ears. Respiratory distress secondary to upper airway obstruction may be present. Many syndromes have the craniofacial features of Pierre Robin sequence. If noncraniofacial primary malformations are present, then other diagnoses should be considered.

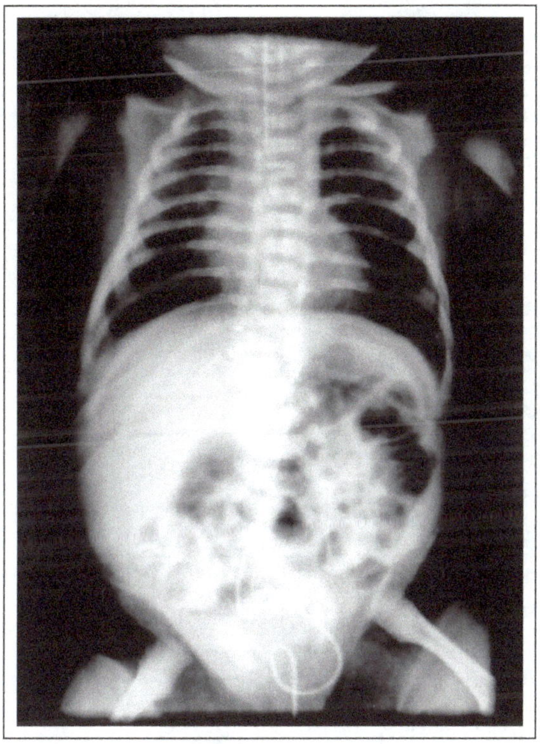

FIGURE 14.16 X-ray of scoliosis

ASSOCIATIONS

Association refers to a nonrandom occurrence of multiple malformations for which no specific or common etiology has been identified.[16] These patterns of morphological anomalies occur together more often than would be expected by chance only. The most usual association is VATER/VACTERL.

VATER/VACTERL Association

VATER/VACTERL is an acronym that includes **V**ertebral anomalies, **A**nal atresia, esophageal atresia with or without **T**racheo**E**sophageal fistula, and **R**adial and/or **R**enal dysplasia. **C**ardiac defects, single umbilical artery, **L**imb abnormalities, and IUGR are also nonrandom features of this pattern of anomalies. VATER/VACTERL occurs in 1 of 5,000 live births, and the etiology is unknown.[14] Diagnosis requires exclusion of other similar disorders, including chromosomal syndromes with the presence of three or more congenital malformations necessary for a VACTERL association diagnosis.[29] Though the causes remain elusive, VACTER/VACTERL is thought to be due to defects in early embryogenesis. Most infants diagnosed with VATER/VACTERL have normal brain function.

TERATOGENS

Although the human embryo is well protected in the uterus, maternal exposure to teratogens may cause developmental disruptions. A teratogen is any agent external to the fetus that causes a structural or functional disability postnatally. Teratogens can be drugs and chemicals, altered maternal metabolic states, or infectious agents. Known teratogenic factors cause 5% to 10% of congenital anomalies. Susceptibility to a teratogen is determined by the embryologic stage of development when exposed. Each part, tissue, and organ of an embryo has a critical period during which development can be disrupted (Figure 14.17). The most critical period in development is when cell division, cell differentiation, and morphogenesis are at their peak.[3]

Fetal Alcohol Spectrum Disorders

Alcohol is thought to be the most common teratogen to which a fetus may be exposed and may result in fetal alcohol syndrome or fetal alcohol spectrum disorder (FASD). FASDs are the group of conditions resulting from fetal alcohol exposure. The most comprehensive disorder is fetal alcohol syndrome. The incidence in the United States is difficult to estimate, but the risk that a pregnant person with a chronic alcohol use disorder will have a child with fetal alcohol syndrome is 30% to 50%.[8] Common features include short palpebral fissures; epicanthal folds; a flat nasal bridge; a long, simple philtrum; a thin upper lip; small hypoplastic nails; irritability in infancy; and growth deficiency. Associated anomalies are cardiac defects, ventricular septal defect being the

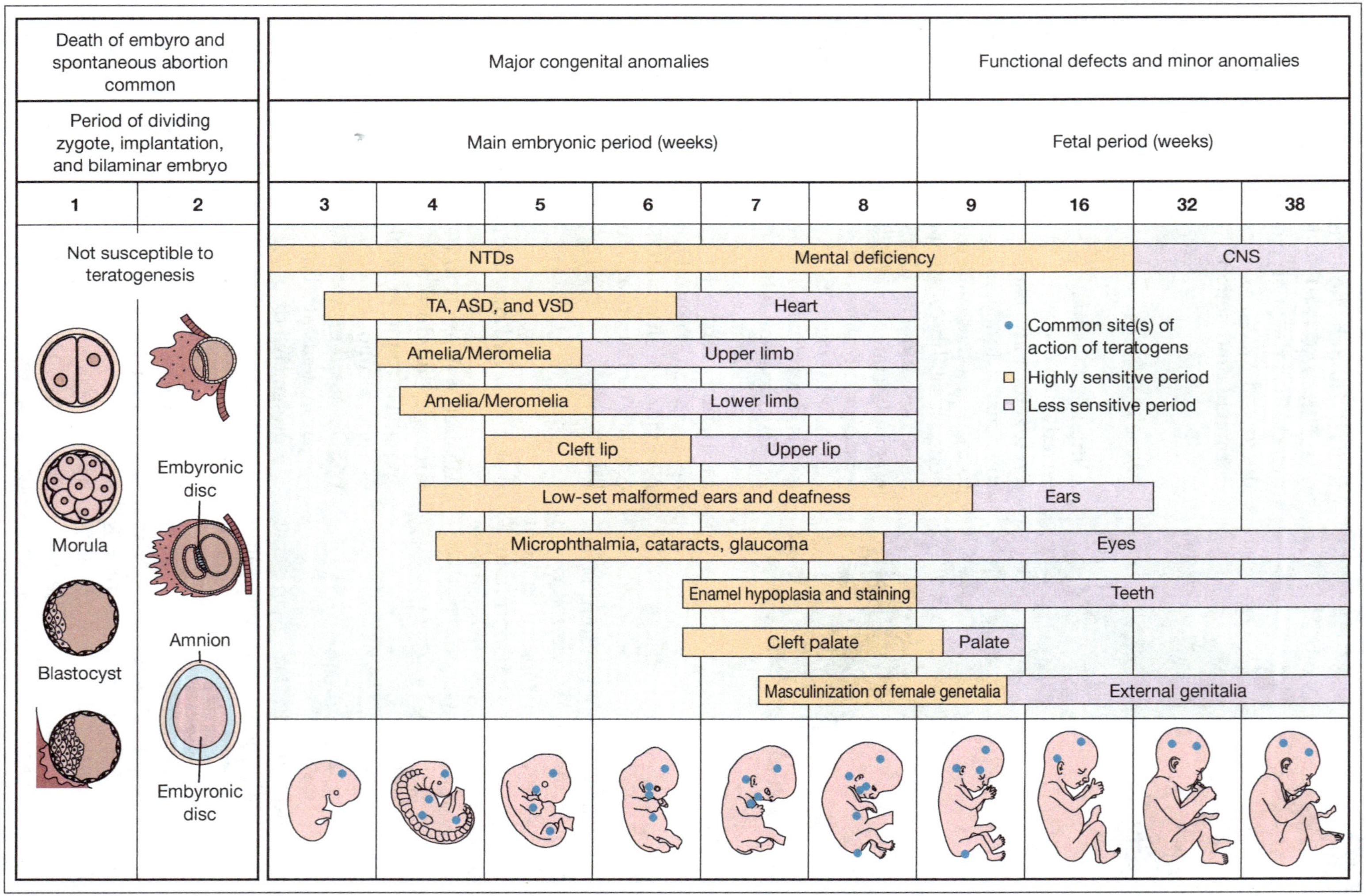

FIGURE 14.17 Embryonic and fetal development

ASD, atrial septal defect; NTD, neural tube defect; TA, truncus arteriosus; VSD, ventricular septal defect

Source: From Moore KL, Persaud TVN, and Torchia MG. 2020. Human birth defects. In *The Developing Human: Clinically Oriented Embryology*, 11th ed. Philadelphia, PA: Elsevier, 901. Reprinted by permission.

most common, and microcephaly. Long-term effects include mental deficiency and behavioral problems.[30]

Fetal Cocaine Exposure

Cocaine has been suggested as a teratogen. Infants exposed to cocaine in utero are more likely to be born prematurely, be characterized as growth restricted, and may present with hyperirritability, feeding problems, and abnormal sleep patterns. Physical findings may include microcephaly and an increased incidence of genitourinary tract anomalies.[8]

Anticonvulsants

Phenytoin (Dilantin) and valproic acid are commonly prescribed for management of maternal epilepsy; however, both are teratogens. Fetal hydantoin syndrome is characterized by atypical facies (broad, low nasal bridge, hypertelorism, epicanthal folds, ptosis, and metopic ridging), low-set hairline, and nail hypoplasia. Cleft lip and palate and umbilical and inguinal hernias are associated anomalies.[30] Fetal valproate syndrome features consist of a prominent or fused metopic suture, epicanthal folds, mid-face hypoplasia, and broad, low nasal bridge with short nose and long philtrum. Congenital heart defects, genitourinary anomalies, and club feet are associated anomalies.[30]

Infants of Diabetic Mothers

Maternal altered metabolic states can increase the risk for abnormalities in the newborn. Poorly controlled maternal diabetes mellitus with persistent hyperglycemia and ketosis, particularly during embryogenesis, is associated with an incidence of birth defects that is up to five times higher than the general population.[2,3] Significant anomalies include holoprosencephaly (failure of the forebrain to divide into hemispheres), meroencephaly (partial absence of the brain), sacral agenesis, vertebral anomalies, congenital heart defects, limb defects, and renal anomalies. Improved diabetic control during gestation dramatically decreases the incidence of diabetes-related malformations but does not reduce it back to the level of incidence for a mother without diabetes. Preconception control may achieve an incidence similar to the general population, emphasizing the importance of preconception counseling.[3]

Infectious Diseases

Congenital anomalies also may be associated with certain infections during pregnancy. The common and best-understood infections are represented by the acronym TORCH, which stands for **T**oxoplasmosis, **O**ther agents (including syphilis), **R**ubella, **C**ytomegalovirus, and **H**erpes simplex. TORCH infections may present with similar clinical findings: IUGR; hepatosplenomegaly; rash; CNS manifestations such as microcephaly, chorioretinitis, and intracranial calcifications; jaundice; and low platelets.[31]

RESOURCES

The internet is a powerful tool to utilize when searching for information regarding birth defects, including specific conditions, diagnosis, prevention, screening, research, and national organizations. An abundance of reliable and up-to-date information from expert sources can be accessed in a short time. Each of the sources listed in the following section provides links to alternate websites if additional information is desired.

Online Resources for Birth Defect Information

Centers for Disease Control and Prevention
www.cdc.gov/ncbddd/birthdefects/index.html

Biomedical and Genomic Information
www.ncbi.nlm.nih.gov

March of Dimes Birth Defects Foundation
www.marchofdimes.org/our-work/health-professionals

Medline Plus
www.nlm.nih.gov/medlineplus/birthdefects.html
National Birth Defects Prevention Network (NBDPN)
www.nbdpn.org
National Human Genome Research Institute
www.genome.gov
Eunice Shriver National Institute of Child Health and Human Development
www.nichd.nih.gov
The Society for Birth Defects Research and Prevention
https://birthdefectsresearch.org/
Online Mendelian Inheritance in Man
www.ncbi.nlm.nih.gov/omim
The Genetic Alliance
www.geneticalliance.org/
Prenatal and Postnatal Diagnosis Support
www.lettercase.org

SUMMARY

The approach to the evaluation of the infant with dysmorphic features is multifaceted and begins with a thorough history and physical examination. With experience, the examiner's identification of physical findings on the continuum of normal to abnormal is enhanced. A general knowledge of genetics and common disorders is helpful when counseling parents. Multiple resources, including geneticists, genetic counselors, and internet websites, are available to healthcare professionals and parents involved in caring for the infant with dysmorphic features.

ADDITIONAL RESOURCES

SPRINGER PUBLISHING CONNECT™

A robust set of resources designed to supplement this text is located at http://connect.springerpub.com/content/book/978-0-8261-4063-0. Qualifying instructors may request access by emailing textbook@springerpub.com.

REFERENCES

1. Almli LM, Ely DM, Ailes EC, Abouk R, Grosse SD, Isenburg JL, Waldron DB, and Reefhuis J. 2020, January 17. Infant mortality attributable to birth defects—United States, 2003–2017. *Morbidity and Mortality Weekly Report* 69(2): 25–29. doi: 10.15585/mmwr.mm6902a1
2. Moore KL, Persaud TVN, and Tochia MG. 2020. Human birth defects. In *The Developing Human: Clinically Oriented Embryology*, 11th ed. Moore KL, Persaud TVN, Torchia MG, eds. Philadelphia, PA: Saunders, 900–961.
3. Mitchell AL. 2020. Congenital Anomalies. In *Fanaroff and Martin's Neonatal–Perinatal Medicine: Diseases of the Fetus and Infant*, 11th ed. Martin RJ, Fanaroff AA, and Walsh MC, eds. Philadelphia, PA: Elsevier Saunders, 489–516.
4. Rose NC, Kaimal AJ, Dugoff L, Norton ME, and American College of Obstetricians and Gynecologists' Committee on Practice Bulletins—Obstetrics Committee on Genetics Society for Maternal-Fetal Medicine. 2020, October. Screening for fetal chromosomal abnormalities: ACOG practice bulletin, number 226. *Obstetrics & Gynecology* 136(4): e48–e69. doi: 10.1097/AOG.0000000000004084
5. D'Antoni AV, Donaldson OI, Schmidt C, Macchi V, De Caro R, Oskouian RJ, Loukas M, and Shane Tubbs R. 2017. A comprehensive review of the anterior fontanelle: Embryology, anatomy, and clinical considerations. *Childs Nervous System* 33(6): 909–914.
6. Arya S, Jain SK, and Richardson CJ. 2017. Facial asymmetry in a crying newborn: A comparison of two cases and review of literature. *Case Reports in Pediatrics* 2017: 1–3.
7. Hunter A, Frias JL, Gillessan-Kaesbach G, Hughes H, Jones KL, and Wilson L. 2009. Elements of morphology: Standard terminology for the ear. *American Journal of Medical Genetics Part A* 149A(1): 40–60.
8. Gomella TL, Cunningham MD, and Eyal FG. 2020. *Neonatology: Management, Procedures, On-Call Problems, Diseases, and Drugs*. McGraw Hill, 673–674.
9. Li TG, Guan CL, Wang J, and Peng MJ. 2021. Comparative study of umbilical cord cross sectional area in fetuses with single umbilical artery and normal umbilical artery. *Journal of Obstetrics and Gynecology* 42(5): 935–940.
10. Kaplan E, and Sepulvada W. 2023. *Single Umbilical Artery*. UpToDate. Levine D, Wilkins-Haug L, and Chakrabarti A, eds. Retrieved from https://www.uptodate.com/contents/single-umbilical-artery
11. Dagklis T, Siargkas A, Apostolopoulou A, Tsakiridis I, Mamopoulos A, Athanasiadis A, and Sotiriadis A. 2022. Adverse perinatal outcomes following the prenatal diagnosis of isolated single umbilical artery in singleton pregnancies: A systematic review and meta-analysis. *Journal of Perinatal Medicine* 50(3): 244–252.

12. Diaz A, and Lipman Diaz EG. 2021. Disorders of sex development. *Pediatrics in Review* 42(8): 414–426. doi: 10.1542/pir.2018-0183
13. Gomella TL, Cunningham MD, and Eyal FG. 2020. Orthopedic and musculoskeletal problems. In *Neonatology: Management, Procedures, On-Call Problems, Diseases, and Drugs*. McGraw Hill, 606–613.
14. Jones KL, Jones MC, and DelCampo M. 2013–2022. Recognizable patterns of malformation. In *Smith's Recognizable Patterns of Human Malformation*, 8th ed. Elsevier, 2022, 1–18, 218–224, 334–336, 356–358, 484–492, 892–894, 898–902, 922–926.
15. McCance KL, and Huether SE. 2019. *Pathophysiology: The Biologic Basis for Disease in Adults and Children*, 8th ed. Philadelphia, PA: Mosby.
16. Verna RP. 2021. Evaluation and risk assessment of congenital anomalies in neonates. *Children* 8(10): 862–874.
17. Halderman-Englert CR, Saitta SC, and Zackai EH. 2018. The dysmorphic infant. In *Avery's Diseases of the Newborn*, 10th ed. Gleason CA, and Juul SE, eds. Philadelphia, PA: Elsevier, 201–210.
18. National Human Genome Research Institute. 2018. *Genetic Disorders*. Retrieved from https://www.genome.gov/10001204/specific-genetic-disorders/
19. Online Mendelian Inheritance in Man. 2017. *Entry #190685 Down Syndrome*. Retrieved from https://www.omim.org/entry/190685?search=Down%20syndrome&highlight=down%20syndromic%20=syndrome#clinicalFeatures
20. Frick TA, and Tejtel KS. 2021. Trisomy 18 trends over the last 20 years. *The Journal of Pediatrics* 239(12): 206–211.
21. Diaz D, Benjamin RH, Navarro Sanchez ML, Mitchell LE, Langlois PH, Canfield MA, Chen H, Scheuerle AE, Schaaf CP, Scott DA, and Northrup H. 2021. Patterns of congenital anomalies among individuals with trisomy 13 in Texas. *American Journal of Medical Genetics Part A* 185A: 1787–1793.
22. Steiner M, and Saenger P. 2022. Turner syndrome: An update. *Advances in Pediatric* 69(1): 177–202.
23. Singh A, and Kumari R. 2019. DiGeorge syndrome—Chromosome 22q11 deletion syndrome: An update and review. *International Journal of Nursing Education* 11(1): 30–34.
24. Online Mendelian Inheritance in Man. 2022. *Entry #188400 DiGeorge Syndrome*. Retrieved from https://www.omim.org/entry/188400?search=22q11%20deletion&highlight=22q11%20deletion
25. Online Mendelian Inheritance in Man. 2022. *Entry #130650 Beckwith Weidemann Syndrome*. Retrieved from https://www.omim.org/entry/130650?search=Beckwith%E2%80%93Wiedemann%20syndrome&highlight=beckwithwiedemann%20syndromic%20wiedemann%20beckwith%20syndrome
26. Online Mendelian Inheritance in Man. 2022. *Entry #214800 CHARGE Syndrome*. Retrieved from https://www.omim.org/entry/214800
27. National Institutes of Health: Genetic and Rare Diseases Information Center. 2017. *Potter Sequence*. Retrieved from https://rarediseases.info.nih.gov/diseases/4462/potter-sequence
28. Gandhi M, Rac MW, and McKinney J. 2019. Amniotic band sequence. *American Journal of Obstetrics and Gynecology* 221(6): B5–B6.
29. Husain M, Dutra-Clarke M, Lemieux B, Wencel M, Solomon BD, and Kimonis V. 2018. Phenotypic diversity of patients diagnosed with VACTERL association. *Americal Journal of Medical Genetics* 176A: 1830–1837.
30. Jones KL, Jones MC, and DelCampo M. 2022. Environmental agents. In *Smith's Recognizable Patterns of Human Malformation*, 8th ed. Philadelphia, PA: Elsevier, 786–815.
31. Moodley A, and Payton KSE. 2021. The term newborn: Congenital infections. *Clinics in Perinatology* 48(3): 485–511. doi: 10.1016/j.clp.2021.05.004

15 PAIN ASSESSMENT IN THE NEWBORN

Christina Baxter

Infants in the neonatal intensive care unit (NICU) experience multiple painful events each day. Simple tasks, such as changing a diaper, can cause significant distress for an infant born at 24 weeks gestation.[1] Unfortunately, these painful events are needed for survival outside of the womb. These painful experiences occur at a critical time of brain development. In neonates, repeated exposures to pain have been shown to cause long-term developmental and behavioral issues.[2] Neonates cannot verbalize their pain, but they do show changes behaviorally and physiologically that can be noted by a care provider to adequately assess levels of pain.[1] It is important for all care providers to be able to recognize and assess pain of infants hospitalized in the NICU to provide appropriate pain-relieving measures.

APPROACH TO PAIN ASSESSMENT

Pain assessment in the newborn and especially the preterm neonate presents a challenge to even the most skilled clinician. Infants needing neonatal intensive care may not respond to pain with clear signals. There are many reasons, such as low energy reserves, sedation, paralysis, and vague or unclear behavioral cues due to illness and/or prematurity.[3] These factors can cause care providers to differ in their assessment of a neonate's pain. A complete approach to assessment is required for the neonatal care provider to adequately determine the presence of pain, interpret the findings, and address pain appropriately. Cong et al. developed a conceptual framework for analyzing and interpreting pain in neonates.[4] It is represented in Figure 15.1.

FACTORS AFFECTING NEONATAL PAIN

There are many factors that can contribute to neonatal pain. It is important for clinicians to identify background information and other factors that might affect the intensity of pain. To begin, gestational age (GA) is one factor that can cause pain to be magnified. New research has suggested the younger the GA the more exaggerated the pain response, due to the immaturity of the neurologic system.[3] The severity of a neonate's illness is another contributing factor to pain, as well as previous pain experiences. Next, the type of procedure being performed changes the severity of a painful event and whether the event is repeated. Finally, infants who have experienced long-term pain may have an amplified response to pain because it has not been properly controlled in the past.[4]

CLINICIAN JUDGEMENT AND ATTITUDES ON PAIN

Pain assessment is an area that can be very subjective depending on the experiences, attitudes, and beliefs of the clinician. Knowledge and clinical judgement about pain together play a role in accurately assessing pain.[5] Clinicians must understand and believe that certain events are painful and stressful to neonates in the NICU. Even as

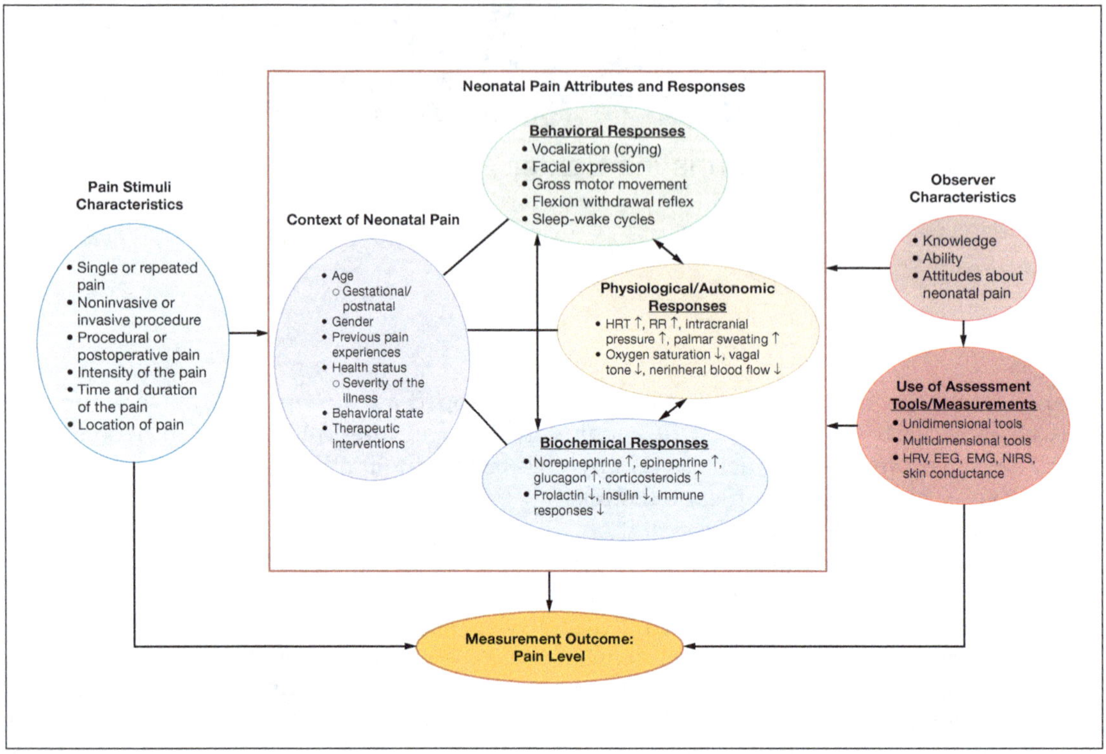

FIGURE 15.1 Conceptual framework of pain measurement in neonates

Source: From Cong X, McGrath JM, Cusson RM, and Zhang D. 2013. Pain assessment and measurement in neonates: An updated review. *Advances in Neonatal Care* 13(6): 379–395. doi: 10.1097/ANC.0b013e3182a41452

recently as 30 years ago, many believed neonates did not feel pain and did not need pain-relieving interventions.[6] Understanding severity of procedures, the immaturity of the neurologic system, and previous painful experiences are all key for a clinician to understand neonatal pain.[5] Utilizing reliable and validated pain assessment tools is necessary to make objective pain assessments and address a neonate's pain in an appropriate manner. A combination of both pain assessment guidelines and staff education is associated with improved neonatal pain management.[7]

TYPES OF PAIN RESPONSES

There are several different types of responses that can be seen with neonates experiencing pain. They include behavioral, physiological, and biochemical responses.[4] Behavioral and physiological responses are used in pain assessment tools to accurately quantify pain in a population that cannot verbalize their pain. Biochemical responses cannot be assessed clinically, so they are not included in current tools; however, there is research being conducted on different ways to measure neonatal pain that include these types of responses.[1]

Behavioral Responses

Behavioral responses can be observed in an infant's facial activity, crying, and body movements. A "cry face" (Figure 15.2) consisting of subtle changes in the infant's facial expressions such as brow bulge, eye squeeze, and nasolabial furrow is the most specific indicator of acute pain in newborns.[8–11] GA and behavioral state (BS) will have a significant impact on the infant's facial expressions, with younger and sleeping infants having a diminished or delayed response.

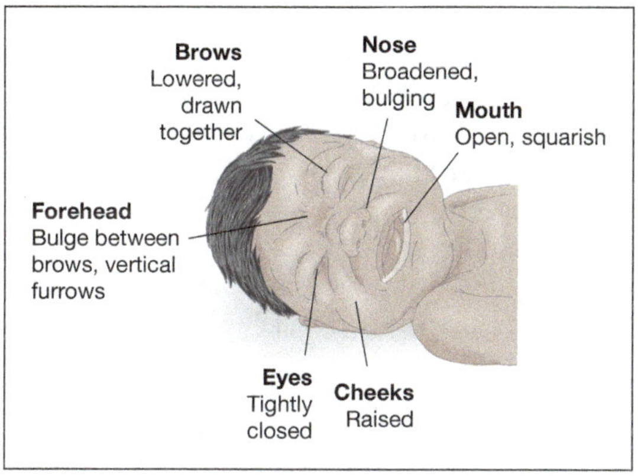

FIGURE 15.2 Characteristic of "cry face"

The clinician can also observe and listen to the infant's cry. Different aspects of cry, such as pitch, harshness, and intensity, may communicate the urgency or severity of distress.[12,13] Absence of cry or objective signs of pain does not necessarily mean that the infant is not in pain; it may only signal that the infant's response capability has been depleted.[11,14–17] Individual body movements can also provide helpful information about the infant's pain experience. Infants, particularly healthy term newborns, may use reflexive limb withdrawal in response to noxious stimuli to signal pain.[18] Because of inadequate muscle strength, posture, tone, and movement compared to term newborns, preterm neonates display less vigorous and robust pain responses.[14,15,19] Other observed behaviors exhibited by preterm neonates include increased flexion and extension of arms, and toe and finger splay.[20–22]

Physiologic Responses

Evidence of pain can also be observed through physiologic changes. The clinician can often observe vital sign changes when pain is experienced by an infant. Neonates will acutely respond to pain of handling or procedures with increases in heart rate (HR) and blood pressure while oxygen saturation decreases.[3,4,23] There can be changes in perfusion, including mottling, decreased capillary refill, and peripheral pulses.[4] These responses may be even more exaggerated in extremely preterm infants, or they can exhibit a "shut down" response as this is their only way to exhibit pain.[4,5] However, in prolonged pain, these physiologic parameters may not be valid indicators for assessment.[24]

Biochemical Responses

Biochemical responses that have been identified in neonates include increases in the secretion of norepinephrine and epinephrine. Often, this is why blood pressure increases are observed. There is also an uptake in glucagon and secretion of cortisol, all characteristics of a stress response. This stress response results in decreased insulin, prolactin, and immune responses placing the infant at higher risk for more severe illness states.[4]

SPECIAL POPULATIONS

Extremely preterm infants (born <28 weeks), neurologically impaired, pharmacologically paralyzed or sedated, and other special populations of infants can be even more challenging to accurately assess pain. They require extensive knowledge and excellent caregiver judgement to adequately assess and address their pain.

Extremely Preterm Infants

Gestation at birth and postmenstrual age both affect pain response, with more robust responses to pain stimuli noted with advancing gestation and postmenstrual age.[25] The extremely preterm infant's lack of response does not necessarily indicate a lack of pain perception, but may be due to factors such as exhaustion, minimal energy reserves, protective apathy (resulting from the infant's repeated attempts to communicate that they are in pain with no response from caregivers), or disease progression.[14,26,27]

Many factors influence healthcare providers effectively recognizing pain in extremely preterm infants. Factors in the NICU include unit culture, workload, experience of the team, patient acuity, process efficiency, and general knowledge of neonatal pain behaviors that evolve with development and maturity. Caregivers express uncertainty in their assessment of extremely preterm infants because of variable and sometimes very subtle indications of pain. More research is needed on pain responses in this special population to assist healthcare staff in recognizing and treating pain in vulnerable infants.[5]

Neurologically Impaired Infants

There are generalized perceptions that, as the level of neurologic impairment increases, the infant experiences progressively less pain compared to infants without impairment.[28,29]

Stevens et al. conducted a study to gain group consensus among 14 pediatric pain experts on pain indicators thought to be characteristic of infants at risk for neurologic impairment (low, moderate, and severe risk). The highest level of agreement among experts on pain indicators in infants at risk for neurologic impairment was on brow bulge, facial grimace, eye squeeze, and inconsolability. The expert panel also agreed that, for the severe risk group, HR changes and decreased oxygen saturation were important indicators of pain.[30]

Another study found infants at a postmenstrual age of approximately 32 weeks with Grade IV intraventricular hemorrhage or cystic periventricular leukomalacia by ultrasound showed no signs of altered pain response compared with matched controls. The infants with parenchymal brain injury demonstrated significantly more tongue protrusion upon heel lance.[31]

In a prospective cohort study, pain was compared in healthy newborn babies to babies with trisomy 21 who had developmental delays. The infants with trisomy 21 expressed pain more slowly, and the response was less clearly defined than in the infants without trisomy 21. Infants with trisomy 21 had significantly lower oxygen saturation levels after the puncture ($p < .001$). When pain was finally detected in these infants, it took twice as long for them to recover to baseline values than the control group ($p < .001$). Oxygen saturation and pain response after a painful procedure was not affected by skin-to-skin contact. Nurses need to keep in mind that infants with trisomy 21 are neither quick nor robust in their response to pain.[32]

It is essential for the clinician to remember that pain control is still necessary for neurologically impaired infants to reduce pain and possibly aid in faster recovery from procedures.

Pharmacologically Paralyzed or Sedated Infants

Infants receiving moderate to heavy sedation or paralytic agents cannot mount a behavioral response to pain. Risk factors for pain should be carefully considered, and physiologic measures of pain should be used in the absence of behavioral indicators.[33,34] Unfortunately, there are no available pain instruments for use with this special NICU population. The Neonatal Pain, Agitation, and Sedation Scale (N-PASS) can be used to help evaluate sedation levels; however, it is not reflective of actual pain scores. There are new and emerging technologies, such as near-infrared spectroscopy (NIRS), amplitude-integrated electroencephalography (EEG), functional magnetic resonance imaging (FMRI), skin conductance, and HR variability assessment, that are being explored and may be future technology used to assess pain in these infants.[2,35]

Infants With Persistent or Chronic Pain

Prolonged or persistent pain is limited in research, especially in the preterm population. Most of the research on neonatal pain consists of acute procedural, and postoperative pain.[1] Neonatal staff often form a general impression when assessing persistent pain in neonates. Indicators most used by staff include physiological parameters, facial expression, body posture and movements, response to handling, sleep patterns, and subjective opinion. Neonatal staff report more difficulty identifying chronic pain and comfort than parents do observing their own infant.[36] One study evaluated chronic pain in ventilated preterm infants. The infants were randomized to receive morphine or a placebo. They were then assessed for persistent pain by clinical staff, including nurses and doctors. Infants on morphine therapy were correctly identified by staff members 71% of the time.[37]

It has been suggested that neonatal pain that lasts longer than 7 days should be treated as chronic pain. Over time, chronic pain can dampen the physiologic response to pain. An infant with acute pain may show dramatic changes in vital signs, such as HR, whereas an infant with chronic pain may have little change in HR variability.[38]

The Échelle Douleur Inconfort Nouveau-Né (EDIN [Scale of Pain and Discomfort Newborn]) scale and N-PASS have shown validity and reliability for chronic pain, but the evidence is not strong.[1,39,40] A study by Ancora et al. showed that GA affected EDIN scores of infants exposed to prolonged pain.[41] EDIN scores were lowest in the extremely low-birth-weight (ELBW) infants as compared to infants who were gestationally more mature. Five behavioral indicators with increasing scores indicating prolonged pain comprise this scale: facial activity, body movements, quality of sleep, quality of nurse–infant interaction, and ability to be consoled (Figure 15.3).

More subdued responses may be seen in infants with chronic pain, or a complete shutdown may become apparent when pain exceeds the infant's ability to respond, as with any overwhelming stimulation.[25,42] These reactions may be caused by the ongoing nature of persistent or chronic pain, during which the usual pain signals do not result in relief, thus resulting in a negative feedback loop.

Indicator	Score/Description	Results
Facial activity	0: Relaxed facial activity 1: Transient grimaces with frowning, lip purse, and chin quiver 2: Frequent grimaces, lasting grimaces 3: Permanent grimaces resembling crying or blank face	
Body movements	0: Relaxed body movements 1: Transient agitation, often quiet 2: Frequent agitation but can becalmed down 3: Permanent agitation with contraction of fingers and toes and hypertonia of limbs or infrequent, slow movements and prostration	
Quality of sleep	0: Falls asleep easily 1: Falls asleep with difficulty 2: Frequent, spontaneous arousals, independent of nursing, restless sleep 3: Sleeplessness	
Quality of contact with nurses	0: Smiles, attentive to voice 1: Transient apprehension during interactions with nurses 2: Difficulty communicating with nurses, cries in response to minor stimulation 3: Refusal to communicate with nurses, no interpersonal rapport, moans without stimulation	
Consolability	0: Quiet, total relaxation 1: Calms down quickly in response to stroking or voice or with sucking 2: Calms down with difficulty 3: Disconsolate, sucks desperately	
	TOTAL SCORE =	

FIGURE 15.3 EDIN pain scale—assessment of prolonged pain in premature infants

Source: Adapted from Debillon T, Zupan V, Ravault N, Magny JF, and Dehan M. 2001. Development and initial validation of the EDIN scale, a new tool for assessing prolonged pain in preterm infants. *Archives of Disease in Childhood: Fetal Neonatal Edition* 85(1): F37. Reprinted by permission.[39]

Infants Exposed to Maternal Medications and Opioids

Infants born to mothers who have taken medications and/or drugs that may lead to withdrawal are another population of infants where pain scoring can be affected due to exposure. Infants exposed prenatally or postnatally through breast milk to selective serotonin reuptake inhibitors (SSRIs) and benzodiazepines demonstrate significantly decreased facial action and less cardiac reactivity during heel lance than those not exposed to psychotropic medications. Mean HR was significantly lower during recovery from heel lance for the SSRI-exposed infants.[43,44]

Infants with neonatal opioid withdrawal syndrome (NOWS) should be evaluated for pain during their weaning process. Pain screening with a validated tool in combination with neonatal abstinence scoring and/or Eat, Sleep, Console scoring can alert the clinician to the presence of pain because some indicators differ among instruments.[45] Iatrogenic withdrawal differs from neonatal abstinence in that dependence results from medications to alleviate pain. Therefore, outside sources of pain, rather than pain from withdrawal, should be considered. Healthcare providers must distinguish between iatrogenic withdrawal and NOWS.[46]

Infants at End of Life

Infants at the end of life warrant specialized pain assessment and care outside standard pain management practices. Currently, there is no appropriate tool sensitive to neonatal pain at the end of life. It is best, if available, to guide pain management with the help of palliative care services. Ethics committees can also be a useful resource for this population. Providing proper education for end-of-life care practices within an institution is necessary for all clinicians that may care for dying infants.[47] A study by Fortney and Steward reported documentation of pain scores and symptoms of discomfort in neonates at end of life is frequently inadequate. Inadequate medical record documentation may lead to undertreatment of pain throughout the dying process.[48]

Special Conditions

Neonates with certain conditions and circumstances have an increased risk for painful experiences. Infants with disorders like epidermolysis bullosa (EB) or osteogenesis imperfecta likely experience higher levels of pain due to the nature of their conditions. They will warrant extra pain-control measures and monitoring.[49,50]

Infants are also at risk of pain during transport to other facilities. A prospective cohort study by Harrison and McKechnie[51] showed higher pain scores for all GAs during road transfer. Pain assessment during transfer and appropriate treatment are critical components of neonatal care.

PAIN ASSESSSMENT TOOLS

Pain assessment is best accomplished using a published pain assessment tool with known reliability and validity that has been demonstrated to be clinically useful and feasible in the clinical setting. Identifying and adapting a single pain assessment tool to be used in practice, depending on the caregiver's population, is necessary to reduce subjectivity and gain consistency.[52] There are a variety of pain assessment tools available for scoring pain in hospitalized neonates. Many of these tools have been studied extensively to show interrater reliability and validity. Consistency in use and excellent comprehension with a pain assessment tool is necessary for addressing pain appropriately. Table 15.1 summarizes commonly used pain scoring tools developed by Perry et al.[3] The most commonly used tools in neonates for daily pain assessment[3] are Neonatal Facial Coding System (NFCS) developed by Grunau and Craig;[9] N-PASS developed by Hummel et al.;[53,54] COMFORTneo Scale by van Dijk et al.;[55] Neonatal Infant Pain Scale (NIPS) developed by Lawrence et al.;[56] and Face, Legs, Activity, Cry, Consolability (FLACC) scale

TABLE 15.1: SUMMARY OF RECOMMENDED PAIN ASSESSMENT SCALES FOR NEONATES

INSTRUMENT	ITEMS/SCORE RANGE	CLINICAL UTILITY	RELIABILITY/ VALIDITY
NFCS (Grunau et al., 1987)	9 items: Brow bulge, eye squeeze, naso-labial furrow, open lips, stretch mouth (vertical), stretch mouth (horizontal), lip purse, taut tongue, and chin quiver Score: 0 to 9 (full-term); 0 to 10 (preterm)	Procedural pain; Preterm, Full-term	InterRR: 0.88 IntraRR: 0.83 Face, content, and construct validity: Yes
FLACC (Merkel et al., 1997)	5 items: FLACC Score: 0 to 10	Postoperative pain; Preverbal/nonverbal children <7 years old	InterRR: 0.94 Content and construct validity: Yes
COMFORTneo—modified from the COMFORT behavior scale (Van Dijk et al., 2009)	7 items: Alertness, calmness/agitation, respiratory response (in mechanically ventilated children), crying (in spontaneously breathing children), body movement, facial tension, (body) muscle tone. Score: 6 to 30	Prolonged pain Sedation level; Preterm, Full-term 24 to 42 weeks GA	InterRR: 0.79 Internal consistency: 0.84 to 0.88 Concurrent validity: Yes
NIPS (Lawrence et al., 1993)	6 items: 5 behavioral items (facial expression, cry, arms, legs, and state of arousal) and 1 physiological item (breathing pattern) Score: 0 to 7	Procedural pain, Postoperative pain; Preterm, Full-term 26 to 47 weeks GA	InterRR: 0.92 to 0.97 Internal consistency: 0.87 to 0.95 Concurrent validity: 0.53 to 0.84
N-PASS (Hummel et al., 2008)	5 items: 4 behavioral items (crying/irritability, behavior/state, facial expression, extremities/tone) and 1 physiological item (vital signs: HR, RR, BP, and SaO 2) Score: 0 to 10	Ongoing pain (Ventilation Sedation level), Procedural pain, Postoperative pain, Preterm, and Full-term 23 to 40 weeks GA	Internal consistency: 0.85 to 0.95 InterRR: 0.88 to 0.93 Test–retest reliability: 0.87

(continued)

TABLE 15.1: SUMMARY OF RECOMMENDED PAIN ASSESSMENT SCALES FOR NEONATES *(continued)*

INSTRUMENT	ITEMS/SCORE RANGE	CLINICAL UTILITY	RELIABILITY/ VALIDITY
PIPP (Stevens et al., 1996) **PIPP-R** (Stevens et al., 2014)	7 items: 3 behavioral items (brow bulge, eye squeeze, and nasolabial furrow), 2 physiological items (HR oxygen saturation), and 2 contextual items (gestational age, behavioral state) Score: 0 to 18 (full-term); 21 (preterm)	Procedural pain, postoperative pain; Preterm, Full-term 28 to 42 weeks GA The most commonly used tools in research studies	InterRR: 0.93 to 0.96 IntraRR: 0.94 to 0.98 Content and construct validity: Yes

FLACC, Face, Legs, Activity, Cry, Consolability; GA, gestational age; HR, heart rate; InterRR, inter-rater reliability; IntraRR, intra-rater reliability; NFCS, Neonatal Facial Coding System; NIPS, Neonatal Infant Pain Scale; N-PASS, Neonatal Pain, Agitation, and Sedation Scale; PIPP, Premature Infant Pain Profile; PIPP-R, Premature Infant Pain Profile—Revised; wks, weeks.

Source: Perry M, Tan Z, Chen J, Weidig T, Xu W, and Cong XS. 2018. Neonatal pain: Perceptions and current practice. *Critical Care Nursing Clinics of North America* 30(4): 549–561. doi: 10.1016/j.cnc.2018.07.013[3]

by Merkel et al.[57] The Premature Infant Pain Profile-Revised (PIPP-R) developed by Stevens et al.[58,59] is recommended for pain measurement in research studies.[3,59] The NFCS, N-PASS, COMFORTneo, NIPS, and PIPP-R are all validated for premature infants as low as 23 weeks gestation.[52]

The NFCS is a tool that is validated and reliable for infants from 25 to 40 weeks gestation. It has nine items that evaluate behavioral indicators of pain. It does not have a physiologic component to the pain scale. Scores range from 0 to 9 for term and 0 to 10 for preterm, as it has a prematurity adjustment.[3,9,52]

The N-PASS measures acute or chronic pain and agitation, and it has a component to evaluate level of sedation in neonates between 23 and 40 weeks GA.[53,54] It has been shown to be reliable and valid in many populations including extremely preterm, post operatively, ventilated, and nonventilated infants.[40] The N-PASS is the pain score recommended by the American Academy of Pediatrics for measuring neonatal pain and sedation.[2,40] The N-PASS contains four behavioral indicators (crying/irritability, behavior state, facial expression, and extremities/tone) and one physiologic indicator (vital signs). Points are added to the pain score based on the infant's GA to compensate for the preterm neonate's limited ability to communicate pain behaviorally or physiologically. Total pain scores vary depending on the infant's GA, but scores greater than or equal to four usually signify pain requiring an intervention. Nonpharmacologic comfort measures should always be utilized first and then move to pharmacologic pain interventions.[52] The sedation portion of the N-PASS requires an assessment of response to stimuli and can be useful in titrating opioid requirements based on level of sedation desired. Sedation is scored between 0 and 2 for each behavioral and physiologic criterion, then summed and noted as a negative score (0 to −10). Scores of −10 to −5 are considered deep sedation, whereas light sedation scores range from −5 to −2. The N-PASS is shown in Figure 15.4.

The COMFORTneo is a tool for infants from 25 to 43 weeks gestation. It can assess acute or chronic pain. The tool also only has behavioral indicators of pain and no physiologic indicators. It can assess prolonged sedation levels as well. Scores range from 6 to 30.[9,52,55]

N-PASS:
Neonatal Pain, Agitation, & Sedation Scale

Assessment Criteria	Sedation		Sedation/Pain	Pain/Agitation	
	−2	−1	0/0	1	2
Crying Irritability	No cry with painful stimuli	Moans or cries minimally with painful stimuli	No sedation/ No pain signs	Irritable or crying at intervals Consolable	High-pitched or silent-continuous cry Inconsolable
Behavior State	No arousal to any stimuli No spontaneous movement	Arouses minimally to stimuli Little spontaneous movement	No sedation/ No pain signs	Restless, squirming Awakens frequently	Arching, kicking Constantly awake or Arouses minimally/no movement (not sedated)
Facial Expression	Mouth is lax No expression	Minimal expression with stimuli	No sedation/ No pain signs	Any pain expression intermittent	Any pain expression continual
Extremities Tone	No grasp reflex Flaccid tone	Weak grasp reflex ↓ muscle tone	No sedation/ No pain signs	Intermittent clenched toes, fists or finger splay Body is not tense	Continual clenched toes, fists, or finger splay Body is tense
Vital Signs HR, RR, BP, SaO_2	No variability with stimuli Hypoventilation or apnea	< 10% variability from baseline with stimuli	No sedation/ No pain signs	↑ 10–20% from baseline SaO_2 76–85% with stimulation – quick ↑	↑ > 20% from baseline SaO_2 ≤ 75% with stimulation – slow ↑ Out of sync/fighting vent

Premature Pain Assessment → +1 if <30 weeks gestation / corrected age

FIGURE 15.4 N-PASS pain assessment tool

BP, blood pressure; HR, heart rate; RR, respiration rate

Source: Hummel P, Puchalski M, Creech SD, and Weiss MG. 2008. Clinical reliability and validity of the N-PASS: Neonatal pain, agitation and sedation scale with prolonged pain. *Journal of Perinatology* 28(1): 55–60.

The NIPS (Figure 15.5) was originally developed to assess procedural pain in preterm and term newborns, but some literature also validates its utility with postoperative pain.[60–62] However, due to the lack of physiologic parameters for HR, blood pressure, or oxygen saturation, some have questioned its ability to completely assess pain in postoperative infants.[2,3,52] The NIPS examines five behavioral parameters (e.g., facial expression, crying, arms, legs, and state of arousal) and one physiologic parameter (e.g., breathing pattern). Total score ranges from 0 to 7.[56] This tool is particularly useful in assessing pain in healthy term and preterm infants. Although guidelines for pain interventions based on total score are not provided by the developers of the NIPS, all pain instruments in neonates are based on the premise of increasing pain intensity. Therefore, in tools without scoring guidelines for pain management, when pain scores reach the midrange of the total possible points for that tool (e.g., approximately 4 or greater with the NIPS), the clinician may infer that the infant is experiencing moderate to severe pain and that an intervention for that pain is warranted.

The FLACC is a scale that addresses behavioral indicators of pain. It consists of five items with scores from 0 to 10. It is clinically used for postoperative pain in children under 7 years old. It has no adjustment for prematurity, so it is not often used in NICUs. It is more likely used in pediatric intensive care settings.[3,57,63]

	Before Time*		During Time*					After Time*		
	1	2	1	2	3	4	5	1	2	3
Facial expression 0: Relaxed 1: Grimace										
Cry 0: No cry 1: Whimper 2: Vigorous										
Breathing patterns 0: Relaxed 1: Change in breathing										
Arms 0: Relaxed/restrained 1: Flexed/extended										
Legs 0: Relaxed/restrained 1: Flexed/extended										
State of arousal 0: Sleeping/awake 1: Fussy										
Total										

* Time is measured in 1-minute intervals.

FIGURE 15.5 Neonatal Infant Pain Scale

The PIPP has been revised (PIPP-R) to address construct validity and feasibility, allowing the caregiver to more easily apply the PIPP-R (Figure 15.6) in the clinical setting.[32] The PIPP-R, which measures acute pain, has undergone rigorous psychometric testing, making it an ideal tool for research studies.[58,59] Although the PIPP-R may be presumed to be valid only with preterm neonates, it has been tested in neonates ranging in age from 24 to 40 weeks GA. The PIPP-R incorporates two contextual factors that may account for an infant's less robust pain responses, which can result from immaturity or BS. By scoring infants who are younger or asleep higher on the PIPP-R, the adjusted scores do not penalize those known to be less capable of mounting a robust response to noxious stimuli. The PIPP-R contains two physiologic indicators (e.g., HR and oxygen saturation) and three facial indicators (e.g., brow bulge, eye squeeze, and nasolabial furrow). Physiologic and behavioral indicators are straightforward to score when scoring procedural pain but are often more challenging if used to score ongoing pain. If no clear 15-second baseline period is available for scoring, the clinician must sometimes judge baseline parameters using either preoperative vital signs or estimated vital signs before the known painful event. Although total scores vary between 18 and 21, depending on the infant's GA, scores between 7 and 12 usually signify mild to moderate pain requiring nonpharmacologic comfort measures and possibly a mild analgesic. Scores greater than 12 indicate moderate to severe pain requiring pharmacologic pain intervention in addition to comfort measures.[3,59]

The CRIES tool (an acronym for the five parameters it measures: **C**rying, **R**equires oxygen to maintain saturation greater than 95%, **I**ncreased vital signs, **E**xpression, and **S**leepless) is another instrument that has

Infant Indicator	Indicator Score				Infant Indicator Score
	0	+1	+2	+3	
Change in HR (bpm) Baseline: ______	0–4	5–14	15–24	>24	
Decrease in oxygen SAT (%) Baseline: ______	0–2	3–5	6–8	>8 or increase in O_2	
Brow bulge (seconds)	None (<3)	Minimal (3–10)	Moderate (11–20)	Maximal (>20)	
Eye squeeze (seconds)	None (<3)	Minimal (3–10)	Moderate (11–20)	Maximal (>20)	
Nasolabial furrow (seconds)	None (<3)	Minimal (3–10)	Moderate (11–20)	Maximal (>20)	
				Subtotal Score:*	
Gestational Age (weeks + days)	>36 weeks	32 weeks–35 weeks, 6 days	28 weeks–31 weeks, 6 days	<28 weeks	
Baseline BS	Active and awake	Quiet and awake	Active and asleep	Quiet and asleep	
				Total Score:**	

*Subtotal for physiological and facial indicators. If subtotal score is >0, add GA and BS indicator scores.

**Total Score should equal Subtotal Score + GA Score + BS Score.

Scoring instructions

Step 1: Observe infant for **15 seconds at rest** and assess vital sign indicators (highest HR and lowest O_2 SAT) and BS.

Step 2: Observe infant for **30 seconds after procedure** and assess **change** in vital sign indicators (maximal HR, lowest O_2 SAT* and duration of facial actions observed).
*If infant requires an increase in oxygen at any point before or during procedure, they receive a score of 3 for the O_2 SAT indicator.

Step 3: Score for corrected gestational GA and BS if the subtotal score >0.

Step 4: Calculate total score by adding **Subtotal Score + BS Score.**

FIGURE 15.6 Premature Infant Pain Profile—Revised

BS, behavioral state; GA, gestational age; HR, heart rate; SAT, saturation.

Source: Adapted from Stevens BJ, Gibbins S, Yamada J, Dionne K, Lee G, Johnston C, and Taddio A. 2014. The premature infant pain profile—Revised (PIPP-R): Initial validation and feasibility. *Clinical Journal of Pain* 30(3): 239.[59]

been used extensively to assess postoperative or prolonged pain in neonates between 32 and 60 weeks gestation age (Figure 15.7).[2,64] Infants previously requiring oxygen are more difficult to score using the CRIES instrument. It provides no specific guideline for infants previously requiring oxygen, so nursing judgment is required to systematically adjust scores in this category to account for increases in oxygen levels above baseline values. In addition, if the CRIES score is used for procedural pain assessment, baseline vital signs taken immediately before the procedure can be used for scoring the category of "increased vital signs." Total scores for CRIES range from 0 to 10, with scores less than 4 indicating mild pain requiring nonpharmacologic pain relief measures and scores 5 or greater consistent with moderate to severe pain requiring pharmacologic intervention in conjunction with comfort measures.[64]

DIFFERENT TYPES OF TECHNOLOGY

There are many different types of technology that have been used in research settings to better objectively assess pain in neonates, in conjunction with validated pain scoring

	Scoring Criteria for Each Assessment			
	0	1	2	Infant's Score
Crying	No	High pitched	Inconsolable	
Requires O_2 for saturation >95%	No	<30%	>30%	
Increased vital signs*	HR and BP within 10% of preoperative value	HR or BP 11–20% higher than preoperative value	HR or BP 21% or more above preoperative value	
Expression	None	Grimace	Grimace/grunt	
Sleepless	No	Wakes at frequent intervals	Constantly awake	
			Total score†	

* BP should be done last.
† Add scores for all assessments to calculate total score.
Key: BP = blood pressure; HR = heart rate.

FIGURE 15.7 CRIES: Neonatal postoperative pain assessment score

Source: Copyright Krechel S, and Bildner J. Neonatal pain assessment tool developed at the University of Missouri-Columbia. Reprinted by permission.

tools. However, many of these are difficult to apply in clinical practice due to feasibility of use and lack of knowledge of how to interpret results. Some of these tools are HR variability, EEG, NIRS, skin conductance, and salivary cortisol levels.[3,52] They all need further research in studies to be able to apply to clinical practice.

DOCUMENTATION

Documentation of pain data should be done in a way that helps the caregiver analyze the infant's current pain responses and trends over time. Pain should also be assessed prior to painful procedures as well as within 30 minutes after a procedure to ensure pain is properly addressed. This information allows the care provider to better communicate with the clinical team to evaluate the trend of pain scores and vital signs over time that may support the need for additional pain management interventions. A single pain score provides immediate information about pain at one moment in time (Figure 15.8) but does not give an overview of fluctuating scores over time; adequacy of pain control; gradually increasing pain; or emerging tolerance to a particular medication, dose, or dose interval. Individual scores are useful when an acute event causes elevated pain scores. However, gradually increasing scores may be missed until the score is high enough to rate intervention. By that time, pain management may be more difficult. A documentation design that can be used in electronic format must be capable of plotting pain scores and vital signs over time (e.g., 12 hours, 24 hours, 1 week). Subtle changes are easier to see if the documentation method allows for an overview of vital signs along with pain scores, as is the case when using a graphic display (Figure 15.9). A care provider that is familiar with the infant's baseline assessment of vital signs and behaviors will be able to note the subtle variations over time, which may lead to better identification and management of pain.

	0800
Vitals	
Temp	98 (36.7)
Temp src	Axillary
Pulse	160
Resp	38
BP	81/56
MAP (mmHg)	61
BP location	Left leg
HeRO documentation	0.45
Oximeter	
SpO2	99
PIPS (Premature Infant Pain Scale)	
Gestational age	1
Behavioral state	1
HR baseline	160
Sat baseline	99
HR max	171
Oxygen sat minimum	99
Heart Rate	1
Oxygen sat	0
Brow bulge	0
Eye squeeze	0
Nasolabial furrow	0
PIPS Score	3
Is PIPS Score >7? If yes a reassessment is needed:	

FIGURE 15.8 Example of a single pain evaluation in an electronic medical record

BP, blood pressure; BS, behavioral state;HR, heart rate; MAP, mean arterial pressure.

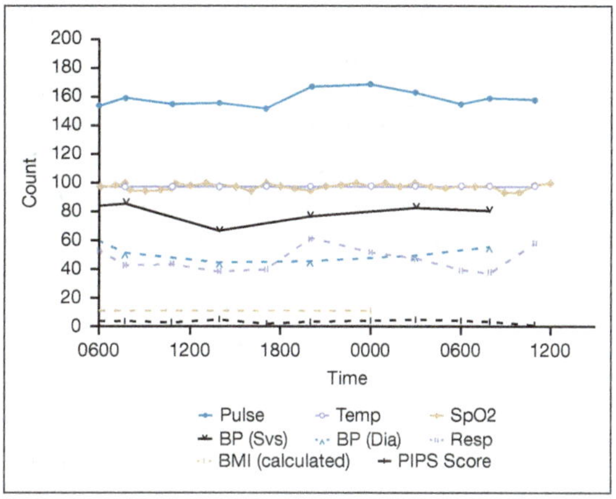

FIGURE 15.9 Graphic display example of 48 hours' trend of pain assessment with vital signs from an EMR

EMR, electronic medical record.

PARENTS' VIEWS ON PAIN

Core concepts central to family-centered care highlight the importance of information sharing and shared decision making between parents and the healthcare team. Over the past decade, parents have voiced an increasing desire for more information about their infant's pain and to have the opportunity to participate in their infant's pain relief.[65–67]

Surveys of parents regarding pain assessment and management for their infant in the NICU provide some guidance concerning their needs associated with neonatal pain. In one survey of 257 parents from nine NICUs in the United Kingdom and the United States, 64% of parents were dissatisfied because they received no information about infant pain. Thirty percent of parents were disappointed with the information they had received and only 18% of parents reported being taught by NICU staff how to identify their infant's pain signals. Seventy percent of parents wrote comments on ways they identified their infant's pain signs, with crying (37%), movements (31%), or facial expression (21%) being the most reported. Very few parents used skin color or cardiorespiratory monitor data for pain assessment.[68]

A study by Franck et al. in 2011 provided parents with written information on pain assessment and comfort techniques. Study findings demonstrated that while maternal satisfaction increased, stress was not reduced.[69] The timing of information received and increased involvement opportunities were important to NICU parents. Consideration of the parents' emotional states, quality of NICU staff communication, and support are positively related to parents' desired level of participation.[70]

Interviews and focus groups with parents show that their infant's pain is a source of stress and that health team members have an important role in alleviating that stress.[71] The ability to participate in parenting their infant seems to provide a coping mechanism that relieved some of the distress associated with the pain their infant endured in the NICU. Parents felt there was a difference between their perceptions of their infant's pain and the perceptions of NICU staff members. This disparity increased their anxiety, as did the concern that staff might not intervene when presented with signs of pain by their infant after the parents left the NICU. These issues heightened parental stress, whereas support by NICU staff, parenting opportunities, and information or resources relieved it.

Parental participation in pain management activities is enhanced when parents are provided with adequate and ongoing information about their infant's medical procedures, knowledge of effective pain management strategies, and knowing how they can be an active partner in providing pain relief to their infant.[65] A family-friendly environment, close communication, and collaboration between parents and the healthcare team may also foster parental participation. In contrast, work culture, unsupportive hospital policies, and paternalistic staff attitudes may hinder parental involvement during painful procedures.[65,67] For the benefit of both families and the infant, it is important for healthcare providers to encourage parents to participate in their infant's care and pain management. They are a vital resource that is often overlooked.[1]

SUMMARY

Pain assessment is an essential prerequisite to optimal pain management. Pain is best assessed when a multidimensional approach is employed using a valid and reliable instrument. Balancing pain assessment data with the infant's risk factors for pain and contextual modifiers that can impact how the infant communicates pain will ensure that pain is recognized early and interventions are implemented in a timely manner.

ADDITIONAL RESOURCES

SPRINGER PUBLISHING CONNECT™

A robust set of resources designed to supplement this text is located at http://connect.springerpub.com/content/book/978-0-8261-4063-0. Qualifying instructors may request access by emailing textbook@springerpub.com.

REFERENCES

1. Maxwell LG, Fraga MV, and Malavolta CP. 2019. Assessment of pain in the newborn: An update. *Clinics in Perinatology* 46(4): 693–707. doi: 10.1016/j.clp.2019.08.005
2. Committee on Fetus and Newborn, and Section on Anesthesiology and Pain Medicine. 2016. Prevention and management of procedural pain in the neonate: An update. *Pediatrics* 137(2): e20154271. doi: 10.1542/peds.2015-4271
3. Perry M, Tan Z, Chen J, Weidig T, Xu W, and Cong XS. 2018. Neonatal pain: Perceptions and current practice. *Critical Care Nursing Clinics of North America* 30(4): 549–561. doi: 10.1016/j.cnc.2018.07.013
4. Cong X, McGrath JM, Cusson RM, and Zhang D. 2013. Pain assessment and measurement in neonates: An updated review. *Advances in Neonatal Care* 13(6): 379–395. doi: 10.1097/ANC.0b013e3182a41452
5. Gibbins S, Stevens B, Dionne K, Yamada J, Pillai Riddell R, McGrath P, Asztalos E, O'Brien K, Beyene J, McNamara P, and Johnston C. 2015. Perceptions of health professionals on pain in extremely low gestational age infants. *Qualitative Health Research* 25(6): 763–774.
6. Allegaert K. 2020. A critical review on the relevance of paracetamol for procedural pain management in neonates. *Frontiers in Pediatrics* 8: 89. Published 2020, March 18. doi: 10.3389/fped.2020.00089
7. Pölkki T, Korhonen A, and Laukkala H. 2018. Nurses' perceptions of pain assessment and management practices in neonates: A cross-sectional survey. *Scandinavian Journal of Caring Sciences* 32(2): 725–733. doi: 10.1111/scs.12503
8. Gibbins S, and Stevens B. 2003. The influence of gestational age on the efficacy and short-term safety of sucrose for procedural pain relief. *Advances in Neonatal Care* 3(5): 241–249.
9. Grunau RV, and Craig KD. 1987. Pain expression in neonates: Facial action and cry. *Pain* 28(3): 395–410.

10. Grunau RV, Johnston CC, and Craig KD. 1990. Neonatal facial and cry responses to invasive and noninvasive procedures. *Pain* 42(3): 295–305.
11. Stevens BJ, Johnston CC, and Horton L. 1993. Multidimensional pain assessment in premature infants: A pilot study. *Journal of Obstetric, Gynecologic, and Neonatal Nursing* 22(6): 531–541.
12. Fuller BF. 1991. Acoustic discrimination of three types of infant cries. *Nursing Research* 40(3): 156–160.
13. Porter FL, Porges SW, and Marshall RE. 1988. Newborn cries and vagal tone: Parallel changes in response to circumcision. *Child Development* 59(2): 495–505.
14. Johnston CC, Stevens BJ, Franck LS, Jack A, Stremler R, and Platt R. 1999. Factors explaining lack of response to heel stick in preterm newborns. *Journal of Obstetric, Gynecologic, and Neonatal Nursing* 28(6): 587–594.
15. Johnston CC, Stevens BJ, Yang F, and Horton L. 1995. Differential response to pain by very premature infants. *Pain* 61(3): 471–479.
16. Stevens BJ, Johnston CC, and Horton L. 1994. Factors that influence the behavioral pain responses of premature infants. *Pain* 59(1): 101–109.
17. Walden M. 2014. Pain in the newborn and infant. In *Comprehensive Neonatal Nursing Care: An Interdisciplinary Approach*, 5th ed. Kenner C, and Lott JW, eds. Philadelphia, PA: Saunders, 571–586.
18. Franck LS. 1986. A new method to quantitatively describe pain behavior in infants. *Nursing Research* 35(1): 28–31.
19. Craig KD, Whitfield MF, Grunau RV, Linton J, and Hadjistavropoulos HD. 1993. Pain in the preterm neonate: Behavioral and physiological indices. *Pain* 52(3): 287–299. (Published erratum in *Pain*, 1993, 54[1]: 111.)
20. Grunau RE, Holsti L, Whitfield MF, and Ling E. 2000. Are twitches, startles, and body movements pain indicators in extremely low birth weight infants? *Clinical Journal of Pain* 16(1): 37–45.
21. Holsti L, Grunau RE, Oberlander TF, and Whitfield MF. 2004. Specific newborn individualized developmental care and assessment program movements are associated with acute pain in preterm infants in the neonatal intensive care unit. *Pediatrics* 114(1): 65–72.
22. Morison SJ, Holsti L, Grunau RE, Whitfield MF, Oberlander TF, Chan HW, and Williams L. 2003. Are there developmentally distinct motor indicators of pain in preterm infants? *Early Human Development* 72(2): 131–146.
23. Sweet SD, and McGrath PJ. 1998. Relative importance of mothers' versus medical staffs' behavior in the prediction of infant immunization pain behavior. *Journal of Pediatric Psychology* 23(4): 249–256.
24. Hummel P, and van Dijk M. 2006. Pain assessment: Current status and challenges. *Seminars in Fetal & Neonatal Medicine* 11(4): 237–245.
25. Ranger M, Johnston CC, and Anand KJ. 2007. Current controversies regarding pain assessment in neonates. *Seminars in Perinatology* 31(5): 283–288.
26. Tronick EZ, Scanlon KB, and Scanlon JW. 1990. Protective apathy, a hypothesis about the behavioral organization and its relation to clinical and physiologic status of the preterm infant during the newborn period. *Clinics in Perinatology* 17(1): 125–154.
27. Gibbins S, Stevens B, McGrath PJ, Yamada J, Beyene J, Breau L, Camfield C, Finley A, Franck L, Johnston C, and Howlett A. 2008. Comparison of pain responses in infants of different gestational ages. *Neonatology* 93(1): 10–18.
28. Breau LM, McGrath PJ, Stevens B, Beyene J, Camfield C, Finley GA, Franck L, Gibbins S, Howlett A, McKeever P, and O'Brien K. 2006. Judgments of pain in the neonatal intensive care setting: A survey of direct care staffs' perceptions of pain in infants at risk for neurological impairment. *Clinical Journal of Pain* 22(2): 122–129.
29. Stevens B, McGrath P, Dupuis A, Gibbins S, Beyene J, Breau L, Camfield C, Allen Finley G, Franck LS, Howlett A, and Johnston C. 2009. Indicators of pain in neonates at risk for neurological impairment. *Journal of Advanced Nursing* 65(2): 285–296.
30. Stevens B, McGrath P, Yamada J, Gibbins S, Beyene J, Breau L, Camfield C, Finley A, Franck L, Howlett A, and Johnston C. 2006. Identification of pain indicators for infants at risk for neurological impairment: A Delphi consensus study. *BMC Pediatrics* 6: 1–9.
31. Oberlander TF, Grunau RE, Fitzgerald C, and Whitfield MF. 2002. Does parenchymal brain injury affect biobehavioral pain responses in very low birth weight infants at 32 weeks postconceptional age? *Pediatrics* 110(3): 570–576.
32. Aguilar Cordero MJ, Mur Villar N, and Garcia Garcia I. 2015. Evaluation of pain in healthy newborns and in newborns with developmental problems (Down syndrome). *Pain Management Nursing* 16(3): 267–272.
33. Walden M, Sudia-Robinson T, and Carrier CT. 2001. Comfort care for infants in the neonatal intensive care unit at end of life. *Newborn and Infant Nursing Reviews* 1(2): 97–105.
34. Walden M. 2015. Pain assessment and management. In *Core Curriculum for Neonatal Intensive Care Nursing*, 5th ed. Verklan MT, and Walden M, eds. Philadelphia, PA: Saunders, 316–330.
35. Holsti L, Grunau RE, and Shany E. 2011. Assessing pain in preterm infants in the neonatal intensive care unit: Moving to a "brain-oriented" approach. *Pain Management* 1(2): 171–179.
36. Boyle EM, Bradshaw J, and Blake KI. 2017. Persistent pain in neonates: Challenges in assessment without the aid of a clinical tool. *Acta Paediatrica* 107(1): 63–67.
37. Boyle EM, Freer Y, Wong CM, McIntosh N, and Anand KJS. 2006. Assessment of persistent pain or distress and adequacy of analgesia in preterm ventilated infants. *Pain* 124(1–2): 87–91.
38. Anand KJS. 2017. Defining pain in newborns: Need for a uniform taxonomy? *Acta Paediatrica* 106(9): 1438–1444.
39. Debillon T, Zupan V, Ravault N, Magny JF, and Dehan M. 2001. Development and initial validation of the EDIN scale, a new tool for assessing prolonged

pain in preterm infants. *Archives of Disease in Childhood: Fetal and Neonatal Edition* 85(1): F36–F41.
40. Morgan ME, Kukora S, Nemshak M, and Shuman CJ. 2020. Neonatal pain, agitation, and sedation scale's use, reliability, and validity: A systematic review. *Journal of Perinatology* 40(12): 1753–1763. doi: 10.1038/s41372-020-00840-7
41. Ancora G, Mastrocola M, Bagnara C, Zola D, Pierantoni L, Rossi G, Corvaglia L, and Faldella G. 2009. Influence of gestational age on the EDIN score: An observational study. *Archives of Disease in Childhood: Fetal and Neonatal Edition* 94(1): F35–F38.
42. Herr K, Coyne PJ, Key T, Manworren R, McCaffery M, Merkel S, Pelosi-Kelly J, and Wild L. 2006. Pain assessment in the nonverbal patient: Position statement with clinical practice recommendations. *Pain Management Nursing* 7(2): 44–52.
43. Oberlander TF, Eckstein Grunau R, Fitzgerald C, Ellwood AL, Misri S, Rurak D, and Riggs KW. 2002. Prolonged prenatal psychotropic medication exposure alters neonatal acute pain response. *Pediatric Research* 51(4): 443–453.
44. Oberlander TF, Grunau RE, Fitzgerald C, Papsdorf M, Rurak D, and Riggs W. 2005. Pain reactivity in 2-month-old infants after prenatal and postnatal serotonin reuptake inhibitor medication exposure. *Pediatrics* 115(2): 411–425.
45. Isaac L, van den Hoogen NJ, Habib S, and Trang T. 2022. Maternal and iatrogenic neonatal opioid withdrawal syndrome: Differences and similarities in recognition, management, and consequences. *Journal of Neuroscience Research* 100(1): 373–395. doi: 10.1002/jnr.24811
46. Cramton REM, and Gruchala NE. 2013. Babies breaking bad: Neonatal and iatrogenic withdrawal syndromes. *Current Opinions in Pediatrics* 25(4): 532–542.
47. Carter BS. 2018. Pediatric palliative care in infants and neonates. *Children (Basel)* 5(2): 21. Published 2018, February 7. doi: 10.3390/children5020021
48. Fortney CA, and Steward DK. 2015. Medical record documentation and symptom management at the end of life in the NICU. *Advances in Neonatal Care* 15(1): 48–55.
49. Prodinger C, Reichelt J, Bauer JW, and Laimer M. 2019. Epidermolysis bullosa: Advances in research and treatment. *Experimental Dermatology* 28(10): 1176–1189. doi: 10.1111/exd.13979
50. Marom R, Rabenhorst BM, and Morello R. 2020. Osteogenesis imperfecta: An update on clinical features and therapies. *European Journal of Endocrinology* 183(4): R95–R106. doi: 10.1530/EJE-20-0299
51. Harrison C, and McKechnie L. 2012. How comfortable is neonatal transport? *Acta Paediatrica* 101(2): 143–147.
52. McPherson C, Ortinau CM, and Vesoulis Z. 2021. Practical approaches to sedation and analgesia in the newborn. *Journal of Perinatology* 41(3): 383–395. doi: 10.1038/s41372-020-00878-7
53. Hummel P, Puchalski M, Creech SD, and Weiss MG. 2008. Clinical reliability and validity of the N-PASS: Neonatal pain, agitation and sedation scale with prolonged pain. *Journal of Perinatology* 28(1): 55–60.
54. Hummel P, Lawlor-Klean P, and Weiss MG. 2010. Validity and reliability of the N-PASS assessment tool with acute pain. *Journal of Perinatology* 30(7): 474–478.
55. van Dijk M, Roofthooft DW, Anand KJ, Guldemond F, de Graaf J, Simons S, de Jager Y, van Goudoever JB, and Tibboel D. 2009. Taking up the challenge of measuring prolonged pain in (premature) neonates: The COMFORTneo scale seems promising. *Clinical Journal of Pain* 25(7): 607–616. doi: 10.1097/AJP.0b013e3181a5b52a
56. Lawrence J, Alcock D, McGrath P, Kay J, MacMurray SB, and Dulberg C. 1993. The development of a tool to assess neonatal pain. *Neonatal Network* 12(6): 59–66.
57. Merkel SI, Voepel-Lewis T, Shayevitz JR, and Malviya S. 1997. The FLACC: A behavioral scale for scoring postoperative pain in young children. *Pediatric Nursing* 23(3): 293–297.
58. Stevens B, Johnston C, Petryshen P, and Taddio A. 1996. Premature infant pain profile: Development and initial validation. *Clinical Journal of Pain* 12(1): 13–22.
59. Stevens BJ, Gibbins S, Yamada J, Dionne K, Lee G, Johnston C, and Taddio A. 2014. The premature infant pain profile-revised (PIPP-R): Initial validation and feasibility. *Clinical Journal of Pain* 30(3): 238–243.
60. Rouss K, Gerber A, Albisetti M, Hug M, and Bernet V. 2007. Long-term subcutaneous morphine administration after surgery in newborns. *Journal of Perinatal Medicine* 35(1): 79–81.
61. Suraseranivongse S, Kaosaard R, Intakong P, Pornsiriprasert S, Karnchana Y, Kaopinpruck J, and Sangjeen K. 2006. A comparison of postoperative pain scales in neonates. *British Journal of Anaesthesia* 97(4): 540–544.
62. Leelanukrom R, Suraseranivongse S, Boonrukwanich V, and Wechwinij S. 2012. Effect of wound infiltration with bupivacaine on postoperative analgesia in neonates and infants undergoing major abdominal surgery: A pilot randomized control trial. *Journal of Anesthesia* 26(4): 541–544.
63. Crellin DJ, Harrison D, Santamaria N, and Babl FE. 2015. Systematic review of the face, legs, activity, cry and consolability scale for assessing pain in infants and children: Is it reliable, valid, and feasible for use? *Pain* 156(11): 2132–2151. doi: 10.1097/j.pain.0000000000000305
64. Krechel SW, and Bildner J. 1995. CRIES: A new neonatal postoperative pain measurement score. Initial testing of validity and reliability. *Paediatric Anaesthesia* 5(1): 53–61. doi: 10.1111/j.1460-9592.1995.tb00242.x
65. Palomaa AK, Korhonen A, and Polkki T. 2016. Factors influencing parental participation in neonatal pain alleviation. *Journal of Pediatric Nursing* 31(5): 519–527.
66. Marfurt-Russenberger K, Axelin A, Kesselring A, Franck LS, and Cignacco E. 2016. The experiences of professionals regarding involvement of parents

in neonatal pain management. *Journal of Obstetric Gynecologic and Neonatal Nursing* 45(5): 671–683.

67. Vazquez V, Cong X, and DeJong A. 2015. Maternal and paternal knowledge and perceptions regarding infant pain in the NICU. *Neonatal Network* 34(6): 337–344.
68. Franck LS, Allen A, Cox S, and Winter I. 2005. Parents' views about infant pain in neonatal intensive care. *Clinical Journal of Pain* 21(2): 133–139.
69. Franck L, Oulton K, Nderitu S, Lim M, Fang S, and Kaiser A. 2011. Parent involvement in pain management for NICU infants: A randomized controlled trial. *Pediatrics* 128(3): 510–518.
70. Franck L, Oulton K, and Bruce E. 2012. Parental involvement in neonatal pain management: An empirical and conceptual update. *Journal of Nursing Scholarship* 44(1): 45–54.
71. Gale G, Franck LS, Kools S, and Lynch M. 2004. Parents' perceptions of their infant's pain experience in the NICU. *International Journal of Nursing Studies* 41(1): 51–58.

16 ASSESSMENT OF THE NEWBORN WITH ANTENATAL EXPOSURE TO DRUGS

Carol M. Wallman

Substance use disorders during pregnancy are a significant health issue. A thorough assessment of a newborn involves the evaluation for possible in utero exposure to tobacco, alcohol, marijuana, and other pharmacologic agents either prescribed or from illicit use. The National Survey on Drug Use and Health (NSDUH) conducted by the Substance Abuse and Mental Health Services Administration (SAMHSA) provides data on the use of tobacco, alcohol, marijuana, and illicit drugs, including the misuse of prescription medications, in the United States. This data has been collected for several years by asking individuals about their use of substances in the month prior to answering the survey questions. The surveys report this data as "past month substance use." In 2020 (SAMHSA 2022), "past month use" among pregnant females aged 15 to 44 varied only slightly from 194,000 or 8.5% in 2017 to 169,000 or 8.3% in 2020 (Table 16.1).[1]

The most common illicit drug consumed during pregnancy remains marijuana followed by opioids and cocaine.[1] While many states have voted to legalize both medicinal and recreational marijuana, it remains illegal at a federal level and is reported as an illicit drug. The misuse of prescription pain relievers and the opioid epidemic in the United States remains a national problem, yet misuse among pregnant women has shown a decrease from 32,000 or 1.4% in 2017 to 8,000 or 0.4% in 2020.[1] Current evidence supports an increased use of nonpharmacologic means and rooming in with parents rather than direct admission to a neonatal intensive care unit to manage neonatal withdrawal and has decreased both the length of stay and use of medications for neonates experiencing withdrawal.[2]

The use of alcohol continues to be a significant health issue among pregnant females aged 15 to 44 (Table 16.1).[1] Although it is difficult to obtain exact data on the number of infants exposed to alcohol in utero who subsequently develop fetal alcohol syndrome (FAS) or fetal alcohol spectrum disorders (FASD), global rates of 0.77% and European/North American rates of 2% to 5% are estimated.[3]

In addition to illicit drug and alcohol use, there is concern for cigarette use during pregnancy. According to the SAMHSA survey, the percentage of pregnant females aged 15 to 44 who used cigarettes decreased from 14.7% in 2017 to 8.4% in 2020, still leaving significant room for improvement (see Table 16.1).

ASSESSMENT AND IDENTIFICATION

The first step in assessing an infant with perinatal substance exposure is accurate identification. Perinatal substance use disorder is a complex diagnosis and crosses socioeconomic and racial lines, making an objective approach to identifying risk factors imperative. The most comprehensive approach to identification of perinatal substance use includes an accurate review of maternal history for self-reported use, risk factors for maternal use, neonatal history and presentation, as well as biologic specimens supporting maternal use or neonatal exposure.[4]

Maternal Risk Factors

Individuals with a diagnosis of a substance use disorder can experience significant stigmatization.[4] However, accurate identification

TABLE 16.1: SUBSTANCE USE IN PAST MONTH AMONG PREGNANT FEMALES AGED 15 TO 44

DRUG	2017 (%)	2018 (%)	2019 (%)	2020 (%)
Illicit drugs (total)	8.5	5.4	5.8	8.3
Marijuana	7.1	4.7	5.4	8
Opioids	1.4	0.9	0.4	0.4
Cocaine	0.4	Precise data not available	0.2	0.3
Tobacco products	14.7	11.6	9.6	8.4
Alcohol	11.5	9.9	9.5	10.6

Source: Center for Behavioral Health Statistics and Quality. 2022. *National Survey on Drug Use and Health: Detailed Tables.* Rockville, MD: Substance Abuse and Mental Health Services Administration. Retrieved from https://www.samhsa.gov/data/sites/default/files/reports/rpt37925/2020NSDUHWomenSlides072522.pdf.[1]

is essential to provide optimal care to the newborn, along with supportive and nonjudgmental care to the mother and family. Ideally prenatal counseling and support addressing perinatal substance use concerns has been provided. If this has not occurred, the neonatal healthcare team is responsible for identifying the neonate who has been exposed. The combination of a structured interview and review of maternal and neonatal history along with the evaluation of a biologic specimen increases the likelihood of identification.[5] A thorough maternal history should include information gathered on substance use, including prescribed and unprescribed medications; childhood adversities; inconsistent, limited, inadequate, or no prenatal care; exposure to violence and unresolved trauma; mental health disorders; perinatal depression; poor nutrition; presence of infectious diseases including HIV and hepatitis C virus infections; and sexually transmitted diseases. Additionally, the family housing needs, food insecurities, and status of significant others should be assessed. Finally, the presence of premature onset of labor, abruptio placentae, intrauterine growth restriction, and congenital malformations should be identified. However, restricting assessment to those only with associated risk factors will not identify all neonates perinatally exposed. For this reason, some advocate for universal testing of all pregnant patients or newborns.[5] Finally, once identified, an ongoing assessment includes assessment of family strengths and needs for a safe discharge plan for the newborn.[5]

Newborn Risk Factors

Newborns born to women with a substance use disorder during pregnancy have an increased risk of complications. Due to the prevalence of polysubstance use, it is difficult to determine a direct cause between a specific substance use during pregnancy and a specific newborn complication. Prematurity, intrauterine growth restriction, jitteriness, hypertonicity, congenital malformations, and signs of withdrawal have all been associated with perinatal substance use.[5] During this time of assessment other diagnoses with similar presentations should be considered; these may include infection, hypocalcemia, hypoglycemia, and other causes of neurologic injury.[5]

BIOLOGIC SPECIMENS

Biologic specimens available to aide in the identification of in utero exposure to nicotine, alcohol, and illicit drugs include urine, hair, meconium, and umbilical cord tissue. Each specimen has its own unique challenges with collection and accuracy of results and only identifies substances within a limited time frame between exposure and collection of a sample.[5] This variability in identification leads to the potential for a false negative test result. Biologic specimens should be considered only one part of a comprehensive evaluation for perinatal substance use. However, even with this combined approach of interviews, a comprehensive review of both maternal and newborn histories, and the evaluation of biologic specimens, some newborns with antenatal exposure may not be identified.[5]

IMPACT ON THE FETUS

An accurate assessment of the neonate with in utero drug exposure requires an understanding of the mechanism of the impact of fetal exposure to drugs. Impact on the fetus is determined by a multitude of factors. Exposure during the embryonic phase of gestation, when a woman may not yet realize she is pregnant, can have teratogenic effects such as seen with FAS. During the next phase of development, the fetal period, major structural development has occurred. Drug exposure during this phase may be more subtle upon examination but can include abnormal growth patterns, as well as alterations in neurotransmitters, receptors, and brain organization. In addition to exposure to substances in utero, maternal lifestyle challenges, including poor nutrition, limited or no access to healthcare, exposure to violence, as well as a history of significant mental illness, can impact fetal growth and development.[5]

Alcohol

Teratogenic effects of maternal alcohol consumption during pregnancy have been well documented since 1973.[3] The impact on the fetus occurs throughout gestation and can include identifiable physical characteristics noted in the neonatal period as well as behavioral problems and learning deficits identified after the neonatal period. The wide range of potential findings are referred to as FASDs. The most impactful end of the FASD spectrum is FAS. A neonate with FAS may exhibit craniofacial abnormalities such as smooth philtrum, thin upper lip, short palpebral fissures, as well as microcephaly, growth restriction, and central nervous system dysfunction.[3]

Nicotine

Fetal nicotine exposure can occur secondary to maternal cigarette smoking, e-cigarettes, vaping, and secondhand smoke. Fetal exposure to maternal smoking has been associated with placental dysfunction, spontaneous abortion, intrauterine growth restriction, preterm birth, and cleft lip and palate.[6] A newborn exposed to in utero cigarette smoke may demonstrate jitteriness and hypertonicity. Potential long-term morbidities related to fetal exposure to nicotine and toxins from cigarette smoke include decreased cognitive functioning, auditory processing deficits, impulsivity, anxiety, depression, attention deficit hyperactivity disorder, reduced lung function, and asthma in offspring and an increased risk for sudden infant death syndrome.[6]

Cocaine

Cocaine alters the norepinephrine, dopamine, and serotonin neurotransmitter pathways and readily crosses the placenta and is excreted into breast milk. Exposure to cocaine can result in tachycardia, arrhythmias, hypertension, vasoconstriction, diaphoresis, and mild tremors when in the bloodstream. Newborns may present with a high-pitched cry, excessive sucking, irritability, and hyperactivity when cocaine is present in the bloodstream as a result of maternal use. These symptoms are often reported on the second or third postnatal day. There is no specific withdrawal syndrome reported in newborns exposed to in utero cocaine. Antenatal exposure to cocaine has a significant impact on fetal growth due to restriction of placental blood flow resulting in decreased birth weight, length, and head circumference in term newborns. The vasoconstriction associated with cocaine has also been correlated with placental abruption, intestinal atresia, and necrotizing enterocolitis in a small series of term and preterm newborns prenatally exposed to cocaine. However, no clear association with a teratogenic effect has been identified with maternal use of cocaine during pregnancy.[5]

Amphetamines

Methamphetamine is a potent sympathomimetic stimulant causing vasoconstriction. Like the use of cocaine during pregnancy, the use of methamphetamine during pregnancy has been associated with premature birth, growth restriction, placental abruption, and fetal distress.[5] There are no clear associations with methamphetamine use during pregnancy and a withdrawal syndrome or congenital malformations, yet there is some concern for long-term cognitive deficits and physical dexterity.[5]

Marijuana

Marijuana is the most frequently used illicit drug among females, yet is consumed less during pregnancy (Table 16.2). The frequency of use during pregnancy continues to rise in correlation with the legalization of marijuana for both medical and recreational use in some states.[1] The active psychogenic component of marijuana is delta-9-tetrahydrocannabinol (THC). THC readily crosses the placenta and may be associated with fetal growth restriction, prematurity, and stillbirth.[7] In addition, patients who used marijuana during their pregnancy had a higher incidence of anemia, and newborns had a lower birth weight and higher NICU admission rate.[7] No clear withdrawal syndrome has been associated with newborns exposed to antenatal marijuana, yet exposure has been associated with abnormal sleep patterns, poor responses to visual stimuli, and high-pitched cries. Furthermore, a long-term association with decreased executive functioning skills, including poor impulse control, poor visual memory, and attention deficit and learning challenges has been reported.[7,8] Finally, it is important to note that the marijuana consumed currently has significantly higher THC levels than the marijuana consumed decades ago when most research data regarding marijuana use during pregnancy and potential fetal/neonatal impacts were reported.[8]

Opioids

Newborns may have been exposed to opioids in utero from either illicit or prescribed maternal use. They may also have been exposed in the NICU for pain management. Maternal illicit opioid use is frequently combined with other substances. Fetal or neonatal exposure can result in unique neurobehavioral findings described as either neonatal abstinence syndrome (NAS) or more recently referred to as neonatal opioid withdrawal syndrome (NOWS). This differentiation has been made to distinguish between withdrawal from non-opioid exposures such as benzodiazepines, NAS, and that from primarily opioid

TABLE 16.2: DAILY OR ALMOST DAILY MARIJUANA USE IN PAST YEAR: AMONG WOMEN AGED 15 TO 44 BY PREGNANCY STATUS

	2017 (%)	2018 (%)	2019 (%)	2020 (%)
Pregnant	3.1	1.5	1.7	2.8
Not Pregnant	3.4	3.6	4.4	4.8

Source: Center for Behavioral Health Statistics and Quality. 2022. *National Survey on Drug Use and Health: Detailed Tables*. Rockville, MD: Substance Abuse and Mental Health Services Administration. Retrieved from https://www.samhsa.gov/data/sites/default/files/reports/rpt37925/2020NSDUHWomenSlides072522.pdf.[1]

exposures, NOWS. The amount and duration of fetal or neonatal opioid exposure may correlate with the degree of NOWS. The longer and higher concentrations of opioid exposure are associated with more severe clinical presentation and a longer duration. Maternal patterns of polysubstance use of cigarettes, benzodiazepines, and gabapentin may also increase the severity and duration of withdrawal symptoms in NAS. Short-term maternal exposures around the time of delivery such as in an epidural do not cause signs of neonatal withdrawal.[9]

Patients receiving treatment for opioid addiction may be treated with a synthetic medication to decrease their cravings for an opioid and to improve healthy lifestyle choices including increased prenatal care, decreased illicit drug use, and improved fetal outcomes. Synthetic medications prescribed for substance use disorders during pregnancy include methadone, buprenorphine, and Suboxone (buprenorphine and naloxone). However, it is important to note that even prescribed medication-assisted treatments can result in the neonate experiencing NOWS.[9] Some patients with opioid use disorders have turned to Kratom which carries a natural herb status but has opioid effects as a treatment for pain. There is limited data related to maternal Kratom use, but it has been associated with a neonatal withdrawal similar to NOWS.[10]

NEONATAL OPIOID WITHDRAWAL SYNDROME

Abrupt discontinuation of prolonged opioid exposure to a fetus or newborn may result in NOWS. The withdrawal experienced by the newborn is a physiologic withdrawal and should be distinguished from an addiction. An addiction includes drug-seeking behavior. Opioid withdrawal is complex and not well understood in adults, and is even more complicated in newborns due to intricate maternal–fetal–placental pharmacokinetics and immature neurologic development of the fetus/newborn. Opioids primarily act through opioid receptors located in the central nervous system, peripheral nervous system, and gastrointestinal system. The lack of exposure to opioids during withdrawal causes an increase in norepinephrine production, triggering the majority of clinical symptoms including loose stools and tremors.[9]

Clinical Presentation

NOWS is complex and its presentation may vary from newborn to newborn depending on the type of opioid exposure, dose and length of exposure, length of time from last exposure to presentation of symptoms, and neurologic maturity of the newborn (Table 16.3). Premature infants tend to exhibit fewer signs of withdrawal, which may be due to decreased amount and length of exposure as well as neurologic immaturity, limiting their ability to demonstrate clinical signs of NOWS or NAS. In general, heroin exposure results in earlier and shorter NOWS symptoms when compared to methadone or buprenorphine.[9]

Clinical signs and symptoms of NOWS or NAS include tremors, jitteriness, myoclonic jerks, irritability, poor sleep patterns, excessive crying, high-pitched crying, poor feeding, poor weight gain, hyperphagia (excessive desire to eat), emesis, diarrhea, sneezing, mottling, tachypnea, tachycardia, temperature instability, and skin excoriation. Perianal excoriation is secondary to gastrointestinal disturbances, whereas excoriation of face and body is secondary to excessive irritation and movements. In general, term newborns, with good birth weights, exposure to more than one substance in utero, and/or cigarette exposure, present with more severe clinical symptoms of NAS with a longer duration of symptoms.[5] Although rarely seen today, in the 1970s seizures were reported in 2% to 11% of neonates with severe NAS.[11] In 1988, a study by Pinto and associates reported abnormal EEG findings in 30% of infants with NAS.[12] Clinical and long-term implications of seizures and abnormal EEG findings are unknown. Withdrawal signs in the neonate can mimic other serious conditions such as infection, hypoglycemia, hypocalcemia, hyperthyroidism, intracranial hemorrhage,

TABLE 16.3: NOWS PRESENTATION ONSET AND DURATION BASED ON DRUG EXPOSURE

DRUG	ONSET IN HOURS AFTER LAST EXPOSURE	DURATION OF NAS IN DAYS
Heroin	24 to 48	8 to 10
Methadone	48 to 72	Up to 30 or more
Buprenorphine	36 to 60	Up to 28 or more
Prescription opioid medications	36 to 72	10 to 30

NAS, neonatal abstinence syndrome; NOWS, neonatal opioid withdrawal syndrome.

Source: Kocherlakota P. 2014. Neonatal abstinence syndrome. *Journal of Pediatrics* 134(2): e547–e561.

hypoxic ischemic encephalopathy, and hyperviscosity (Table 16.4).[13] Therefore, a complete assessment and evaluation are always necessary when an infant presents with any of the findings mentioned here.

ANTIDEPRESSANTS AND BENZODIAZEPINES

Women with perinatal depression are at increased risk for substance use disorders. In addition, antidepressants and benzodiazepines when used as prescribed have been associated with NAS. Selective serotonin reuptake inhibitors (SSRIs), selective norepinephrine reuptake inhibitors (SNRIs), and tricyclic antidepressants (TCAs) have all been associated with NAS, especially with long-term high-dose maternal use. The neonatal withdrawal can present as late as 7 to 21 days in exposed neonates due to the long half-life of these medications.[5]

ASSESSMENT TOOLS

When NAS was first recognized, a standardized, objective, and comprehensive approach to assessment became critical to guide treatment. Assessment should be ongoing and obtained when the infant is in a

TABLE 16.4: CAUSES OF THE CLINICAL PRESENTATION OF NAS

CENTRAL NERVOUS DISTURBANCES	METABOLIC/VASOMOTOR/ RESPIRATORY DISTURBANCES	GASTROINTESTINAL DYSFUNCTION
Excessive/continuous high-pitched cry	Sweating	Excessive sucking
Poor sleep patterns/ excessive wakefulness	Temperature instability/fever	Poor feeding
Hyperactive Moro reflex	Mottling	Emesis
Tremors	Yawning	Loose/watery stools
Increased muscle tone	Nasal stuffiness	Excoriation of skin
Myoclonic jerks	Sneezing	
Seizures	Nasal flaring, tachypnea	

NAS, neonatal abstinence syndrome.

Source: Jones HE, et al. 2012. Maternal opioid treatment: Human experimental research (MOTHER) approach, issues and lessons learned. *Addiction* 107: 28–35.[13]

low-stimulation environment using a standardized and validated tool.[7] The predominant NAS scoring tool studied for validity and reliability and historically utilized in the United States is the Finnegan Neonatal Abstinence Scoring System.[14] Based on this early work by Finnegan, a variety of infant withdrawal assessment tools have been developed and utilized over the past several decades.[5]

Current evidence supports a comprehensive approach to managing perinatal substance use disorders to maximize pregnancy outcomes and minimize clinical presentation of NAS and NOWS. Incorporating prenatal counseling and empowerment of parent involvement, along with a simplified newborn functional assessment, has shown a significant reduction in both the need for newborn pharmacologic treatment and hospital length of stay. The simplified functional assessment includes assessing the newborn's ability to either breastfeed successfully or take greater than or equal to 1 ounce from a bottle per feed, sleep undisturbed for greater than or equal to 1 hour, and, if crying, be consoled within 10 minutes. This approach to management of the neonate is often referred to as the Eat, Sleep, Console (ESC) approach.[15] Effective utilization of any scoring tool or functional assessment approach includes ongoing education and training for staff and providers regarding objective scoring and interpretation and a team approach to family-centered care, objective assessments, a supportive and low-stimulation environment, maximization of nonpharmacologic techniques, and pharmacologic treatment only when indicated.

SUMMARY

Substance use disorders during pregnancy continue to be a significant health issue impacting the fetus and newborn. A thorough assessment of a newborn involves the systematic, objective evaluation for possible in utero exposure to nicotine, alcohol, marijuana, opioids, and other illicit drugs. Recognizing varying risks associated with specific substances used in utero will aid the provider in offering appropriate nonjudgmental support and care for each newborn and family impacted by substance use disorders.

ADDITIONAL RESOURCES

SPRINGER PUBLISHING CONNECT™

A robust set of resources designed to supplement this text is located at http://connect.springerpub.com/content/book/978-0-8261-4063-0. Qualifying instructors may request access by emailing textbook@springerpub.com.

REFERENCES

1. Center for Behavioral Health Statistics and Quality. 2022. *National Survey on Drug Use and Health: Detailed Tables*. Rockville, MD: Substance Abuse and Mental Health Services Administration. Retrieved from https://www.samhsa.gov/data/sites/default/files/reports/rpt37925/2020NSDUHWomenSlides072522.pdf
2. Grossman MR, Berkwitt AK, Osborn RR, Citarella BV, Hochreiter D, and Bizzaro MJ. 2020. Evaluating the effect of hospital setting on outcomes for neonatal abstinence syndrome. *Journal of Perinatology* 40: 1483–1488. doi: 10.1038/s41372-020-0621-5
3. Wozniak JR, Riley EP, and Charness ME. 2019, August. Clinical presentation, diagnosis, and management of fetal alcohol spectrum disorder. *Lancet Neurology* 18(8): 760–770. doi: 10.1016/S1474-4422(19)30150-4. Epub 2019 May 31. PMID: 31160204; PMCID: PMC6995665.
4. Nichols TR, Welborn A, Gringle MR, and Lee A. 2021. Social stigma and perinatal substance use services: Recognizing the power of the good mother ideal. *Contemporary Drug Problems* 48(1): 19–37. doi: 10.1177/0091450920969200
5. Hudak ML. 2020. Infants of substance-using mothers. In *Neonatal—Perinatal Medicine Diseases of the Fetus and Infant*, 11th ed. Martin RJ, Fanaroff AA, and Walsh MA, eds. Elsevier, vol. 1, 735–750.
6. Falck AJ, Mooney SM, and Bearer CF. 2019. Adverse exposures to the fetus and neonate. In *Neonatal—Perinatal Medicine Diseases of the Fetus and Infant*, 11th ed. Martin RJ, Fanaroff AA, and Walsh MC, eds. Elsevier, vol. 1, 239–259.
7. Ryan SA, Ammerman SD, O'Connor ME, Committee on Substance Use and Prevention; Section on

Breastfeeding, Gonzalez L, Patrick SW, Quigley J, Walker LR, Meek JY, Johnston M, Stellwagen L, Thomas J, and Ware J. 2018. Committee on substance use and prevention, section on breastfeeding. Gonzalez L et al. Marijuana use during pregnancy and breastfeeding: Implications for neonatal and childhood outcomes. *Pediatrics* 142(3): e20181889. doi: 10.1542/peds.2018-1889

8. Wallman C, Baessler C, and Hoffman JM. 2020. National association of neonatal nurses. Marijuana, breastfeeding, and the use of human milk position statement #3071. *Advances in Neonatal Care* 21(3): 176–177. doi: 10.1097/ANC.0000000000000904
9. Patrick SW, Barfield WD, Poindexter BB, Committee on Fetus and Newborn, Committee on Substance Use And Prevention, Cummings J, Hand I, Adams-Chapman I, Aucott SW, Puopolo KM, Goldsmith JP, MD, Kaufman D, Martin C, Mowitz M, Gonzalez L, Camenga DR, Quigley J, Ryan SA, and Walker-Harding L. 2020. Committee on fetus and newborn, committee on substance use and prevention. Cummings J, et al. Neonatal opioid withdrawal syndrome. *Pediatrics* 146 (5): e2020029074. doi: 10.1542/peds.2020-029074
10. Davidson L, Rawat M, Stojanovski S, and Chandrasekharan P. 2018. Natural drugs, not so natural effects: Neonatal abstinence syndrome secondary to 'kratom'. *Journal of Neonatal—Perinatal Medicine* 12(1): 109–112. doi: 10.3233/NPM-1863
11. Herzlinger RA, Kandall SR, and Vaughan HG. 1971. Neonatal seizures associated with narcotic withdrawal. *Journal of Pediatrics* 91(4): 638–641.
12. Pinto F, Torrioli MG, Gasella G, Tempesta E, and Fundarò C. 1988. Sleep in babies born to chronically heroin addicted mothers: A follow up study. *Drug and Alcohol Dependency* 21(1): 43–47.
13. Jones HE, Fischer G, Heil SH, Kaltenbach K, Martin PR, Coyle MG, Selby P, Stine SM, O'Grady KE, and Arria AM. 2012. Maternal opioid treatment: Issues and lessons learned. *Addiction* 107: 23–28.
14. Finnegal LP, Connaughton Jr. JF, Kron RE, and Emich JP. 1974. Neonatal abstinence syndrome: Assessment and management. *Addiction Management* (1–2): 141–158.
15. Grossman MR, Berkwitt AK, Osborn RR, Xu Y, Esserman DA, Shapiro ED, and Bizzaro MJ. 2017. An initiative to improve the quality of care of infants with neonatal abstinence syndrome. *Pediatrics* 139(6): e1–e8.

A ANTEPARTUM TESTS AND INTRAPARTUM MONITORING

Kimberly M. Horns and Julie A. Javernick

COMMON ANTEPARTUM SCREENING TESTS

Sequential or Integrated Screen—Ultrasound and Biochemical Assay

A mainstay of aneuploidy testing in maternal fetal medicine is the sequential screen offered to all low-risk pregnant women and birthing people. Specifically, this test screens for Patau (trisomy 13), Edwards (trisomy 18), and Down (trisomy 21) syndromes. Between 11 and 13 weeks an ultrasound is performed to measure the nuchal translucency (fluid in the nape of the neck). A measurement >3 mm is related to an abnormal collection of fluid in this area and is associated with trisomy 21. Maternal blood is also drawn and evaluated for pregnancy-associated plasma protein-A and total human chorionic gonadotropin (hcCG). If this evaluation shows an increased risk of trisomy 21, 18, or 13, a diagnostic test is offered. If this first sequence does not show an increased risk, between 15 and 17 weeks maternal serum is drawn to evaluate alpha-fetoprotein, total hcCG, unconjugated estriol, and dimeric inhibin-A. The sequential screen can detect 90% to 95% of babies with trisomy 21 with a 5% false positive rate. The nuchal fold thickness is also increased in cases of Turner syndrome (karyotype XO) due to webbing of the neck, when a cystic hygroma is present in this area, and with congenital heart disorders of the great arteries.[1,2]

Alpha-Fetoprotein Level

Alpha-fetoprotein is evaluated at 15 to 18 weeks of gestation to screen for neural tube defects, which are associated with elevated levels of this protein. Maternal serum or amniotic fluid (AF) can be used to determine levels. High levels are also associated with multiple gestation, congenital nephritis, exstrophy of the bladder, omphalocele, gastroschisis, intrauterine growth restriction, and fetal death. A lower than normal level is associated with trisomy 1, 18, and 13.[3]

Triple and Quadruple Noninvasive Screen

In the late 1970s, pregnancies were monitored by examining the AF for optical density. A low serum alpha-fetoprotein level and advanced maternal age alerted the prenatal provider to a positive risk for fetal chromosomal abnormalities.[3] The triple screen may indicate that trisomy 21 (Down syndrome) is present in the fetus and suggests the need for further evaluation. The triple screen markers of aneuploidy include alpha-fetoprotein, hcCG, and unconjugated estriol.[4] Later, the addition of inhibin-A created the "quadruple screen" increasing trisomy 21 and 18 positive screening rates to 80%.[5] This test is currently only offered to women and birthing people who enter prenatal care late and miss first trimester screening.

Noninvasive Prenatal Screening

Noninvasive prenatal screening (NIPS) utilizes a cell-free DNA analysis to screen for aneuploidies and specific genetic copy number variations (CNV), also known as *microdeletions*. Examples of these genetic disorders include trisomy 13, trisomy 18, and trisomy 21 syndromes; Turner syndrome (XO syndrome); Klinefelter syndrome (46, XXY); and microdeletions, 22q 11.2 deletion (DiGeorge syndrome), 1p36 deletion, and 15q11.2-13 deletion.[6] This noninvasive test needs only 1 mL of the mother's blood to detect the fetal DNA; DNA fractions of greater than 4% of fetal DNA found in the mother's blood are accurate for aneuploidy detection by NIPS. The NIPS is highly sensitive and specific toward the end of the first trimester and typically drawn as early as 10 weeks gestation.[7]

Genetic Carrier Screening

If women and birthing people have not previously undergone genetic carrier screening, this is offered in the first trimester. The goal of screening is to identify individuals/parents who are carriers of autosomal recessive or sex-linked disorders. Many labs now offer expanded genetic carrier screening regardless of ethnicity. While most women and birthing people only consider this screening test, during pregnancy, it can be offered prepregnancy.[8]

COMMON ANTEPARTUM DIAGNOSTIC TESTS

Amniocentesis

Amniocentesis is advised for mothers with known hereditary disorders or carrier states (e.g., cystic fibrosis) to identify a potential genetic/chromosomal disorder in the fetus and for those over 35 years of age to screen for chromosomal abnormalities. Other indications for amniocentesis for chromosomal analysis are known consanguinity in the parents, a previous child with a chromosomal or hereditary disease, or an abnormal first trimester screening test. Amniocentesis ideally is performed between 15 and 17 6/7 weeks gestation. For chromosomal analysis, the cells acquired from the AF can take from 10 to 14 days for karyotyping. At later gestational ages, amniocentesis can be used to evaluate fetal lung maturity.[9]

Chorionic Villus Sampling

Chorionic villus sampling is indicated for suspected chromosomal or biochemical defects in the fetus. It has the advantage of earlier diagnostic analysis than when amniocentesis is used. Sampling can be by the transabdominal or transcervical approach.[10,11] Chorionic tissue has the same genotype as the fetus, and testing can be performed at 10 to 12 weeks. Results are available within 24 hours because living tissue is analyzed.

OTHER ANTEPARTUM ASSESSMENTS OF FETAL WELL-BEING

Assessment of Fetal Activity

Assessment of fetal activity, or kick counts by the mother, is a noninvasive technique for monitoring fetal well-being and is recommended if there is concern for decreased fetal movement. This is thought to be an effective method of reducing fetal stillbirth.[3] Usually, monitoring begins at 28 weeks gestation.[11,12] For this evaluation, the mother rests for 1 hour daily at the same time each day in a quiet room. During that rest period, she records the fetal movements on an activity chart. Most practitioners consider a baseline of four fetal movements per hour acceptable.[11] If fewer than four fetal movements are detected, further testing is indicated.

Biophysical Profile

The biophysical profile is a more extensive evaluation of the fetus using ultrasound and the nonstress test (NST). Scoring and recommended management approaches are explained in Tables A.1 and A.2.[13] In addition to NST, ultrasound evaluations of the AF index, fetal breathing, gross and fine movement, and tone are obtained.[10,14]

Doppler Velocimetry

Doppler velocimetry evaluates blood flow in the umbilical arteries during diastole. The

TABLE A.1: BIOPHYSICAL PROFILE SCORING: VARIABLES AND SCORING CRITERIA

BIOPHYSICAL VARIABLE	NORMAL (SCORE = 2)	ABNORMAL (SCORE = 0)
FBM	At least one episode of FBM of at least 20 seconds' duration in 30 minutes of observation	Absent FBM or no episodes of >20 seconds in 30 minutes
Gross body movements	At least two discrete body/limb movements in 30 minutes (episodes of active continuous movement are considered to be a single movement)	Less than two episodes of body/limb movements in 30 minutes
Fetal tone	At least one episode of active extension with return to flexion of fetal limb(s) or trunk; opening and closing of hand considered normal tone	Either slow extension with return to partial flexion or movement of limb in full extension or absent fetal movement or partially open fetal hand
Qualitative pockets of AFV	At least one pocket of AF that measures at least 2 cm in vertical axis	Either no pockets or a pocket of <2 cm in vertical axis
Reactive FHR episodes	At least two episodes of FHR accelerations of at least 15 bpm and of >15 seconds' duration associated with fetal movement in 20 minutes	Fewer than two accelerations of FHR or accelerations of <15 bpm in 20 minutes

AF, amniotic fluid; AFV, amniotic fluid volume; bpm, beats per minute; FBM, fetal breathing movements; FHR, fetal heart rate.

Source: Adapted from Manning FA. 1999. The fetal biophysical profile. *Obstetrics and Gynecology Clinics of North America* 26(4): 560. Reprinted by permission.[13]

flow study is performed on the fetal umbilical arteries to evaluate the placental perfusion and vascular resistance of flow. Fetal deterioration and sudden critical fetal and neonatal outcome characteristics, such as growth restriction and progressively worsening placental perfusion, can be correlated with the overall measure. A decrease in diastolic flow indicates an increase in downstream placental resistance. Absent or reversed flow is an ominous sign and may indicate uteroplacental insufficiency.[10,15] It has been estimated that the use of Doppler flow velocimetry has been associated with a 29% decrease in perinatal mortality.[10] This test is used to detect a compromised fetus in diabetic, chronic hypertensive, and preeclamptic pregnancies. Doppler velocimetry is also used to detect twin-to-twin transfusion in utero.

Contraction Stress Test

A contraction stress test is a method of determining fetal well-being by evaluating the response of fetal heart rate (FHR) to uterine contractions. It is a nonspecific test of placental reserve and may be used to determine if labor induction is valid if fetal compromise is suspected. Uterine contractions normally increase FHR variability and can result in increased fetal movement. Uterine contractions are induced by oxytocin (Pitocin) or by nipple stimulation. Three contractions in a 10-minute period are evaluated. A negative test indicates the absence of late deceleration in FHR with contractions. A positive test shows late deceleration in FHR with contractions. In cases of positive stress tests and suspicious or technically poor tests, a biophysical profile may be ordered or providers may move to cesarean section.[11,16,17]

Fetal Fibronectin Levels

Fetal fibronectin is the "glue" that helps to attach the membranes surrounding the infant to the lower part of the uterus. Shortly before labor (or sometimes during labor),

TABLE A.2: INTERPRETATION OF FETAL BIOPHYSICAL PROFILE SCORE RESULTS AND RECOMMENDED CLINICAL MANAGEMENT

SCORE	INTERPRETATION	RISK OF FETAL DEATH/1,000/WEEK UNDELIVERED	MANAGEMENT
10 of 10	Nonasphyxiated	0.565	Conservative
8 of 10; normal AFV	Nonasphyxiated	0.565	Conservative
8 of 8 (NST not done)	Nonasphyxiated	0.565	Conservative
8 of 10; decreased AFV	Chronic compensated asphyxia	20 to 30	If mature (≥37 weeks): deliver
			If immature: serial testing twice a week
6 of 10; normal AFV	Possible acute fetal asphyxia	50	If mature (≥37 weeks): deliver
			If immature: repeat test in 24 hours and deliver if score remains ≤6 of 10
6 of 10; decreased AFV	Chronic asphyxia, with possible acute asphyxia	>50	If ≥32 weeks: deliver If ≤32 weeks: test daily
4 of 10; normal AFV	Acute asphyxia likely	115	If ≥32 weeks: deliver If ≤32 weeks: test daily
4 of 10; decreased AFV	Chronic asphyxia, with acute likely	>115	If ≥26 weeks: deliver
2 of 10; normal AFV	Acute asphyxia almost certain	220	If ≥26 weeks: deliver
0 of 10	Gross severe asphyxia	550	If ≥26 weeks: deliver

AFV, amniotic fluid volume; NST, nonstress test.

Source: Adapted from Manning FA. 1999. Fetal biophysical profile. *Obstetrics and Gynecology Clinics of North America* 26(4): 564. Reprinted by permission.[13]

this lower part of the uterus begins to change shape, causing the membranes to separate from the uterine wall. When this happens, fibronectin is released and mingles with a woman's cervical and vaginal secretions. The fetal fibronectin test measures the absence or presence of fibronectin levels in these secretions. When a positive fetal fibronectin value is found and added to the clinical sign of cervical shortening, the combined findings are a powerful positive predictor of preterm labor and impending birth.[18]

Lecithin-Sphingomyelin Ratio

The lecithin-sphingomyelin ratio (L/S ratio) is used to determine fetal lung maturity and is done on AF. Levels of 2 or higher indicate fetal lung maturity. Falsely high levels are seen if blood, meconium, or vaginal secretions contaminate the AF. Mature L/S ratios are not always accurate in the diabetic pregnancy and in those affected by erythroblastosis fetalis. Use of a lung profile with a phosphatidylglycerol (PG) level (see the next section) is more accurate in determining fetal lung maturity in these pregnancies.[10,16,17]

Lung Profile

The lung profile evaluates AF for the L/S ratio and for PG and phosphatidylinositol levels. PG appears in the AF as phosphatidylinositol begins to fall. The presence of PG indicates mature lungs and is not affected by a diabetic or erythroblastotic pregnancy. Contamination of the AF does not alter test accuracy. Some institutions use the lung profile for the L/S ratio and PG measurement only.[10,13]

A commercial test, the **AmnioStatFLM-PG** (Irvine Scientific Products, Santa Ana, California), is available and detects PG in a sample of AF. The test takes approximately 15 minutes and is not affected by contamination with blood or meconium. A positive test indicates pulmonary maturity.

The **TDx FLx FLM II assay** (Abbott Laboratories, Abbott Park, Illinois) is an automated fetal lung maturity test that also can be performed in less than an hour. This test determines the relative concentrations of surfactant and albumin in a sample of AF. The manufacturer's recommended interpretation of the surfactant/albumin values is as follows:[19,20]

- A value less than 30 mg/g is considered definitely immature.
- A value of 30 to 50 mg/g is considered transitionally immature and risky.
- A value of 50 to 70 mg/g is considered transitionally mature and should be treated with caution.
- A value greater than 70 mg/g indicates lung maturity.

Nonstress Test

The NST is an indirect test of placental function that assesses FHR acceleration and variability. External fetal monitoring is done, and uterine activity is monitored. Observations of the baseline FHR, accelerations, and decelerations are made. Fetal movements and changes in FHR with movement are assessed. Generally, patients are monitored for 20 minutes.[11,16] Fetal movements can be spontaneous, or they can be induced by manipulation or vibroacoustic stimulation to the mother or birthing person's abdomen.[11] Accelerations in the FHR of at least 15 bpm above baseline for 15 seconds correlate positively with fetal well-being in the term infant. At less than 32 weeks, an increase of 10 bpm above baseline for at least 10 seconds is acceptable. The results are classified as reactive, which indicates that two accelerations in FHR occurred with fetal movement in a 20-minute period, or nonreactive, which indicates that no or fewer than two periods of FHR acceleration occurred. If test results are nonreactive, testing time may be continued for another 20 minutes, or the test may be repeated later the same day.[11] In some cases, a contraction stress test or a biophysical profile will be the next step.

Ultrasound

Ultrasound examination is used throughout pregnancy for a variety of reasons. It is useful in helping to determine the gestational age, for detecting altered or abnormal growth, to monitor for changes in AF volume (AFV), and for identifying the presence of malformations. In the first trimester, it can be used to locate the gestational sac and the embryo or embryos and to determine crown-to-rump length. Pregnancy can be detected by ultrasound as early as 5 weeks from the last menstrual period. In the second and third trimesters, ultrasound can be used to evaluate for fetal loss; fetal age; a four-chamber heart; and abnormalities of the bladder, kidneys, brain, spine, and extremities. Placental maturity can be determined by grading the placenta from Grade 0 to Grade III. The status of AFV can be evaluated, and the umbilical cord can be inspected.[10] Hydrops fetalis can also be detected and monitored.

Another ultrasound finding of Down syndrome is short, long bones (femur and humerus). The nuchal fold thickness is also increased in cases of Turner syndrome (karyotype XO) due to webbing of the neck, when a cystic hygroma is present in this area, and with congenital heart disorders of the great arteries.[2]

INTRAPARTAL MONITORING

Cord Blood Gases

Cord blood gases are often obtained following delivery of depressed neonates and those with abnormal monitoring results during the intrapartum period. Information from the cord blood gases often aids understanding of the events surrounding the birth of a neonate with low Apgar scores. Cord blood gases are routinely obtained in many institutions.[2,10,21] Normal values are listed in Table A.3.

FHR Monitoring

FHR monitoring is commonly used during labor to identify fetal distress. Both continuous electronic fetal monitoring and intermittent auscultation can be used in low-risk women and birthing people. In intermittent auscultation, the fetal heartbeat is evaluated periodically with a handheld doppler before, during, and after a contraction. If any variable or late decelerations are noted, conversion to continuous electronic fetal monitoring is initiated. In continuous electronic fetal monitoring, the beat-to-beat FHR is recorded, with simultaneous recording of uterine activity. The normal baseline FHR is 110 to 160 bpm and should be accompanied by good baseline FHR variability. The following FHR abnormalities may occur:

Decreased or lost beat-to-beat variability can result from fetal hypoxia. It is also seen when narcotics, sedatives, or analgesic drugs have been administered to the mother. A decrease in variability can be seen with fetal sleep. Other factors that can lead to decreased or lost variability are administration of magnesium sulfate to the mother, fetal immaturity, and fetal tachycardia.[10,14,22]

Fetal tachycardia, indicated by a FHR greater than 160 bpm, can be associated with maternal fever, chorioamnionitis, and administration of certain medications to the mother, such as atropine, terbutaline, and others that may cause a decrease in uterine blood flow. A small percentage of fetuses whose mothers are hyperthyroid demonstrate tachycardia. Rates of 200 to 300 bpm are seen with fetal supraventricular tachycardia. Tachycardia is frequently seen in the recovery phase following fetal bradycardia related to a hypoxic episode but can also be seen with the gradual onset of fetal hypoxemia.

Fetal bradycardia is indicated by a heart rate less than 110 bpm. It is often referred to as physiologic, not related to hypoxemia, if accompanied by good baseline variability. Sustained low heart rates with normal variability can also be seen with fetal heart block, fetal central nervous system anomalies, and administration of beta-adrenergic receptor blocking drugs, such as propranolol, to the mother. Loss of variability with bradycardia can be associated with fetal hypoxia.

TABLE A.3: NORMAL ARTERIAL UMBILICAL BLOOD GAS VALUES FOR TERM AND PREMATURE INFANTS

VALUE	TERM (*N* = 3,520)	PREMATURE (*N* = 1,015)
pH	7.25 ± 0.07	7.28 ± 0.089
PCO2 (mmHg)	50.30 ± 11.1	50.20 ± 12.3
HCO3 (mmol/L)	22.00 ± 3.6	22.40 ± 3.5
BE (mmol/L)	−2.70 ± 2.8	−2.50 ± 3.0

BE, base excess.

Source: Adapted from Riley RJ, and Johnson JWC. 1993. Collecting and analyzing cord blood gases. *Clinical Obstetrics and Gynecology* 36(1): 13. Reprinted by permission.[23]

Early FHR decelerations are a benign response to uterine pressure on the fetal head. Baseline FHR and variability are normal.

Variable decelerations of FHR are caused by umbilical cord compression as uterine contraction activity peaks. Transient fetal hypoxemia and acidosis occur with compression of the arteries.

Late decelerations reflect fetal hypoxemia. Initially, the late deceleration pattern may be mediated by the vagus nerve, but with continued, prolonged hypoxia, the heart rate is low because of myocardial depression. Other factors leading to this pattern are maternal hypotension; hypercontractility of the uterus due to oxytocin; regional anesthesia; and major maternal emergencies such as hemorrhage, seizures, or respiratory arrest.[10,22]

Sinusoidal patterns of FHR appear as baseline oscillations of FHR similar to a sine wave, with fixed periodicity and loss of variability. They are associated with severe fetal anemia and are seen with Rh-sensitized fetuses and with large fetofetal transfusion; fetomaternal transfusion; and fetal hemorrhage, as into a cavernous hemangioma.[10,22]

REFERENCES

1. Lowdermilk DL, Perry SE, Cashion K, Alden KR, and Olshansky EF. 2019. *Maternity & Women's Health Care*, 12th ed. St. Louis, MO: Elsevier.
2. Kuller JA, Strauss RA, and Cefalo RC. 2001. Preconceptional and prenatal care. In *Obstetrics and Gynecology: Principles for Practice Study Guide*, Ling FW, and Duff P, eds. New York, NY: McGraw-Hill, 48–49.
3. Merkatz, IR, Nitowsky, HM, Macri, JN, Johnson, WE. 1984. An association between low maternal serum alpha-fetoprotein and fetal chromosomes. *American Journal of Obstetrics and Gynecology* 148: 886–894.
4. Wald NJ, Cuckle HS, Densem JW, Nanchahal K, Royston P, Chard T, Haddow JE, Knight GJ, Palomaki GE, and Canick JA. 1988. Maternal serum screening for down's syndrome in early pregnancy. *British Medical Journal* 297: 883–887.
5. Wald NJ, Hackshaw AK, Walters J, Mackinson AM, Rodeck C, and Chitty L. 2003. First and second trimester antenatal screening for down's syndrome: The results of the serum, urine, and ultrasound screening study (SUR-USS). *Journal of Medical Screening* 10: 56–104.
6. Gregg AR, Skotko, BG, Benkendorf JL, Monaghan, KG, Bajaj, K, Best RG, Klugman S, and Watson MS. 2016. Noninvasive prenatal screening for fetal aneuploidy, 2016 update: A position statement of the American College of Medical Genetics and Genomics. *Genetics in Medicine* 16: 1058–1065.
7. Norwitz ER, and Levy B. 2013. Noninvasive prenatal testing: The future is now. *Reviews in Obstetrics & Gynecology* 6(2): 48–62.
8. Committee on Genetics. 2017. Committee opinion no. 691: Carrier screening for genetic conditions. *Obstetrics & Gynecology* 129: e41–e55. Reaffirmed 2019.
9. American College of Obstetricians and Gynecologists' Committee on Practice Bulletins—Obstetrics, Committee on Genetics, Society for Maternal–Fetal Medicine. 2016. Practice bulletin no. 162: Prenatal diagnostic testing for genetic disorders. *Obstetrics & Gynecology* 127(5): e108–e122. doi: 10.1097/AOG.0000000000001405
10. Kaimal AJ. 2023. Assessment of fetal health. In *Creasy and Resnick's Maternal–Fetal Medicine: Principles and Practice*. Lockwood CJ, Copel JA, Dugoff L, Louis J, Moore TR, Silver RM, Resnick R, eds. Philadelphia, PA: Elsevier, 2988–3034.
11. Gomella TL, Eyal FG, and Bany-Mohammed F, eds. 2020. *Gomella's Neonatology: Management, Procedures, On-Call Problems, Diseases, and Drugs*, 8th ed. New York, NY: McGraw-Hill.
12. Shaffer BL, and Parer JT. 2012. Antepartum fetal monitoring. In *Queenan's Management of High-Risk Pregnancy: An Evidence-Based Approach*, 6th ed. Queenan JT, Spong CY, and Lockwood CJ, eds. Oxford, UK: Wiley-Blackwell. doi: 10.1002/9781119963783
13. Manning FA. 1999. Fetal biophysical profile. *Obstetrics and Gynecology Clinics of North America* 26(4): 557–577.
14. Chavira E, and Goodwin TM. 2012. Fetal lung maturation, the respiratory distress, and antenatal steroid therapy. In *Management of Common Problems in Obstetrics and Gynecology*, 5th ed. Goodwin TM, Montoro MN, Muderspach LI, Paulson RJ, and Roy S, eds. Malden, MA: Wiley-Blackwell Science, 216–219.
15. Farmakides G, Weiner Z, Mammapoulos M, and Nikolaides P. 1994. Doppler velocimetry. Where does it belong in evaluation of fetal status? *Clinics in Perinatology* 21(4): 849–861.
16. Berkley E, and Abuhamad A. 2012. Sonographic dating and standard fetal biometry. In *Queenan's Management of High-Risk Pregnancy: An Evidence-Based Approach*, 6th ed. Queenan JT, Spong CY, and Lockwood CJ, eds. Malden, MA: Wiley-Blackwell. doi: 10.1002/9781119963783
17. Bahadue FL, and Gecsi KS. 2020. Antenatal and intrapartum care of the high-risk neonate. In *Klaus and Fanaroff's Care of the High-Risk Neonate*, 7th ed. Fanaroff AA, and Fanaroff JM, eds. Philadelphia, PA: Saunders, 61–178.
18. Tekesin I, Wallweiner D, and Schmidt S. 2005. The value of quantitative ultrasound tissue characterization of the cervix and rapid fetal fibronectin in predicting preterm delivery. *Journal of Perinatal Medicine* 33(5): 383–391.
19. Herbert WNP, Chapman JF, and Schnoor MM. 1993. Role of the TDx FLM assay in fetal lung maturity.

American Journal of Obstetrics and Gynecology 168(3 Part 1): 808–812.

20. Russell JC, Cooper CM, Ketchum CH, Torday JS, Richardson DK, Holt JA, Kaplan LA, Swanson JR, and Ivie WM. 1989. Multicenter evaluation of TDx test for assessing fetal lung maturity. *Clinical Chemistry* 35(6): 1005–1010.
21. Victory R, Penava D, Da Silva O, Natale R, and Richardson B. 2004. Umbilical cord pH and base excess values in relation to adverse outcome events for infants delivering at term. *American Journal of Obstetrics and Gynecology* 191(6): 2021–2028.
22. Miller LA, Miller DA, and Cypher RL. 2022. *Mosby's Pocket Guide to Fetal Monitoring: A Multidisciplinary Approach*, 9th ed. St. Louis, MO: Elsevier, 112–115.
23. Riley RJ, and Johnson JWC. 1993. Collecting and analyzing cord blood gases. *Clinical Obstetrics and Gynecology* 36(1): 13.

GLOSSARY

Abduction: Drawing a limb or limbs away from the midline of the body or the digits away from the axial line of the limb. The lower the neonate's gestational age, the greater the amount of hip abduction seen.

Acetabulum: The cup-shaped cavity in which the femoral head articulates.

Achondroplasia: Congenitally shortened lower extremities, seen when the ratio of upper body length to lower body length exceeds 1.7:1.

Acrocyanosis: Bluish discoloration of the palms of the hands and the soles of the feet. This condition is normal in otherwise normal neonates immediately after birth but should not persist longer than 48 hours. Sometimes called *peripheral cyanosis.*

Active alert state: A wakeful state of infant consciousness characterized by increased motor activity and sensitivity to stimuli. The eyes are less attentive than in the quiet alert state, and periods of fussiness may be seen. In this state, preterm infants may become distressed and unable to focus.

Active sleep: A sleeping state of infant consciousness characterized by low activity but with some response to external stimuli (startle, brief crying noises). Rapid eye movements may be seen.

Adduction: Drawing a limb or limbs toward the midline of the body or the digits toward the axial line of the limb. In the neonate, hip adduction increases with gestational age.

Adventitious breath sounds: Abnormal breath sounds or sounds not normally found within the lungs.

Agenesis: Absence or failure of development of any organ or part.

Allis sign: A procedure for observing femoral length. With the infant's feet flat on the bed and the big toes and femurs aligned, flex the infant's knees. Face the feet and observe the height of the knees. A positive Allis sign is present if one knee is higher than the other.

Anal wink: Reflexive contraction of the anal sphincter in response to gentle stroking of the anal area. This reflex aids inspection of sphincter placement and tone in the newborn. Also called *anocutaneous reflex.*

Anencephaly: A defect in the newborn's skull (beginning at the vertex and extending, in some cases, to the foramen magnum) resulting from defective closure of the anterior neural tube. Hemorrhagic and fibrotic cerebral tissue protrudes, uncovered, through the defect. Generally, anencephaly involves the forebrain and some amount of the upper brainstem. The infant displays an underdeveloped cranial vault, shallow orbits, and protruding eyes. Abnormalities of other systems are also seen.

Anomaly: A deviation from normal, especially a defect of congenital or hereditary origin. A **minor anomaly** is one that is of little cosmetic significance and requires minimal or no intervention. Many deformations fall into this category. A **major anomaly** is medically or cosmetically significant and requires medical intervention. Most malformations and disruptions are categorized as major anomalies. The greater the number of minor anomalies seen in an infant, the higher the risk of a major anomaly also being present.

Anterior axillary line: A reference line (used to describe the location of physical findings) that passes vertically through the anterior axillary fold.

Anterior vascular capsule of the lens: Within the first 24 to 48 hours of life, transient embryologic vascular systems that nourish the eye during active intrauterine growth can be seen on the anterior vascular capsule of the preterm infant's lens using an ophthalmoscope. Because these systems appear at week 27 and disappear by the end of week 34 of gestation, the degree of their presence in the neonate's lens can be used to determine gestational age.

Aphonia: Loss of the voice.

Apical impulse: The forward thrust of the left ventricle during systole, usually seen in the newborn in the fourth intercostal space at or left of the midclavicular line. An apical impulse downward and to the left suggests left ventricular dilatation. A very sharp apical impulse indicates high cardiac output or left ventricular hypertrophy.

Aplasia cutis congenita (ACC): A congenital abnormality of unknown cause, ACC most often appears on the scalp (over the parietal bones or near the sagittal suture) and is characterized by the absence of some or all layers of the skin. It may be an isolated defect or may be associated with chromosomal disorders such as trisomy 13.

Apnea: A lapse of 20 seconds or more between respiratory cycles, with bradycardia or color changes. Apnea is commonly seen in premature neonates and is outgrown as the infant approaches term. It is abnormal in late preterm or term infants.

Appropriate for gestational age (AGA): An infant whose weight, length, and/or occipital–frontal circumference (OFC) falls between the 10th and the 90th percentiles for gestational age when plotted on a standard growth chart.

Areola: The darkened area surrounding the nipple. In a full-term infant, it is raised and stippled, with 0.75 to 1 cm of palpable breast tissue. The distance between the outside of the two areolae should be less than 25% of the chest circumference.

Arnold-Chiari malformation: A congenital anomaly marked by inferior displacement of the medulla and fourth ventricle into the upper cervical canal and elongation and thinning of the upper medulla and lower pons, along with interior displacement of the lower cerebellum through the foramen magnum into the lower cervical canal. It is generally associated with hydrocephalus and myelomeningocele.

Arrhythmia: An irregularity in the heart rhythm. Arrhythmias are common—and usually benign—in the newborn. **Sinus arrhythmia** is characterized by irregularity of the R-R interval with an otherwise normal cardiac cycle. **Premature atrial beat**, seen in perhaps a third of healthy term and premature infants, is an early beat arising from a supraventricular focus, with normal ventricular conduction. **Premature ventricular beat** is an early beat arising from an irritable ventricular focus, with abnormal ventricular conduction producing a wide QRS complex.

Arthrogryposis: Congenital limitation of movement of limbs due to nonprogressive contracture of the joint.

Ascites: Accumulation of serous fluid in the peritoneal cavity.

Asphyxia, perinatal: Acidosis, hypoxia, and hypercapnia caused by lack of oxygen and carbon dioxide exchange and decreased perfusion in the fetus or the newborn. It may result in hypoxic-ischemic encephalopathy.

Association: A combination of defects that occur together more frequently than would be normal by chance, but that is less fixed than the pattern seen in a syndrome. Associations are generally named by acronyms formed from the initial letter of each defect in them.

Atelectasis: Incomplete expansion of all or part of a lung.

Atresia, anal: Congenital absence of the anal canal and/or orifice, indicated by lack of stool passage, progressive abdominal distention, and finally vomiting. Also called *imperforate anus.*

Atresia, bilateral choanal: Obstruction of the posterior nasal passages. Infants affected are cyanotic at rest and pink when crying because they are breathing through an open mouth.

Atresia, esophageal: Congenital lack of continuity of the esophagus, characterized by excessive salivation.

Auscultation: A physical assessment technique involving listening for body sounds—chiefly those of the heart and lungs, but also those of the pleura and abdomen. *Direct* auscultation is performed without the aid of a stethoscope; *indirect* (*mediate*) auscultation involves use of the stethoscope.

Avulsion: A tearing away.

Ballotable: Use of palpation to detect movement of objects suspended in fluid, such as a fetus in amniotic fluid.

Barrel chest: An abnormality of the bony structure of the chest in which the anterior–posterior diameter of the chest is greater than normal. It is seen with transient tachypnea of the newborn (TTN), meconium aspiration, and hyperinflation.

Behavioral assessment: Evaluation of the infant's ability to interact with the environment; includes assessment of organization, changes in state of consciousness, response to stimuli, and evaluation of motor maturity, muscle tone, strength, and coordination.

Behavioral cues: Signs infants give to indicate their physical, psychological, and social needs. **Signs of attention** (also called *signs of approach*) indicate a readiness to interact. These cues include an alert, focused gaze, and regular breathing; they may also include grasping, sucking, or hand-to-mouth movements. **Time-out signals** (also called *avoidance behaviors*) indicate the need for a respite from interaction. These cues include an averted gaze, frowning, sneezing, yawning, vomiting, and hiccups, sometimes accompanied by finger splaying, arching, and stiffening. Color changes, apnea, irregular breathing, and decreased oxygen saturation levels may also be seen.

Bell palsy: Paralysis of the facial nerve with a resultant characteristic distortion of the face with a unilateral presentation.

Bones, cranial: There are four cranial bones: *frontal, occipital, parietal,* and *temporal.* See Figure 6.2 for locations.

Bowel sounds: Metallic, tinkling sounds heard every 15 to 20 seconds when the four abdominal quadrants are auscultated beginning within 15 minutes after birth. Hyperactive sounds immediately after feeding, with the intensity of the sounds diminishing as the next feeding approaches, are normal. Auscultation of *friction rubs* (resembling the sound of rubbing a finger over a cupped hand held near the ear) may indicate peritoneal irritation. When heard in the newborn over the lung fields, bowel sounds are likely referred sounds from the abdomen. If they persist, however, they could indicate diaphragmatic hernia.

Brachial plexus palsy: A functional paralysis of part or all of the arm, resulting from birth trauma and more common in large babies. It is caused by stretching injuries to the components of the brachial plexus during delivery. The upper arm is more commonly affected than the lower or the entire arm. The Moro reflex is absent on the affected side, but the grasp reflex remains. If the nerve roots are not injured, neurologic function returns within several days of birth as hemorrhage and edema resolve.

Brachycephaly: Broad skull shape caused by craniosynostosis (premature fusion) of the coronal suture, limiting forward growth of the skull.

Bradycardia, sinus: A heart rate less than 80 beats per minute in a newborn. Transient bradycardia, with origin in the sinus node, is commonly seen in both full-term and premature newborns, generally in response to vagal stimulation.

Bradypnea: Excessively slow respirations. In the neonate, persistent respirations of less than 40 per minute are associated with central nervous system depression from such factors as maternal drug ingestion, asphyxia, or birth injury.

Branchial sinus: An abnormal opening seen anywhere along the sternocleidomastoid muscle. It may communicate with deeper structures, with potential for infection.

Bronchial breath sounds: Seldom heard in the neonate, bronchial sounds are the loudest of the normal breath sounds. They are found over the trachea and are marked by a short inspiration and a longer expiration.

Bronchopulmonary dysplasia (BPD): *See* Chronic lung disease (CLD).

Broncho vesicular breath sounds: Normally found over the manubrium and the intrascapular regions, bronchovesicular sounds are intermediate in intensity between bronchial and vesicular breath sounds. In these sounds, inspiration and expiration are equal in quality, intensity, pitch, and duration.

Bruit: (a) A murmurlike sound auscultated over the fontanels or the lateral skull. It may signify intracranial arteriovenous malformation in an infant with congestive heart failure. (b) A sound, resembling a systolic murmur, heard with dilated, tortuous, or constricted vessels during auscultation of the skull. It is produced by the vibration of vessel walls within the skull, caused by flow disturbances that interfere with the normal laminar flow through the vessels. Bruits may be heard with Sturge–Weber syndrome. (c) If heard over the newborn's abdomen and not eliminated by changing the infant's position, bruits may indicate umbilical vein or hepatic vascular system abnormalities, renal artery stenosis, or hepatic hemangiomas.

Brushfield spots: White specks scattered linearly around the circumference of the iris. These spots are associated with Down syndrome, but may also be seen as a normal variant.

Bulla: An elevation of the skin filled with serous fluid (a vesicle) greater than 1 cm in diameter.

Café au lait spot (patch): A tan or light-brown macule or patch with well-defined borders. One patch is found in up to 19% of normal children, and these patches are of no pathologic significance when they are less than 3 cm in length and less than six in number. A greater number of patches or patches larger than 3 cm may indicate cutaneous neurofibromatosis, an autosomal dominant genetic disorder.

Candida diaper dermatitis: A moist, erythematous rash caused by or associated with *Candida albicans* and consisting of small white or yellow pustules over the buttocks and perianal region (and occasionally the thighs).

Canthus: The angle at either end of the opening between the eyelids. The eye has two canthi, the inner (adjacent to the nose) and the outer.

Capillary filling time: A measurement used to assess cardiac perfusion in the newborn. Press the infant's skin with a finger until it blanches; then count the seconds required for the color to return. This should take no more than 3 to 4 seconds in a normal infant. Check filling time in both a central and a peripheral area.

Caput: Referring to the head.

Caput succedaneum: Edema occurring in and under the presenting part of the fetal scalp during delivery, generally due to pressure restricting venous and lymph flow. The edema has poorly defined edges, pits on pressure, and usually crosses suture lines. It typically resolves within a few days. Caput succedaneum is the most common form of birth trauma to the head.

Cephalhematoma: Collection of blood (hemorrhage) between the periosteum and the skull, generally resulting from birth trauma. The edges are clearly demarcated and bounded by suture lines. Cephalhematomas are most commonly seen over the parietal and occipital bones. Over time, a cephalhematoma may liquefy and become fluctuant on palpation; resolution can take weeks to months.

Chordee: Ventral bowing of the penis, which produces a downward curvature on erection. It is often seen with hypospadias.

Chromosomal aneuploidy: Too many or too few chromosomes, resulting in a genetic malformation. Normal infants have 46 chromosomes (22 pairs of autosomes and two sex chromosomes). Forms of aneuploidy include monosomy and trisomy.

Chronic lung disease: A chronic respiratory problem characterized by bronchiolar metaplasia and interstitial fibrosis. It affects neonates born before 30-weeks gestation who have previously received mechanical ventilation and/or supplemental oxygen. Also known as BPD.

Clavicle: One of the pair of bones linking the sternum with a scapula. Commonly called the *collarbone*.

Cleft lip: A congenital defect in the upper lip.

Cleidocranial dysostosis: Syndrome characterized by congenital complete or partial absence of the clavicles. Defective cranial ossification, large fontanels, and delayed suture closure are often seen with complete absence of clavicles. This anomaly is characterized by excessive scapulothoracic motion.

Clonic: Relating to or characterized by clonus.

Clonus: Involuntary repetitive muscle contraction and relaxation.

Clubfoot (*talipes equinovarus*): One of the common congenital deformities of the foot, seen more often in male infants than in female, and varying in severity. The forefoot is adducted and points medially, there is pronounced varus of the heel, and the foot and toes point downward. In unilateral presentation, the affected foot is smaller, with thickened joints.

Coloboma: A malformation characterized by absence of or a defect in the tissue of the eye. It is sometimes seen as a keyhole shaped pupil and associated with other anomalies.

Congenital absence of the radius: A bilateral anomaly in half the infants who exhibit it, radial absence presents with a deviated hand and wrist, a shortened forearm with a bowed ulna, an absent or hypoplastic thumb, and limited elbow movement. The condition may require surgery.

Congenital absence of the tibia or fibula: This unusual anomaly more frequently affects the fibula than the tibia and is more often unilateral than bilateral. There may be partial or complete absence of the bone. Foot deformity and leg length discrepancies are generally seen in the absence of either long bone.

Congenital constricting bands (Streeter dysplasia): Bands of tissue (thought to be amniotic in origin) encircling one or more extremities of the newborn. These bands can produce shallow indentations of the soft tissue or constrictions severe enough to cause partial or complete amputation of the extremity. Treatment depends on severity; a surgical consultation may be required.

Congenital heart disease (CHD): A spectrum of cardiac anomalies present at birth. There is increased risk of CHD in infants of mothers with CHD, in infants with an older sibling who has CHD, and in low-birth-weight infants. An increased incidence of CHD is also associated with extracardiac anomalies, including those of the gastrointestinal, renal, and urogenital systems; tracheoesophageal fistulas; and diaphragmatic hernias.

Consolability: An infant's ability to quiet themselves when in the crying state or to respond to attempts by a caregiver to quiet them. An infant with well-developed organization generally exhibits self-consoling behaviors, including bringing the hands to the mouth, sucking on the fist or tongue, or using environmental stimuli as a distraction.

Consolidation: An area of increased lung tissue density.

Cost of attention: A term used by T. B. Brazelton to describe the amount of energy an infant must expend to maintain an alert state of consciousness. The cost of attention depends on both the health and maturity of the infant.

Crackles: Adventitious breath sounds involving a series of brief crackling or bubbling sounds. (Crackles were previously termed *rales*.) **Fine crackles**, usually heard at the end of inspiration, resemble the sound made by rubbing a lock of hair. They may be associated with respiratory distress syndrome (RDS) or BPD. **Medium crackles** sound like carbonated fizz. They are believed to reflect the passage of air past sticky surfaces, as found with pneumonia or TTN. **Coarse crackles** (also called *rhonchi*) are loud, bubbly sounds associated with mucus or fluid accumulation in the large airways.

Craniosynostosis: Premature fusion of one or more sutures, stopping bone growth perpendicular to the suture, but permitting it parallel to the suture.

Craniotabes: Areas of soft (demineralized) bone in the skull, usually in the occipital and parietal bones along the lambdoidal suture. Craniotabes is sometimes seen with hydrocephalus.

Cremasteric reflex: Contraction of the cremaster muscle resulting in a drawing up of the ipsilateral testis when the inner thigh is stroked or stretched longitudinally.

Cri du chat syndrome: A chromosomal disorder in which the short arm of the fifth chromosome is missing. It presents with a catlike cry in the newborn and other associated anomalies.

Crust: Dried serous exudate, blood, or pus.

Crying: A wakeful state of infant consciousness characterized by crying (in term infants), increased motor activity, color changes, and exaggerated response to unpleasant stimuli. Some term infants console themselves by returning to a lower state of consciousness. Preterm infants may have a very weak (or even absent) cry, but exhibit the other signs of stress indicative of this state.

Cryptorchidism: Failure of one or both testes to descend into the scrotum. It can be unilateral (most often occurring on the right side) or bilateral. In full-term infants who present with undescended testes at birth, about half show descent by 6 weeks of age; in 75% of preterm infants, the testes descend by 3 months of age. Testes do not usually descend spontaneously after 9 months of age. Inguinal hernia is commonly seen with cryptorchidism.

Cutis marmorata: Bluish mottling or marbling of the skin in response to chilling, stress, or overstimulation, usually disappearing when the infant is warmed.

Cyanosis, central: Bluish discoloration of the skin and mucous membranes due to significant arterial oxygen desaturation. It presents when at least 5 g of unbound (to oxygen) hemoglobin are present per 100 mL of blood. An important indicator of CHD, cyanosis due to cardiac causes does not improve on administration of 100% oxygen and also increases with crying. In cyanotic infants without increased respiratory effort, the cause of the cyanosis is most likely CHD. Central cyanosis may also occur in the presence of persistent pulmonary hypertension, lung disease, sepsis, or neurologic disease. Central cyanosis must be differentiated from acrocyanosis (peripheral cyanosis) and circumoral cyanosis, both of which are normally seen in the first few days after birth.

Cyanosis, circumoral: Bluish discoloration of the lips and area surrounding the mouth.

Darwinian tubercle: A normal variant appearing as a small nodule on the upper helix of the ear.

Deep sleep state: A sleeping state of infant consciousness characterized by closed eyes, regular breathing, and lack of spontaneous activity. Response to external stimuli is delayed.

Defect, single-gene: A genetically caused malformation. The form of inheritance may be dominant (carried by one gene from one parent), recessive (requiring one gene from each parent), or X-linked (carried on the X chromosome and expressed in male offspring, with female offspring being carriers).

Deformation: A congenital abnormality caused by pressure exerted by mechanical forces on the fetus generally late in gestation after the major organ systems are formed. The source of the pressure is generally uterine constraint (maternal or fetal). Most deformations occur to the musculoskeletal system.

Depigmentation lesion: A white, macular lesion with an irregular, leaflike border. These lesions may be early indicators of tuberous sclerosis, a progressive degenerative neurologic disease.

Dermis: Inner, vascular layer of the skin containing fibrous and elastic tissues, sweat and sebaceous glands and ducts, hair follicles and shafts, blood vessels, and nerves.

Developmental dysplasia of the hip: An abnormality in which the hip joint develops abnormally, causing instability of the hip ranging from minimal to dislocation. The causes of congenital hip dysplasia may include lack of acetabular depth, laxity of the ligaments, and/or intrauterine breech position. Congenital hip dysplasia is more often seen in Caucasian than in African American or Asian infants, it is more common in females than in males, and the left hip is affected more often than the right. In multiple births, it is more common in the first born. A positive Allis sign may indicate congenital hip dysplasia. It is associated with other orthopedic anomalies and deformities.

Diaphragmatic hernia: Protrusion of abdominal contents through an opening in the diaphragm.

Diastasis recti: A palpable midline gap between the rectus muscles of the abdominal wall. Bulging may be seen when the infant cries. Diastasis recti is often seen in otherwise normal infants and is benign unless a hernia is present.

Diastole: Dilation of the heart (particularly of the ventricles), coincident with the interval between the second heart sound (S2) and the first heart sound (S1).

Disorders of sexual development (DSDs): A heterogeneous array of innate conditions secondary to abnormal development of sex chromosomes, as well as atypical growth of the gonads and genital anatomy.

Disruption: A congenital abnormality caused by the breakdown of normal tissue in utero. Most disruptions result from amniotic bands wrapping around fetal extremities or entering the fetus's mouth.

Doll's eye maneuver: Used to evaluate movement of the eyes as the head is turned. The infant's head is gently rotated from side to side; the eyes should deviate away from the direction of rotation, that is, turning the head to the right, the eyes should deviate to the left.

Dorsiflexion: Flexion toward the back, as in flexion of the foot so that the forefoot is higher than the ankle.

Drowsiness: The transitional state of infant consciousness between sleep and wakefulness. The infant exhibits a variable activity level, with dull, heavy-lidded eyes that open and close periodically. Movements are smooth, and there is a response to stimuli, but not immediately.

Dysmorphogenesis: Abnormal development of form or structure, as seen in congenital malformations. Dysmorphic features are also called anomalies.

Early term: An infant born between 37 0/7 and 38 6/7 weeks gestation.

Ecchymosis (plural: ecchymoses): A nonblanching area of subepidermal hemorrhage, initially bluish black in color, then changing to greenish brown or yellow. Ecchymoses may be seen on the labia of female infants and the scrotal area of male infants after breech deliveries.

Edema: Abnormally large amounts of fluid in the intercellular tissue spaces of the body, usually the subcutaneous tissues. Most newborns have some edema around the face and eyes due to excess fluid volume after delivery. After difficult deliveries, edema of the scalp or in dependent areas is often seen. In *pitting edema,* indentations produced by pressure remain for prolonged periods.

Ejection click: A snappy, high-frequency heart sound normal during the first 24 hours of life; after that, it is considered abnormal. If present, it is best heard just after S1 and resembles in timing, but not in quality, a widely split S1.

Embryonic period: The third to the eighth week of pregnancy, the period during which differentiation and major organ system development take place. Insults to the embryo during this period can result in major anomalies in the newborn.

Encephalocele: A restricted disorder of anterior neural tube closure producing a defect in the skull called *cranium bifidum.* In some cases, a skin-covered protrusion (sac) containing meninges and cerebrospinal fluid (and sometimes cerebral tissue) is present. In other cases, the defect appears as a small tissue-covered opening (often surrounded by tufts of abnormal hair) on the skull, with no protrusion of skull contents. The most common location for encephaloceles is the midline of the occipital bone, but they are also seen in the parietal, temporal, or frontal nasopharyngeal areas. Size varies from tiny to massive; severity depends on location, size, and the contents of the protrusion. Skull x-rays can identify the cranium bifidum, and transillumination and ultrasound help identify the contents of the protrusion.

Encephalopathy, hypoxic-ischemic: A syndrome resulting from perinatal asphyxia. It can be categorized as **mild** (associated with irritability, jitteriness, and hyperalertness), **moderate** (characterized by lethargy, hypotonia, decreased spontaneous movement, and seizures), or **severe** (characterized by coma, flaccidity, disturbed brainstem function, and seizures). The pattern of limb weakness displayed by an affected infant reflects the area of the brain injured by the asphyxia. In term neonates, injury to the parasagittal areas (resulting in weakness of the shoulder girdle and proximal upper extremities) or the middle cerebral artery (presenting as hemiparesis) predominates. In the premature newborn, injury is often to the periventricular area, resulting in weakness in the lower extremities.

Epicanthal fold: A vertical fold of skin on either side of the nose that covers the lacrimal caruncle. These folds are normal in Asian infants but suggestive of Down syndrome in neonates of other races.

Epidermis: Outermost layer of the skin, itself composed of five layers. The top layer is the *stratum corneum* (dead cells that are constantly being sloughed off and replaced); lower layers contain keratin-forming cells and melanocytes.

Epispadias: Location of the urethral meatus on the *dorsal* surface of the penis. It is a less common abnormality than hypospadias. In **balanic epispadias**, the meatus is found at the base of the balanus (glans); in **penile epispadias**, it is on the penile shaft; and in **penopubic epispadias**, it is found not on the penis at all, but directly below the symphysis pubis.

Epstein pearls: Epidermal inclusion cysts seen in the newborn at the junction of the hard and soft palates of the mouth and on the gums. They usually disappear by a few weeks of age.

Erb palsy: Damage (generally due to birth trauma) to the upper spinal roots C5 and C6, resulting in paralysis of an arm (but usually without involvement of the hand). *See also* **Brachial plexus palsy**.

Erythema toxicum neonatorum: A benign rash consisting of small white or yellow papules or vesicles with an erythematous base. Seen in up to 70% of term infants between 24 and 48 hours of age, the rash occurs most often on the face, trunk, or extremities.

Everted: Turned out and away from the midline of the body.

Exophthalmos: *Synonym, Proptosis.* Abnormal anterior displacement (protrusion) of the eye. It may be associated with hyperthyroidism.

Expected date of confinement (EDC): Delivery due date. Generally 280 days (40 weeks) from the onset of the mother's last menstrual period.

Exstrophy of the bladder: A visible fissure between the anterior abdominal wall and the urinary bladder. In male infants, it is commonly accompanied by epispadias.

Extension: The straightening of a limb at a joint.

Familial traits: Atypical features (subtle or significant) identified by a family as characteristic of its phenotype.

Fasciculation: The spontaneous localized contraction of a group of fibers in a motor unit, visible through the skin. In Werdnig–Hoffmann disease, these continuous and rapid twitching movements can be seen by observing the tongue.

Fetal period: The ninth week of pregnancy through birth. The fetus becomes more and more resistant to teratogens as this period progresses.

Fibrils: Tiny fibers or filaments connecting the dermis and the epidermis.

Fistula, rectourethral: An abnormal connection between the rectum and the urethra, indicated by the presence of meconium in the urethral orifice.

Fistula, rectovaginal: An abnormal connection between the rectum and the vagina, indicated by the presence of meconium in the vaginal orifice.

Flexion: The act of bending or the condition of being bent. The bending of a limb at a joint. In the neonate, the degree of arm, knee, and hip flexion is indicative of gestational age.

Flexion contracture: Resistance of a muscle to passive flexion. The newborn's hips generally have a flexion contracture; when the right hip is flexed to stabilize the pelvis and flatten the lumbar spine, a flexion contracture of the left hip may be seen. The infant's elbow also shows a flexion contracture for the first few weeks of life, making it difficult to examine.

Fontanel: A membrane-covered space (soft spot) in the infant's skull reflecting incomplete ossification of the skull. Fontanels occur where two sutures meet. The **anterior fontanel** occurs at the intersection of the metopic, coronal, and sagittal sutures. The **posterior fontanel** occurs where the sagittal and lambdoidal sutures meet. The **sphenoid fontanel** is at the juncture of the coronal and squamosal sutures. The **mastoid fontanel** occurs at the intersection of the squamosal and lambdoidal sutures. A defect of the parietal bone along the sagittal suture may appear to be—but is not—a true fontanel (third fontanel). It may be a normal variant or may be associated with Down syndrome or congenital hypothyroidism.

Forcep marks: Red, bruised, or abraded areas on the cheeks, scalp, and face of infants born after application of forceps. Observation of forcep marks calls for examination for facial palsy, fractured clavicles, skull fractures, or other complications of birth trauma.

Frog leg position: A resting posture, normal in premature neonates of 36 or fewer weeks gestation, in which the legs are abducted and the lateral thigh rests against the bed surface. This position is abnormal if seen in newborns older than 36-weeks gestational age.

Funnel chest (pectus excavatum): An abnormality of the bony structure of the chest in which the sternum is indented. It is seen in infants with Marfan syndrome and rickets.

Galactorrhea: Milky secretions engorging the breasts of some infants at birth, due to the influence of maternal estrogen. The secretions generally disappear in 1 to 2 weeks, and the enlargement subsides over several months. Also referred to as *Witch's milk*.

Gastroschisis: Protrusion of abdominal contents and other organs through an abdominal wall defect lateral to the midline; the protrusion is not covered by a membrane. A gastroschisis is associated with fewer congenital malformations than is an omphalocele.

Gestational age: The length of time between fertilization of the egg and birth of the infant.

Glabella: The area above the nose and between the eyebrows (bridge of the nose).

Growth parameters: Measurements used to determine whether an infant is small, appropriate, or large for gestational age (LGA). The three parameters are weight, length, and occipital–frontal head circumference.

Habituation: A newborn's ability to alter his response to a repeated stimulus, decreasing and finally eliminating the response on repetition of the stimulus. Habituation is a defense mechanism.

Hamstring: In human anatomy, the **hamstring** is any one of a group of six tendons contracted by three posterior thigh muscles (semitendinosus, semimembranosus, and biceps femoris). The term is sometimes used to refer to the muscles themselves.

Harlequin sign: A sharply demarcated red color in the dependent half of the body, with the superior half of the body appearing pale, when the infant is placed on his side. Rotating the infant to the other side reverses the coloring. Harlequin color change occurs in both healthy and sick infants but is more common in low-birth-weight infants. It has no pathologic significance.

Heart rate: The normal heart rate for a full-term neonate is 80 to 160 beats per minute.

Heart sounds: **S1**, the first heart sound, is best heard at the mitral or tricuspid area. It is usually loud at birth, but decreases in intensity by 2 days of life. **S2**, the second heart sound, is best heard at the aortic or pulmonic area. It is usually single at birth but is split in two-thirds of infants by 16 hours of age and in 80% by 48 hours of age. Wide splitting of S2 is abnormal. **S3**, commonly heard in premature infants with a patent ductus arteriosus (PDA), is best heard at the apex of the heart during early diastole. **S4**, a pathologic sound, is heard at the apex of the heart in infants with conditions characterized by decreased compliance.

Heave: A point of maximum impulse that is slow rising and diffuse, generally associated with ventricular dilation or volume overload. Also called a *lift*.

Helix: The upper and outer margin of the pinna of the ear.

Hemangioma, cavernous: A raised, lobulated, soft and compressible bluish-red tumor, with poorly defined margins. The cavernous hemangioma consists of large, mature vascular elements lined with endothelial cells and involves the dermis and subcutaneous tissues of the skin. It increases in size during the first 6 to 12 months of life, and then involutes spontaneously. Two syndromes—Kasabach–Merritt and Klippel–Trenaunay–Weber—may be associated with cavernous hemangiomas.

Hemangioma, infantile: A raised, lobulated, soft and compressible bright-red tumor, with sharply demarcated margins, on the head, neck, trunk, or extremities. (Tumors occurring in the throat can obstruct the airway.) Caused by dilated capillaries, with associated endothelial proliferation in the dermal and subdermal layers of the skin, the infantile hemangioma occurs in up to 10% of newborns. It gradually increases in size for about 6 months and then spontaneously regresses over a period of up to several years.

Hemiparesis: Muscle weakness or partial paralysis affecting one half of the body.

Hepatomegaly: Enlargement of the liver.

Hernia, epigastric: Protrusion of fat through a defect on the midline above the umbilicus and below the sternum, presenting as a firm palpable mass. Palpation may elicit a pain response. Surgical intervention is necessary.

Hernia, femoral: A small bulge adjacent and medial to the femoral artery. It is more common in females than in males.

Hernia, inguinal: Muscle wall defect in the inguinal area through which bowel loops or gonads enter the scrotal sac (in males) or the soft tissues (in females). The hernia usually presents as bulging in the groin area and is more common in male than in female infants.

Hernia, umbilical: Skin- and subcutaneous-tissue-covered protrusion of part of the intestine at the umbilicus. It is seen with some frequency in low-birth-weight and African American male infants and in infants of other races with hypothyroidism. The hernia usually reduces by 2 years of age, but intervention is required with strangulation of abdominal contents or large size.

Holosystolic: Occurring throughout systole. Also called *pansystolic.*

Hydranencephaly: Partial or complete absence of the cerebral hemispheres, with the space being filled with cerebrospinal fluid.

Hydrocele: A circumscribed collection of clear fluid in the scrotum, which may resolve spontaneously by 6 months of age. A hydrocele may communicate with the inguinal canal, however, and may be associated with a hernia. **Hydrocele of the cord** presents as a palpable, sausage-shaped, smooth bulge above the testes.

Hydrocephalus: Accumulation of cerebrospinal fluid (often under increased pressure) within the skull, due to obstruction of the cerebrospinal fluid pathways causing dilation of the cerebral ventricles. It may be congenital or may develop after birth and is characterized by head enlargement, forehead prominence, brain atrophy, mental deterioration, and convulsions. The skull is often globular in shape.

Hydrometrocolpos: Collection of secretions in the vagina and uterus due to an imperforate hymen. It may be palpated as a small midline lower abdominal mass or a cystic movable mass as the quantity of secretions increases.

Hygroma, cystic: The most commonly seen neck mass in newborns, a cystic hygroma is soft, fluctuant, and can range from only a few centimeters in size to massive. It is usually seen laterally or over the clavicle and transilluminates well.

Hymenal tag: A small appendage or flap on the hymen, normal in female infants. It disappears in several weeks.

Hyperpigmented macule: A large gray or blue-green macule or patch caused by melanocyte infiltration of the dermis. This pigmented lesion (generally found on the buttocks, flanks, or shoulders) is seen in up to 90% of African American, Asian, and Hispanic and up to 10% of Caucasian infants.

Hyperplasia, sebaceous gland: Numerous white or yellow papules (<0.5 mm in size) on the nose and upper lips. These enlarged sebaceous glands spontaneously decrease in size with age and require no treatment.

Hypertelorism: Widely spaced eyes—those with greater than a palpebral fissure length between them.

Hypertonia: Increased resistance of the skeletal muscles to passive stretching. In the presence of hypertonia, passive manipulation of the limbs often increases the tone.

Hypertrophy: Enlargement or overgrowth of an organ or part.

Hypertrophy of the clitoris: The most common genitourinary abnormality in female infants. When significant, consider an evaluation for a disorder of sexual development.

Hypoplastic nails: Nails that are incompletely developed. Edema of the hands can give the appearance of hypoplastic nails.

Hypospadias: Location of the urethral meatus on the **ventral** surface of the penis. In **balanic (glanular) hypospadias**, the meatus is located at the base of the balanus (glans). In **penile hypospadias**, the meatus is found between the glans and the scrotum. It is often accompanied by chordee, flattening of the glans, and an absent ventral foreskin. In **penoscrotal (perineal) hypospadias**, the meatus is found at the penoscrotal junction. Gender ambiguity is associated with penoscrotal hypospadias, as is bifid scrotum, small penis with a large meatus, and undescended testes.

Hypotelorism: Closely spaced eyes—those with less than a palpebral fissure length between them.

Hypotonia: Depressed postural muscle tone.

Inner canthal distance: The measurement between the inner canthi of the two eyes. If the eyes are normally spaced, this distance should be equal to the length of the palpebral fissure.

Inspection: A physical assessment technique involving careful visual attention to, measurement of, and notation of the status of external body parts and systems, for the purpose of forming a judgment.

Intersex: Anomalous differentiation of the gonads, with presence of both ovarian and testicular tissue and ambiguous morphologic sex criteria. A disorder of sexual development may be suspected when only one testis is confirmed in a male-appearing infant or in the presence of clitoral hyperplasia.

Intrauterine growth restricted (IUGR) neonate: A newborn who did not grow in utero at the expected rate for weight, length, or occipital–frontal head circumference. Although the term is often used synonymously with *small for gestational age* (*SGA*), the two terms do not necessarily mean the same thing. A neonate may have been growth restricted in utero but may not fall below the 10th percentile for gestational age.

Inverted: Turned inward toward the midline of the body.

Jaundice: Yellow coloring of the skin and whites of the eyes, generally appearing first on the head and face and then progressing toward the feet. Jaundice is due to excess bilirubin in the blood (hyperbilirubinemia).

Jitteriness: A series of movements seen at times in normal preterm neonates and in normal term neonates with vigorous crying. (Persistent jitteriness may indicate a disorder.) Jitteriness is characterized by rapid movements of equal amplitude in alternating directions, generally occurs in response to a stimulus, can be stopped by flexing and holding the involved extremity, and is not associated with abnormal eye movements or other signs of seizure. Jitteriness must be distinguished from seizure activity. *See also* **Seizure**.

Karyotype: Representation by diagram of the chromosomal characteristics of an individual or species.

Karyotyping: Chromosomal evaluation.

Keratin: An insoluble, fibrous protein that is the main component of certain protective and/or supportive elements of the body, including the nails, hair, and epidermis.

Klippel–Feil syndrome: Defects of the cervical vertebrae, resulting in a shorter-than normal neck with limited motion and asymmetry in rotation and lateral flexion.

Klumpke palsy: Damage (generally due to birth trauma) resulting in paralysis of the forearm. *See also* **Brachial plexus palsy**.

Kyphosis: A spinal abnormality in which the curvature of the thoracic spine is excessively convex. Commonly called *hunchback.*

Lacrimal caruncle: The red area at the inner canthus of the eye.

Lanugo: A fine, soft, downy hair covering the fetus in utero and sometimes the neonate. It first appears at about 20 weeks gestation, covering most of the body including the face. Most of it disappears by 40 weeks gestation.

Large for gestational age: An infant whose weight falls above the 90th percentile for gestational age when plotted on a standard growth chart.

Late term: An infant born 41 weeks 0 days' gestation through 41 weeks 6 days' gestation.

Late preterm: An infant born between 34 0/7 and 36 6/7 weeks gestation.

Lesion: Any discontinuity of tissue or change in the structure or function of an organ or part due to disease or trauma.

Leukoplakia: A white spot or patch on the tongue or mucous membranes in the mouth, which cannot be wiped off and that does not clinically represent any other condition.

Light sleep state: See **Active sleep**.

Lipoma: A benign tumor composed of fat cells.

Lordosis: A spinal abnormality in which the curvature of the lumbar and cervical spine is excessively concave. Commonly called *swayback.*

Low birth weight: An infant who weighs less than 2,500 g at birth.

Macrocephaly: Excessive head size (an OFC above the 90th percentile for gestational age, with otherwise normal weight and length percentiles). Macrocephaly can be familial or it may be due to hydrocephalus or associated with dwarfism or osteogenesis imperfecta.

Macrodactyly: An enlarged finger or toe. It is seen in otherwise normal infants, or it may indicate neurofibromatosis.

Macroglossia: An abnormally large tongue.

Macrostomia: An abnormally large oral opening.

Macule: A discolored, flat, nonpalpable spot or patch less than 1 cm in diameter.

Malacia: Abnormal softening of tissues.

Malformation: A congenital defect arising from abnormal tissue. The cause of the tissue abnormality may be intrinsic (genetic) or extrinsic (environmental).

Manubrium: Uppermost portion of the sternum.

Mediastinum: A space within the chest cavity containing the heart, esophagus, trachea, mainstem bronchi, thymus, and major blood vessels.

Melanosis, transient neonatal pustular: Small pigmented macules (often surrounded by very fine white scales) caused by the rupture of superficial vesiculopustular lesions 12 to 48 hours after birth. The condition—seen in up to 5% of African American and about 0.2% of Caucasian infants—is benign and generally resolves by 3 months of age.

Meningocele: A lesion associated with spina bifida in which more than one vertebra is involved. The meninges protrude through the bony defect and are covered by a thin atrophic skin. The spinal roots and nerves are normal.

Metatarsus adductus: A common congenital foot anomaly caused by intrauterine positioning. It may be positional (flexible) or structural (fixed). In the structural type (with bony abnormalities), there is limited abduction of the forefoot, and the heel is in a valgus position. In the positional type, the forefoot abducts easily, and the heel is in a varus or neutral position.

Microcephaly: Abnormal smallness of the head (an OFC below the 10th percentile for gestational age), generally due to poor brain growth.

Micrognathia: An abnormally small lower jaw, seen in Robin sequence and other syndromes.

Micropenis: Abnormally small penis. Micropenis suggests congenital hypopituitarism when seen with certain other anomalies or conditions. Also called *penile hypoplasia.*

Microstomia: An abnormally small oral opening. It may be seen with some trisomies.

Midclavicular line: A reference line (used to describe the location of physical findings) passing vertically through the clavicle.

Midsternal line: A reference line (used to describe the location of physical findings) bisecting the suprasternal notch.

Milia: Multiple yellow or pearly white papules about 1 mm in size. These epidermal cysts (found on the brow, cheeks, and nose of up to 40% of newborns) are caused by accumulation of sebaceous gland secretions and spontaneously resolve during the first few weeks of life.

Miliaria: Changes in the skin caused by obstruction of the sweat ducts. Miliaria is generally associated with excessive warmth and/or humidity and is classified into four types, based on severity. **Miliaria crystallina** occurs when sweat escapes into the epidermal stratum corneum, causing formation of clear, thin vesicles 1 to 2 mm in diameter. **Miliaria rubra**, commonly called *prickly heat,* presents as small erythematous papules and occurs when continued obstruction of the sweat ducts causes release of sweat into adjacent tissues of the epidermis. **Miliaria pustulosa** occurs with continued occlusion of the sweat ducts, as leukocytes infiltrate the vesicles. Unresolved miliaria pustulosa can lead to **miliaria profunda**, secondary infection of the deeper dermal portions of the sweat glands.

Morphogenesis: Differentiation of cells and tissues in the early embryo that establishes the form and structure of the various organs and parts of the body.

Mottling: Blotchy skin showing areas of different color. It may indicate cardiogenic shock in the neonate.

Mucocele: A mucous retention cyst (distended cavity containing mucus) presenting as a translucent or bluish swelling under the tongue.

Murmur: A prolonged heart sound caused by turbulent blood flow. Documenting the timing, location, intensity, radiation, quality, and pitch are all important to the evaluation of the origin of a murmur, as is the age of the newborn. There are two types of murmurs: *innocent* and *pathologic*; see **Murmurs, innocent** and **Murmurs, pathologic**.

Murmur, continuous: A pathologic murmur, heard through both systole and diastole, present in about a third of premature infants with a PDA and also in full-term or premature infants with arteriovenous fistulas.

Murmur, continuous systolic (crescendo systolic): An innocent murmur heard in up to 15% of newborns, beginning within the first 8 hours of life. It is best heard in the upper-left sternal border.

Murmur, early soft midsystolic ejection: An innocent murmur often heard in premature infants, beginning within the first or second week of life and disappearing by the eighth week. Medium to high pitched, it is best heard in the upper-left sternal border, with wide radiation.

Murmur, loud systolic ejection: A pathologic murmur that presents within hours of birth, generally due to aortic or pulmonary stenosis or coarctation of the aorta.

Murmur, systolic ejection: An innocent murmur heard in more than half of all newborns, beginning within the first day of life and lasting up to a week. It can be described as "vibratory" and is best heard along the mid- and upper-left sternal border.

Murmurs, innocent: Innocent murmurs have no pathologic cause within the heart or great vessels. They are generally systolic, symptomless, and common in normal newborns during the first 48 hours of life when they are associated with decreasing pulmonary vascular resistance and with closure of the PDA. They include systolic ejection murmurs, continuous systolic (crescendo systolic) murmurs, and early soft midsystolic ejection murmurs.

Murmurs, pathologic: Pathologic murmurs are due to cardiovascular disease. When they present is dependent on their cause and on normal changes associated with transitional circulation. Many do not appear until pulmonary vascular resistance falls. Absence of a murmur does not rule out CHD; as many as a fifth of the infants who die from CHD by 1 month of age do not have murmurs. Pathologic murmurs include **loud systolic ejection murmurs** and **continuous murmurs.**

Muscle tone, phasic: The brief, forceful contraction of a muscle in response to a short duration, high-amplitude stretch. In the newborn, phasic tone is evaluated by testing the resistance of the extremities to movement (scarf sign and arm and leg recoil) and by assessing the activity of the deep tendon reflexes (biceps and patellar reflexes).

Muscle tone, postural: The long-duration, low-amplitude stretch of a muscle in response to gravity. In the newborn, the traction response (pull-to-sit maneuver) is used to evaluate postural tone. Depressed postural tone is called *hypotonia.*

Myelomeningocele: A lesion associated with spina bifida in which bilateral broadening of the vertebrae or absence of the vertebral arches is seen. The lesion is most often seen in the lumbar spine and is characterized by protrusion of meninges and spinal roots and nerves, along with fusion of remnants of the spinal cord and an exposed neural tube. The higher the defect on the spine, the greater the degree of paralysis. Hydrocephalus is frequently seen with a myelomeningocele, especially in the Arnold–Chiari malformation.

Necrosis, subcutaneous fat: A hard, nonpitting, sharply circumscribed subcutaneous nodule that appears during the first weeks of life, grows larger over several days, and then resolves spontaneously over several weeks. Color will vary. Possible causes include trauma, cold, or asphyxia. Intervention may be necessary if the condition is associated with hypercalcemia.

Neonatal Behavioral Assessment Scale (NBAS): An examination tool developed by T. B. Brazelton to assess behavior in the term infant.

Neonatal torsion of the testis: A condition in which a testis and its tunica vaginalis rotate in the scrotal sac, inguinal canal, or abdomen. Torsion of a descended testis presents with reddish to bluish coloring of the scrotal skin and a nontender or mildly tender mass. Torsion is difficult to identify if the testis has not descended.

Nevus, pigmented: A dark-brown or black macule commonly seen on the lower back or buttocks. Although pigmented nevi are generally benign, malignant changes occur in up to 10% of these lesions.

Nevus, port wine: A flat, nonblanching pink or reddish-purple lesion with sharply delineated edges directly beneath the epidermis. The port wine nevus generally appears on the face, consists of dilated capillaries, and varies in size from small to covering almost half the body. Although usually unilateral, on occasion it crosses the midline. It neither grows in size nor resolves spontaneously. Port wine nevi located over the branches of the trigeminal nerve may be associated with Sturge–Weber syndrome.

Nevus, sebaceous: A small yellow or yellowish-orange papule or plaque consisting of immature hair follicles and sebaceous glands. It is commonly found on the scalp or face.

Nevus simplex: An irregularly bordered pink macule that blanches with pressure and becomes more prominent with crying. Found most often on the nape of the neck, the upper eyelids, the bridge of the nose, or the upper lip, the nevus simplex is composed of dilated capillaries and is seen in up to 50% of newborns. It is commonly called *stork bite.*

Nipple line: A reference line (used to describe the location of physical findings) passing horizontally through the nipples.

Nipples, supernumerary: Accessory nipples—raised or pigmented areas 5 to 6 cm below the normal nipples. In Caucasian infants, they may be associated with congenital anomalies.

Nodule: An elevated palpable lesion, solid and circumscribed (a papule), greater than 1 cm in diameter.

Normal variants: Minor differences in the appearance of the features between races, but that are normal for the race. Also called *minor variants.*

Nuchal cord: An umbilical cord that has become wrapped around the fetus's neck.

Nystagmus: A rapid, searching movement of the eyeballs seen in some newborns until 3 to 4 months of age. Occasional nystagmus is normal in the otherwise normal neonate; persistent is abnormal and may indicate loss of vision.

Observation: A physical assessment technique involving careful visual attention to, and notation of the status of, external body parts and systems, for the purpose of forming a judgment. Also called *inspection.*

Occipital–frontal circumference: Measurement of the neonate's head taken over the occipital, parietal, and frontal prominences, avoiding the ears. This growth parameter is used, with the infant's gestational age, to determine whether the infant's head is small, appropriate, or LGA. In the term infant, the normal OFC is 31 to 38 cm.

Oligohydramnios: The presence of less than 500 mL of amniotic fluid at term or 50% of normal volume at any time during pregnancy. The intrauterine compression caused by the lack of fluid may produce unusual flattening of the facial features in the newborn.

Omphalocele: Protrusion of abdominal contents through a defect at the umbilicus. A thin, translucent membrane covers the protrusion, and may rupture at delivery. Omphalocele is seen more often in male infants, especially premature males, and is usually associated with trisomies 13, 18, and 21; Beckwith–Wiedemann syndrome; or CHD.

Omphalomesenteric duct: Persistence in the newborn of this embryological duct between the ileum and the umbilicus, with seepage of ileal liquid from the opening.

Ophthalmoscope: A hand-held device, containing lenses and a mirror, that produces a beam of light for inspection of the interior of the eye. In physical examination of the newborn, it is used to assess pupillary constriction and the red reflex. It can also be used to inspect the anterior vascular capsule of the lens to determine gestational age.

Opisthotonus: Marked extensor hypertonia, with arching of the back. It may be seen with bacterial meningitis, severe hypoxicischemic brain damage, and massive intraventricular hemorrhage.

Orchiopexy: Surgical fixation of an undescended testis in the scrotum. Generally done between 9 and 18 months of age.

Organization: An infant's ability to integrate physiologic (heart rate, respiratory rate, oxygen consumption, and digestion) and behavioral (state, motor activity) systems in response to the environment. Preterm infants show decreased organizational abilities.

Ortolani maneuver: A procedure for evaluating hip stability in the newborn. After flexing the infant's knee and hip, grasp the thigh and first abduct with a lifting motion and then adduct the leg. If a clunk is felt as the femoral head passes over the acetabulum, the infant may have congenital hip dysplasia.

Osteoblast: A cell that arises from a mesenchymal stem cell and works with other osteoblasts to synthesize bone.

Otoscope: A device used to inspect the ears. Due to the presence of vernix in the neonate's ear canal, the device is normally not used in newborn examinations.

Outer canthal distance: The measurement between the outer canthi of the two eyes.

Pallor: Paleness of the skin in the newborn may indicate compromised cardiac status. The paleness may be due to vasoconstriction and to shunting of blood away from the skin to vital organs or anemia.

Palpation: A physical assessment technique involving application of pressure to the skin with the fingertips or part of the palm to assess the condition of underlying body parts.

Palpebral fissure: The eye opening.

Papule: An elevated palpable lesion, solid and circumscribed, less than 1 cm in diameter.

Patch: A discolored, flat, nonpalpable spot (a macule) greater than 1 cm in diameter.

Patent ductus arteriosus: A cardiac abnormality marked by failure of the ductus arteriosus to close after birth. In a left to-right shunt, blood flows from the aorta to the pulmonary artery, resulting in recirculation of arterial blood through the lungs.

Patent urachus: Persistence of an embryological communication between the urinary bladder and the umbilicus, with passage of urine through the umbilicus.

Percussion, direct: A physical assessment technique involving striking the body surface sharply and listening to the sound produced, to determine the condition of an underlying body part. In *indirect* (*mediate*) percussion, the examiner places the middle finger of the left hand on the area to be assessed and then strikes the finger with the middle finger of the other hand. Although not generally employed in examination of the abdomen, percussion can distinguish areas of tympanic (resonant or bell-like) sound from areas of dull sound. Tympanic sounds are present over the organs that contain air; increased tympany suggests abnormal amounts of air. Dull sounds are percussed over the liver, spleen, and bladder. Extended areas of dullness suggest organ enlargement; dullness in unusual areas may indicate masses. Shifting dullness is heard with ascites. It is of limited value in examination of the neonate's chest due to its small size, but can be useful in distinguishing among air, fluid, and solid tissue in some situations. Changes in resonance indicate changes in the consistency of the underlying tissue.

Perfusion, peripheral: Cardiac perfusion to the skin.

Perinatal history: Record of occurrences in the life of the mother, the fetus, and the newborn.

Perinatal period: Definitions of the length of the perinatal period vary; it extends from about week 20 or 28 of gestation until 1 week to 1 month after birth.

Perineum: Area between the scrotum and anus in the male and the vulva and anus in the female. It should be smooth in newborns. Dimpling suggests genetic anomalies or fistulas.

Periodic breathing: A series of respirations followed by a pause of up to 20 seconds.

Periosteum: Fibrous membrane covering the bones of the skull.

PERL: A notation that means "pupils equal and reactive to light."

Petechia (plural: petechiae): A pinpoint-sized hemorrhagic spot on the skin.

Phimosis: An irretractable foreskin. It may not be diagnosed until the infant reaches 3 months of age.

Pigeon chest: An abnormality of the bony structure of the chest in which the sternum protrudes. It is seen in infants with Marfan syndrome and rickets.

Pinna: The part of the ear that projects from the head. Formation, amount of cartilage present, and recoil when folded and released are considered indicators of gestational age.

Pit, ear: A slight depression anterior to the tragus. It may lead to a congenital preauricular sinus or fistula. Ear pits may be familial or associated with other anomalies.

Plagiocephaly: Asymmetrical skull shape caused by craniosynostosis (premature fusion) of the sutures on one side of the skull.

Plantar flexion: Flexing the foot toward the plantar surface.

Plantar surface: The sole of the foot. Creases appear on the plantar surface of the foot between 28 and 30 weeks gestation and cover the surface at or near term. Therefore, plantar surface creasing is one indicator of gestational age.

Plaque: A fusion or coalescence of several papules (solid, circumscribed, elevated palpable lesions <1 cm in diameter).

Plethora: Ruddy appearance of the skin in a newborn. Plethora may indicate a high level of red blood cells to blood volume.

Pleural cavities: Two potential spaces (left and right) within the chest cavity enclosed by a serous membrane called the pleura. A portion of the pleura called the **parietal pleura** lines the walls of the thoracic cavity; the portion called the **visceral pleura** envelops the lungs.

Pneumothorax: Accumulation of air or gas in the pleural space.

Polycythemia: A condition in which the infant's central hematocrit is greater than 65. An infant with polycythemia is pink at rest but plethoric to purplish when crying. The ruddy coloring can sometimes be mistaken for cyanosis (because the unsaturated hemoglobin in the blood of the infant may mask the saturated hemoglobin, making the infant appear purplish).

Polydactyly: A congenital anomaly marked by one or more extra digits on the hands or feet. There appears to be a familial tendency to polydactyly, and it is more common in African American infants than in those of other races. The extra digit may be only a skin tag or a floppy appendage or it may appear normal.

Ponderal index: Cube root of body weight times 100 divided by height in centimeters.

Popliteal angle: The angle between the lower leg and the thigh posterior to the knee.

The popliteal angle decreases with advancing gestational age.

Positional deformity: A flexible deformity of an extremity with no bony abnormality involved. It is caused by intrauterine positioning and generally corrects without treatment.

Postterm: An infant born at 42 0/7 or more weeks gestation.

Precordium: The area of the anterior chest over the heart. In the full-term newborn after the first few hours of life, the precordium should be quiet; a bounding precordium is characteristic of left-to-right shunt lesions (PDA or ventricular septal defect). In premature infants, the precordium is more active due to decreased subcutaneous tissue.

Preterm: An infant born at less than 38-weeks gestation.

Priapism: Constant erection of the penis, an abnormal finding that may indicate a spinal cord lesion.

Pronation: The turning of the body or a body part face down, as of the hand so that the palm is facing down.

Prone: Positioned face down.

Proptosis: Abnormal protrusion or bulging of the eyeball. Also called *exophthalmos.*

Prune belly syndrome: Also referred to as *Eagle–Barrett syndrome* or *Triad syndrome.* A rare clinical triad presenting with poorly developed abdominal muscles appearing as a thin-walled abdomen covered with wrinkled skin, undescended testes, and renal and urinary tract abnormalities. It occurs more frequently in males.

Pseudostrabismus: The appearance of strabismus (crossed eyes) due to a flat nasal bridge or the presence of epicanthal folds.

Ptosis: Paralytic drooping of the eyelid in which the upper lid droops when the eyes are fully open.

Pulse deficit: A difference between the heart rate counted by a peripheral pulse and that counted by auscultation. A pulse deficit is frequently seen with ectopic rhythms.

Pulse pressure: The difference between the systolic and the diastolic blood pressure. For term infants, the average difference is 25 to 30 mmHg; for premature infants, it is 15 to 25 mmHg. Wide pulse pressures can indicate large aortic runoff, as in PDA. Narrow pulse pressures are seen with peripheral vasoconstriction, heart failure, and low cardiac output.

Pupillary reflex: Contraction of the pupil when the eye is exposed to bright light.

Pustule: An elevation of the skin filled with cloudy or purulent fluid.

Q-switched ruby laser: Laser used in removal of nevi or tattoos. Emits a short pulse of intense red light that is selectively absorbed by melanin located in the epidermal and dermal skin layers. The laser energy causes the melanin to break down into smaller pigment particles that are removed by the body's immune system.

Quiet alert state: A wakeful state of infant consciousness characterized by interaction with the environment. The infant focuses on stimuli and presents an alert appearance, especially in the eyes. Motor activity is minimal. In this state, preterm infants may show hyperalertness (inability to terminate fixation on a stimulus).

Rachitic rosary: In a newborn with rickets, a series of small lumps can be felt along the edge of the sternum during palpation. The lumps are enlarged costal cartilages.

Radiation: The transmission of a body sound to another location.

Rales: See **Crackles**.

Ranula: A cystic tumor, presenting as a translucent or bluish swelling beneath the tongue, caused by obstruction of a salivary duct or a mucous gland.

Recoil, arm or leg: Test used to evaluate phasic muscle tone. The infant's arm or leg is gently extended. In premature infants of 28 or fewer weeks gestation, minimal resistance is normal. Resistance increases with gestational age.

Red retinal reflex: Reflection of a clear red color from the retina when a bright light is directed at the newborn's lens. The reflex is a pale color in dark-skinned infants.

Reflex, anocutaneous: An autonomic nervous system reflex. *Stimulus*: Cutaneous stimulation of the perianal skin. *Normal response*: Contraction of the external sphincter. Also called *anal wink.*

Reflex, Babinski: A developmental reflex. *Stimulus*: Stroke the sole of the infant's foot. *Positive response*: Extension of the great toe and spreading of the other toes.

Reflex, biceps: A motor reflex that is most active during the first 2 days after birth and when the newborn is alert. *Stimulus*: Place thumb over insertion of infant's biceps tendon, flex newborn's arm, and tap thumb with reflex hammer. *Normal response*: Infant flexes biceps muscle.

Reflex, corneal: A peripheral sensory reflex. *Stimulus*: Blow air on the infant's eye or touch the cornea gently with a piece of cotton. *Normal response*: The infant blinks.

Reflex, Moro: A developmental reflex that is normally completely present at birth only in term neonates. This reflex may be elicited by sudden movement of surface infant is on, loud noise, or causing the head to drop approximately 30°. *Stimulus*: Hold infant supine, supporting head a few centimeters above bed, withdraw supporting hand and allow the infant to "fall back" to it. *Normal response*: As infant's head falls, infant extends and abducts arms and opens hands; then adducts and partially flexes arms, and makes fists. Infants greater than 32 weeks gestation may cry out. Premature infants do not complete the reflex by adducting and flexing the extremities, nor do they cry. Complete lack of the reflex is abnormal; asymmetric response may indicate a localized neurologic defect (such as a brachial plexus injury).

Reflex, palmar grasp: A developmental reflex that is normally present at birth in both term and preterm infants. *Stimulus*: Stroke infant's palm with a finger. *Normal response*: Infant grasps finger and tightens grasp on attempt to withdraw finger.

Reflex, patellar (knee jerk): A motor reflex that is most active during the first 2 days after birth and when the newborn is alert. *Stimulus*: Tap infant's patellar tendon just below kneecap, with newborn's knee flexed and supported. *Normal response*: Infant extends knee and contracts quadriceps.

Reflex, rooting: A developmental reflex that is normally present at birth in both term and preterm infants. *Stimulus*: Stroke infant's cheek and corner of mouth. *Normal response*: Infant turns head toward stimulus and opens mouth.

Reflex, startle: Resembles Moro reflex but is more limited. See **Reflex, Moro**.

Reflex, stepping: A developmental reflex that becomes more active 72 hours after birth. *Stimulus*: Hold infant upright with soles of feet touching a flat surface. *Normal response*: Alternate stepping movements.

Reflex, sucking: A developmental reflex that is normally present at birth in both term and preterm infants. (It is weaker in preterm neonates.) *Stimulus*: Touch infant's lips. *Normal response*: Infant opens mouth and makes sucking movements.

Reflex, tonic neck: A developmental reflex that is normally present at birth only in term neonates. *Stimulus*: With infant supine, turn infant's head to one side. *Normal response*: Extension of upper extremity on side to which head is turned and flexion of upper extremity on opposite side. Lack of response or a marked response with minimal head turning is abnormal. Also called *fencing position.*

Reflex, truncal incurvation (Galant): A developmental reflex. *Stimulus*: Suspend infant ventrally, supporting anterior chest wall in palm of hand. Apply firm pressure parallel to spine in thoracic area with thumb or cotton swab. *Positive response*: Infant flexes pelvis toward side of stimulus.

Reflexes, developmental: Reflexes that do not require functional brain above the diencephalon. Those present in most newborns include the sucking, rooting, palmar grasp, tonic neck, Moro, stepping, truncal incurvation, and Babinski reflexes. Also called *primary* or *primitive* reflexes.

Respiratory distress syndrome: A condition of the newborn most often occurring in premature infants, but may be seen at term, marked by breathing difficulties and cyanosis and having as its origin a deficiency of surfactant and structural immaturity.

Retinoblastoma: A retinal tumor. Lack of a red reflex in a newborn could indicate its presence.

Retractions: Drawing in of the chest during respiration. Immediately after birth, substernal or intercostal retractions are common; if they persist, they may indicate respiratory problems. Suprasternal retraction, especially with gasping or stridor, may indicate obstruction of the upper airway.

Rhonchi: Adventitious breath sounds lower in pitch and more musical than crackles. Although seldom heard in the neonate, they may be auscultated if secretions or aspirated foreign matter are present in the large airways.

Rotation, neck: Turning of the face to the side.

Rub: Adventitious breath sound resembling the rubbing of a finger over a cupped hand held near the ear. Rubs are often heard in newborns during mechanical ventilation; they are also associated with inflammation of the pleura.

Ruga (plural: rugae): A ridge, wrinkle, or fold. Rugae first appear on the front of the scrotal sac at about 36 weeks gestation, covering the sac by 40 weeks gestation. In the term male infant, the scrotum is fully rugated; the preterm male has few or no rugae.

Scale: Exfoliation of dead or dying bits of skin. Scale can also result from excess keratin production.

Scaphocephaly: Long, narrow head shape caused by craniosynostosis (premature fusion) of the sagittal suture, limiting lateral growth of the skull.

Scapula: One of the pair of triangular bones at the back of the shoulder articulating with a clavicle. Commonly called the *shoulder blade.*

Scarf sign: A test for newborn gestational age involving gently pulling the arm of a supine infant across the chest and around the neck as far as possible posteriorly. The older the infant, the greater the resistance to this maneuver.

Sclera: The white portion of the eyeball.

Sclera, blue: Unusual blue coloring of the white portion of the eyeball. It is seen with a variation of osteogenesis imperfecta and certain other abnormalities.

Scoliosis: A congenital deformity of the spine in which vertebrae fail to form and/or segment. It is embryonic in origin. If undetected, it can affect neurologic function as well as appearance. Congenital scoliosis may be associated with genitourinary tract anomalies, Klippel–Feil syndrome, and Sprengel deformity.

Seizure: An abnormal series of movements (neurologic in origin) characterized by alternate muscular contraction and relaxation of unequal amplitude. The movements are less rapid than those seen in jitteriness. They do not occur in response to stimuli and cannot be stopped by flexing and holding the affected limb; may be accompanied by abnormal eye movements. *See also* **Jitteriness**.

Sensory threshold: An infant's level of tolerance for stimuli. Infants who exceed their sensory thresholds (are overstimulated) exhibit signs and symptoms of stress. Low sensory thresholds are generally seen in preterm infants and in infants with neurologic impairment.

Sequence: A single defect as the cause for other anomalies (the "snowball" effect).

Single transverse palmar crease: May be found in normal newborns, but when seen with short fingers, an incurved little finger, and a low-set thumb, it is suggestive of Down syndrome.

Sinus, dermal: A posterior neural tube defect occurring along the midline of the back, frequently in the lumbar region. It may present as a dimple surrounded by tufts of hair or lipomas or may terminate in subcutaneous tissue, a cyst, or a fibrous band. It may also extend into the spinal cord and be associated with spina bifida.

Sinus, preauricular: An abnormal channel located in front of the pinna (auricle) of the ear. If it communicates with the internal ear or the brain, chronic infection is likely.

Skin tag: A small skin outgrowth. Those occurring anterior to the tragus are thought to be embryological remnants of the first branchial arch. Skin tags may be familial or associated with other anomalies.

Small for gestational age: An infant whose weight falls below the 10th percentile for gestational age when plotted on a standard growth chart.

Spina bifida: The mildest form of posterior neural tube defect, with the malformation arising from lack of or incomplete closure of the posterior portion of the vertebrae. The meninges and spinal cord are normal. The defect is covered with skin (which may be dimpled), and it is most common in the lower lumbar and lumbosacral area. *See also* **Sinus, dermal**.

Split: Term describing a heart sound in which two components can be heard. The "splitting" is caused by the asynchronous closure of the two valves that create the sound. The rapid newborn heart rate makes splitting difficult to auscultate. In newborns splitting is usually not heard in S1. S2 is generally single at birth but is split in two-thirds of infants by 16 hours of age and in four-fifths by 48 hours of age. Wide splitting of S2 is abnormal, however.

Sprengel deformity: A congenital anomaly of the shoulder girdle, marked by some hypoplasia and malrotation of the scapula, which gives it an elevated appearance. Shoulder abduction and flexion are limited. This deformity is more often unilateral, but can be bilateral. It is often associated with congenital spinal anomalies, Klippel–Feil syndrome, and renal anomalies.

State (of consciousness): One of six levels of consciousness seen in infants. There are two sleep states (*deep* and *light*), one transitional state (*drowsiness*), and three awake states (*quiet alert, active alert*, and *crying*). Behavioral assessment evaluates the newborn's ability to control his state, move smoothly from one state to another, and maintain alertness when in an awake state. Term infants may use changes in state to control environmental input.

Stenosis, anal: Constriction or obstruction of the anorectal canal. Signs include passage of small, thin stools; progressive abdominal distention; and finally, vomiting.

Stenosis, pyloric: Obstruction of the pyloric orifice of the stomach, usually presenting about 3 weeks of age, rarely before the fourth or fifth day of life. If present, it is palpable immediately after feeding or vomiting as an ovoid mass between the umbilicus and the right lower costal margin. Signs of pyloric stenosis (upper-quadrant distention and visible peristalsis) in the absence of a palpable mass may indicate duodenal or jejunal obstruction in the neonate.

Sternocleidomastoid muscle: The muscle that flexes the vertebral column and rotates the head.

Stethoscope: An acoustical device used to auscultate (listen to) sounds within the body. In the neonate, these include heart, lung, venous, arterial, and intestinal sounds. A neonatal stethoscope generally has a double head composed of a flat diaphragm (for auscultating high-frequency sounds) and a bell (for auscultating low frequency sounds). It does not magnify sound but simply eliminates environmental noise.

Stippling: A speckling of fine dots.

Strabismus: The appearance of crossed eyes in the newborn due to muscular incoordination.

Stridor: A high-pitched hoarse adventitious breath sound heard during inspiration or expiration at the larynx or upper airways. In the newborn, stridor indicates partial obstruction of the airway. It may also be heard in infants with edema of the upper airway after extubation.

Structural deformity: A fixed (or rigid) deformity involving bony abnormalities. It generally requires surgical intervention.

Subcutaneous tissue: Layer of fatty tissue underlying the dermis, which insulates the body, protects the internal organs, and stores calories.

Sucking blister: Intact or ruptured vesicle or bulla sometimes seen on the lips, fingers, or hands of the newborn. The cause is vigorous sucking, in utero or after birth.

Sunset sign: Eyelid retraction and a downward gaze in which the sclera is visible above the iris. The sign is often seen in infants with hydrocephalus.

Supination: Turning of the body or a body part face up, as of the hand so that the palm is facing up.

Supine: Positioned face up.

Suprasternal notch: An indentation on the upper border of the sternum.

Suture: A fibrous joint between bones of the skull. The **metopic suture** extends midline down the forehead between the two frontal bones and intersects with the **coronal suture**, which separates the frontal and parietal bones. The **sagittal suture** extends midline between the two parietal bones to the back of the head, where it intersects with the **lambdoidal suture**, which separates the parietal and occipital bones. The **squamosal suture** extends above the ear and separates the temporal from the parietal bone.

Sutures, overriding: Head molding may cause the edge of the bone on one side of a suture to feel as if it is on top of (overriding) the edge of the opposite bone. Overriding is commonly seen in the lambdoidal suture, with the parietal bone on top of the occipital. Overriding sutures must be differentiated from craniosynostosis (premature fusion of a suture).

Symmetrically growth restricted: An infant who has not grown at the expected rate—that is, who ranks at less than the 10th percentile for gestational age on standard growth charts—for *all three* growth parameters: weight, length, and occipital–frontal head circumference.

Symphysis, pubis: Midline cartilaginous joint connecting the pubic bones.

Syndactyly: Congenital webbing of the fingers and toes, frequently familial in origin. The more severe the webbing, the greater the likelihood of underlying bony abnormalities.

Syndrome: A recognizable pattern of anomalies, often of more than one system, that is historically based and leads to a diagnosis.

Systole: The period of contraction of the heart, particularly of the ventricles.

Tachycardia, sinus: A heart rate greater than 180 to 200 beats per minute in the newborn. Simple tachycardia, originating in the sinus node of the heart, normally occurs in response to a stimulus that increases demand on the heart. When the stimulus is removed, the rate gradually returns to normal.

Tachycardia, supraventricular (SVT): A heart rate greater than 200 to 300 beats per minute in the newborn. Without immediate intervention, it can lead to cardiovascular collapse.

Tachypnea: Excessively rapid and shallow respirations. In the neonate, persistent respirations of greater than 60 per minute may indicate TTN, RDS, meconium aspiration, pneumonia, hyperthermia, or pain.

Tap: A sharp, well-localized point of maximum cardiac impulse, usually associated with pressure overload or hypertrophy.

Temperament: The way in which an infant interacts with the environment. Typically three categories of temperament are recognized: easy, difficult, and slow to warm.

Teratogenic agent: An extrinsic factor—either environmental or maternal—that causes abnormalities in fetal development. Examples include infection; metabolic disorders; and exposure to drugs or alcohol, heavy metals, many chemicals, and radiation.

Term: An infant born between 39 0/7 and 40 6/7 weeks of gestation.

Testicular torsion: See **Neonatal torsion of the testis**.

Thorax: The chest. The thoracic cavity is bound by the sternum, 12 thoracic vertebrae, 12 pair of ribs, and the diaphragm.

Thrill: A low-frequency, palpable murmur that resembles holding one's hand on a purring cat. Thrills are uncommon in the newborn. If present, their location can aid in identification of cardiac problems.

Thrush: An oral fungal infection characterized by adherent white patches on the tongue and mucous membranes and caused by *Candida albicans*.

Thyroglossal duct cyst: A cyst on the embryological duct between the thyroid and the back of the tongue.

Tonic: Of or relating to or producing normal tone or tonus in muscles or tissue.

Torticollis: An anomaly affecting the sternocleidomastoid muscle, more often on the right side. It is not usually seen until about 2 weeks of age, when it can be palpated as a firm, immobile mass 1 to 2 cm in diameter in the midportion of the muscle. Undetected, it produces facial asymmetry and limited neck rotation.

Traction response (pull-to-sit maneuver): Tests the ability of the infant's muscles to resist the pull of gravity. When the normal-term infant's hands are grasped and he is slowly pulled from a supine to a sitting position, the infant contracts the shoulder and arm muscles, and then flexes the neck, with the head lagging behind the body only minimally. The infant also flexes the elbows, knees, and ankles. When the infant reaches the sitting position, the head remains erect briefly before falling forward. Neck flexion is not seen in infants of less than 33-weeks gestation.

Tragus: A small cartilaginous flap in front of the external opening of the ear.

Transient tachypnea of the newborn: A condition of the newborn marked by excessively rapid respirations. The underlying pathology is usually retained fetal lung fluid; tachypnea subsides as fluid is absorbed or expelled.

Transillumination: A physical assessment technique involving shining light through body tissues. The area being examined is placed between the light and the observer. If a pneumothorax is suspected in the neonate, transillumination can allow comparison of the left, right, upper, and lower aspects of the chest and illuminate air pockets with a lantern-like glow. If the infant's head is an unusual size or shape or if the neurologic examination is abnormal, transillumination can help identify the reason. It is useful for identification of abnormal findings in the scrotum. Masses filled with clear fluid appear translucent with illumination; solid or blood-filled masses do not transilluminate.

Trisomy: A form of chromosomal aneuploidy characterized by the presence of 47 chromosomes. It is generally caused by nondisjunction (failure of the egg or sperm to divide the genetic material equally). The most common autosomal trisomies are of chromosome 21 (Down syndrome), chromosome 18, and chromosome 13.

Urethral meatus: Opening of the urethra on the body surface, located directly below the clitoris in female infants and at the center of the end of the penile shaft in males.

Uvula, bifid: A split uvula. This may be associated with other congenital anomalies.

Valgus: Bent outward or twisted away from the midline of the body.

Varus: Turned inward.

Vernix caseosa: A greasy white or yellow material, composed of sebaceous gland secretions and exfoliated skin cells, that covers the newborn infant's skin. Vernix develops during the third trimester of intrauterine growth, gradually decreasing in amount as the fetus approaches 40 weeks gestation. Because vernix may be present in the newborn's auditory canal, otoscopic examination is not done immediately after birth.

Very low birth weight (VLBW): An infant who weighs less than 1,500 g at birth.

Vesicle: An elevation of the skin filled with serous fluid and less than 1 cm in diameter.

Vesicular breath sounds: Normally found over the entire chest, except over the manubrium and the trachea. During expiration, vesicular sounds are soft, short, and low-pitched; during inspiration, they are louder, longer, and higher pitched.

Werdnig–Hoffmann disease: A disorder of the lower motor neurons, causing flaccid weakness of the extremities as well as tongue fasciculation.

Wheal: A reddened, solid elevation of the skin caused by a collection of fluid in the dermis.

Wheezes: Adventitious breath sounds, usually louder on expiration than on inspiration, that are higher in pitch than rhonchi. They are usually heard only in newborns with CLD.

Whorl, hair: Spiral hair growth pattern commonly seen in the posterior parietal region of the newborn's scalp. Absence of or abnormal location of a whorl can indicate abnormal brain growth.

Xiphoid process: Sword-shaped cartilaginous projection at the end of the sternum.

GLOSSARY COMPILED AND VERIFIED USING THE FOLLOWING SOURCES

- Blackburn ST, ed. 2018. *Maternal, Fetal, and Neonatal Physiology: A Clinical Perspective*, 5th ed. St. Louis, MO: Elsevier.
- *Dorlands Medical Dictionary*, 33rd ed. 2019. Philadelphia, PA: Saunders.
- Diaz A, and Lipman Diaz EG. 2021. *Pediatrics in Review* 42(8): 414–426.
- Gleason CA, and Juul, SE, eds. 2018. *Avery's Diseases of the Newborn*, 10th ed. Philadelphia, PA: Elsevier.
- Kenner C, Altimier L, and Boykova MV, eds. 2019. *Comprehensive Neonatal Nursing Care*, 6th ed. New York, NY: Springer Publishing Company.
- *Miller–Keane Encyclopedia and Dictionary of Medicine, Nursing, and Allied Health*, 7th ed. 2005. Philadelphia, PA: Saunders.
- *Mosbys Medical, Nursing and Allied Health Dictionary*, 9th ed. 2012. Philadelphia, PA: Mosby.
- *Pediatrics* 2019; 144(5): e20192760. doi: 10.1542/peds.2019-2760
- Polin RA, Abman SH, et al. eds. 2021. *Fetal and Neonatal Physiology*, 6th ed. Philadelphia, PA: Elsevier.
- *Stedman's Medical Dictionary*, 28th ed. 2013. Baltimore, MD: Lippincott Williams & Wilkins.
- VanPutte C, et al., eds. 2022. *Seeleys Anatomy and Physiology*, 13th ed. New York, NY: McGraw-Hill Education.

INDEX

Note: Page numbers followed by *t* or *f* indicate tables or figures, respectively